Exercise Prescription: Physiological Foundations

For Felix and my family.

For Elsevier:

Commissioning Editor: Dinah Thom
Associate Editor: Claire Wilson
Project Manager: Joannah Duncan
Design Direction: George Ajayi
Illustration Buyer: Gillian Murray
Illustrator: Jane Fallows

Exercise Prescription: Physiological Foundations

A Guide for Health, Sport and Exercise Professionals

Kate Woolf-May PhD

*Research Fellow and Lecturer, Department of Sport Science, Tourism and Leisure,
Canterbury Christ Church University College, Canterbury, Kent, UK*

With contribution from

Steve Bird PhD FIBiol FBASES
Director, Centre for Population Health, Sunshine Hospital, St Albans, Victoria, Australia

Foreword by

Polly Davey PhD

*Senior Lecturer and Director, Human
Performance Centre, London South Bank University, London, UK*

Illustrations by

Jane Fallows

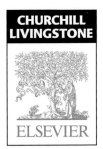

CHURCHILL LIVINGSTONE

ELSEVIER

EDINBURGH   LONDON   NEW YORK   OXFORD   PHILADELPHIA   ST LOUIS   SYDNEY   TORONTO   2006

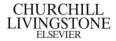

The right of Kate Woolf-May to be identified as author of this work has been asserted by her in accordance with the Copyright, Designs and Patents Act 1988

First published 2006

ISBN: 0443 10017 9
ISBN-13: 978 0 443 10017 8

British Library Cataloguing in Publication Data
A catalogue record for this book is available from the British Library

Library of Congress Cataloging in Publication Data
A catalog record for this book is available from the Library of Congress

Notice
Neither the Publisher nor the Authors assume any responsibility for any loss or injury and/or damage to persons or property arising out of or related to any use of the material contained in this book. It is the responsibility of the treating practitioner, relying on independent expertise and knowledge of the patient, to determine the best treatment and method of application for the patient.

The Publisher

Working together to grow
libraries in developing countries

www.elsevier.com | www.bookaid.org | www.sabre.org

ELSEVIER   BOOK AID International   Sabre Foundation

your source for books,
journals and multimedia
in the health sciences
www.elsevierhealth.com

The
publisher's
policy is to use
**paper manufactured
from sustainable forests**

Printed in China

Contents

Foreword   vii
Preface   ix

Chapter 1   Introduction: physical activity, fitness and health   1

Chapter 2   Individuals with existing heart and vascular disease   9

Chapter 3   Blood lipids and hyperlipidaemia   33

Chapter 4   Diabetes and insulin resistance/insensitivity   57

Chapter 5   Blood pressure and hypertension   81

Chapter 6   Overweight and obese adults   95

Chapter 7   Coagulation, fibrinolysis and risk of thrombosis   113

Chapter 8   Adults with asthma   **Steve Bird and Kate Woolf-May**   127

Chapter 9   Chronic obstructive pulmonary disease   139

Chapter 10   Adults with arthritis   159

Chapter 11   Adults with osteoporosis   173

Chapter 12   Adults with and surviving from cancer   191

Chapter 13   Exercise and the older adult   **Steve Bird**   203

Chapter 14   Therapeutic medications: influences with regard to physical activity and exercise   219

Appendix A Screening and assessment for prescription of physical activity and exercise   237
Appendix B Physical activity and exercise: intensity, endurance and progression   247
Glossary of terms   249
Index   261

Foreword

It is both a privilege and an honour to be able to introduce the first edition of *Exercise Prescription: Physiological Foundations, A Guide for Health, Sport and Exercise Professionals*. It is well known that physical activity has earned its place in contemporary medicine, providing both preventative and therapeutic benefits to the patient and client. Nevertheless, despite increasing knowledge of the benefits that physical activity/exercise brings to those suffering from chronic diseases such as hypertension, stroke, certain cancers, non-insulin dependent diabetes mellitus, obesity and the heart and vascular diseases, there is a dearth of knowledge on the prescriptive advice that should be given by clinicians and practitioners to patients and clients.

The author, Dr Kate Woolf-May, has provided a unique approach in the way in which she has innovatively incorporated both the aetiology and pathology of the disease alongside the physical activity/exercise prescription. Previous texts have separated these two main areas and this text benefits from a more joined-up approach which enables the clinician and practitioner to develop an understanding of the background to the disease and the way it manifests itself, as well as providing descriptive physical activity/exercise prescription.

The chapters are clearly set out and easy to follow, each covering material on underlying aetiology, pathophysiology of chronic diseases, and treatment through conventional pharmacological intervention and the prescription of physical activity/exercise. Exercise prescription is further detailed by the mechanistic effects it has on the body alongside the different modes (resistance circuit and weight training, eccentric exercise, weight bearing versus non-weight bearing activities, aerobic and interval training); durations (acute bouts and regular bouts, continuous versus interval); frequency; intensity of physical activity; and training respectively. However it has also

been recognized that individuals suffering from chronic disease respond differently from healthy individuals with respect to physical activity/exercise. The needs, limitations, contraindications and absolute contraindications of the different disease conditions have been covered succinctly enabling the formulation of both a safe and effective physical activity/exercise programme. Later on in the text the author provides the reader with both a useful and comprehensive guide to the interaction between therapeutic medications and physical activity/exercise, and the potential internal and external limitations that this might pose upon functional performance. Not only is the aforementioned information of use to both the individual concerned and the clinician and practitioner whilst the individual is performing the physical activity/exercise, but it is also of utmost importance to the practitioner and clinician in the interpretation of results from screening and exercise stress testing.

In the current climate patients and clients are increasingly becoming more demanding of the medical profession. One of the main areas in which the profession can be seen to develop is through the application of a more interdisciplinary approach to the management of chronic diseases. The author has reviewed resources from a broad range of current literature, producing a book with a sound research basis, proving a widely accepted belief that physical activity/exercise can have a hand to play in the prevention and management of chronic diseases. This book is not only excellent reference material for any exercise practitioner or clinician working in the field of exercise prescription for clients or patients, but would also provide a useful and informative core text for final-year degree and Masters level medical, health and sports science students. The challenge is for the reader to apply this relatively novel information and understanding of the aetiology and pathophysiology of the chronic diseases wisely and to improve both functional capacity and prognosis of the patient/client. I hope you enjoy this book as much as I have done.

Dr Polly Davey

Preface

It is becoming more widely accepted that for most individuals physical activity can not only reduce the risk of ill health, but can also be an effective tool for improving the health of both asymptomatic and symptomatic people. Increasingly, therefore, symptomatic individuals are being referred to health professionals and exercise practitioners for advice and prescription of appropriate physical activity and exercise. Consequently the demand for qualified and knowledgeable staff to carry out this work has risen.

The objective of this book is not to provide descriptive exercise prescription but rather to enable the reader to develop an understanding of the underlying aetiology and pathophysiology of commonly occurring chronic diseases in adult individuals. The available current literature regarding the impact of these disorders upon physical activity and exercise ability has been reviewed, as has the effect that physical activity/exercise might have on the symptoms of these disorders. Specific considerations and contraindications regarding physical activity/exercise in these special populations have also been highlighted.

Since the prescription of physical activity/exercise in this field is relatively novel, there is still a great deal to be determined with regard to appropriate physical activity/exercise prescription. Notwithstanding this, the aim is to provide a reference, in order to assist the exercise practitioner in prescribing appropriate physical activity/exercise for individual clients or patients.

Canterbury 2006   Kate Woolf-May

Chapter 1

Introduction: physical activity, fitness and health

CHAPTER CONTENTS

Epidemiological evidence   1
   Physical activity   1
   Energy expenditure   2
   Aerobic fitness   2
   Physical activity/exercise intensity   2
   Current physical activity guidelines and physical
   inactivity   2
Adaptations to physical activity/exercise   3
   Central adaptations   4
   Peripheral adaptations   4
Aerobic capacity   4
   Genetic predisposition   4
   Aerobic capacity and physical work   4
Moderate intensity physical activity/exercise   5
Summary   5
Suggested readings, references and bibliography   6

EPIDEMIOLOGICAL EVIDENCE

PHYSICAL ACTIVITY

In the past 50 years our understanding has increased regarding the relationship between a sedentary lifestyle and many chronic degenerative disorders, particularly heart and vascular disease. This understanding has come from a wealth of epidemiological studies. One of the earliest was a retrospective study of bus conductors and drivers carried out by William Morris in the 1950s, which revealed that the more physically active conductors had a lower incidence of coronary heart disease (CHD) and lower rates of early mortality from disease than bus drivers (Morris & Crawford 1958). Indeed the bus drivers were found to have one and a half times the incidence of CHD with greater serum cholesterol and blood pressure than the conductors (Morris et al 1966). These findings were supported by Paffenbarger et al (1971), who prospectively followed the work-time physical activity levels of 59 401 longshoremen (dock workers), and found that those men who expended around 8500 kcal per week had, at any age, reduced risk of fatal CHD compared to those men whose jobs require less energy expenditure. These findings have been echoed by several large epidemiological studies, such as that carried out by Taylor et al (1962) on US railroad workers, which found death rates to be lower among physically active than among sedentary employees, and that by Morris et al (1973) on UK civil servants, where those who were most physically active had a lower incidence of CHD and lower rates of mortality from disease. The influence that leisure-time physical activity had upon these findings and/or whether those with poorer health selected themselves into more sedentary occupations is difficult to determine. Nonetheless, considering the number of subjects involved in these studies it is difficult not to accept the link between physical activity and health. This is especially so, as numerous studies have demonstrated that being physically active can reduce an individual's risk of hypertension (Paffenbarger et al 1983), stroke (Paffenbarger et al 1984), colon and breast cancer (Vena et al 1985), non-insulin-dependent diabetes mellitus (Helmrich et al 1991) and obesity (Tremblay et al 1990). However, much still remains to be determined regarding the influence that physical activity (PA)/exercise intensity, aerobic fitness and the dose of PA/exercise has upon an individual's health.

ENERGY EXPENDITURE

It is clear that being more physically active is beneficial to an individual's health and research suggests this may be as a result of an increase in the amount of energy expenditure. A study carried out on 16 936 Harvard alumni between 1962 and 1972 (Paffenbarger & Wing 1978) looked into leisure-time physical activity and that carried out at work. They found that those who expended >2000 kcal per week had a reduced risk of CHD. This was regardless of whether the physical activity was performed at work or during leisure time. Additionally, a review of 43 studies (Powell et al 1987) involving physical activity in relation to coronary artery disease (CAD) found that overall the greater the physical activity, expressed in kcal per week, the lower the risk of CAD. Furthermore, more recent research, also carried out on the Harvard alumni (7303 men, mean age 66.1 years), found that men who expended >4000 kcal per week in physical activity had a 30–40% lower risk of CHD compared to those who expended <1000 kcal per week (Lee et al 2000). This suggests that energy expenditure through physical activity is indeed important in reducing risk of CAD and CHD.

AEROBIC FITNESS

Although energy expenditure through physical activity is shown to be important in reducing risk of disease there is some debate as to whether it is enhanced aerobic fitness that conveys these benefits. In the 1970s a study from the Cooper Center (Cooper et al 1976) in Dallas, on 2924 middle-aged men, demonstrated an inverse relationship between aerobic fitness and risk factors for CHD, such as body mass, per cent body fat, blood cholesterol and triglycerides, and systolic blood pressure. A prospective study, also from the same centre, carried out by Blair et al (1989) looking at the aerobic capacity ($\dot{V}O_2$max) of 10 224 men and 3120 women, also found that at 8 years follow-up, the higher the physical fitness the lower the rates of all-cause mortality, with the lower rates being primarily due to lower rates of CHD and cancer (Fig. 1.1). However, reported improvements in aerobic capacity can range from 0% to 50%, from up to one year of aerobic training, signifying that some individuals are highly responsive to aerobic training and others are not, a response that is likely to be determined by genetics (Wilmore 2003). Hence, it is difficult to determine to what extent genetic predisposition may have influenced these findings.

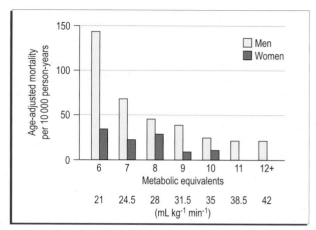

Figure 1.1 Age-adjusted all-cause mortality rates per 10000 person-years of follow up by physical fitness categories in 3120 women and 10224 men in the Aerobics Center Longitudinal Study. Physical fitness categories are expressed here as maximal metabolic equivalents (work metabolic rate/resting metabolic rate) achieved during the maximal treadmill exercise test. One metabolic equivalent equals 3.5 ml kg^{-1} min^{-1}. The estimated maximal oxygen uptake for each category is also shown. (From Blair et al 1989, Journal of the American Medical Association 262(17):2395–2401, with permission. Copyright © 1989, American Medical Association. All rights reserved.)

PHYSICAL ACTIVITY/EXERCISE INTENSITY

Even though research supports the role of increased levels of physical activity and reduced risk of certain diseases, the findings from some studies suggest that greater protection from CHD may be gained from regular vigorous forms of physical activity (Morris et al 1980, 1990, Yu et al 2000). Paffenbarger et al (1986) observed from a 12–16-year survey of all-cause mortality rates that those individuals who carried out between one and two hours per week of vigorous sports had lower death rates than regular walkers or stair climbers (49.1, 66.7 and 62.7 deaths per 10 000 person-years, respectively). Williams (1998) also found from 7059 male recreational runners (who 5 years retrospectively self-reported their average weekly running distance and best marathon and 10 km race times) that those who ran faster had lower blood pressures, triglyceride levels and ratio of total cholesterol to high-density lipoprotein cholesterol. However, there is much debate regarding the effect of PA/exercise intensity upon the health of the general population, and for sedentary and symptomatic individuals a regimen of regular vigorous PA/exercise may be contraindicated; given the findings from national surveys (NHS 2001), it may also be an unrealistic target for the majority of the population (Prior 1998). Hence, moderate-intensity PA/exercise is generally recommended.

CURRENT PHYSICAL ACTIVITY GUIDELINES AND PHYSICAL INACTIVITY

The optimal frequency, intensity, type and duration of physical activity to achieve optimal health still remain to be determined. Furthermore, the findings from research regarding the frequency of various bouts of PA/exercise are often conflicting (Hardman 2001) and whether more vigorous the intensity confers additional health benefits is debatable (Lee & Skerrett 2001). Moreover, the intensity threshold necessary to induce a training response varies with age and initial fitness and is lower for older individuals (Dehn & Bruce 1972). Nonetheless, in terms of health, the appropriateness of the traditionally recommended vigorous exercise (60–90% of $\dot{V}O_2$max, Appendix B, Table B.3) for around 15–60 minutes, three times per week (ACSM 1978, 1990), has been brought into question, in part due to its vigorous nature but also due to poor adherence (Dishman 1994). Therefore, on the basis of the numerous epidemiological studies, governments in the US and UK now recommend the daily accumulation of 30 minutes or more of moderate-intensity physical activity (40–60% $\dot{V}O_2$max), which for most healthy adults is the equivalent of brisk walking at around 3 to 4 miles per hour (Pate et al 1995). This is still a modest amount of physical activity, which is around 1050 to 1400 kcal per week. However, since a significant proportion of the US population are sedentary (King 1994) this section of the population have most to gain in terms of disease prevention and health promotion, through even modest increases in physical activity levels (Leon et al 1987). Additionally, in the UK 4316 men and women were interviewed as part of the Allied Dunbar National Fitness Survey (1992). The findings revealed that two-thirds of all women were unable to sustain a walking speed of 3 miles per hour up a slight incline, and walking at a 'normal pace' would be extremely difficult for more than half of the women and one-third of the men aged 55 to 74 years. Additionally, more recently figures from the *World Health Report* indicated that around 60% of the world's population are still not active enough to benefit their health (WHO 2002).

Inactivity is thus a major public health problem in many Western societies and a major cause of heart and vascular diseases, hypertension, obesity, hyperlipidaemia, non-insulin-dependent diabetes mellitus (type II diabetes), osteoporosis and some forms of cancer, and is also linked to mental health problems (DoH 1995, USA-DHHS 1996, WHO 1996). Therefore, the promotion of physical activity has now been written into many government strategies in an effort to increase the physical activity of the general population.

Schemes within Western societies have developed, most extensively within the last decade, where individuals who need to increase their levels of physical activity are referred to exercise practitioners for appropriate PA/exercise prescription. These schemes have been an important provider of PA/exercise opportunity for those who would not normally undertake such activity (Biddle et al 1994, Riddoch et al 1998, NHS 2001), such as sedentary and elderly people. Furthermore, since research is increasingly finding that appropriate PA/exercise intervention is beneficial to certain symptomatic individuals, PA/exercise referral has extended to accommodate those with more complicated medical conditions. However, with the increase in individuals with more complex medical conditions comes the need for more highly trained and qualified staff to be able to appropriately prescribe PA/exercise to these individuals. This has, in some countries, proved to be problematic, in part due to lack of staff expertise, where some individuals have either been prescribed inappropriate and potentially harmful PA/exercise or where symptomatic individuals have been unable to take up PA/exercise. Nonetheless, courses to train staff to deal with these more complicated clients are developing, thus further increasing the PA/exercise opportunities for members of the population who a few years ago would not have had the opportunity to carry out such activities.

ADAPTATIONS TO PHYSICAL ACTIVITY/EXERCISE

The benefits to health from habitual PA/exercise are outlined above and, for specific medical conditions, detailed in the various chapters within this book. Although it is not the intention of this chapter to go into great depth regarding adaptations to training (refer to Bird 1992, McArdle et al 2000), it is relevant to consider briefly the physiological adaptations that take place in the healthy individual.

Adaptation to endurance/aerobic training is the result of various physiological changes, most of which are considered to be beneficial to the individual in terms of enhanced performance and health. Aerobic exercise, when performed regularly, can result in a range of adaptive physical responses, namely the training effect or training response. Haskell (1994) describes the training response as:

A temporary or extended change in structure or function that results from performing repeated bouts of exercise and is independent of the immediate or short-term effects produced by a single bout of exercise. (Haskell 1994, p. 655)

The extent of these adaptations will depend on the type, frequency, intensity, duration and mode of exercise undertaken (Astrand & Rodahl 1977, ACSM 1991). These adaptations within the body collectively result in an enhanced ability to perform both maximal and submaximal exercise. They include cardiovascular changes and changes in skeletal and cardiac muscle morphology and biochemistry. These adaptations are generally categorized into *peripheral* adaptations or specific local changes and changes in cardiac performance, most notably ventricular contractility, usually referred to as *central adaptations*. However, changes in the periphery influence central changes, reflecting the integrated nature of skeletal muscle and the cardiovascular system (Rowell 1986, Mitchell & Victor 1996).

CENTRAL ADAPTATIONS

Central adaptations, such as changes in cardiac function and structure, contribute toward an increase in aerobic capacity ($\dot{V}O_2$max), and these have been found to be greatest following aerobic training of large muscle groups (Clausen et al 1973). The most notable of these adaptations is the often-observed increase in cardiac output (heart rate × stroke volume). Initially this is found without an increase in heart size (Brooks & Fahey 1984). During exercise the increase in venous return causes enhanced end-diastolic filling. This produces a higher stroke volume through the Starling mechanism (Blomqvist & Saltin 1983) and greater emptying of the left ventricle. Over time adaptations take place, which in some individuals result in an enlargement in the left ventricle, namely left ventricular hypertrophy (Puffer 2001). The stimulus for this adaptation is thought to be related to volume load on the heart (Blomqvist & Saltin 1983, Di Bello et al 1996), although the exact mechanism has still to be determined. Other cardiac parameters are often observed in those who have undergone many years of endurance training, such as an increase in transverse right ventricular cavity and left atrial transverse dimensions (Johnson & Lombardo 1994). Whereas in contrast, strength trained athletes tend to show normal ventricular volume, but an increase in septum wall thickness and mass (Snoeckx et al 1982).

PERIPHERAL ADAPTATIONS

Peripheral adaptations are generally specific to the muscle groups being used during training. The adaptations that occur enhance the ability of the trained muscle to generate, aerobically, the substance involved in the production of energy, i.e. adenosine triphosphate (ATP). Training induces peripheral adaptations such as an increase in capillarization of the specific skeletal muscle through the processes of angiogenesis and arteriogenesis (Prior et al 2003), an increase in the muscle mitochondria (Hollowszy & Coyle 1984), enhanced muscle myoglobin content (Pattengale & Holloszy 1967), greater fat metabolism (Mole et al 1971) and oxidization of carbohydrate (Gollnick & Hermansen 1973), and metabolic adaptations in different muscle types (Gollnick et al 1972), which jointly result in enhanced aerobic metabolism. Other adaptations that have also been found to occur are selective hypertrophy of different muscle fibres specific to the overload (Gollnick et al 1972, Thorstensson et al 1976) and adaptations to the anaerobic system, if vigorous PA/exercise is undertaken. The latter may include increases in resting levels of anaerobic substrates (Karlsson et al 1972), increases in the quantity and activity of key enzymes controlling the anaerobic phase of glucose breakdown (Thorstensson et al 1975), and increased capacity for blood lactic acid during all-out exercise (MacDougall et al 1977) (see McArdle et al 2000, pp. 368–377).

AEROBIC CAPACITY

Measures of aerobic capacity are the most commonly applied measurement used to assess training-induced improvements in fitness, with numerous studies reporting increases in $\dot{V}O_2$max as a result of aerobic training. Hence, the exercise practitioner will be required to carry out assessments of this factor. A target $\dot{V}O_2$max in terms of 'optimal' health for older members of the population (40–60 years) has been suggested to be around 35.0 ml kg^{-1} min^{-1} and 32.5 ml kg^{-1} min^{-1} for men and women, respectively, where this level of aerobic fitness for the older age group has been associated with a plateau in mortality risk (Blair et al 1989). The range of training-induced increase in $\dot{V}O_2$max can be from 0% to 50% (Wilmore 2003) or more (Saltin et al 1968). However, the magnitude of any change in $\dot{V}O_2$max will depend on the total training stimulus, initial training status, age and genetic predisposition of an individual. An oft-cited classic study carried out by Saltin et al (1968), on five males aged between 10 and 21 years, demonstrated that after 3 weeks of bed-rest there was a 28% reduction in $\dot{V}O_2$max. However, following 50 days of endurance training, $\dot{V}O_2$max values increased by 60%, thus indicating how the training status of an individual can affect aerobic capacity. These observed improvements in $\dot{V}O_2$max may appear rather extreme; however, they were probably due to the low initial training status after the prolonged bed-rest of the individuals.

GENETIC PREDISPOSITION

The genetically determined upper limit to an individual's $\dot{V}O_2$max needs to be considered when looking at changes in this factor. Nonetheless, although early studies on monozygous and dizygous twins observed that hereditary factors accounted for about 93% of the difference between individuals in $\dot{V}O_2$max (Klissouras 1971), more recent research has found the genetic contribution toward aerobic capacity to be more modest, at around 25–40% (Bouchard & Perusse 1994). These studies do, however, indicate that increases to a genetically determined aerobic capacity may not be exceeded. This poses questions regarding the relationship between aerobic capacity and health.

AEROBIC CAPACITY AND PHYSICAL WORK

There is a strong, almost linear relationship between $\dot{V}O_2$ and work rate (Fig. 1.2), which means that an increase in $\dot{V}O_2$max will allow for a greater maximal exercise capacity

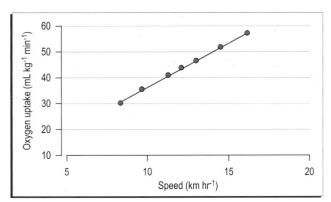

Figure 1.2 General linear relationship between work rate and oxygen uptake (ml kg^{-1} min^{-1}).

(Saltin 1969). This was demonstrated by Sjodin & Svedenhag (1985), who observed that in addition to improvements in $\dot{V}O_2$max, trained individuals were able to exercise at a higher percentage of their $\dot{V}O_2$max and could maintain this intensity for longer than their less active counterparts. In trained individuals this has been shown by a reduction in blood lactate concentration (Hurley et al 1984, Seals et al 1984, Ramsbottom et al 1995) and heart rate values (Hanne-Paparo & Kellerman 1981, Schmidt et al 1988) at the same relative and absolute submaximal exercise intensity. The combined effects of these adaptations are a reduced disturbance to the homeostasis of the body at any given submaximal PA/exercise intensity. In practical terms this would mean that a pre-training physical task, such as stair climbing, would be less physically stressful post-training. Thus, for elderly individuals this might have a considerable effect on their physical independence.

MODERATE INTENSITY PHYSICAL ACTIVITY/EXERCISE

Whilst the majority of the above-stated adaptations have been observed as a result of vigorous PA/exercise, similar adaptations have been found to result from moderate-intensity activities. For example, a study carried out by Pollock et al (1971) on 16 previously sedentary middle-aged men found that after 20 weeks of brisk walking, at between 63% and 76% of maximal heart rate (HRmax) (see Appendix B, Table B.3), four times a week for 40 minutes each session, improvements in $\dot{V}O_2$max of around 28% were observed. Pollock et al (1975) repeated this study on a group of younger adults, but the magnitude of the increase in $\dot{V}O_2$max was only around 9.6%. Another study by Jette et al (1988), on previously sedentary men and women aged 35–53 years, also showed a 14.9% increase in $\dot{V}O_2$max after only 12 weeks of walking at around 60% $\dot{V}O_2$max, thus indicating that adaptations to training may be achieved from moderate as well as vigorous physical activity. However, it is important to note that the intensity of PA/exercise is relative. Therefore, whilst most of these studies em-

ployed brisk walking as a moderate-intensity intervention, for some individuals, who might have a low initial aerobic capacity, brisk walking may indeed be a vigorous aerobic activity. Nonetheless, a study carried out by Santiago et al (1995) on a group of previously sedentary women observed that although they increased their initial $\dot{V}O_2$max by around 22% after 20 weeks of walking at between 68% and 71% of their HRmax, they failed to show increases in this factor after a further 20 weeks of walking at an increased exercise intensity of 76% of their HRmax. These findings imply that there may be a need for more vigorous activity for further improvements in $\dot{V}O_2$max to occur. However, not all studies employing moderate-intensity PA/exercise interventions have found improvements in $\dot{V}O_2$max. For example, Stensel et al (1994) observed no significant change in aerobic capacity, compared to controls, in a group of 65 previously sedentary middle-aged men (50.8 ± 5.3 years), after 12 months of brisk walking at 68% HRmax for 28 minutes per day. This indicates the diversity in changes in aerobic capacity as a result of training.

SUMMARY

- Fifty years of epidemiological research has increased our understanding regarding the relationship between a sedentary lifestyle and many chronic degenerative disorders.
- Numerous epidemiological studies have demonstrated that being physically active can reduce an individual's risk of heart and vascular diseases, hypertension, stroke, colon and breast cancer, non-insulin-dependent diabetes mellitus and obesity.
- Much still remains to be determined regarding the influence that PA/exercise intensity, aerobic fitness and the dose of PA/exercise has upon an individual's health.
- A significant proportion of the Western population are sedentary and these individuals have most to gain in terms of disease prevention and enhancement of health, through even modest increases in physical activity.
- Adaptation to endurance/aerobic training is the result of various physiological changes, most of which are considered to be beneficial to the individual in terms of enhanced performance and health.
- The extent of an individual's adaptation to training may be dependent upon the total training stimulus, initial training status, age and their genetic predisposition.
- Increases in aerobic capacity and energy expenditure through physical activity have been linked to enhanced health.
- In practical terms an increase in aerobic capacity can mean greater physical independence, especially for older and symptomatic individuals.

Suggested readings, references and bibliography

Suggested readings

Allied Dunbar National Fitness Survey 1992 Sports Council and Health Education Authority, UK

Bird S R 1992 Exercise physiology for health professionals. Chapman & Hall, London

McArdle W D, Katch F I, Katch V L 2000 Essentials of exercise physiology, 2nd edn. Lippincott Williams & Wilkins, Philadelphia

National Health Service (NHS) 2001 Exercise referral systems: a national quality assurance framework. NHS, London

References and bibliography

ACSM (American College of Sports Medicine) 1978 The recommended quantity and quality of exercise for developing and maintaining fitness in healthy adults. Medicine and Science in Sports and Exercise 10(3):vii–x

ACSM 1990 The recommended quantity and quality of exercise for developing and maintaining cardiorespiratory and muscular fitness in healthy adults. Medicine and Science in Sports and Exercise 22:265–274

ACSM 1991 Guidelines for exercise testing and prescription, 4th edn. Lea & Febiger, Philadelphia

Allied Dunbar National Fitness Survey 1992 Sports Council and Health Education Authority, UK

Astrand P O, Rodahl K 1977 Textbook of work physiology. McGraw Hill, London

Biddle S J, Fox K, Edmunds L 1994 Physical activity promotion in primary health care in England. Routledge, London

Bird S 1992 Exercise physiology for health professionals. Chapman & Hall, London

Blair S N, Kohl III H W, Paffenbarger Jr R S et al 1989 Physical fitness and all-cause mortality: a prospective study of healthy men and women. Journal of the American Medical Association 262(17):2395–2401

Blomqvist C G, Saltin B 1983 Cardiovascular adaptations to physical training. Annual Review of Physiology 45:169–189

Bouchard C, Perusse L 1994 Heredity, activity level, fitness, and health. In: Bouchard C, Shepherd R J, Stephens T (eds) Physical activity, fitness and health: international proceedings and consensus statement. Human Kinetics, Champaign, IL

Brooks G A, Fahey T D 1984 Exercise physiology: human bioenergetics and its applications. John Wiley, New York

Clausen J P, Klausen K, Rasmussen B et al 1973 Central and peripheral circulatory changes after training of the arms and legs. American Journal of Physiology 225:675–682

Cooper K H, Pollock M L, Martin R P et al 1976 Physical fitness levels vs. selected coronary risk factors. Journal of the American Medical Association 236:166–169

Dehn M M, Bruce R A 1972 Longitudinal variations in maximal oxygen intake with age and activity. Journal of Applied Physiology 33(6):805–807

Di Bello V, Santoro G, Talarico L et al 1996 Left ventricular function during exercise in athletes and sedentary men. Medicine and Science in Sports and Exercise 28:190–196

Dishman R K 1994 Advances in exercise adherence. Human Kinetics, Champaign, IL

DoH (Department of Health) 1995 More people, more active, more often. Physical activity in England: a consultation paper. DoH, London

Gollnick P, Hermansen L 1973 Biochemical adaptation to exercise: anaerobic metabolism. In: Wilmore J (ed) Exercise and sports science reviews, vol 1. Academic Press, New York

Gollnick P D, Armstrong R B, Saubert C W 4th et al 1972 Enzyme activity and fibre composition in skeletal muscle of untrained men. Journal of Applied Physiology 33(3):312–319

Hanne-Paparo N, Kellerman J J 1981 Long-term Holter ECG monitoring of athletes. Medicine and Science in Sports and Exercise 13:294

Hardman A E 2001 Issues of fractionization of exercise (short versus long). Medicine and Science in Sports and Exercise 33(6):S421–S427

Haskell W L 1994 Health consequences of physical activity: understanding and challenges regarding dose-response. Medicine and Science in Sports and Exercise 26(6):649–660

Helmrich S P, Ragland D R, Leung R W et al 1991 Physical activity and reduced occurrence of non-insulin-dependent diabetes mellitus. New England Journal of Medicine 325(3):147–152

Hollowszy J O, Coyle E F 1984 Adaptations of skeletal muscle to endurance exercise and their metabolic consequences. Journal of Applied Physiology 58:492

Hurley B F, Hagber J M, William K A et al 1984 Effect of training on blood lactate levels during submaximal exercise. Journal of Applied Physiology 56(5):1260–1264

Jette M, Sidney K, Cambell J 1988 Effects of a twelve-week walking programme on maximal and submaximal work output indices in sedentary middle-aged men and women. Journal of Sports Medicine and Physical Fitness 28(1):59–66

Johnson R J, Lombardo J (eds) 1994 Current reviews of sports medicine. Imago, Singapore, p 164–165

Karlsson J, Nordesjo L O, Jorfeldt L, Saltin B 1972 Muscle lactate, ATP, and CP levels during exercise after physical training in man. Journal of Applied Physiology 33(2):199–203

King A C 1994 Clinical and community interventions to promote and support physical activity participation. In: Dishman R K Advances in exercise adherence. Human Kinetics, Champaign, IL, p 186

Klissouras V 1971 Habitability of adaptive variation. Journal of Applied Physiology 31:338–344

Lee I M, Skerrett P L 2001 Physical activity and all-cause mortality: what is the dose response relation? Medicine and Science in Sports and Exercise 33(6):S459–S471

Lee I M, Sesso H D, Paffenbarger R S Jr 2000 Physical activity and coronary heart disease as risk in men: does the duration of exercise episodes predict risk? Circulation 102(9):981–986

Leon A S, Connett J, Jacobs D R Jr et al 1987 Leisure-time physical activity levels and risk of coronary heart disease and death: the multiple risk factor intervention trial. Journal of the American Medical Association 258:2388–2394

McArdle W D, Katch F I, Victor L K 2000 Essentials of exercise physiology, 2nd edn. Lippincott William & Wilkins, Philadelphia

MacDougall J D, Ward G R, Sale D G et al 1977 Biochemical adaptation of human skeletal muscle to heavy resistance training and immobilization. Journal of Applied Physiology 43(4):700–703

Mitchell J H, Victor R G 1996 Neural control of the cardiovascular system: insights from muscle sympathetic nerve recordings in humans. Medicine and Science in Sports and Exercise 10(suppl):S60–S69

Mole P A, Oscai L B, Holloszy J O 1971 Adaptation of muscle to exercise. Increase in levels of palmityl Co A synthetase, carnitine palmityltransferase and palmityl Co A dehydrogenase, and in capacity to oxidize fatty acids. Journal of Clinical Investigation 50(11):2323–2330

Morris J N, Crawford M D 1958 Coronary heart disease and physical activity of work; evidence of a national necropsy survey. British Medical Journal 30(5111):1485–1496

Morris J N, Kagan A, Pattison D C et al 1966 Incidence and prediction of ischemic heart disease in London busmen. Lancet 2(7463):553–559

Morris J N, Chave S P W, Adam C et al 1973 Vigorous exercise in leisure-time and the incidence of coronary heart disease. Lancet 1(7799):333–339

Morris J N, Pollard R, Everitt M G et al 1980 Vigorous exercise in leisure-time: protection against coronary heart disease. Lancet 2(8206):1207–1210

Morris J N, Clayton D G, Everitt M G et al 1990 Exercise in leisure time: coronary attack and death rates. British Heart Journal 63:325–334

NHS (National Health Service) 2001 Exercise referral systems: a national quality assurance framework. NHS, UK

Paffenbarger R S, Wing A L 1978 Chronic disease in former college students XVI. Physical activity as an index of death attack risk in college alumni. American Journal of Epidemiology 108:165–175

Paffenbarger R S, Gima A S, Laughlin M E et al 1971 Characteristics of longshoremen related to fatal coronary heart disease and stroke. American Journal of Public Health 61(7):1362–1370

Paffenbarger R S, Wing A L, Hyde R T et al 1983 Physical activity and incidence of hypertension in college alumni. American Journal of Epidemiology 117(3):245–257

Paffenbarger R S Jr, Hyde R T, Wing A L et al 1984 A natural history of athleticism and cardiovascular health. Journal of the American Medical Association 252(4):491–495

Paffenbarger R S, Hyde R T, Wing A et al 1986 Physical activity, all-cause mortality, and longevity of college alumni. New England Journal of Medicine 314:605–613

Pate R R, Pratt M, Blair S N et al 1995 Physical activity and public health: a recommendation from the Centers of Disease Control and Prevention and the American College of Sports Medicine. Journal of the American Medical Association 273:402–407

Pattengale P K, Holloszy J O 1967 Augmentation of skeletal muscle myoglobin by programs of treadmill running. American Journal of Physiology 213(3):783–785

Pollock M L, Miller H S, Janeway R et al 1971 Effects of walking on body composition and cardiovascular function of middle aged men. Journal of Applied Physiology 30:126–130

Pollock M L, Dimmick J, Miller H S et al 1975 Effects of mode of training on cardiovascular function and body composition of adult men. Medicine and Science in Sports 7:139–145

Powell K E, Thompson P D, Caspersen C J et al 1987 Physical activity and the incidence of coronary heart disease. Annual Reviews of Public Health 8:253–287

Prior B M, Pamela G L, Yang H T et al 2003 Exercise-induced vascular remodelling. Exercise and Sport Sciences Reviews 31(1):26–33

Prior G 1998 Physical activity. Health Survey of England. Online. Available: http://www.archive.official-documents.co.uk May 2002

Puffer J C 2001 Overview of the athletic heart syndrome. Exercise and sports cardiology. McGraw-Hill, New York

Ramsbottom R, Williams C, Fleming N et al 1995 Training induced physiological and metabolic changes associated with improvements in running performance. British Journal of Sports Medicine 23(3):171–176

Riddoch C, Puig-Ribera A, Copper A 1998 Effectiveness of physical activity promotion schemes in primary care: a review. HEA, London

Rowell L B 1986 Human circulation regulation during physical stress. Oxford University Press, New York

Saltin B 1969 Physiological effects of physical training. Medicine and Science in Sport 1:50

Saltin B, Blomqvist B, Mitchell J H et al 1968 Response to submaximal and maximal exercise after bed rest and training. Circulation (Supplement 7):38

Santiago M C, Leon A S, Serfass R C 1995 Failure of 40 weeks brisk walking to alter blood lipids in normolipemic women. Canadian Journal of Applied Physiology 20(4):417–428

Schmidt W, Maassen T, Trost F, Boning D 1988 Training induced effects on blood volume erythrocyte turn over and haemoglobin oxygen binding properties. European Journal of Applied Physiology and Occupational Physiology 57(4):490–498

Seals D R, Hurley B F, Schultz J, Hagberg J M 1984 Endurance training in older men and women II. Blood lactate response to submaximal exercise. Journal of Applied Physiology 57:1030–1033

Sjodin B, Svedenhag J 1985 Applied physiology of marathon running. Sports Medicine 2:83–99

Snoeckx L H E H, Abeling H F M, Lambregts J A C et al 1982 Echocardiographic dimensions in athletes in relation to their training programs. Medicine and Science in Sports and Exercise 14(6):428–434

Stensel D J, Hardman A E, Brooke-Wavell K et al 1994 The influence of brisk walking on endurance fitness in previously sedentary middle-aged men. European Journal of Applied Physiology 68:513–537

Taylor H L, Klepetar E, Keys A et al 1962 Death rates among physically active and sedentary employees in the railroad industry. American Journal of Public Health 52(10):1697

Thorstensson A, Sjodin B, Karlsson J 1975 Enzyme activities and muscle strength after sprint training in man. Acta Physiologica Scandinavica 94(3):313–318

Thorstensson A, Hulten B, von Dobeln W et al 1976 Effect of strength training on enzyme activities and fibre characteristics in human skeletal muscle. Acta Physiologica Scandinavica 96(3):392–398

Tremblay A, Despres J-P, Leblanc C et al 1990 Effect of intensity of physical activity on body fat and fat distribution. American Journal of Clinical Nutrition 52:153–157

USA-DHHS (US Dept of Health and Human Services) 1996 Physical activity and health: a report of the surgeon general. Centers for Disease Control, Atlanta

Vena J E, Graham S, Zielezny M et al 1985 Lifetime occupational exercise and colon cancer. American Journal of Epidemiology 122(3):357–365

WHO (World Health Organization) 1996 The Heidelberg guidelines for promoting physical activity among older persons. WHO, Geneva

WHO 2002 World Health Report 2002. Reducing risks, promoting healthy life. Online. Available: http://www.who.int/whr/2002/en August 2003

Williams P T 1998 Relationships of heart disease risk factors to exercise quantity and intensity. Archives of International Medicine 158:237–245

Wilmore J H 2003 Applied exercise physiology: a personal perspective of the past, present and future. Exercise and Sport Science Reviews 31(4):159–160

Yu S, Yarnell J, Murray L et al 2000 Physical activity and the risk of CHD: nine-year follow up in the Caerphilly prospective study. European Heart Journal 21(suppl):694

Chapter 2

Individuals with existing heart and vascular disease

CHAPTER CONTENTS

Introduction   9
Prevalence   10
Aetiology   10
    Primary risk factors   10
        Cigarette smoking   10
    Secondary risk factors   11
    Non-modifiable risk factors   11
Function of the vascular endothelium   11
Pathology of atherosclerosis   11
    Modified response-to-injury theory   12
Treatments   13
Pharmacological treatment   13
    Alpha-blockers   13
    Beta-blockers   13
    Nitrates   13
    Calcium channel blockers   14
    Angiotensin-converting enzyme (ACE) inhibitors   14
    Angiotensin receptor antagonists   14
    Diuretics   14
    Anti-arrhythmia drugs   14
Physical activity and exercise   14
    Exercise and atherosclerosis   15
        Exercise and endothelium   15
        Exercise and T cells   16
        Endothelium and T-cell relationship   16
    Myocardial infarction   16
    Coronary artery bypass graft and angioplasty   17
    Angina and silent ischaemia   17
    Pacemakers   17
    Peripheral vascular disease   17
    Chronic heart failure   18
Single bout of physical activity/exercise   18
Adaptations to regular physical activity/exercise   18
    Peripheral adaptations   18
    Central adaptations   18
        Myocardial adaptations   19

    Catecholamines   19
    Aerobic capacity   20
Adverse cardiac events in response to exercise   20
Pre-exercise prescription   21
Physical activity/exercise prescription   21
Physical intensity   24
Aerobic activities   24
Resistance circuit training and weight training   24
Interval training   25
Water-based activities   25
Warming up and cooling down   25
    Flexibility and stretching   26
Considerations and contraindications   26
    Absolute contraindications for exercise   26
    Considerations   26
    Upright and supine exercise   27
    Medications   27
Summary   27
Suggested readings, references and bibliography   28

INTRODUCTION

The focus of this chapter will be primarily on individuals with existing heart and vascular disease arising predominantly as a result of atherosclerosis. Coronary heart disease (CHD), coronary artery disease (CAD) and cardiovascular disease (CVD) are complex multifactorial diseases and the terms are often used interchangeably although their meanings are different (see Glossary). Since the causes of these diseases are highly related to other diseases and disorders, the reader will be directed to other related areas within this book.

PREVALENCE

Heart disease has no geographic, gender or socio-economic boundaries. Yet despite the decline in CVD death rates over the past 10 years in countries such as the USA (AHA 2003a) and the UK (BHF 1999), CHD/CVD is still the most common cause of death in most Western societies, and is a major health and economic burden throughout the world (AIHW 2002). In 1999 CVD contributed to a third of global deaths and by 2010 it is predicted to be the leading cause of death in developing countries (WHO 2002).

AETIOLOGY

Although CHD, CAD and CVD have slightly different meanings, generally the causes of these diseases are similar. The factors that are currently known to result in these diseases are commonly known as CHD risk factors. These have been divided into two categories known as *primary* and *secondary* risk factors. A primary risk factor is one that is individually capable of producing clinical complications associated with CHD/CAD/CVD, whereas a secondary risk factor can evoke clinical complications only in conjunction with one or more of the primary factors. Currently primary risk factors have been identified as hypercholesterolaemia (Ch. 3), high-density lipoprotein cholesterol (HDL-C) less than 1.0 mmol/l (40 mg/dl) (NCEP 2001), cigarette smoking and hypertension (Ch. 5). Secondary risk factors have been identified as diabetes mellitus (Ch. 4), obesity (Ch. 6) and physical inactivity. Other factors such as age, gender (male) and genetic predisposition (a family history of heart and related diseases) are also considered as factors of risk. However, whereas the listed *primary* and *secondary* risk factors may be altered through lifestyle and/or medical intervention (known as *modifiable* or *influenceable* risk factors), this latter group cannot and are therefore non-modifiable risk factors (Table 2.1). Furthermore, although there can be several

sources of heart and vascular disease, in the majority of cases atherosclerosis is the main cause (Lilly 1997).

In recent years scientists have recognized that some of the risk factors for heart and vascular disease cluster in certain people. These include central obesity, glucose intolerance, dyslipidaemia and high blood pressure. This has been termed syndrome X or metabolic syndrome. It is believed that this syndrome is closely linked to insulin resistance and may be genetically determined. However, more study is required to determine fully the underlying cause and whether intervention, such as physical activity (PA)/exercise, has any beneficial effect on those with this syndrome as they are especially prone to heart and vascular disease (AHA 2003b).

PRIMARY RISK FACTORS

The contribution to heart and vascular disease of hypercholesterolaemia and low levels of HDL will be discussed in Chapter 3 (p. 33), and that of hypertension in Chapter 5 (p. 81).

Cigarette smoking

Cigarette smoking is one of the most preventable of all the risk factors, and although it is difficult to directly relate the number of cigarettes smoked with the risk of atherosclerosis, it does appear that smokers' risk of dying from CHD is increased (Kawachi et al 1993). Furthermore, smoking low tar cigarettes does not appear to reduce one's risk of myocardial infarction (MI) compared to smoking regular cigarettes (Tavani et al 2001), though there does appear to be a dose–response relationship between total amount of tar consumed and risk of MI (Sauer et al 2002). The mechanisms relating cigarette smoking to risk of heart and vascular disease are not totally understood. However, it is known that smoking reduces circulating HDL, possibly by affecting the cholesteryl ester transfer protein (CETP) (Dullaart et al 1994) (Ch. 3). Cigarette smoking is also known to inappropriately stimulate the sympathetic nervous system (SNS) causing a transient rise in blood pressure. Cigarette constituents also cause endothelial dysfunction by altering or decreasing prostacyclin and/or increasing platelet adhesiveness. Research carried out on the acute and chronic effects of smoking on endothelium-dependent dilation of the peripheral arteries found that smokers' resting blood flow-mediated dilation was significantly reduced and their intima-media thickness was greater compared to matched controls. These impairments in the smokers were also related to the duration and number of cigarettes smoked (Poredos et al 1999). After approximately 5 or more years of smoking cessation one's risk of heart and vascular disease is similar to someone who has never smoked (Pyorala et al 1994). However, it is still not known if damage incurred to the endothelium is reversible.

Table 2.1 Risk factors for heart and vascular disease

Classification	Risk factors
Primary	Hypercholesterolaemia (p. 34)
	HDL-C <1.0 mmol/l (40 mg/dl) (p. 40)
	Cigarette smoking (p. 10)
	Hypertension and high blood pressure (p. 81)
Secondary	Diabetes mellitus (p. 58)
	Obesity (p. 95)
	Physical inactivity
Non-modifiable	Increasing age
	Gender (male) (p. 44)
	Genetic predisposition (p. 42)

SECONDARY RISK FACTORS

The contribution of the secondary risk factors diabetes mellitus (p. 57) and obesity (p. 81) to heart and vascular diseases is discussed elsewhere. Despite physical inactivity being generally defined as a secondary risk factor, it is arguably a primary factor since a sedentary lifestyle is deemed a major cause of the rise in the rates of heart and vascular diseases (WHO 2002). The links between heart and vascular diseases and lack of physical fitness (Blair et al 1989) and a sedentary lifestyle (Morris et al 1953) are well documented and are outlined in Chapter 1 (p. 1).

NON-MODIFIABLE RISK FACTORS

Risk factors such as age, gender and genetic predisposition are unalterable and as one increases in age the risk of developing heart and vascular disease is augmented. However, whether this is due to ageing per se or change in lifestyle is debatable. It is clear that males are at greater risk of these diseases than premenopausal women, which is mainly due to the effect of oestrogen upon HDL-C levels (Wallace et al 1979) resulting in a more favourable blood lipid profile (Henderson et al 1991, Freedman 1996) (p. 44).

An individual's risk of certain diseases is to some extent determined by their genetic predisposition and this is true for heart and vascular diseases. Individuals with genetic diseases such as Tangier disease, which is characterized by the virtual absence of circulating plasma HDL (Ordovas 2000), and those with low levels of low-density lipoprotein (LDL) receptors leading to high levels of plasma LDL-C (Brown & Goldstein 1986), are obviously at increased risk, since low HDL and high LDL-C are primary risk factors for heart and vascular disease. Nonetheless, despite these risk factors being *non-modifiable*, appropriate PA/exercise prescription may reduce some of the other modifiable risk factors, thereby attenuating the overall health risk.

FUNCTION OF THE VASCULAR ENDOTHELIUM

The endothelium plays an important role in the atherosclerotic process and in response to exercise. The vascular endothelium consists of a single-celled layer of smooth endothelial cells that line the entire cardiovascular system from the heart to the smallest capillaries, which are only endothelium. Endothelial cells are also present in other parts of the body and have a large number of active functions as well as serving as a physical lining to the heart and blood vessels. Endothelial cells secrete endothelium-derived relaxation factors, which mediate vascular smooth muscle responses to many chemical agents and to mechanical force. Endothelial cells also secrete substances that stimulate angiogenesis (vascular growth), and regulate transport of macromolecules and other substances between plasma and interstitial fluid. They regulate blood coagulation and fibrinolysis; synthesize active hormones from inactive precursors; extract and degrade hormones and other mediators; undergo contractile activity, which regulates capillary permeability; and influence vascular smooth muscle proliferation in atherosclerosis (Vander et al 1990).

The vascular endothelium plays an important role in vasoconstriction and vasodilatation, which are important determinants of blood pressure, and in myocardial oxygen supply in the coronary arteries. A study on the aortic endothelium of the rabbit showed that acetylcholine induced vasodilation. However, in the absence of the endothelium the acetylcholine-induced dilation was attenuated (Furchgott & Zawadzki 1980), thus indicating the importance of the vascular endothelium in vasoregulation (Libonati et al 2001). One of the most potent endothelial-derived vasodilators is nitric oxide (NO). The endothelial cells produce NO in response to several physiological stimuli including platelet products, thrombin, changes in oxygen tension and shear stress. An increase in blood flow appears to activate shear-sensitive calcium-dependent potassium channels that result in NO release. Furthermore, inhibitors of NO synthesis are known to cause vasoconstriction and hypertension (Vallance et al 1989). Nitric oxide also inhibits platelet aggregation in response to serotonin, adenosine diphosphate (ADP) and thrombin (Lusher et al 1988) and inhibits leukocyte adhesion (Ohara et al 1993). Oxidation of LDLs may also suppress the action of NO, impairing the NO reactivity which is associated with arteriosclerosis. Nitric oxide induces vasodilation by increasing intracellular cyclic 3',5'-guanosine monophosphate (cGMP) in smooth muscle cells (SMC) and is regulated by NO synthase (NOS). Other vasodilation factors such as prostacyclin and endothelium-derived hyperpolarizing factor are also secreted by the vascular endothelium. The vascular endothelium also secretes vasoconstriction substances such as endothelin and angiotensin II (Libonati et al 2001) and regulates fibrinolysis (p. 117).

PATHOLOGY OF ATHEROSCLEROSIS

The word atherosclerosis is derived from the Greek words *athere* meaning gruel, *oma* meaning mass and *skleros* meaning hard, and they aptly describe the nature of the lesions which characterize this degenerative disease of the blood vessels (Thompson 1989). In order to understand how the atherosclerosis develops it is important first to understand the basic construction of the arterial blood vessel. The arterial blood vessels consist of an inner layer of endothelial cells known as the *intima* that rests on connective tissue. The endothelium forms a barrier against the circulating blood and also serves many very important additional metabolic and signalling functions that help maintain the integrity of the vessel walls (p. 11). It is in

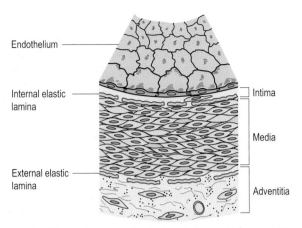

Figure 2.1   Basic structure of arterial blood vessel (adapted from http://rx.stlcop.edu/pathophysiology/LIPIDS/sld004.htm)

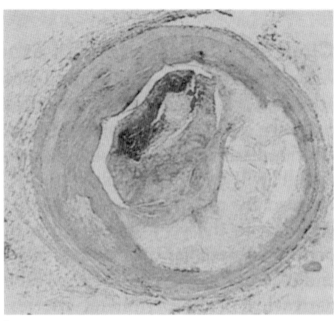

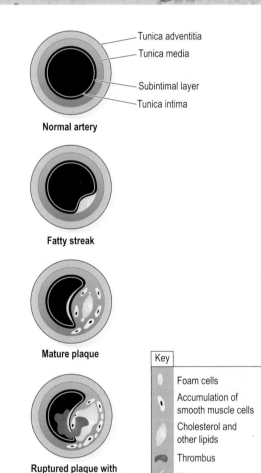

Figure 2.2   (a and b) Fibrous plaques of arterial blood vessel. (Part a from Lindsay & Gaw 2003; part b from Ross & Wilson 2001.)

the *intima* where the atherosclerotic lesions develop. The *media*, the thickest layer of the artery, is separated from the *intima* and the *adventitia* (the outermost layer of the artery wall) by elastic type laminae. The laminae contain openings between elastic fibres that allow cells to pass through. The *media* itself is composed mainly of SMCs in a matrix of collagen, elastin and proteoglycans. The *adventitia* consists of fibroblasts, collagen, blood vessels, nerves and lymphatics and is thought not to be directly involved or affected by the atherosclerotic lesions (Fig. 2.1).

Atherosclerosis is the most common underlying cause of heart and vascular disease, and has been defined as a variable combination of changes in the intima consisting of the focal accumulation of lipids, other blood constituents and fibrous tissue, accompanied by changes in the media of the vessel (Thompson 1989) (Fig 2.2). The exact mechanism by which atherosclerosis develops remains incompletely understood and despite there being several non-exclusive theories regarding the development of atherosclerosis, such as chemical factors, molecular mechanisms and/or infectious agents, such as bacteria (Brown 1996), the modified *response-to-injury* hypothesis is at present the most widely accepted theory (Lilly 1997).

MODIFIED RESPONSE-TO-INJURY THEORY

Initially the process by which atherosclerosis was thought to develop was as a result of irritation and/or injury to the endothelial cells of the intima. There are many possible causes of this, such as shear stress, hypertension, diabetes, toxins, nicotine from tobacco smoke and plasma cholesterol. Nonetheless, prime causes have been identified as raised plasma cholesterol and the influence of blood pressure (Thompson 1989). Cholesterol is transported in the blood via lipoproteins (p. 35). Low-density lipoprotein is nearly half cholesterol and is the major cholesterol carrier (Levy 1981). The problem is thought to start when the endothelium is irritated and/or damaged by these LDLs and/or the above-mentioned factors (Brown 1996, Lilly

1997). The original *response-to-injury theory* was based on the premise that injury to the endothelium allowed entry of blood platelets into the arterial wall, followed by proliferation of SMCs in the media. However, this theory was

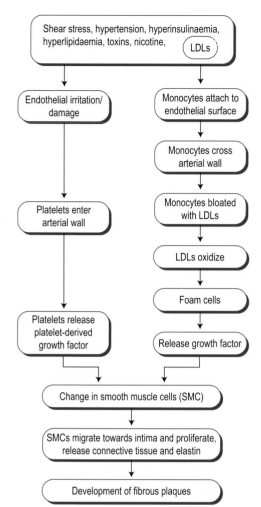

Figure 2.3   Simplified diagrammatic representation of the response-to-injury theory.

later modified as research showed that after only a few weeks of diet-induced hypercholesterolaemia (Ross 1986) clusters of monocytes become attached to the endothelial surface of arteries that had become irritated by the increase in circulating LDL-C. Irritated and/or damaged endothelium releases substances that attract white blood cells (monocytes and T lymphocytes) and platelets that bind to the endothelium, which then cross the arterial wall. The macrophages, which are related to monocytes but are situated in connective tissue, become bloated with lipid from LDLs, oxidize and turn into foam cells (Aqel et al 1984). The release of growth factor from the monocytes and the platelets (platelet-derived growth factor) causes a change in the SMCs, which then migrate toward the intima and proliferate. Further damage is also caused by the oxidization of the LDL particle. Over time visible fatty streaks develop where the platelets have adhered and thrombus formation starts. The release of connective tissue and elastin from the SMC also contributes toward fibrosis and hardening of the area and the development of fibrous plaques (Fig. 2.3). Complications occur when a plaque ruptures, providing a site for thrombosis (p. 113) and potential embolism and/or sudden occlusion of an arterial

lumen, which can lead to conditions such as MI, stroke and/or pulmonary embolism. Complications may also occur when there is insidious narrowing of the arterial lumen, which may under certain circumstances, such as physical exertion, result in intermittent claudication, angina and/or MI, or when a vessel wall weakens, resulting in an aneurysm.

TREATMENTS

After a cardiac event, most cardiac patients will be treated through pharmacological and non-pharmacological interventions. The non-pharmacological intervention will generally take the form of cardiac rehabilitation, which usually includes some type of exercise programme (p. 21).

PHARMACOLOGICAL TREATMENT

There are numerous medications that can be prescribed for those with heart or vascular problems. The most common types are alpha- and beta-blockers, nitrates, calcium channel blockers, angiotensin-converting enzyme (ACE) inhibitors, angiotensin receptor antagonists, diuretics and the anti-arrhythmia drugs. The effects of these drugs on PA/exercise ability are outlined in Chapter 14 (p. 223).

ALPHA-BLOCKERS

An alpha-blocker is generally prescribed for hypertension when no other hypertensive medications are being prescribed. They work by preventing the release of noradrenaline (norepinephrine) from the postganglionic adrenergic neurons. However, since these drugs do not control supine blood pressure they may cause postural hypotension, and have largely fallen from general use (p. 226) (BMA, RPS GB 2005).

BETA-BLOCKERS

Beta-blockers are generally used to treat those with hypertension, angina, tachycardia and arrhythmias. These drugs work by blocking the beta-adrenoreceptors in the heart, peripheral vasculature, bronchi, pancreas and liver. A wide variety of beta-blockers are now available, and some are more specific with regard to the beta-adrenoreceptors that they block (BMA, RPS GB 2005).

NITRATES

Nitrates are prescribed for relief and prevention of angina. They are potent coronary vasodilators, and their principal effect is in the reduction in venous return, which reduces left ventricular work. However, their use is often accompanied by side effects, such as, flushing, headache and postural hypotension (BMA, RPS GB 2005).

CALCIUM CHANNEL BLOCKERS

Calcium channel blockers are generally prescribed for those with hypertension and angina and for the control of arrhythmias. These drugs work by interfering with the inward displacement of calcium ions through the slow channels of the active cell membranes. They affect the specialized conducting cells of the myocardium and the cells of the vascular smooth muscle. Thus, they cause a reduction in both myocardial contraction and the formation and propagation of electrical impulses within the heart, as well as a reduction in the coronary and systemic vascular tone. These drugs may cause side effects such as palpitations, headaches, constipation, mild swelling of the ankles and facial flushing (BMA, RPS GB 2005).

ANGIOTENSIN-CONVERTING ENZYME (ACE) INHIBITORS

Angiotensin-converting enzyme (ACE) inhibitors, most commonly known as ACE inhibitors, are generally prescribed for hypertension, heart failure and the prevention of a cardiovascular event in MI patients. ACE inhibitors work by inhibiting the conversion of angiotensin I to angiotensin II, which is a strong vasoconstrictor (p. 83). Potential side effects include a dry cough, hypotension, skin rash, metallic taste, reduced kidney function and oedema of the lips and tongue (BMA, RPS GB 2005).

ANGIOTENSIN RECEPTOR ANTAGONISTS

Angiotensin receptor antagonists are prescribed for hypertension, heart failure and the prevention of a cardiovascular event in MI patients. They have many of the properties of ACE inhibitors. However, unlike ACE inhibitors, they do not inhibit the breakdown of bradykinin and other kinins, and thus do not tend to cause the persistent dry cough that is often seen with ACE inhibitors. Angiotensin receptor antagonists are therefore used as an alternative for those who discontinue ACE inhibitors (BMA, RPS GB 2005).

DIURETICS

Diuretics are prescribed to assist in the treatment of hypertension and acute heart failure, and on a short-term basis for those with mild heart failure. There are many different types of diuretics, and not all are used to treat cardiovascular conditions. These are categorized into carbonic anhydrase inhibitors, loop diuretics, thiazide diuretics, osmotic and potassium sparing diuretics. Generally, they allow for an increase in the excretion of urine, which reduces the blood volume thereby taking pressure out of the cardiovascular system. There are differing side effects depending on the type/s of diuretic taken (BMA, RPS GB 2005).

ANTI-ARRHYTHMIA DRUGS

There are different types of anti-arrhythmia drugs and in the UK they are classified according to their effect. For example, some are specific for treating supraventricular arrhythmias, and some act on both supraventricular and ventricular arrhythmias. Amiodarone is most commonly prescribed for supraventricular tachycardia and atrial fibrillation, and can sometimes be used to treat heart failure. This drug is often used when other medication is ineffective or contraindicated. The possible side effects are also dependent upon the type of drug used.

Inotropic drugs, such as cardiac glycosides, can be classified as anti-arrhythmic drugs. Cardiac glycoside increases the force of myocardial contraction and reduces conductivity within the atrioventricular node. These drugs are seen as most useful in the treatment of supraventricular tachycardias, especially in persistent atrial fibrillation. Potential side effects of any of the anti-arrhythmic drugs include nausea, loss of appetite, vomiting, fatigue, slow heart rate, photosensitivity, metallic taste and nightmares (BMA, RPS GB 2005).

PHYSICAL ACTIVITY AND EXERCISE

The promotion of PA/exercise as part of the cardiac rehabilitation (CR) is increasing and it is becoming a prominent aspect of many CR programmes. The critical goals for any cardiac programme are to (i) maintain or improve the patient's functional capacity, (ii) improve the patient's quality of life, and (iii) prevent recurrent cardiac events (Thompson 2001a). Compelling data have shown exercise CR (ECR) to result in reductions in all-cause and cardiac mortality of about 20–25% compared to cardiac patients receiving conventional care (Oldridge et al 1988, US DHHS 1996). Moreover, meta-analysis carried out on studies involving MI patients undertaking ECR revealed a significant decrease in total mortality at 2- and 3-year follow-up, although total mortality at 1-year follow-up was not changed, and a 37% reduction in sudden death (O'Connor et al 1989). Animal studies suggest that physical training reduces ventricular fibrillation (Noaks et al 1983) and enhances the myocardial ischaemic tolerance (Libonati et al 1997), thereby reducing risk of a cardiac event.

Early ECR programmes originally focused primarily on medically stable, low-risk, middle-aged post-MI and coronary artery bypass graft men and tended to exclude women, the elderly and those with greater cardiac complications (Jolliffe et al 2000). However, it has been recognized that those with atrial fibrillation (Vanhees et al 2000), extensive myocardial damage, left ventricular dysfunction or failure and ongoing myocardial ischaemia may also benefit from undertaking exercise. Therefore,

ECR programmes now include a wider patient category (Todd et al 1992, Gohlke & Gohlke-Barwolf 1998). It is known that substantial improvements in functional capacity can occur 11 weeks after MI in patients not taking any exercise (Savin et al 1981), simply as a result of the recovery process. Nonetheless, patients that do undertake light exercise in the early stages of recovery have shown greater reductions in resting heart rate and improvements in aerobic capacity ($\dot{V}o_2$max) (Dressendorfer et al 1995). Additionally, those that undertake ECR tend to achieve greater scores in terms of self-efficacy (Gulanick 1991) and reduction in depression (Milani et al 1996).

The benefits of exercise for cardiac patients continue to be discovered, especially for less well patients such as those with heart failure (Hambrecht et al 2000a, Schulze et al 2002). Physical activity/exercise helps to reduce the morbidity and mortality associated with atherosclerotic heart disease through direct (cardiovascular) and indirect (i.e. risk factor modification) mechanisms. The mechanisms by which habitual and acute PA/exercise influence the pathophysiology of those with heart and vascular disease is complex, encompassing many physiological processes. Indirectly, regular PA/exercise modifies cardiovascular disease risk factors, such as blood lipids, hypertension, obesity and haemostasis and directly, by affecting haemodynamics and metabolic and physiological processes and mechanisms.

EXERCISE AND ATHEROSCLEROSIS

Evidence suggests that for those with existing atherosclerosis, exercise training (Franklin & Khan 1996) and leisure-time energy expenditure in excess of 1533 ± 122 kcal·per week (Hambrecht et al 1993) may help to slow the progression of atherosclerotic CAD. Although the precise mechanisms are yet to be fully known, it appears that regular PA/exercise has a beneficial effect on both the endothelial cells and T-cell function (a class of white blood cell that coordinates the immune system) (Smith 2001).

Exercise and endothelium

There is substantial evidence supporting the beneficial effect of exercise training on the reduction in endothelial dysfunction for both CAD and chronic heart failure (CHF) patients (Gielen et al 2001, 2002). This is important in that it reduces vasoconstriction and consequently peripheral vascular resistance, also lowering blood pressure. In normal individuals physical activity or mental stress results in coronary artery vasodilation as a result of the activation of the sympathetic nervous system and the release of NO in response to an increase in blood flow and shear stress. This outweighs the direct alpha-adrenergic constriction effect of catecholamines on arterial SMC. However, in patients with endothelial dysfunction (e.g.

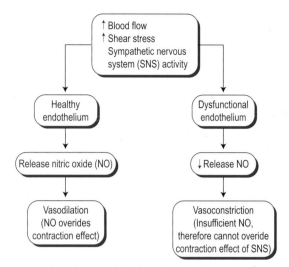

Figure 2.4 Functional and dysfunctional endothelium (adapted from Vander et al 1990).

atherosclerosis) the direct effect on the endothelium is unopposed, leading to vasoconstriction and a decrease in coronary blood flow and myocardial oxygen supply, and contributing to ischaemia (Sabatine et al 1997) (Fig. 2.4).

A study looking into endothelium-dependent vasodilation of coronary vessels was carried out on 19 CAD patients of about 70 years of age. Ten subjects underwent 4 weeks of exercise intervention (six times per day for 10 minutes on a cycle ergometer at 80% of maximum heart rate during peak oxygen uptake) with nine matched controls (Hambrecht et al 2000b). The results of the study showed a reduction in coronary vasoconstriction and improved blood flow in response to acetylcholine. The coronary vascular response to acetylcholine depends on the integrity of the endothelium and endothelium NO pathway. Hence these findings suggest an improvement in endothelial function in the exercise group. Additionally, coronary blood flow was also increased after administration of adenosine, indicating improved function of the smooth muscle of the coronary microvasculature.

Arterial shear stress also appears to play a role in the endothelial atheroprotective process. In the normal artery, shear stress of $>15\,\text{dyne/cm}^2$ tends to induce an atheroprotective effect. However, at atherosclerotic sites shear stress is generally low ($<4\,\text{dyne/cm}^2$) (Malek et al 1999). It is possible therefore that an increase in shear stress as a result of exercise training may help to stimulate this atheroprotective process. For instance, a study carried out on stable CAD patients found that after 4 weeks of exercise training acetylcholine-induced vasodilation was closely related to shear stress-induced activation of factors that result in NO, which is known to be atheroprotective (Hambrecht et al 2003). Additionally, findings from the cell culture of animal experiments indicate that shear stress enhances the endothelial L-arginine uptake; this enhances NOS activity and expression, and upregulates the production of extracellular substances which prevent premature NO breakdown, all of which leads to a reduction of myocardial ischaemic events in CAD and decreased afterload in CHF (Gielen et al 2002).

Exercise and T cells

There are different subsets of T cells (also known as lymphocytes) that are categorized according to their function, such as cytotoxic (which attack a specifically targeted cell), helper (which enhance antibody and cytotoxic T production) and suppressor T cells (which inhibit antibody and cytotoxic T production) (Vander et al 1990). Research indicates that some of these functions may be influenced by exercise intervention. A study carried out on 43 subjects, at risk of ischaemic heart disease, who underwent 6 months of varied moderate-intensity aerobic exercise (not including water based activities) found a highly significant reduction (58.3%) in atherogenic cytokines (which are the protein messengers secreted by macrophages and monocytes and lymphocytes) and increase (35.9%) in the production of atheroprotective cytokines, which could not be attributed to the modification of other risk factors. These changes also correlated with the total number of hours that the subjects spent doing exercise (Smith et al 1999).

Endothelium and T-cell relationship

The relationship between the endothelium and the various types of T cells is important in the atherogenic or atheroprotective process. Once these processes are initiated they appear to be self-sustaining. For instance, the atherogenic endothelial cells express adhesion molecules and produce chemokines that favour the acceptance of T-helper cells and monocytes, which in turn produce cytokines that further activate the endothelium. However, for individuals who exercise, training appears to stimulate an atheroprotective process in the endothelial cells and T cells. In the healthy individual, the atheroprotective T cells inhibit endothelial cell activation and apoptosis by suppressing the production of atherogenic cytokines produced by macrophages. In turn, the healthy endothelium restricts its expression of molecules that invite the influx of atherogenic T cells and monocytes and also minimizes its production of cytokines that inhibit the development of atheroprotective T cells (Smith 2001). This process may also operate in individuals with atherosclerosis who undertake exercise training and may be a possible mechanism for the atheroprotective effect.

MYOCARDIAL INFARCTION

Myocardial infarction generally affects the left ventricle (LV) and is associated with permanent loss of contractile function in the area of the infarction and impaired contractility in the surrounding muscle tissue. Infarctions

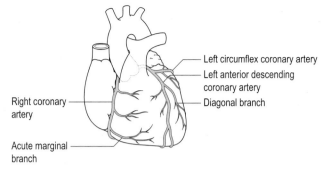

Figure 2.5   Coronary arteries (adapted from Lilly 1997).

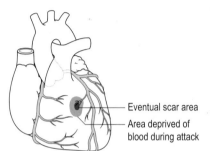

Figure 2.6   Sites of myocardial infarction (adapted from BACR 2002).

can, however, occur in various areas of the heart dependent upon the affected coronary artery. The most common infarct sites are lateral, posterior and septal. Infarcts involving larger sections of the left ventricle may be referred to as anteroseptal or inferolateral, for example (Figs 2.5 and 2.6). Future risk of morbidity and mortality is generally determined by the degree of residual myocardial ischaemia and extent of LV damage and/or dysfunction, which is illustrated by the ejection fraction (Franklin 1997).

After an acute MI these patients may have altered cardio-respiratory and haemodynamic responses to submaximal and maximal physical exertion. Those who have suffered a previous MI may have an aerobic capacity of 50–70% of that predicted for healthy individuals of their age and gender. The reduction in oxygen transport capacity is primarily due to reduced cardiac output (stroke volume and/or heart rate) as peripheral oxygen extraction is generally unaffected. In some MI patients this is due to a reduction in contractile force of the left ventricle as a result of residual ischaemia or scarring causing a decrease in ejection fraction and stroke volume. This may lead to a decrease in systolic blood pressure (SBP) with progressive exercise (exertional hypotension). In other MI patients, cardiac output may be reduced by the heart's inability to increase heart rate, as a result of physical exertion, due to chronotropic impairment and/or angina symptoms (Franklin 1997). Furthermore, medications (Ch. 14) and co-morbidities will have additional effects.

CORONARY ARTERY BYPASS GRAFT AND ANGIOPLASTY

Coronary artery bypass graft (CABG) is employed under circumstances when pharmacological therapy fails to relieve anginal symptoms, when percutaneous transluminal coronary angioplasty (PTCA) is contraindicated and when there is severe occlusion of the coronary vessels and/or severe LV dysfunction. Individuals who undergo CABG generally have an ejection fraction of about 38%, whilst those who undergo PTCA have an ejection fraction of around 55% (normal average ejection fraction is around 62%) (Franklin 1997).

Successful revascularization increases the blood flow and oxygen supply to the myocardium beyond the region of the obstructive coronary lesion (Fig. 2.7). Therefore, during exertion there can be a reduction or elimination of ischaemia and anginal symptoms. This may also be reflected in electrocardiographic changes (p. 245). Improvement in the relation between myocardial oxygen supply and demand may also enhance ventricular contractility and wall motion, enhancing haemodynamic response to physical exertion. Furthermore, chronotropic impairment and/or exertional hypotension may be less apparent following revascularization (Franklin 1997).

The benefits and limitations of physical training are similar for post-MI patients. Revascularized patients who have not previously had an MI tend to commence inpatient ECR earlier than MI patients, since their myocardium has not recently undergone acute damage, and tend to progress at a faster rate. Many patients begin to resume normal activities, such as walking, within 24 to 48 hours after PTCA (Franklin 1997).

ANGINA AND SILENT ISCHAEMIA

Angina and ischaemia occur when the obstructed artery cannot supply the myocardium with adequate oxygen to meet its demand. Symptoms of angina have been described as discomfort in the chest that may radiate to the arm, neck and jaw. This may be accompanied by shortness of breath, nausea and/or sweating. Angina that predictably occurs during physical exertion is termed 'stable'. 'Unstable' angina occurs when an individual experiences a noticeable increase in frequency of angina or begins to experience angina at rest. Ischaemia may be symptomatic or silent. Initially ischaemia occurs only during intense physical exertion or stress; however, as plaque builds up the occlusion may increase and symptoms may occur with minimal activity or at rest. It is inadvisable for those with unstable angina to carry out exercise until their symptoms have improved. Those with stable angina respond well to physical training and the aim is to raise their ischaemic threshold and the point when symptoms of angina occur (Friedman 1997).

PACEMAKERS

In patients who lose normal cardiac sequencing, such as atrial and ventricular filling and contraction, there may be deterioration in haemodynamics. Pacing techniques are therefore sometimes employed for those with sinus node dysfunction and those with life-threatening ventricular dysrhythmias. The benefits of physical training in such patients are the same as for other cardiac patients and they benefit from an improved heart rate response to exercise. However, patients with an implantable cardioverter defibrillator are at risk of receiving inappropriate shocks during exercise, which can occur when the sinus heart rate exceeds the programmed threshold rate or if an exercise-induced supraventricular tachycardia develops. Therefore these patients need to be closely monitored during physical exertion to ensure that their heart rate does not approach the activation rate for the device (West et al 1997).

PERIPHERAL VASCULAR DISEASE

Peripheral vascular disease (PVD) occurs as a result of stenosis and occlusion of the arteries of the lower extremities, generally as a result of the build-up of atherosclerotic plaques, which result in a reduction in blood flow beyond the obstruction. During physical exertion, pain may be felt in the active muscles that have occluded blood flow, and is termed claudication. This is generally felt in the lower leg during walking and the time and/or distance to onset of maximal pain are used as criteria for assessing the functional severity of this disease. Since exercise training enhances blood flow to the leg through an increase in aerobic metabolism (thus reducing the production of anaerobic metabolites), improves walking economy, and produces a more favourable redistribution of blood flow, patients who suffer from *intermittent claudication* (so called because claudication usually diminishes upon rest) generally respond well to physical training, as it increases their exercise tolerance and point to onset of pain (Gardener 1997).

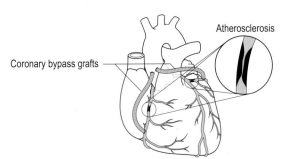

Figure 2.7 Revascularization of coronary arteries (adapted from BACR 2002).

CHRONIC HEART FAILURE

Chronic heart failure (CHF) is the inability of the heart to adequately deliver oxygen to the metabolizing tissues. The majority of patients with CHF have depressed LV systolic function as a result either of loss of myocardial function due to an MI or of reduced contractility. These patients also nearly always have reduced diastolic function, indicated by abnormal diastolic filling of the left ventricle as a result of poor compliance. They commonly display reduced cardiac output during exercise, and in severe cases at rest. They also display increased LV filling pressures, compensatory ventricular volume overload and elevated pulmonary and central venous pressures. Peripheral secondary abnormalities also occur in skeletal muscle metabolism, impaired vasodilation and renal changes, which result in fatigue, breathlessness and reduced exercise tolerance. Poor cardiac output underlies the mismatch of ventilation to perfusion in the lung, causing an increase in physiological dead space resulting in breathlessness. Although breathlessness on physical exertion is indicative of CHF, about two-thirds of these patients will be limited by leg fatigue (Myers 1997). This is related to the heart's inability to supply adequate blood flow and oxygen to the working muscles (Matsui et al 1995). Lactate accumulates in the blood at relatively low work rates, which contributes to hyperventilation in response to physical exertion and early fatigue. Other abnormalities also occur in these individuals, such as peripheral changes in muscle, which result in greater glycolysis, reduced oxidative phosphorylation and greater acidosis, mainly due to histological changes in skeletal muscle and a reduction in mitochondria. Physical training improves exercise capacity as a result of peripheral rather than central adaptations, and appears to have no effect on ventricular function (Myers 1997).

Supervised physical training has proven to be effective (Gielen et al 2001, 2002) in lessening the symptoms and improving exercise capacity. Therefore enhancing patients' ability to sustain low-level activities leads to improved independence and quality of daily life. Nonetheless, complications may occur in these patients, as they tend to deteriorate regardless of medical or physical therapy. Hence regular re-evaluation of these patients is required (Myers 1997).

SINGLE BOUT OF PHYSICAL ACTIVITY/EXERCISE

There is little research to indicate that a single bout of PA/exercise will have any beneficial indirect or direct long-term effect upon heart and vascular disease risk factors. Nevertheless, a single bout of PA/exercise will have transient physiological effects. For instance, a single bout of PA/exercise enhances insulin sensitivity and glucose transport into muscles and assists in the control of diabetes (Lutoslawska 2000) (p. 69). Additionally it has transient effects on blood pressure and blood triglycerides, and for those unfit individuals a single bout of PA/exercise may increase their risk of thrombosis (Gibbs et al 2001). Research, however, indicates that it is habitual aerobic exercise training that appears to be most beneficial to those with existing heart and/or vascular diseases.

ADAPTATIONS TO REGULAR PHYSICAL ACTIVITY/EXERCISE

Those with heart and vascular disease adapt to PA/exercise intervention in a similar way to healthy individuals. These adaptations are often segregated into central (cardiac) or peripheral (skeletal muscle) adaptations (p. 4). However, peripheral adaptations, such as a reduction in vascular resistance, may contribute to a central increase in cardiac output during exercise (Rowell 1986). Furthermore, skeletal muscle is richly endowed with afferent nerves that help to regulate the cardiovascular response to exercise (Mitchell & Victor 1996), demonstrating the integrated nature of skeletal muscle and the cardiovascular system.

Exercise intervention in those with existing heart and vascular disease has been found to do little to improve serious ventricular arrhythmias or collateral circulation (Wenger et al 1995, Franklin & Saunders 2000, Gielen & Hambrecht 2001). Exercise intervention has, however, been found to act on the sympathetic and parasympathetic nervous systems to decrease rate pressure product (RPP) (p. 87), and associated myocardial oxygen demands at any given submaximal work rate. Furthermore, there appears to be a reduction in the signs and symptoms of myocardial ischaemia at matched RPP after exercise training (Balady et al 1994).

PERIPHERAL ADAPTATIONS

Peripheral adaptations from habitual aerobic PA/exercise upon skeletal muscle include a small increase in strength, an increase in capillary density, mitochondrial number, size and function. An increase in capillary density and mitochondrial number, size and function allows for greater aerobic metabolism resulting in enhanced arterial-venous (a-v) oxygen (O_2) difference, which is considered to be the main physiological mechanism for the improvement in CAD patients' performance after exercise training (Detry et al 1971, Thompson 2001b).

CENTRAL ADAPTATIONS

In healthy individuals one of the initial adaptations to aerobic training is an increase in maximum cardiac output without any cardiac structural changes, mainly as a result of the *Starling mechanism* (Blomqvist & Saltin 1983).

During aerobic exercise, higher peak transmitral inflow velocity results in enhanced end-diastolic filling (Di Bello et al 1996), which produces a higher stroke volume and consequently greater emptying of the left ventricle. Numerous years of endurance exercise influence cardiac function and structure and in some instances result in an enlarged heart, allowing for a further increase in maximum cardiac output (MacFarlane et al 1991). This normal adaptation to strenuous aerobic training is different from the pathological enlargement of the heart sometimes observed in those with heart disease, which may be as a consequence of conditions such as heart failure, cardiomyopathy, chronic hypertension and/or valvular disease (Lilly 1997). However, whereas the endurance athletes' ratio of LV radius to wall thickness has been found to be normal, this ratio is increased in those with aortic regurgitation and dilated cardiomyopathy (Sugishita et al 1983).

In healthy individuals, years of extensive endurance training cause an increase in LV end-diastolic dimensions, stroke volume and increase in mean fibre shortening velocity and a small decrease in end-systolic dimension (DeMaria et al 1978), with a possible slight increase in LV volume mass (Di Bello et al 1996) and wall thickness (DeMaria et al 1978). Although the exact stimulus for these adaptations is not clear, these changes may be related to the volume load on the heart (Blomqvist & Saltin 1983, Di Bello et al 1996). Despite these adaptations generally resulting from intense aerobic exercise, changes in LV diastolic function have been observed in healthy, previously less active individuals after only 18 weeks of brisk walking at around 68% of their aerobic capacity (~74% maximum heart rate) (Woolf-May et al 1997). This was detected using a method of echocardiography not commonly employed in this setting (Woolf-May et al 1999). There is therefore the suggestion that central adaptations may also occur in cardiac patients after moderate intensity PA/exercise intervention but have yet to be detected. Studies have found central adaptations to occur in cardiac patients but generally as a result of high intensity exercise. For instance, a study carried out on 18 ischaemic heart disease patients (aged 51 ± 3 years, mean $\pm$ SE) observed that after 12 months of exercise, at $89.7 \pm 2\%$ of peak aerobic capacity, there was a significant increase in stroke volume and an improved ejection fraction. This was found both at rest and during exercise, with no change in LV volume (Ehsani 1987b). These and findings from other research (Rinder et al 1999) indicated that the training-induced increase in stroke volume was probably due to enhanced LV function, through an improved contractile state (Ehsani et al 1986) as a result of enhanced inotropic sensitivity to catecholamines (Spina et al 1998).

Cardiac parameters that are commonly observed in healthy endurance athletes are an increase in transverse right ventricular cavity (Johnson & Lombardo 1994) and left atrial transverse dimension (Snoeckx et al 1982, Johnson & Lombardo 1994). By comparison, individuals who engage in years of resistance training, such as strength athletes, tend to show normal ventricular volume, but greater increase in septum wall thickness and mass (Snoeckx et al 1982). Whether cardiac patients show similar adaptations has yet to be fully determined. Additionally, for those with existing heart and vascular disease aerobic training appears to have no effect on blood vessel wall thickness; however, the animal model has shown an increase in the vessel lumen area (Amaral et al 2000), which may allow for greater coronary blood flow.

Myocardial adaptations

In the animal model, habitual aerobic training has been found to increase the sensitivity of the beta-adrenergic receptors of the myocardium to catecholamines from both swimming and running (Wyatt et al 1978, Hammond et al 1988). However, the literature regarding alterations in cardiac beta-receptor (Moore et al 1982) number, density and affinity are conflicting (Mazzeo 1991). Research on healthy older individuals, however, indicates that the probable mechanism for the increase in stroke volume in response to the training is enhanced inotropic sensitivity to catecholamines (Spina et al 1998).

CATECHOLAMINES

Circulating levels of catecholamines are seen as a reference indicator for SNS activity, and have been found to change after exercise intervention. Although the exact mechanism for this change has yet to be fully elucidated, several studies have shown reductions in catecholamines after exercise intervention for those with existing heart disease. For example, after one year of controlled exercise a group of 18 male post-MI patients (aged 56 ± 9 years) showed reductions in maximal and resting mean arterial blood pressure, related to reduced concentrations of catecholamines during exercise and rest (Lehmann et al 1984). An earlier study also found that at the same relative exercise intensity, levels of noradrenaline but not adrenaline were reduced after 27 weeks of jogging in a group of post-MI males (aged 34–54 years) (McCrimmon et al 1976). In another study, a group of 20 male MI patients (aged 57 ± 11 years) were treated by coronary angioplasty, after which 10 of the group underwent 2 weeks of cycle ergometry at 80% of their anaerobic threshold for 10 minutes twice a day. Post-intervention resting levels of serum and urinary noradrenaline were significantly reduced compared to the control group ($n = 10$), who showed no significant change, indicating that autonomic nervous system adaptations may occur early on in physical training (Fujimoto et al 1997).

Neurohormonal stimulation is an important compensatory mechanism to a reduction in cardiac output which is most pronounced in those with CHF (p. 18). A fall in cardiac output and subsequently systolic blood pressure

(SBP) is sensed by the carotid sinus and aortic arch, which stimulate SNS outflow of adrenaline (epinephrine) and noradrenaline (norephinephrine) to the heart and peripheral circulation, with a corresponding decrease in parasympathetic activity (acetylcholine). This results in an increase in heart rate and ventricular contractility and peripheral vasoconstriction, as the catecholamines stimulate the β_1, β_2 and α receptors, respectively. The renin–angiotensin system (p. 83) is also stimulated due to reduced renal artery perfusion as a result of the decreased cardiac output, as is the production of antidiuretic hormone (ADH). All serve to maintain blood pressure. However, ultimately over time this compensatory response proves to be deleterious to the failing heart. For instance, the increase in heart rate may increase myocardial oxygen demand and the increase in arteriolar resistance increases afterload. Additionally, the enhanced circulating volume (as a consequence of the stimulation of the renin–angiotensin system and production of ADH) and subsequent augmentation in venous return to the heart may also worsen engorgement of the vasculature of the lungs. Over time, continually high resting levels of circulating catecholamines also lead to a downregulation of cardiac beta-adrenergic receptors, which causes a decrease in the myocardium's sensitivity and may be detrimental to health (Lilly 1997).

AEROBIC CAPACITY

Research shows that those with a high aerobic capacity have a significantly reduced risk of heart disease and all-cause mortality (Blair et al 1989). In asymptomatic and healthy individuals aerobic exercise intervention leads to an increase in maximum aerobic capacity (Mitchell & Blomqvist 1971). The extent of adaptation varies according to an individual's genetic predisposition, baseline aerobic capacity and age, and with training can increase by as much as 20% (Brooks et al 1996). Individuals with heart and vascular diseases adapt to PA/exercise intervention in a similar way to healthy individuals and published studies have shown improvements to range from 11% to 56% (Thompson 1988). However, the severity of disease and length and type of intervention influences the response (Thompson 2001a). Improvements in the functional capacity of cardiac patients after moderate intensity PA/exercise training have primarily been thought to be due to peripheral rather than central adaptations (Ehsani 1987a). It is only when these individuals undergo a longer period of intense exercise training, a type not suitable for the majority of cardiac patients, that central adaptations have been observed (Hagberg et al 1983). Individuals with only CAD and no CHD often have an aerobic capacity that is within the normal range for their age and sex. These individuals may be those who have had an MI aborted by thrombolytic therapy or primary coronary angioplasty and sustained no permanent myocardial injury. Conversely individuals with CHD

generally demonstrate a reduction in maximal exercise capacity, the magnitude of which is related to the severity of existing myocardial damage, which can limit the ability of the heart to increase cardiac output during physical exertion. Some individuals with angina pectoris may have no detectable myocardial damage but limited exercise capacity due to exercise-limited discomfort. Individuals with angina pectoris tend to experience this discomfort at highly reproducible relative workload or RPP, which corresponds with the point where myocardial oxygen demand cannot be adequately supplied by coronary blood flow as a result of the coronary lesion. However, numerous individuals show considerable variation in the workload that produces symptoms. Some of this diversity in physical exertion-induced symptoms is thought to be due to variation in coronary artery vaso-motion (Thompson 2001b). Coronary arteries can alter their internal diameter in response to various stimuli, and whilst exercise induces arterial dilation in healthy individuals, in areas of atherosclerosis it can induce vasoconstriction (p. 15) (Gordon et al 1989), thus leading to ischaemia.

The physiological rationale for employing aerobic activities as a treatment for those with heart and vascular disease is that it enhances aerobic capacity with no known adverse effects on LV function; it also decreases myocardial oxygen demand at a given submaximal workload. The functional outcome is that the cardiovascular system is more efficient, responding to a higher workload with less effort (Cox 1997). Individuals with angina and post-MI who undertake aerobic training may decrease myocardial ischaemia by a decrease in myocardial oxygen demand at a given submaximal workload. Studies carried out on individuals with angina pectoris have shown onset of angina to occur at the same RPP despite exercise capacity being higher at the onset (Clausen & Trap-Jensen 1976). The mechanism for this change is thought, in the early stages, not to be as a result of structural changes but due to enhance coronary blood flow due in part to a reduction in artery vasoconstriction during physical exertion. The relative contribution of increases in stroke volume and a-v O_2 difference in relation to an increase in aerobic capacity varies between individuals and can depend upon the severity of the disease and duration of training. Individuals with considerable myocardial damage may only be able to augment the a-v O_2, thus attenuating an increase in aerobic capacity (Thompson 2001b).

ADVERSE CARDIAC EVENTS IN RESPONSE TO EXERCISE

For those with existing atherosclerosis, the major cardiac problems arising from a bout of exercise are sudden cardiac death and MI (Libonati & Glassberg 2002). When participating in supervised ECR, the absolute risk of sudden cardiac death is low, at around 1 event for every 784 000 patient-hours of exercise, and risk of MI at around

Table 2.2 Risk stratification for cardiac patients (adapted from AACVPR 1999)

Criteria	Risk
Uncomplicated MI, CABG, PTCA or atherectomy Functional capacity ≥6 Metabolic equivalents (METs) 3 or more weeks after clinical event No resting or exercise-induced myocardial ischaemia manifested as angina and/or ST–segment displacement No resting or exercise-induced complex arrhythmias No significant LV dysfunction (ejection fraction ≥50%)	Low
Functional capacity <5–6 METs three or more weeks after clinical event Mild to moderately depressed LV function (ejection fraction 31–49%) Failure to comply with exercise prescription Exercise-induced ST–segment depression of 1–2 mm or reversible ischaemic defects (echocardiography or nuclear radiography)	Moderate
Severely depressed LV function (ejection fraction ≤30%) Complex ventricular arrhythmias at rest or appearing or increasing with exercise Decrease in SBP of >15 mmHg during exercise or failure to rise consistent with exercise workloads (usually determined during exercise stress test) MI complicated by CHF, cardiogenic shock, and/or complex ventricular arrhythmias Patients with severe CAD and marked (>2 mm) exercise induced ST–segment depression Survivor of cardiac arrest	High

1 for every 294 000 patient hours; and in the event of a cardiac arrest 85% of patients are successfully resuscitated (Van Camp & Peterson 1986). However, the risks are far greater when patients undertake vigorous exercise or exceed their recommended exercise intensity (Haskell 1978, Thompson 2001b). Despite this, cardiac arrest during exercise is still two to seven times greater in MI patients than in healthy individuals (Siscovick et al 1991), which is probably due to myocardial scarring increasing the risk of fibrillation (Libonati & Glassberg 2002). For these reasons such individuals should be discouraged from strenuous competitive sporting activities.

Although heart patients are at a greater risk of a cardiac event during or soon after a bout of physical exertion (Rautaharju & Neaton 1987, McCance & Forfar 1992, Piepoli et al 1993), this may be limited by the patient being aware of strategies that help prevent this from occurring, and the exercise practitioner or other members of the CR team should reinforce these. The exercise practitioner may assist in reducing risk by appropriate screening, assessment (Appendix A), risk stratification (Table 2.2) and exercise prescription for the patient. However, the exercise

practitioner should be trained to deal with an emergency if one should occur, and regularly review emergency procedures (Table 2.3).

PRE-EXERCISE PRESCRIPTION

It is strongly recommended that initially exercise should be within a CR programme. Nonetheless, these programmes often cease after around 12 weeks and patients may require exercise prescription outside this setting. Therefore when prescribing to those with existing heart and vascular diseases it is advisable to work within an outpatient community-based programme or consult with the patient's cardiac rehabilitation team before carrying out any prescription. It is also important to be fully aware of the patient's medical history, current physical status and medications, in addition to their attitudes toward their lifestyle. It is not always possible due to data protection to have full access to a patient's medical notes. Therefore it is important that the patient be appropriately screened and assessed (Appendix A). It is also important to risk-stratify the patient, which may not be as clear-cut as one might imagine as risk stratification criteria have been set by numerous organizations (Table 2.2). Moreover, the ability of the risk stratification guidelines to predict complications has been found to fail and it has been suggested that further work needs to be carried out (Labrador et al 1999). Medications (Ch. 14) and co-morbidities such as insulin-dependent diabetes mellitus, morbid obesity, severe pulmonary disease, complicated pregnancy, debilitating neurological or orthopaedic conditions also need to be considered in conjunction with the stratification guidelines, as these may constitute contraindications for exercise or warrant closer patient supervision (Thompson et al 1994).

PHYSICAL ACTIVITY/EXERCISE PRESCRIPTION

Physical activity/exercise can commence at varying stages of a patient's recovery from a cardiac event or surgery. The stage of recovery is generally phased, which can be confusing when reviewing the literature as phase II in the USA is similar to stage III in the UK. Nonetheless, activity such as general mobilization can start after only a few days for some patients while others may be required to wait until several weeks into rehabilitation. A patient's suitability to undertake any form of physical activity can therefore be determined by undergoing pre-participation screening, risk stratification (Table 2.2) and assessment (Appendix A). Assessment of maximal aerobic capacity is useful in determining a patient's maximal ability and ischaemic threshold for the prescription of PA/exercise. However, improvements in maximal aerobic capacity can be proportionally less than the improvements in submaximal physical activity. For example, a study carried

Table 2.3 Action plan for instructors in the event of incidents that may occur when cardiac patients undertake PA/exercise (adapted from BACR 2002)

Problem	Signs and symptoms	Immediate action	Further action
Hypotension	Dizziness	Lie patient down Elevate feet Check blood pressure (BP) Reassure patient	Ensure recovery before travelling home Send written details to general practitioner (GP) and ask patient to see GP soon
Hypertension	Usually none, generally detected on random BP check or when already diagnosed	(i) If resting BP unusually high for patient, recheck and if still high (ii) Resting BP values of systolic BP >200 mmHg or diastolic BP >115 mmHg is considered a contraindication for exercise, and attaining SBP >250 mmHg or DBP >120 mmHg during exercise session would indicate that the exercise session shold be terminated (ACSM 1993)	(i) Send letter to their GP for advice (ii) Do not exercise
Arrhythmias	*Tachycardia* Consistent pre-exercise heart rate (HR) of ≥100 beats/min	Common in post-surgery patients; if apparent at community-based exercise phase (i.e. phase IV in UK) it is a contraindication	Refer to their GP
	Pre-exercise ↑ HR from normal	Adjust exercise programme	Monitor
	Pre-exercise ↑ from initial high HR	Adjust exercise programme, monitor HR	Refer to their GP
	Bradycardia HR of 40–60 beats/min not normal for patient	Check medications	Monitor
	Irregular New to patient; faint; dizzy; lethargic	Monitor	Refer to their GP
	New to patient or uncontrolled	Do not exercise	Refer to their GP
	If treated and normal for patient	Exercise as normal to patient	Monitor regularly
Cardiac arrest	Absence of pulse and respiration	Proceed with cardiopulmonary resuscitation Send for help Someone to call emergency services and to inform paramedics that patient has a cardiac history	Confirm details of incident, patient's medications and contact for relatives Reassure others present
Angina	Chest pain Dyspnoea Shoulder/arm pain	Cease exercise Sit patient down on floor, back against the wall, knees up to chest. If patient uses glyceryl trinitrate (GTN), request that patient takes a dose. If pain relieved If not, repeat GTN at 5-minute intervals (up to 3 times) If no relief	Reassure others present Rest for 5 minutes Send for emergency service

Table 2.3 Action plan for instructors in the event of incidents that may occur when cardiac patients undertake PA/exercise (adapted from BACR 2002) (*con't*)

Problem	Signs and symptoms	Immediate action	Further action
Myocardial infarction (MI)/heart attack	Central chest pain may be prolonged and severe and not relieved by GTN. Patient pale, sweaty, shocked	Reassure patient Sit on floor as for angina Someone to call emergency services and to inform paramedics of MI and that patient has a cardiac history	Confirm details of incident, patient's medications and contact for relatives Reassure others present
Deterioration of LV function or progression of CHD	Increased symptoms or frequency of angina/dyspnoea on minimal exertion	Determine frequency and severity of attacks of angina Check whether medication has changed and/or patient is complying with medication prescription	Refer to their GP
	Loss of effectiveness of long-acting nitrates, which previously controlled angina	*Ask patient:* Whether GTN is working If their medication has changed	If unclear refer to their GP
	Reduced exercise capacity with no concurrent change in medication despite apparent compliance with PA/exercise prescription	*Ask patient:* Whether they have noticed a change in their physical capacity Whether they have complied with their PA/exercise prescription	Reduce PA/exercise intensity If unclear refer to their GP
Collapse	*Sudden faint or loss of consciousness, pale, sweaty with rapid pulse*		
	Diabetic and conscious	Administer sweet drink or oral glucose	
	Diabetic unconscious	Place in recovery position	Send for emergency service
	Epileptic	Protect from injury and do not move	
	Epileptic seizures repeated or more than every 5 minutes	Protect from injury and do not move	Send for emergency service

out on 45 cardiac patients (aged 62–82 years) found that exercise training improved aerobic capacity by only 16% compared to a 37% increase in time to exhaustion walking on a treadmill at 80% of their pre-intervention aerobic capacity (Ades et al 1993). This indicates that assessing maximal effort only can underestimate many of the benefits of exercise function on daily activities (Thompson 2001b). Nonetheless, assessment of patients' functional capacity can be useful in establishing their metabolic equivalent (MET) (Appendix B) and is a useful tool for prescription of a range of appropriate physical activities. However, MET values can be confounded by many factors such as changing external environment (Haymes et al 1982) and clothing worn. According to the ACSM guidelines (1995) patients with two or more CHD risk factors and/or a functional capacity of ≤8 METs should exercise under supervised conditions. At and above 8 METs patients

are at a level where their functional capacity allows for them to carry out the majority of daily activities and exercise at a moderate intensity level without putting their health at risk. Even so, it is difficult to determine how patients are going to respond to physical training, and findings have been variable (Myers & Froehlicher 1990). Furthermore, the complexity relating to these patients renders it extremely difficult to determine an optimal training programme, since the exercise dose–response relationship still remains inconclusive. Hence until this is clarified, patients should work at a level that will not trigger symptoms (Cox 1997). The exercise practitioner should be aware of these confounding factors and of the need for individualized PA/exercise prescription. This also poses a challenge to the practitioner since these patients, at some stage of their rehabilitation, will exercise within a group environment.

The physical status of those with heart and vascular disease tends to fluctuate, which may be due to changes in disease progression/regression, exercise and/or medical interventions and/or co-morbidities. Consequently they require regular reassessment so that adaptations to their activity regimen can be made.

PHYSICAL INTENSITY

It is important that each patient works at an appropriate intensity and in healthy individuals this is usually determined using a percentage of their maximum oxygen uptake ($\dot{V}O_2$max) or HRmax. However, following acute MI, CABG or other acute cardiac illness, HR response to physical exertion may be affected by a variable degree of chronotropic dysfunction (Frick et al 1973, Powles et al 1979) due to intrinsic disease of the sinoatrial or atrioventricular node, and possibly additional modification due to medication (Gobel et al 1991). Furthermore, their maximal heart rate achieved by a symptom-limited maximal exercise test may fall far below that expected from any formula devised for predicting maximal heart rate for normal subjects. Consequently, determining a training heart rate value from the usual formulas is not advisable. Therefore, physical intensity is generally determined through the use of ratings of perceived exertion (RPE). Perception of effort during physical activity is complex and still not totally understood (Hampson et al 2001), and for cardiac patients RPE values may not always correlate with the intensities from the Borg scale (Borg 1970, APHD 1999). Nonetheless, intra-subject RPE is a fairly reliable indicator of a subject's exercise intensity even for those taking beta-blockers (Eston & Connolly 1996). Hence, RPE is generally employed. In a supervised situation patients should also be regularly asked how they feel and supervisors should observe how they are performing. It is essential that there is a high supervisor-to-patient ratio so that patients can be effectively monitored. For those patients who are considered stable enough to exercise unsupervised, to minimize risk of a cardiac event or other injury, exercise principles and rationales should be enforced. Therefore, patients should understand why, for example, it is not a good idea to work beyond the feeling of 'slightly breathless and slightly sweaty' and why they should warm up and cool down (p. 25) after a brisk walk.

Prescribed exercise intensity for cardiac patients may range from 40% to 85% of their peak aerobic capacity ($\dot{V}O_2$ peak) and this will vary between patients depending on their physical status (see ACSM 1997 for guidelines). Vigorous intensity activities are discouraged and until research clearly demonstrates that the benefits of performing vigorous intensity exercise outweigh the risks involved, moderate intensity exercise is recommended (Franklin et al 1992) (relates to around 60% of an individual's aerobic capacity, roughly equivalent to a rating of 13 (somewhat hard) on the 6–20 RPE Borg scale) (Appendix B, Table B.3).

AEROBIC ACTIVITIES

The physiological benefits from current and regular aerobic physical activity are described elsewhere (p. 2–3). Aerobic activities generally involve using large muscle groups carried out at a sustainable rate. These activities include walking, jogging and cycling. Water-based aerobic activities may be problematic for some cardiac patients and are not initially recommended (p. 25). Given that symptomatic or silent myocardial ischaemia may precipitate malignant ventricular arrhythmias (Hoberg et al 1990), if employed, the prescribed heart rate for endurance activities should be set at least 10 beats per minute below the ischaemic or anginal threshold (ACSM 2000), which is usually determined by an exercise stress test and determined by the ST segment displacement (Appendix A, Fig. A.4).

RESISTANCE CIRCUIT TRAINING AND WEIGHT TRAINING

In the past, resistance training was deemed inappropriate for those with existing heart disease. However, light resistance training for those with heart and vascular disease is now recommended as it improves functional capacity (ACSM 1997). During resistance work, the rise in heart rate is less than it is during aerobic exercise with a lower RPP (p. 87) than aerobic activities of the same metabolic demand (ACSM 2001). However, weight training, isometric or high anaerobic activities are still not recommended as an initial physical therapy for those with hypertension, and/or cardiovascular disease. Isometric and any static component tends to increase afterload (Leutholtz & Ripoll 1999), and these activities can also increase heart rate, blood pressure and RPP, potentially resulting in an ischaemic event. Alternatively resistance training consisting of low weights and high repetitions has been shown to improve upper and lower body strength and the patient's ability to perform daily tasks that require moderate amounts of strength (Vescovi & Fernhall 2000). An increase in muscle strength may also reduce RPP, as a given amount of muscular work will be proportionally less of the maximal voluntary muscle contraction. Hence, there will also be a corresponding reduction in peripheral resistance, SBP and RPP (Franklin 2002). Patients should, however, avoid the *Valsalva manoeuvre* (p. 90), which can cause systolic blood pressure to rise to values in excess of 200 mmHg (Childs 1999, James & Potter 1999), placing some individuals at risk of stroke (Narloch & Brandstater 1995). Furthermore, upper body resistance training is not recommended for CABG patients who have recently had surgery as their wound may have not healed and/or causes them discomfort, and for those with implanted pacemakers as this may aggravate the site of implantation (ACSM 1997).

INTERVAL TRAINING

Some ECR programmes adopt an interval approach, which involves bouts of physical exertion combined with short periods of active recovery. The advantage of this type of activity is that the total amount of work achieved can be greater than that through continuous physical exertion. The rationale is that the change in work, usually from legs to arms, produces less localized fatigue and allows more work to be achieved at a lower heart rate, and less stress on the heart and skeletal muscles. Hence a greater amount of aerobic power is attained with less demand upon the myocardium (Mostardi et al 1981). It is important, however, that during 'active recovery' the patient keeps the lower extremities moving to maintain venous return and avoid blood pooling and orthostastic hypotension (p. 85). The active recovery can take the form of light resistance work and/or simply keeping the lower extremities moving, such as the feet or toes. Whilst the 'active' section generally takes the form of aerobic activities, for some patients it might consist of light resistance work. However, the type of interval programme prescribed will depend on the patient's individual needs and ability.

WATER-BASED ACTIVITIES

Despite the many benefits of water-based exercise, this type of activity may be potentially hazardous to cardiac patients and caution should be taken when prescribing (Jones 2003). Immersion in water results in haemodynamic changes that affect the cardiovascular system (Table 2.4). Upright immersion in water, for instance, causes blood to shift towards the upper body, resulting in an increase in central blood volume leading to engorgement of the

vasculature of the thoracic region (Lin 1988, Jones 2003). There is therefore an increase in blood return to the heart and consequently an increase in stroke volume of around 30% (Jones 2003) as a result of the Starling mechanism. These resting changes in the healthy individual generally do not cause a problem. However, for the cardiac patient this increase in cardiac blood volume will cause a rise in blood pressure and myocardial oxygen demand that may potentially be a problem. Moreover, during water-based exercise the demands for an increase in cardiac output may be beyond a cardiac patient's maximal Starling mechanism; hence the increase in cardiac output will need to be met by an increase in heart rate; and an increase in heart rate will require an increase in myocardial oxygen demand. Furthermore, heart rate response during water-based exercise is different to that on land. For instance, during facial immersion heart rate is generally lower (Journeay et al 2003); however, this does not mean that the physiological demands of the exercise are lower and this should be considered during exercise prescription (Jones 2003). It has been suggested that a reduction of 10 beats per minute should be made to account for the water to land difference (Koszuta 1989). However, this is only a generalization and caution is needed. Conversely, if one's face is not immersed in water, resting heart rate does not appear to be altered, particularly at a thermoneutral temperature, although at higher and lower temperatures heart rate has been found to change (Weston et al 1987). Resting heart rate also tends to drop as the depth of water increases (Jones 2003) and ischaemic symptoms are harder to identify (Magder et al 1981). This makes appropriate prescription difficult and is additionally problematic since RPE has also been found unreliable during immersion in water, as patients tend to underestimate their exercise intensity during water-based activities (Fernhall et al 1992). Nonetheless, there is limited research in this area and the demands of swimming and upright water-based activities may yield different responses in cardiac patients, which warrants further investigation.

WARMING UP AND COOLING DOWN

As a consequence of endothelial dysfunction those with existing heart and vascular disease do not respond in the same way to the initiation of physical exertion as those without these diseases. Hence prior to the onset of anything other than mild physical exertion it is advisable for these patients to warm up for around 10 minutes or more (ACSM 1997, BACR 2002), and the intensity should be no more than an RPE of 10 or 11 on the 6–20 Borg scale (Borg 1970). In healthy individuals the onset of activity generally results in vasodilation of the coronary arteries, initially as a result of a rise in SNS activity. In those with CAD, however, the mechanisms involved in vasodilation do not effectively respond and can result in vasoconstriction (p. 15). Failure to warm up adequately

Table 2.4 Cardiovascular changes due to immersion in water (adapted from Jones 2003)

Parameter	Immersion in water
Right arterial blood pressure	↑ 8–12 mmHg
Mean pulmonary artery pressure	↑ 12 mmHg
Heart blood volume	↑ 180–250 ml
Cardiac output	↑ ≥25%
Central venous pressure	↑ 300–700 ml
Stroke volume	↑ 30–50%
Heart rate	Same or slightly ↓
Systemic blood pressure	Same or slightly ↓
Left ventricular end-diastolic pressure	↑

before strenuous activity, even in healthy individuals, can potentially result in ischaemia, arrhythmias (McCance & Forfar 1992) and reduction in LV ejection fraction (BACR 2002). With an extended warm-up, local metabolites, such as adenosine, adenosine triphosphate and potassium which have a local vasodilatory effect (the vasodilatory effect of hydrogen, lactate, nitric oxide and prostacyclin during PA/exercise are less certain) (Lott & Sinoway 2004), have time to build up, causing an increase in blood flow (Deshmukh et al 1997) to the working muscles including the heart. Other factors such as an increase in aortic pressure also divert an enhanced amount of blood into the coronary circulation (Tune et al 2002), increasing coronary blood flow.

The cool-down also needs to be extended for those with heart and vascular diseases and it has been suggested that it be around 10 minutes in length (BACR 2002). These patients are at increased risk of hypotension, due to the side effect of their medication (Ch. 14) and/or reduced baroreceptor responsiveness. Abrupt cessation of physical exertion may therefore result in increased risk of blood pooling and subsequent lack of venous return, potentially leading to hypotension (p. 85) and risk of arrhythmias (McCance & Forfar 1992, Piepoli et al 1993). Furthermore, heart rate tends to take longer to return to pre-exertion levels in these individuals (Koike et al 1998). Hence by increasing the length of the cool-down, venous return is enhanced and the heart rate is given more time to settle back to pre-exertion levels.

FLEXIBILITY AND STRETCHING

Increasing a patient's flexibility is important in that it reduces the risk of injury, not just during physical exertion but also during daily activities (Fattirolli et al 2003). This is usually done as part of the warm-up and cool-down, which should start with gentle mobilization and progressively build up to more muscle specific stretches. In order for these stretches to be effective, especially for those over 65 years, stretches need to be held for around 15 seconds (Feland et al 2001), and for longer (Feland et al 2001) during the cool-down when developmental stretches are carried out. However, during stretching in healthy individuals heart rate has been shown to increase, with a subsequent increase in blood pressure (Feland et al 2001). Therefore, for those with heart and vascular diseases caution should be taken during stretching so that heart rate and blood pressure remain within appropriate boundaries. This is an area that requires greater investigation, as some patients may be advised not to hold a stretch for too long.

CONSIDERATIONS AND CONTRAINDICATIONS

Any physical exertion is potentially hazardous for those with existing heart disease. Hence instructors should be familiar with the signs and symptoms of over-exertion and a cardiac event, and be up to date in emergency and resuscitation techniques. Similarly, those patients who exercise unsupervised should also be aware of these signs and symptoms and be sufficiently aware of the importance of warming up and cooling down (p. 25) and appropriate intensity and types of physical activity (p. 24).

ABSOLUTE CONTRAINDICATIONS FOR EXERCISE

Absolute contraindications may vary according to the phase at which the cardiac patient is during their rehabilitation. Nevertheless, the ACSM (1991) have listed certain criteria that contraindicate entry into inpatient and outpatient exercise programmes (Table 2.5), as these factors, in combination with physical exertion, increase risk to the patient's health. Additionally any other co-morbidity that a patient may have also needs to be fully considered as well as any potential effects of their medications, as these too may contraindicate exercise.

CONSIDERATIONS

During physical exertion, consideration should also be given to co-morbidities, conditions such as heat and humidity and changes in BP. For instance exercise should cease if SBP and/or diastolic BP (DBP) rise above 250 mmHg or 120 mmHg, respectively (ACSM 1993) (as this increases the risk of stroke and/or aneurysm) and if there is a sudden drop in BP ≥20 mmHg (indicating LV dysfunction). However, on a practical note it is unlikely, unless the patient is hypertensive and investigations have been carried out during exercise, that anyone will know of any detrimental changes in BP occurring during physical exertion. Furthermore, increases in heart rate and perhaps BP are possible whilst stretching

Table 2.5 Contraindications for inpatient and outpatient entry into an exercise programme (adapted from ACSM 1991, 1993)

Unstable angina
Resting systolic BP >200 mmHg or resting diastolic BP >115 mmHg
Orthostastic blood pressure drop ≥20 mmHg
Moderate to severe aortic stenosis
Acute illness or fever
Uncontrolled atrial or ventricular dysrhythmias
Uncontrolled sinus tachycardia (≥120 beats/min)
Uncontrolled CHF
3°A-V heart block
Active pericarditis or myocarditis
Recent embolism
Thrombophlebitis
Resting ST displacement (>3 mm)
Uncontrolled diabetes
Orthopaedic problems that would prohibit exercise

(Feland et al 2001) and may be problematic for some patients.

Cardiac patients who have uncontrolled hypertension (SBP >160 mmHg or DBP >100 mmHg, stage II hypertension, see Table 5.1) should also avoid any heavy resistance circuit training (p. 24) and contraindications for such activities include CHF, uncontrolled arrhythmias, severe valvular disease and aerobic capacity <5 METs; for light resistance training, contraindications are abnormal haemodynamic responses to physical exertion, ischaemic changes during graded exercise, poor LV function, uncontrolled hypertension or arrhythmias, and aerobic capacity <6 METs (ACSM 1997, BACR 2002). Furthermore, weight training, isometric or high anaerobic activities are not recommended as an initial physical therapy for those with hypertension or cardiovascular disease, and upper body resistance training is not recommended for the CABG patient whose wound has not healed and/or causes discomfort, or for those with implanted pacemakers as this may aggravate the site of implantation (ACSM 1997). Patients who are stable and well enough to undertake resistance training should also avoid the *Valsalva manoeuvre*. Water-based activities are also potentially hazardous to cardiac patients and need to be carefully considered before prescription (p. 90). Patients with heart and vascular disease will also require a longer warm-up and cool-down compared to healthy individuals (p. 25).

UPRIGHT AND SUPINE EXERCISE

Supine activities, such as sit-ups, are not recommended if carried out within an aerobic workout. Not only are postural changes from supine to upright problematic as they may cause orthostatic/postural hypotension (p. 85), but supine exercise also increases preload on the heart (Mildenberger & Kattenbach 1989) resulting in greater myocardial work and the potential for arrhythmias (Shibuya et al 1985).

MEDICATIONS

The physical status of those with heart and vascular disease tends to change with time and so may their medication. The exercise practitioner and instructor therefore need to be aware of this as different medications and their dose may have variable effects upon a patient's ability to carry out certain physical activities. Consequently a constant update on medications should be made. Furthermore, patients with angina who are prescribed nitrates should be made aware that they should have this available during any physical exertion and those on diuretics that they consume sufficient water during exercise, especially during hot and humid weather. Additionally, beta-blockers also impair the ability of the body to regulate temperature. Therefore, patients/clients should be made aware of the potential to develop 'heat illness' when exercising (Ch. 14).

SUMMARY

- CHD/CVD is a major cause of morbidity and death in Western society.
- The terms CHD/CAD/CVD have slightly different meanings but generally the causes are similar, the most common cause being atherosclerosis.
- The factors that are currently known to result in these diseases are commonly known as CHD risk factors (Table 2.1).
- Appropriate PA/exercise can have a positive effect upon the health of those with existing heart and vascular diseases.
- Moderate intensity PA/exercise that can be carried out on a regular daily basis is generally recommended.
- The precise dose of PA/exercise required to produce optimal responses has yet to be determined.
- Weekly energy expenditure through PA/exercise of ~1400 kcal has been shown to result in improvements in aerobic fitness, 1500 kcal to slow the progression of CAD, and 2200 kcal to show regression in CAD.
- Habitual appropriate PA/exercise intervention can result in:
  ↑ aerobic fitness

  ↓ RPP
  ↑ myocardial ischaemic tolerance
  ↑ endothelium function
  ↓ ventricular fibrillation
  modification of CHD risk factors, diabetes and insulin resistance, obesity, blood lipids, blood pressure
  ↓ risk of mortality and sudden cardiac death
  positive adaptations to the sympathetic nervous system
  ↑ self-efficacy
  ↓ depression.
- Physiological changes are mainly the result of peripheral adaptations. More research is required to clearly determine central adaptations.
- Cardiac patients require a longer than normal pre-PA/exercise warm-up to avoid vasoconstriction, and a longer cool-down to avoid orthostatic hypotension.
- Vigorous intensity PA/exercise or heavy weight training is not recommended, and care should be taken when prescribing water-based activities.
- For absolute contraindications to PA/exercise see Table 2.5

Suggested readings, references and bibliography

Suggested reading

ACSM (American College of Sports Medicine) 1997 Exercise management for persons with chronic diseases and disabilities. Human Kinetics, Champaign, IL

Lilly L S 1997 The pathophysiology of heart disease, 2nd edn. Lippincott Williams & Wilkins, Philadelphia

Thompson P D (ed) 2001 Exercise and sports cardiology. McGraw-Hill, New York

References and bibliography

AACVPR (American Association of Cardiovascular and Pulmonary Rehabilitation) 1999 Guidelines for cardiac rehabilitation and secondary prevention. Human Kinetics, Champaign, IL

ACSM (American College of Sports Medicine) 1991 Guidelines for exercise testing and prescription. Lea and Febiger, Philadelphia

ACSM 1993 ACSM position stand: PA, physical fitness, and hypertension. Medicine and Science in Sports and Exercise 25(10):i–x

ACSM 1995 ACSM's guidelines for exercise testing and prescription, 5th edn. Williams & Wilkins, Baltimore

ACSM 1997 Exercise management for persons with chronic diseases and disabilities. Human Kinetics, Champaign, IL

ACSM 2000 ACSM's guidelines for exercise testing and prescription, 6th edn. Lippincott Williams & Wilkins, Philadelphia

ACSM 2001 ACSM's resource manual for guidelines for exercise testing and prescription, 4th edn. Lippincott Williams & Wilkins, Philadelphia

Ades P A, Waldmann M L, Peohlman E T et al 1993 Exercise conditioning in older coronary patients: submaximal lactate response and endurance capacity. Circulation 88:572–577

AHA (American Heart Association) 2003a Heart disease and stroke statistics – 2003 update. Online. Available: http://www.americanheart.org/downloadable/heart/10461207852 142003hdsstatsbook.pdf July 2003

AHA 2003b Syndrome X or metabolic syndrome. Online. Available: http://www.americanheart.org/presenter November 2003

AIHW (Australian Institute of Health and Welfare) 2002 Australia's Health 2002.

Amaral S L, Zorn T M, Michelini L C 2000 Exercise training normalizes wall-to-wall ratio of the gracilis muscle arterioles and reduces pressure in spontaneously hypertensive rats. Journal of Hypertension 18(11):1563–1572

APHD (Australian Public Health Division) 1999 Best practice guideline for cardiac rehabilitation and secondary prevention. APHD, Australia

Aqel N M, Ball R Y, Waldmann H et al 1984 Monocytic origin of foam cells in human atherosclerotic plaques. Atherosclerosis 53:265–271

BACR (British Association of Cardiac Rehabilitation) 2002 British Association of Cardiac Rehabilitation Phase IV training module, 3rd edn. Human Kinetics, Leeds

Balady G J, Fletcher B J, Froelicher E S et al 1994 Cardiac rehabilitation programs: a statement for healthcare professionals from the American Heart Association. Circulation 90(3):1602–1610

BHF (British Heart Foundation) 1999 Coronary heart disease statistics 8. BHF, London

Blair S N, Kohl III H W, Paffenbarger Jr R S et al 1989 Physical fitness and all-cause mortality: a prospective study of healthy men and women. Journal of the American Medical Association 262(17):2395–2401

Blomqvist C G, Saltin B 1983 Cardiovascular adaptations to physical training. Annual Review of Physiology 45:169–189

BMA, RPS GB (British Medical Association, Royal Pharmaceutical Society of Great Britain) 2005 British national formulary. Pharmaceutical Press, London

Borg G 1970 Perceived exertion as an indicator of somatic stress. Scandinavian Journal of Rehabilitative Medicine 2:92–98

Brooks G, Fahey T D, White T P 1996 Exercise physiology: human bioenergetics and its applications. Mayfield Publishing, Mountain View, CA, p 281–299

Brown M S, Goldstein J L 1986 A receptor-mediated pathway for cholesterol homeostasis. Science 232(4):34–47

Brown P 1996 Can you catch a heart attack? New Scientist June: 38–42

Childs J D 1999 One to one: the impact of the Valsalva manoeuvre during resistance exercise. Strength and Conditioning Journal 21(2):54–55

Clausen J P, Trap-Jensen J 1976 Heart rate and arterial blood pressure during exercise in patients with angina pectoris. Effects of training and of nitro-glycerine. Circulation 53:436–442

Cox M H 1997 Exercise in coronary artery disease: a cornerstone of comprehensive treatment. The Physician and Sports Medicine 25(12):27–32, 34

DeMaria A N, Neumann A, Lee G et al 1978 Alterations in ventricular mass and performance induced by exercise training in man evaluated by echocardiography. Circulation 57:237–244

Deshmukh R, Smith A, Lilly L S 1997 Hypertension. In: Lilly L S The pathophysiology of heart disease, 2nd edn. Lippincott Williams & Wilkins, Philadelphia, p 267–301

Detry J-M R, Rousseau M, Vandenbroucke G et al 1971 Increase in arteriovenous oxygen difference after physical training in coronary heart disease. Circulation 44:109–118

Di Bello V, Santoro G, Talarico L et al 1996 Left ventricular function during exercise in athletes and sedentary men. Medicine and Science in Sports and Exercise 28:190–196

Dressendorfer R H, Franklin B A, Cameron J L et al 1995 Exercise training frequency in early post-infarction cardiac rehabilitation. Influence on aerobic conditioning. Journal of Cardiopulmonary Rehabilitation 15(4):269–276

Dullaart R P, Hoogenberg K, Dikkeschel B D et al 1994 High plasma lipid transfer protein activities and unfavourable lipoprotein change in cigarette-smoking men. Arteriosclerosis and Thrombosis 14(10):1581–1585

Ehsani A A 1987a Cardiovascular adaptations to endurance exercise training in ischaemic heart disease. Exercise and Sport Science Reviews 15:53–66

Ehsani A A 1987b Mechanisms responsible for enhanced stroke volume after exercise training in coronary heart disease. European Heart Journal 8(suppl G):9–14

Ehsani A A, Biello D R, Schultz J et al 1986 Improvement of left ventricular contractile function by exercise training in patients with coronary artery disease. Circulation 74(2):350–358

Eston R, Connolly D 1996 The use of ratings of perceived exertion for exercise prescription in patients receiving beta-blocker therapy. Sports Medicine 21(3):176–190

Fattirolli F, Cellai T, Burgisser C 2003 Physical activity and cardiovascular health and close link. Monaldi Archives for Chest Disease 60(1):73–78

Feland J B, Myrer J W, Schulthies S S et al 2001 The effect of duration of stretching of the hamstring muscle group for increased range of motion in people ages 65 years or older. Physical Therapy 81(5):1110–1117

Fernhall B, Manfredi T, Congdom K 1992 Prescribing water-based exercise from treadmill and arm ergometry in cardiac patients. Medicine and Science in Sports and Exercise 24:139–143

Franklin B A 1997 Myocardial infarction. In: American College of Sports Medicine. Exercise management for persons with chronic diseases and disabilities, Human Kinetics, Champaign, IL, p 19–25

Franklin B 2002 Resistance training for persons with and without heart disease: rationale, safety and prescriptive guideline. British Association of Cardiac Rehabilitation Newsletter 2(2):2

Franklin B A, Khan J K 1996 Delayed progression or regression of coronary atherosclerosis with intensive risk factor modification: effects of diet, drugs and exercise. Sports Medicine 22:306–320

Franklin B A, Saunders W 2000 Reducing the risk of heart disease and stroke. The Physician and Sports Medicine 28(10):19–20, 26

Franklin B A, Gordon S, Timmis G C 1992 Amount of exercise necessary for the patient with coronary artery disease. American Journal of Cardiology 69(17):1426–1432

Freedman M 1996 Postmenopausal hormone replacement therapy and cardiovascular disease risk. Medicine and Science in Sports and Exercise 28(1):17–18

Frick M H, Huttunen J K, Harkonen M 1973 Impaired chronotropic response to beta stimulation in chronic coronary artery disease. American Journal of Medicine 55:571–575

Friedman D 1997 Angina and silent ischaemia. In: American College of Sports Medicine. Exercise management for persons with chronic diseases and disabilities, Human Kinetics, Champaign, IL, p 32–36

Fujimoto S, Uemura S, Tomoda Y et al 1997 Effects of physical training on autonomic nerve activity in patients with acute myocardial infarction. Journal of Cardiology 29:85–93

Furchgott R F, Zawadzki J V 1980 The obligatory role of endothelial cells in the relaxation of arterial smooth muscle by acetylcholine. Nature 288:373–376

Gardener A W 1997 Peripheral arterial disease. In: American College of Sports Medicine. Exercise management for persons with chronic diseases and disabilities. Human Kinetics, Champaign, IL, p 64–68

Gibbs C R, Blann A D, Edmunds E et al 2001 Effects of acute exercise on hemorheological, endothelial and platelet markers in patients with chronic heart failure in sinus rhythm. Clinical Cardiology 24(11):724–729

Gielen S, Hambrecht R 2001 Effects of exercise training on vascular function and myocardial perfusion. Cardiology Clinics 19(3):357–368

Gielen S, Schuler G, Hambrecht R 2001 Exercise training in coronary artery disease and coronary vasomotion. Circulation 103(1):E1–E6

Gielen S, Erbs S, Schuler G et al 2002 Exercise training and endothelial dysfunction in coronary artery disease and chronic heart failure. From molecular biology to clinical benefits. Minerva Cardioangiologica 50(2):95–106

Gobel A J, Hare D L, MacDonald P S et al 1991 Effect of early programmes of high and low intensity exercise on physical performance after transmural acute MI. British Heart Journal 65:126–131

Gohlke H, Gohlke-Barwolf C 1998 Cardiac rehabilitation: where are we going? European Heart Journal 19(suppl O):5–12

Gordon J B, Ganz P, Nabel E G et al 1989 Atherosclerosis influences the vasomotor response of epicardial coronary arteries to exercise. Journal of Clinical Investigation 83:1946–1952

Gulanick M 1991 Is phase 2 cardiac rehabilitation necessary for early recovery of patients with cardiac disease? A randomised, controlled study. Heart and Lung 21(1):9–15

Hagberg J M, Ehsani A A, Holloszy J O 1983 Effect of 12 months of intense exercise training on stroke volume in patients with coronary artery disease. Circulation 67(6):1194–1199

Hambrecht R, Niebauer J, Marburger C et al 1993 Various intensities of leisure time physical activity in patients with coronary artery disease: effects on cardiorespiratory fitness and progression of coronary atherosclerotic lesions. Journal of the American College of Cardiology 22:468–477

Hambrecht R, Gielen S, Linke A et al 2000a Effects of exercise training on left ventricular function and peripheral resistance in patients with chronic heart failure: a randomised trial. Journal of the American Medical Association 283(23):3095–3101

Hambrecht R, Wolf A, Gielen S et al 2000b Effect of exercise on coronary endothelial function in patients with coronary artery disease. New England Journal of Medicine 342(7):454–460

Hambrecht R, Adams V, Erbs S et al 2003 Regular physical activity improves endothelial function in patients with coronary artery disease by increasing phosphorylation of endothelial nitric oxide synthase. Circulation 107(25):3152–3158

Hammond H K, Ransna L A, Linsel P A 1988 Noncoordinate regulation of cardiac G_s protein and beta adrenergic receptors by a physiological stimulus, chronic dynamic exercise. Journal of Clinical Investigation 82:2168–2171

Hampson D B, St Clair Gibson A, Lambert M I et al 2001 The influence of sensory cues on the perception of exertion during exercise and central regulation of exercise performance. Sports Medicine 31(13):935–952

Haskell W L 1978 Cardiovascular complications during exercise training of cardiac patients. Circulation 57(5):920–924

Haymes E M, Dickinson A L, Malville N et al 1982 Effects of wind on thermal and metabolic responses to exercise in cold. Medicine and Science in Sports and Exercise 14(1):41–45

Henderson B E, Paginini-Hill A, Ross R K 1991 Decreased mortality in users of oestrogen replacement therapy. Archives of International Medicine 151:75–78

Hoberg E, Schuler G, Kunze B L et al 1990 Silent myocardial ischemia as a potential link between lack of premonitoring symptoms and increased risk of cardiac arrest during physical stress. American Journal of Cardiology 65(9):583–589

James M A, Potter J F 1999 Orthostastic blood pressure changes and arterial baroreflex sensitivity in elderly subjects. Age and Ageing 28(6):522–530

Johnson R J, Lombardo J (eds) 1994 Current review of sports medicine. Imago, Singapore, p 164–165

Jolliffe J A, Rees K, Taylor R S et al 2000 Exercise-based rehabilitation for coronary heart disease. Cochrane Database of Systematic Reviews (4):CD001800

Jones J 2003 Treading a fine line? CHD and water-based exercise. SportEx Health 16:28–31

Journeay W S, Reardon F D, Kenny G P 2003 Cardiovascular responses to apnoeic facial immersion during altered cardiac filling. Journal of Applied Physiology 94(6):2249–2254

Kawachi I, Colditz G A, Stampfer M J et al 1993 Smoking cessation in relation to total mortality rates in women. A prospective cohort study. Annals of International Medicine 119(10):992–1000

Koike A, Hiroe M, Marumo F 1998 Delayed kinetics of oxygen uptake during recovery after exercise in cardiac patients. Medicine and Science in Sports and Exercise 30(2):185–189

Koszuta L E 1989 From sweats to swimsuits: is water exercise the wave of the future? The Physician and Sports Medicine 17:203–206

Labrador P M, Vongvanich P, Merz C N 1999 Risk stratification for exercise training in cardiac patients: do the proposed guidelines work? Journal of Cardiopulmonary Rehabilitation 19(2):118–125

Lehmann M, Berg A, Keul J 1984 Changes in sympathetic activity in 18 postinfarct patients following a year of exercise therapy. Eitschrift für Kardiologies 73(12):756–759

Leutholtz B C, Ripoll I 1999 Exercise and disease management. CRC Press, Boca Raton, FL

Levy R I 1981 Cholesterol, lipoproteins, apolipoproteins and heart disease: present status and future prospects. Clinical Chemistry 27(5):653–662

Libonati J R, Glassberg H L 2002 Exercise and coronary artery disease. The Physician and Sports Medicine 30(11):23–29

Libonati J R, Gaughan J P, Hefner C A et al 1997 Reduced ischaemia and reperfusion injury following exercise training. Medicine and Science in Sports and Exercise 29(4):509–516

Libonati J R, Glassberg H L, Balady G J 2001 Coronary artery disease. In: Thompson P D (ed) Exercise and sports cardiology. McGraw-Hill, New York

Lilly L S 1997 The pathophysiology of heart disease, 2nd edn. Lippincott Williams & Wilkins, Philadelphia

Lin Y C 1988 Applied physiology of diving. Sports Medicine 5:41–56

Lindsay G, Gaw A 2003 Coronary heart disease prevention. Churchill Livingstone, Edinburgh

Lott M E J, Sinoway L I 2004 What has microdialysis shown us about metabolic milieu within exercising skeletal muscle? Exercise and Sport Science Reviews 32(2):69–74

Lusher T F, Diederich D, Siebenbaum R et al 1988 Difference between endothelium-dependent relaxation in arterial and in venous coronary bypass graft. New England Journal of Medicine 319:462–467

Lutoslawska G 2000 The influence of physical exercise on glucose transport into the muscle. Medicina Sportiva 5(1):9–15

McCance A J, Forfar J C 1992 Myocardial ischaemia and ventricular arrhythmias precipitated by physiological concentrations of adrenaline in patients with coronary heart disease. British Heart Journal 67(5):419–420

McCrimmon D R, Cunningham D A, Rechnitzer P A et al 1976 Effect of training on plasma catecholamines in post myocardial infarction patients. Medicine and Science in Sports and Exercise 8(3):152–156

MacFarlane N, Northridge D B, Wright A R et al 1991 A comparative study of left ventricular structure and function in elite athletes. British Journal of Sports Medicine 2:45–48

Magder S, Linnarsson D, Gullstrand L 1981 The effect of swimming on patients with ischemic heart disease. Circulation 63(5):979–986

Malek A M, Alper S L, Izumo S 1999 Hemodynamic shear stress and its role in atherosclerosis. Journal of the American Medical Association 282:2035–2042

Matsui S, Tamura N, Hirakawa T et al 1995 Assessment of working skeletal muscle oxygenation in patients with chronic heart failure. American Heart Journal 129(4):690–695

Mazzeo R S 1991 Catecholamine responses to acute and chronic exercise. Medicine and Science in Sports and Exercise 23(7):839–845

Milani R V, Lavie C J, Cassidy M M 1996 Effects of cardiac rehabilitation and exercise training programs on depression in patients after major coronary events. American Heart Journal 132(4):726–732

Mildenberger V D, Kattenbach M 1989 Life threatening complications with ergometry. Fortschritte der Medizin 107(27):569–571

Mitchell J H, Blomqvist G 1971 Maximum oxygen uptake. New England Journal of Medicine 284(18):1018–1022

Mitchell J H, Victor R G 1996 Neural control of the cardiovascular system: insights from muscle sympathetic nerve recordings in humans. Medicine and Science in Sports and Exercise 10(suppl):S60–S69

Moore R L, Reidy M, Gollnick P D 1982 Effect of training on beta-adrenoreceptor number in rat heart. Journal of Applied Physiology: Respiratory and Environmental Exercise Physiology 52(2):1133–1137

Morris J N, Heady J A, Raffle P A B et al 1953 Coronary heart disease and physical activity at work. Lancet 265(6795):1053–1057, 265(6796):1111–1120

Mostardi R A, Gandee R N, Norris W A 1981 Exercise training using arms and legs versus legs alone. Archives of Physical Medicine and Rehabilitation 62(7):332–335

Myers J 1997 Congestive heart failure. In: American College of Sports Medicine. Exercise management for persons with chronic diseases and disabilities. Human Kinetics, Champaign, IL

Myers J, Froehlicher V F 1990 Predicting outcome in cardiac rehabilitation. Journal of the American College of Cardiology 15:983–985

Narloch J, Brandstater M 1995 Influence of breathing technique on arterial blood pressure during heavy weight lifting. Archives of Physical Medical Rehabilitation 76(5):457–462

NCEP (National Cholesterol Education Program), Executive Summary of the Third Report 2001 Expert panel on detection, evaluation, and treatment of high blood cholesterol in adults. Journal of the American Medical Association 285:2486–2497

Noaks T D, Higginson L, Opie L H 1983 Physical training increases ventricular fibrillation thresholds of isolated rat hearts during normoxia, hypoxia and regional ischaemia. Circulation 67(1):24–30

O'Connor G T, Buring J E, Yusuf S et al 1989 An overview of randomised trials of rehabilitation with exercise after myocardial infarction. Circulation 80(2):234–244

Ohara Y, Peterson T E, Harrison D G 1993 Hypercholesterolemia increases endothelial superoxide anion production. Journal of Clinical Investigation 91(6):2546–2551

Oldridge N B, Guyatt G H, Fischer M E et al 1988 Cardiac rehabilitation after myocardial infarction. Combined experience of randomised clinical trials. Journal of the American Medical Association 260(7):945–950

Ordovas J M 2000 ABC1: the gene for Tangier disease and beyond. Nutrition Reviews 58(3 Pt 1):76–79

Piepoli M, Lombardi F, Bigoli M et al 1993 Hypotension following maximal physical exercise. Evaluation of hemodynamic and humoral mechanism. Minerva Cardioangiologica 41(10):445–449

Poredos P, Orehek M, Tratnik E 1999 Smoking is associated with dose-related increase of intima-media thickness and endothelial dysfunction. Angiology 50(11):959–961

Powles A C P, Sutton J R, Wicks J R et al 1979 Reduced heart rate response to exercise in ischaemic heart disease. The fallacy of the target heart rate in exercise testing. Medicine and Science in Sports and Exercise 11:227–233

Pyorala K, Backer G, Graham J et al 1994 Prevention of coronary heart disease in clinical practice: recommendations of the task force of the European Society of Cardiology European Atherosclerosis Society and European Society of Hypertension. European Heart 1300–1331

Rautaharju P M, Neaton J D 1987 Electrocardiographic abnormalities and coronary heart disease mortality among hypertensive men in the Multiple Risk Factor Intervention Trial. Clinical and Investigative Medicine 10(6):606–615

Rinder M R, Miller T R, Ehsani A A 1999 Effects of endurance exercise training on left ventricular systolic performance and ventriculoarterial coupling in patients with coronary artery disease. American Heart Journal 138(1 Pt 1):169–174

Ross R 1986 The pathogenesis of atherosclerosis – an update. New England Journal of Medicine 314:488–500

Rowell L B 1986 Human circulation regulation during physical stress. Oxford University Press, New York

Sabatine M S, O'Gara P T, Lilly L S 1997 Ischemic heart disease. In: Lilly L S (ed) The pathophysiology of heart disease. Lippincott Williams & Wilkins, Philadelphia, p 119–143

Sauer W H, Jessa A, Strom B et al 2002 Cigarette yield and the risk of myocardial infarction in smokers. Archives of International Medicine 162(3):300–306

Savin W M, Haskell W L, Houston-Miller N et al 1981 Improvements in aerobic capacity soon after myocardial infarction. Journal of Cardiac Rehabilitation 1:337–342

Schulze P C, Gielen S, Schuler G et al 2002 Chronic heart failure and skeletal muscle catabolism: effects of exercise training. International Journal of Cardiology 85(1):141–149

Shibuya T, Kimuram M, Oda E et al 1985 Ventricular arrhythmia with postural dependency. Journal of Electrocardiology 18(3):303–308

Siscovick D S, Ekelund L G, Johnson J L et al 1991 Sensitivity of exercise electrocardiography for acute cardiac events during moderate and strenuous physical activity: the Lipid Research Clinic Coronary Primary Prevention Trial. Archives of International Medicine 151(12):325–330

Smith J K 2001 Exercise and atherogenesis. Exercise and Sport Sciences Reviews 29(2):49–53

Smith J K, Dykes R, Douglas J E et al 1999 Long-term exercise and atherogenic activity of blood mononuclear cells in person at risk of developing ischemic heart disease. Journal of the American Medical Association 281:1722–1727

Snoeckx L H E H, Abeling H F M, Lambregts J A C et al 1982 Echocardiographic dimensions in athletes in relation to their training programs. Medicine and Science in Sports and Exercise 14(6):428–434

Spina R J, Turner M J, Ehsani A A 1998 Beta-adrenergic-mediated improvement in left ventricular function by exercise training in older men. American Journal of Physiology 271(2 Pt 2):H397–H404

Sugishita Y, Koseki S, Matsuda M et al 1983 Myocardial mechanics of athletic hearts in comparison with diseased hearts. American Heart Journal 105:273–280

Tavani A, Bertuzzi M, Negri E et al 2001 Alcohol, smoking, coffee and risk of non-fatal acute myocardial infarction in Italy. European Journal of Epidemiology 17(12):1131–1137

Thompson G R 1989 A handbook of hyperlipidaemia. Current Science, London

Thompson P D 1988 The benefits and risks of exercise training in patients with chronic coronary artery disease. Journal of the American Medical Association 259(10):1537–1540

Thompson P D 2001a Exercise rehabilitation for cardiac patients: a beneficial but underused therapy. The Physician and Sports Medicine 29(1):69–75

Thompson P D 2001b Exercise for patients with coronary artery and/or coronary heart disease. In: Thompson P D (ed) Exercise and Sports Cardiology. McGraw Hill, USA, p 354–370

Thompson P D, Klocke F J, Levine B D et al 1994 26th Bethesda Conference: Recommendations for determining eligibility for competition in athletes with cardiovascular abnormalities. Task Force 5: coronary artery disease. Medicine and Science in Sports nd Exercise 26(10 suppl):S271–S272

Todd I C, Worsornu D, Stewart I et al 1992 Cardiac rehabilitation following myocardial infarction. A practical approach. Sports Medicine 14(4):234–259

Tune J D, Yeh C, Setty S et al 2002 Coronary blood flow control is impaired at rest and during exercise in conscious diabetic dogs. Basic Research in Cardiology 97(3):248–257

US DHSS (Department of Health and Human Services) 1996 PA and health: a report of the surgeon general. Centers for Disease Control and Prevention, National Center for Chronic Disease Prevention and Health Promotion, US DHHS, Atlanta

Vallance P, Collier J G, Moncada S 1989 Effect of endothelium-derived nitric oxide on peripheral arteriolar tone in man. Lancet 2(8670):997–1000

Van Camp S P, Peterson R A 1986 Cardiovascular complications of outpatient cardiac rehabilitation programs. Journal of the American Medical Association 256:1160–1163

Vander A J, Sherman J H, Luciano D S 1990 Human physiology. McGraw-Hill, New York

Vanhees L, Schepers D, Defoor J et al 2000 Exercise performance and training in cardiac patients with atrial fibrillation. Journal of Cardiopulmonary Rehabilitation 20(6):346–352

Vescovi J, Fernhall B 2000 Cardiac rehabilitation and resistance training: are they compatible? Journal of Strength and Conditioning Research 14(3):350–358

Wallace R B, Hoover I, Barrett-Connor E et al 1979 Altered plasma lipid and lipoprotein levels associated with oral contraceptive and oestrogen use. Lancet :2(8134):112–115

Waugh A, Grant A 2001 Ross and Wilson anatomy and physiology in health and illness, 9th edn. Churchill Livingstone, Edinburgh

Wenger N K, Froelicher E S, Smith L K et al 1995 Cardiac rehabilitation. Clinical Practice Guideline No. 17. Rockville, MD: US Department of Health and Human Services, Public Health Service Agency for Health Care Policy and Research and the National Heart, Lung, and Blood Institute. AHCPR Publication No. 96–0672

West M, Johnson T, Roberts S O 1997 Pacemakers and implantable cardioverter defibrillators. In: American College of Sports Medicine. Exercise management for persons with chronic diseases and disabilities. Human Kinetics, Champaign, IL

Weston C F M, O'Hara J P, Evans J M et al 1987 Haemodynamic changes in man during immersion at different temperatures. Clinical Science 73(6):613–616

WHO (World Health Organization) 2002 World Health Report. Online. Available: http://www.who.int/whr/2002/en August 2003

Woolf-May K, Bird S, Owen A 1997 Effects of an 18 week walking programme on cardiac function in previously sedentary or relatively inactive adults. British Journal of Sports Medicine 31(1):48–53

Woolf-May K, Owen A, Davison R et al 1999 The use of Doppler and atrioventricular plane motion echocardiography for the detection of changes in left ventricular function after training. European Journal of Applied Physiology and Occupational Physiology 80(3):200–204

Wyatt H L, Chuck L, Rabinowitz B et al 1978 Enhanced cardiac response to catecholamines in physically trained cats. American Journal of Physiology 234:(5): H608–H613

Chapter 3

Blood lipids and hyperlipidaemia

CHAPTER CONTENTS

Introduction 34
Prevalence 34
Blood lipid profile 34
Structure of blood lipids, lipoproteins and
    apolipoproteins 35
    Plasma lipids 35
    Transport 35
    Free fatty acids 36
    Triglycerides 36
    Phospholipids 37
    Cholesterol 37
    Apolipoproteins (apos) 38
    Chylomicrons 39
    Very low-density lipoproteins (VLDL) 39
    Metabolism of chylomicrons and VLDL 39
    Intermediate-density lipoprotein (IDL) 'remnant
    particle' 39
    Low-density lipoprotein (LDL) 39
    Cholesterol delivery and LDL receptors 40
    High-density lipoprotein (HDL) 40
    High-density lipoprotein reverse cholesterol
    transport 40
    Lipoprotein(a) (Lp(a)) 41
    Intravascular lipid metabolism 41
Aetiology 41
    Familial hyperlipidaemia 42
    Secondary hyperlipidaemia 42
        Body weight 42
        Diet 42
        Tobacco 43
        Illness and disease 43
        Age 44
        Gender 44
        Race 45
        Seasonal and day-to-day variation 45
    Medications and secondary hyperlipidaemia 45
        Beta-adrenergic receptor blockers (beta-blockers) 45

        Diuretics 45
        Oral hypoglycaemic agents 46
        Thyroid treatments 46
        Sex hormones 46
Treatment 46
    Pharmacological 46
        Bile-acid binders 46
        Fibrates 46
        Statins 46
    Regular physical activity and exercise 46
        Mechanism 46
        Energy expenditure 47
        Intensity 47
        Duration 47
        Frequency 47
        Age 47
        Gender 47
    Single bout of physical activity/exercise 48
        Intensity 48
        Duration 48
        Training status 48
        Gender 49
        Prior physical activity 49
Pre-exercise prescription 49
Regular physical activity and exercise prescription 49
    Physical activity/exercise intensity 49
    Energy expenditure 49
    Low-density lipoprotein cholesterol 49
Aerobic activities 49
Resistance circuit training and weight training 50
Interval training 50
Considerations and contraindications 50
    Medications 50
    Absolute contraindications for exercise 51
Summary 51
Suggested readings, references and bibliography 51

INTRODUCTION

Hyperlipidaemia is characterized by increased levels of serum lipids, such as triglycerides, cholesterol and fatty acids, and is a primary risk factor for heart and vascular disease (AHA 1990) (Ch. 2). Thus it is important to understand the significance of a healthy blood lipid profile (BLP) and the types of physical activity (PA)/exercise that bring this about. This chapter will therefore describe the various constituents that make up the BLP, and the structure and metabolism of the various lipids, lipoproteins and apolipoproteins. Additionally, the influence of PA/exercise intervention upon BLP and lipid metabolism will be discussed, and an overview of the known aetiology for hyper- and dyslipidaemia will be provided.

Higher rates of hyperlipidaemia are found in obese individuals (Ch. 6), and hyperlipidaemia is also worsened by diabetes (Ch. 4), alcoholism and hyperthyroidism (Medline plus 2004). Findings from the Multiple Risk Factor Trial study (which involved more that 360 000 men aged between 35 and 57 years who were followed over a 6-year period, during which 24 000 died) found that both plasma and serum cholesterol concentrations correlated with coronary heart disease (CHD). It was suggested that the risk to health was reasonably continuous over the whole range of serum cholesterol. However, risk of CHD rose appreciably when serum cholesterol levels exceeded 6.5 mmol/l (250 mg/dl), and even more steeply when they rose above 7.8 mmol/l (300 mg/dl). The lowest rates of CHD occurred in men with serum cholesterol levels below 5.2 mmol/l (200 mg/dl) (Martin et al 1986) (Table 3.1). Although high levels of cholesterol are primarily seen as the major lipid risk factor for cardiovascular disease (CVD), triglycerides have also been found to play a contributing role. However, the pathophysiological significance of triglyceride remains largely unclear, though elevated levels have proven to be an independent risk factor for peripheral arterial occlusive disease and fatal coronary heart disease (Hartmann & Stahelin 1981, Malloy & Kane 2001, Kuhar 2002).

Table 3.2 Total blood cholesterol classifications (NCEP 1988, AHA 2004)

Classification	Values
Desirable	<5.2 mmol/l (200 mg/dl)
Borderline high risk	5.2–6.2 mmol/l (200–239 mg/dl)
High risk	≥6.2 mmol/l (240 mg/dl)

PREVALENCE

Hyperlipidaemia is endemic in Western societies and although the cause can be heredity it is also related to lifestyle. Since hyperlipidaemia is a primary risk factor for CVD it is likely that a high proportion of those individuals who died from CVD were hyperlipidaemic during their lifetime (Thompson 1989). Epidemiological data from the UK, from nearly 8000 men, showed that around 75% of heart disease deaths occurred in the 50% of the population with serum total cholesterol levels of 5.2–8.0 mmol/l (200–310 mg/dl) (Shaper et al 1985). In the USA it has been estimated that around 105 million adults have a total blood cholesterol of 5.2 mmol/l (200 mg/dl) and of these about 42 million have levels above 6.2 mmol/l (240 mg/dl) (NHANES III 1988–1994). Whilst total blood cholesterol levels of 5.2 mmol/l (200 mg/dl) or less are currently considered desirable, in the USA (AHA 2004) it is clear that even this 'desirable' level of 5.2mmol/l (200 mg/dl) still conveys some health risk (Table 3.2).

BLOOD LIPID PROFILE

The composition of the BLP, in terms of the various lipoproteins (p. 35), is important in terms of health risk. Epidemiological studies have shown positive correlations between triglyceride (TG), low-density lipoprotein cholesterol (LDL-C), apolipoprotein (apo) B and CHD (Castelli et al 1986, Wallace & Anderson 1987), with less CHD being observed in those with high concentrations of high-density lipoprotein cholesterol (HDL-C) and apo

Table 3.1 Classifications for different serum blood lipoprotein cholesterol levels, mmol/l (mg/dl); age and gender not considered (adapted from NCEP 1988)

Lipoproteins	Desirable	Borderline	Abnormal
Total cholesterol	<5.2 (200)	5.2–6.5 (200–252)	>6.5 (252)
LDL cholesterol	≤3 (116)[a]	4.0–5.0 (155–194)	>5.0 (194)
HDL cholesterol	>1.0 (38.7)	0.9–1.0 (34.8–38.7)	<0.9 (34.8)
Triglyceride	<2.0 (177)	2.0–2.5 (177–221)	>2.5 (221)

[a]South African Medical Association and Lipid and Atherosclerosis Society of South African Working Group (2000).

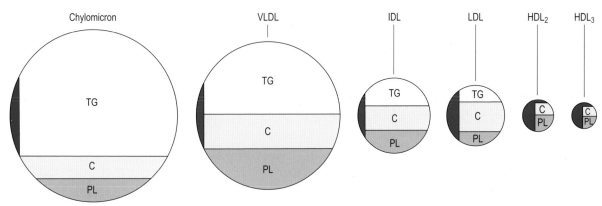

Figure 3.1   Diagrammatic representation of the various lipoprotein constituents, not to scale (adapted from Lewis 1976).

A-I (Wood & Stefanick 1990). Research has also shown that HDL-C levels lower than 1.0 mmol/l (40 mg/dl) (NCEP 2001) are a significant risk factor for heart and vascular diseases, and high levels of LDL-C are of risk to health, since LDL is the main cholesterol-carrying protein within the blood.

STRUCTURE OF BLOOD LIPIDS, LIPOPROTEINS AND APOLIPOPROTEINS

The basic structure, function and metabolism of the various lipids, lipoproteins and apos are described below.

PLASMA LIPIDS

The major lipids in human plasma are TGs, phospholipids and cholesterol esters and together they comprise the lipid components of lipoproteins. Fatty acids also exist in plasma in the free (non-esterified) form (Thompson 1989). Lipids are by definition not readily soluble in water. Their transport in plasma is therefore dependent upon the existence of complexes of soluble proteins (lipoproteins). Lipoproteins are composed of specific polypeptides, the apos, TG, cholesteryl ester, cholesterol

and phospholipid (Lewis 1976, Levy 1981, Spector 1984, Thompson 1989). Human plasma lipoproteins of normal subjects have traditionally been divided into five basic classes: chylomicrons, very low-density lipoproteins (VLDL), intermediate-density lipoproteins (IDL), LDLs and HDLs, and each of these are heterogeneous with respect to protein constituents, namely the apos, and cholesterol content (Jackson et al 1976) (Fig. 3.1 and Table 3.3).

TRANSPORT

All lipids, except free fatty acid (FFA), are transported in plasma in the form of lipoproteins. These macromolecular complexes contain specific apos, which interact with phospholipids and free cholesterol to form the water-soluble or polar, outer shell of lipoprotein particles, encompassing a non-water-soluble or non-polar core, containing TG and cholesterol esters (Fig. 3.2).

Low-density lipoprotein carries most of the cholesterol in the plasma of fasted normal individuals, with much smaller portions being found in VLDL and HDL. In contrast, VLDL carries most of the endogenous TG. Chylomicrons transport dietary TG for a few hours after each meal but are virtually absent from normal plasma after a 12-hour fast. Changes in serum lipids usually reflect changes in lipoprotein concentration and/or lipoprotein

Table 3.3   Approximate lipid composition of plasma lipoproteins (adapted from Thompson 1989)

| Lipoproteins | % of total lipoprotein | | % of total lipids | | | % Cholesterol ester |
	Protein	Lipid	Triglyceride	Cholesterol	Phospholipid	
Chylomicrons	1–2	98–99	88	3	9	46
VLDL	10	90	56	17	19	57
IDL	18	82	32	41	27	66
LDL	25	75	7	59	28	70
HDL$_2$	40	60	6	43	42	74
HDL$_3$	55	45	7	38	41	81

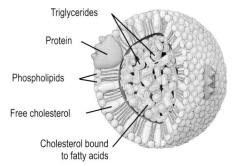

Figure 3.2   Lipoprotein structure. (From Anderson DM, Keith J, Novak PD et al (eds) Mosby's medical, nursing and allied health dictionary, 6th edn. Mosby, St Louis, with permission of Mosby.)

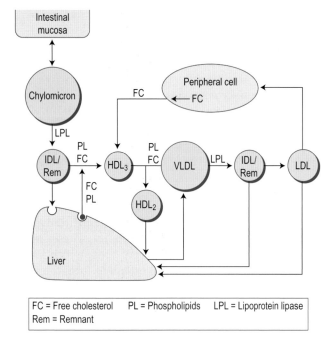

FC = Free cholesterol   PL = Phospholipids   LPL = Lipoprotein lipase
Rem = Remnant

Figure 3.3   Lipid metabolism (adapted from Thompson 1989).

composition. Under normal conditions the concentration of IDL (also known as a remnant particle) in plasma is relatively low and is usually ignored but it can be a major determinant of the concentration of both serum cholesterol and TG in certain forms of hyperlipidaemia (Thompson 1989) (Fig. 3.3).

FREE FATTY ACIDS

FFAs are the form in which fatty acids are transported from their storage site, in adipose tissue, to their sites of utilization in the liver and muscle. Fatty acids are stored in adipose tissue as TGs. The rate-limiting step in the mobilization of TG is the enzyme lipoprotein lipase (LPL) (Vander et al 1990). Lipolysis results in release of FFA and glycerol into plasma and is promoted by acute stress, prolonged fasting and lack of insulin. The concentration of FFA in human plasma ranges from 0.4 to 0.8 mmol/l (35.4–70.8 mg/dl). In the resting state the major sites of oxidation are the liver and heart and

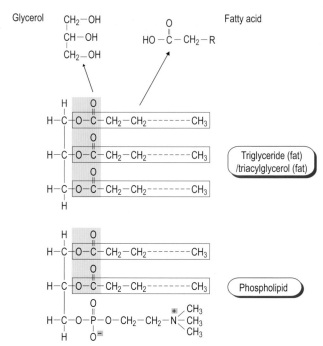

Figure 3.4   Fatty acids, glycerol, triglyceride (triacylglycerol) and phospholipid structure.

during exercise skeletal muscle, when the proportion oxidized rises from 20% to 60%. Much of the FFA taken up by the liver undergoes re-esterification, mainly to TG but also to phospholipid (Thompson 1989) (Fig. 3.4).

TRIGLYCERIDES

TGs are simple fat compounds, of fatty acid esters, consisting of three molecules of fatty acid and glycerol (Fig. 3.4). Dietary TGs are absorbed mainly in the form of chylomicrons, which cross the intestinal lymphatics and enter the systemic circulation via the thoracic duct. Normally, over 90% of TG is absorbed, with around 80–170 mmol (70–150 g) of exogenous TG entering the circulation per day. Triglycerides derived from endogenous fatty acid also originate in the small intestine but their chief source is the liver, where they are secreted in the form of VLDL. The fatty acid content of TG in both chylomicrons and VLDL is markedly influenced by the fatty acid composition of dietary TG. For example, if the diet is poor in the fatty acid linoleic acid, fatty acid deficiency may occur, especially in patients with malabsorption (Jackson & Gotto 1974). Processes involving hydrolysis and uptake by various organs, notably adipose tissues, remove TGs (lipolytic enzymes mediate these). Triglyceride levels remain elevated for several hours after ingestion of a fatty meal, but normally chylomicron TG should be cleared within 12 hours. Thus, measurement of plasma levels in the fasting stage reflects the amount of endogenous TG in the circulation. Normal values for men range from 0.5 to 2.0 mmol/l (44.3–177.0 mg/dl) and up to 1.5 mmol/l (133 mg/dl) in premenopausal women (Thompson 1989, Vander et al 1990) (Table 3.4).

Table 3.4   Mean serum blood lipid levels in US population (aged ≥20 years) 1988–1991 (includes racial and ethnic groups) (adapted from Johnson et al 1993)

Lipid/lipoprotein	Age (years)	Men	Women
Total cholesterol, mmol/l (mg/dl)	≥20	5.30 (205)	5.35 (207)
	20–34	4.89 (189)	4.78 (185)
	35–44	5.35 (207)	5.04 (195)
	45–54	5.64 (218)	5.61 (217)
	55–64	5.72 (221)	6.13 (237)
	65–74	5.64 (218)	6.05 (234)
	≥74	5.30 (205)	5.95 (230)
LDL-C, mmol/l (mg/dl)	≥20	3.39 (131)	3.26 (126)
	20–34	3.10 (120)	2.84 (110)
	35–44	3.47 (134)	3.03 (117)
	45–54	3.57 (138)	3.41 (132)
	55–64	3.67 (142)	3.75 (145)
	65–74	3.65 (141)	3.80 (147)
	≥74	3.41 (132)	3.80 (147)
HDL-C, mmol/l (mg/dl)	≥20	1.22 (47)	1.45 (56)
	20–34	1.22 (47)	1.45 (56)
	35–44	1.19 (46)	1.40 (54)
	45–54	1.22 (47)	1.47 (57)
	55–64	1.19 (46)	1.45 (56)
	65–74	1.16 (45)	1.45 (56)
	≥74	1.22 (47)	1.47 (57)
VLDL-C, mmol/l (mg/dl)	≥20	0.67 (26)	0.62 (24)
	20–34	0.57 (22)	0.49 (19)
	35–44	0.67 (26)	0.54 (21)
	45–54	0.75 (29)	0.62 (24)
	55–64	0.79 (30)	0.78 (30)
	65–74	0.80 (31)	0.75 (29)
	≥74	0.67 (26)	0.72 (28)
TG, mmol/l (mg/dl)	≥20	1.61 (143)	1.42 (126)
	20–34	1.26 (112)	1.14 (101)
	35–44	1.59 (141)	1.28 (113)
	45–54	2.25 (199)	1.42 (128)
	55–64	1.85 (163)	1.90 (126)
	65–74	1.80 (159)	1.75 (155)
	≥74	1.51 (134)	1.77 (157)

PHOSPHOLIPIDS

Plasma phospholipids (Fig. 3.4) are derived mainly from the liver; however, the small intestine makes a contribution. Most of the phospholipid entering the small intestine in the diet undergoes hydrolysis by pancreatic lipase, which probably explains why oral supplements do not exert any great effect upon the content of plasma phospholipids. Phospholipids are integral components of all cell membranes and considerable exchange takes place between plasma and red cells. Phospholipids derived both from the liver and from the diet exist in plasma as constituents of lipoproteins, where they play a key role in maintaining non-polar lipids, such as TGs and cholesterol esters in a soluble state. This property reflects the amphipathic nature of phospholipid molecules, in that their non-polar fatty acyl chains are able to interact with a lipid environment whereas their polar head groups can interact with an aqueous environment (Jackson & Gotto 1974, Thompson 1989) (Fig. 3.2). As with plasma TGs, the fatty acid composition of phospholipids is markedly influenced by the nature of the fat in the diet. Serum phospholipid levels have been found to range from 2.3 to 3.9 mmol/l (204–345 mg/dl) in healthy individuals, and are higher in females than in males. Marked elevations occur in patients with gall bladder (biliary) obstruction (Thompson 1989, Vander et al 1990).

CHOLESTEROL

Cholesterol is a sterol possessing a four-ringed nucleus and a hydroxyl group (Fig. 3.5) In humans it occurs both as free sterol and esterified.   Free cholesterol is a

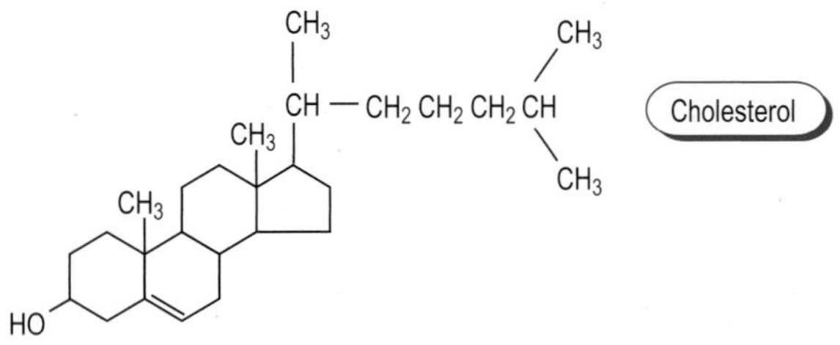

Figure 3.5   Structure of cholesterol (Thibodeau & Patton 1999).

component of all cell membranes and is the principal form in which cholesterol is present in most tissues. Exceptions are the adrenal cortex, the plasma and atheromatous plaques (p 12), where cholesterol esters predominate, and the intestinal lymph and liver. Most tissues have the capacity to synthesize cholesterol but under normal conditions virtually all newly synthesized cholesterol in the body originates from the liver and distal part of the small intestine. The rate-limiting enzyme in the regulation of cholesterol synthesis is β-hydroxy-β-methylglutaryl-coenzyme A reductase (HMG CoA reductase), which is subject to feedback suppression by its final end product, cholesterol (Thompson 1989), meaning that when cholesterol levels are high HMG CoA reductase activity is reduced and therefore so is the synthesis of cholesterol.

More than two-thirds of the cholesterol in plasma is esterified. Esterification is carried out in plasma predominately by the action of the enzyme lecithin:cholesterol acyltransferase (LCAT); small amounts of esterification may take place in the small intestine and the liver by the action of another enzyme. The nature of the cholesterol ester is largely determined by the fatty acid composition, thus the diet. In contrast to cholesterol ester, plasma free cholesterol readily exchanges with cholesterol in cell membranes. Plasma cholesterol is normally in the range 4.0–6.5 mmol/l (155–252 mg/dl) (Table 3.4) but unlike TGs, cholesterol levels do not rise acutely after a fatty meal (Thompson 1989, Vander et al 1990).

APOLIPOPROTEINS (APOS)

Apos are proteins that protrude from the surface of the lipoproteins (Fig. 3.2) and have three main functions: (1) to help solubilize cholesterol ester and TG by interacting with phospholipids, assisting in the structural stability of the lipoprotein's sphere; (2) to act as cofactors by regulating the reaction of these lipids with enzymes, such as LCAT, LPL and hepatic lipase; and (3) to bind to cell surface receptors and thus determine the sites of uptake and rates of degradation of other lipoprotein constituents, most notably cholesterol (Thompson 1989). Around eight or more apos have been discovered and the role of some of these have still to be determined (Levy 1981) (Table 3.5). Increases in apos B_{100} and E and lipoprotein(a) (Lp(a)) have been associated with greater risk of CHD, whereas a greater proportion of apo A-I and associated subclasses

Table 3.5   The function of the major apolipoproteins (apos) (adapted from Woolf-May 1998)

Apos	Major location	Minor location	Function
A-I	HDL	Chylomicrons, VLDL, LDL	Synthesis increases during lipid absorption and is activated by LCAT; also enhances cholesterol efflux out of the adipose cell
A-II	HDL	Chylomicrons, VLDL, LDL	Enhances the lipid-binding property of apo A-I
A-I and A-II	HDL	Chylomicrons, VLDL, LDL	When both apos exist together in HDL, apo A-II enhances the lipid-binding properties of apo A-I
B_{48}	Chylomicrons		Represents the amino-terminal half of apo B_{100} and does not contain the ligand for the LDL receptor
B_{100}	Chylomicrons, VLDL, IDL, LDL, Lp(a)		Essential for cholesterol absorption and contains the ligand for the LDL receptor
C-I	Chylomicrons, VLDL	LDL, HDL	Cofactor for LPL and HDL functions
C-II	Chylomicrons, VLDL	LDL, HDL	When not yet matured chylomicrons and VLDL enter circulation, C-II is transferred to them from HDL to return later as a component of surface remnants during catabolism of TG-rich particles and is an activator for enzyme LPL
C-III	Chylomicrons. VLDL	LDL, HDL	
D		HDL	Helps transfer the ester to chylomicron remnant and IDL which ferry cholesterol to the liver
E	Chylomicrons, IDL, VLDL	LDL, HDL	Has several functions, one of which is the receptor mediated transfer of cholesterol between tissues and plasma

has been identified with reduced risk (Wood & Stefanick 1990, Huang et al 1995, Lagrost et al 1995). Therefore, measuring some of these blood components has been used clinically in identifying those individuals most at risk.

CHYLOMICRONS

Chylomicrons are synthesized in the mucous membrane of the small intestine during fat absorption and compared to the other lipoproteins are relatively big (Fig. 3.1). They consist mainly of TG with lesser amounts of phospholipids, free cholesterol, cholesteryl ester and protein, and they also carry fat-soluble vitamins (Table 3.3). Almost all absorbed dietary fat is transported by chylomicrons derived from the intestinal origin into the lymph, which flows into the systemic circulation via the thoracic duct. The fatty acids of plasma chylomicrons are released, mainly into adipose tissue by the action of endothelial LPL. The remaining chylomicron remnants proceed to the liver (which is the major site for the synthesis anddegradation of phospholipids) where VLDL (derived from hepatic origin) carries TG from the liver to the rest of the body. Triglyceride levels remain elevated for several hours after ingestion of a fatty meal, but normally chylomicron TG should be cleared within 12 hours. Therefore, the presence of chylomicrons in the fasted state is indicative of hypertriglyceridaemia (Lewis 1976, Spector 1984, Thompson 1989), which may contribute towards thrombosis, since TG-rich lipoproteins have been found to stimulate coagulation (Marckmann et al 1992) (Ch. 7).

VERY LOW-DENSITY LIPOPROTEINS (VLDL)

The structure of VLDL is similar to that of chylomicrons and the main differences between them are their sites of synthesis and the source of transported TG. Very low-density lipoproteins are mainly synthesized in the liver, but they contain less TG and more cholesterol, phospholipid and protein, and are smaller in particle size and density than chylomicrons (Fig. 3.1). Much of the VLDL lipid is of endogenous origin and the majority of the TG is derived from plasma FFA, which has its origin in adipose tissue. Triglycerides tend not to accumulate in the blood like cholesterol, though large amounts of VLDL in blood plasma are an indication of hyper-triglyceridaemia (Spector 1984, Thompson 1989).

METABOLISM OF CHYLOMICRONS AND VLDL

Chylomicrons and VLDL are initially metabolized in the peripheral tissues, chiefly muscle and adipose tissue. The rate of catabolism of these TG-rich lipoproteins appears to be regulated by the activity of enzyme LPL, whose activity in adipose tissue rises in the fed state and is increased by insulin. The TG of chylomicrons and VLDL are hydrolysed by LPL and the fatty acids stored. One of

the apos of chylomicrons and VLDL is apo C-II, which is an activator for LPL (Table 3.5). Hence, the presence of apo C-II on these particles determines their sites of catabolism, i.e. those tissues rich in LPL (Spector 1984, Thompson 1989). All plasma lipoproteins are influenced directly or indirectly by LPL, which is modulated by the hormones insulin, thyroxine, cortisol and the oral contraceptive, affecting the rate of lipoprotein catabolism.

The catabolism of TG-rich lipoproteins takes place within the circulation, yielding a series of particles which are progressively depleted of TG and are consequently denser, smaller in diameter and proportionally enriched in cholesteryl ester. These are termed 'remnant particles' (Fig. 3.3).

INTERMEDIATE-DENSITY LIPOPROTEIN (IDL) 'REMNANT PARTICLE'

The IDL is a remnant particle. It is normally low in concentration within the plasma as it is avidly taken up and metabolized by other organs in the abdominal cavity, predominantly the liver. Intermediate-density lipoproteins carry less TG than chylomicrons or VLDL but are still considered to be relatively TG-rich.

The metabolism of VLDL initially yields a denser form of VLDL and IDL. These lipoproteins are further catabolized in the liver, resulting in the major end product LDL (Lewis 1976, Spector 1984, Thompson 1989).

LOW-DENSITY LIPOPROTEIN (LDL)

Low-density lipoprotein is the major cholesterol carrier and differs from its precursor VLDL in that it has a much lower TG content and is greater in density. Low-density lipoprotein is nearly half cholesterol, greater than any other lipoprotein, and is seen as the 'villain' in the cholesterol drama, since it carries cholesterol from its sites of origin into the blood vessels (Lewis 1976, Spector 1984, Thompson 1989). It also plays a significant role in the development of atherosclerosis (Ch. 2). Thus, increases in levels of serum of LDL-C predispose an individual toward heart and vascular disease.

Low-density lipoproteins transport approximately three-quarters of total blood cholesterol and deliver it to the tissues of the body. At LDL concentration greater than 3.36 mmol/l (130 mg/dl) some cholesterol is deposited into the arterial walls, a primary cause of atherosclerosis. The rate of production and removal determine the blood concentration of LDL, and a diet high in saturated fat and cholesterol will increase the liver's production of VLDL, some of which will transform into LDL within the circulation. Saturated fat and cholesterol also suppress withdrawal of LDL, causing a reduction in LDL receptors by the liver, which boosts LDL levels even further (Lewis 1976, Brown & Goldstein 1984, Spector 1984, Thompson 1989) (Fig. 3.6).

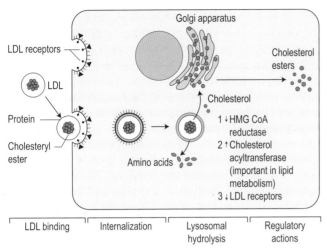

Figure 3.6 LDL receptor endocytosis. Lipoprotein receptors that bind to the LDL are located on the surfaces of certain cells. They internalize the lipoprotein and deliver it to lysosomes where its cholesteryl esters are hydrolyzed. The liberated cholesterol can then be used by the cell or stored in the form of cytoplasmic cholesteryl ester droplets. This process is regulated by HMG CoA reductase (adapted from Thompson 1989).

CHOLESTEROL DELIVERY AND LDL RECEPTORS

Packaging of cholesterol esters into lipoproteins enables transport of lipids that are insoluble within the blood. However, it creates a problem of delivery. Cholesterol esters are unable to pass unaided through membranes. This problem is solved by lipoprotein receptors strategically located on the surfaces of certain cells that bind to the LDL. These receptors operate by receptor-mediated endocytosis (Fig. 3.6), which internalizes the lipoprotein and delivers it to lysosomes where its cholesteryl esters are hydrolyzed. The liberated cholesterol can then be used by the cell for the synthesis of plasma membranes, bile acids and steroid hormones, or stored in the form of cytoplasmic cholesteryl ester droplets. This process is regulated by HMG CoA reductase, which works by negative feedback. For example, when LDL-C is high the activity of HMG CoA is increased, resulting in an increase in LDL receptors, thus increasing cholesterol uptake by the cell. However, when LDL-C is reduced the activity of HMG CoA also becomes reduced (Brown & Goldstein 1986). Apo B_{100} is the main apo of LDL; it fits into a three-dimensional structure of the LDL receptor (like a lock and key). The number of LDL receptor cells displayed varies according to the cell's need for cholesterol. The liver, dense with LDL receptors, removes LDL and IDL from the circulation. The uptake of cholesterol by the cells via the receptors reduces the amount of circulating LDL particles, and one of the major causes of elevated levels of LDL is a decrease in LDL receptor activity (Lithell et al 1982, Brown & Goldstein 1984) (Fig. 3.6).

HIGH-DENSITY LIPOPROTEIN (HDL)

Where LDL is seen as the 'villain' in the cholesterol drama HDL is seen as the 'hero', as it carries cholesterol out of the blood vessels and back to the liver (Levy 1981). High-density lipoprotein is mostly assembled in the extracellular space, where it undergoes continuous remodelling, and can be generated within the circulation from VLDL and chylomicrons (Fig. 3.3). The liver and intestine can also synthesize HDLs. However, HDLs of hepatic origin appear discoid in shape, whereas intestinal HDLs are more spherical in shape (Lewis 1976, Miller 1984, Superko 1991). Numerous studies have found that individuals who have a high proportion of HDLs have a lower risk of heart disease (Castelli et al 1986, Drexel et al 1992). The probable rationale of this is partly related to its role in reverse cholesterol transport (Grundy 1984, Miller 1984) and its promotion of prostacyclin, a substance that inhibits clotting along the inner walls of the arteries (Scanu et al 1984), thus protecting against the development of atherosclerosis.

High-density lipoprotein is divided primarily into subclasses HDL_2 and HDL_3. HDL_3 is relatively cholesterol poor and dense in comparison to HDL_2 (Lippel et al 1981). In circulation HDL_2 and HDL_3 interconvert into one another by enzymes (Eckardstein et al 1994) (Fig. 3.3). The HDL subclasses can be further identified as those that contain only apo A-I and those that contain both apos A-I and A-II. The majority of A-I may be found on HDL_2 and apos A-I and A-II on HDL_3 (Mowri et al 1994). Research has shown that apo A-I reacts to a greater extent to LCAT than apos A-I and A-II together (Fruchart & Ailhaud 1991, Eckardstein et al 1994, James & Pometta 1994), resulting in greater cholesterol efflux (Mahlberg et al 1991, Rothblat et al 1992), whereas the combination of A-I and A-II is thought to inhibit apo A-I and is affected more by hepatic lipase, thereby being more effective at offloading cholesterol to the liver (Fruchart & Ailhaud 1991, Eckardstein et al 1994, James & Pometta 1994). However, these functions may depend upon the stimulating effect of different cells (Rothblat et al 1986, Mahlberg et al 1991, Eckardstein et al 1994).

HIGH-DENSITY LIPOPROTEIN REVERSE CHOLESTEROL TRANSPORT

The efflux of unesterified (free) cholesterol from the tissues, including the arterial walls, to acceptor lipoproteins represents an important process by which cells maintain cholesterol homeostasis. This reaction is the first step in the transport of cholesterol from cells to the liver for excretion, termed 'reverse cholesterol transport' (Glomset 1968, Rothblat et al 1992). Apo A-I on the HDL_2 surface triggers LCAT to convert free cholesterol, taken from plaques, into cholesterol ester, which prevents it from re-entering the arterial wall. The esterification of cholesterol by LCAT and the acquisition of phospholipids, mediated by phospholipid transfer protein, converts the newly formed HDL_3

into HDL_2. The hydrolysis of TG-rich lipoproteins by LPL produces remnants that are transferred to HDL_3, thus contributing to the generation of HDL_2. The export of cholesteryl esters by cholesteryl ester transfer protein (CETP) and the hydrolysis of TGs and phospholipids by hepatic lipase, of the liver, generate HDL_3 at the expense of HDL_2. The additional action of CETP, found to be apo D in humans (Fielding & Fielding 1984), allows the transfer of the newly formed cholesteryl esters from HDL_2 and reduces the rate at which they accumulate in the core of the lipoprotein. This slows the increase in the HDL_2 particle size, thereby delaying the end product, the inhibition of LCAT. The CETP enables the ester to transfer to chylomicron and VLDL remnants (IDL), which also ferry cholesterol to the liver (Miller 1984), and allows for continued reverse cholesterol transport. For a more detailed discussion on HDL and reverse cholesterol transport, refer to Miller (1984).

The liver has the ability to selectively remove cholesterol from HDL_2, allowing for continued uptake of cholesterol from the arteries and tissues, whereas other lipoproteins are completely absorbed (Lewis 1976, Thompson 1989). Furthermore, a proportion of cholesteryl ester is delivered by the receptor-mediated endocytosis of the whole HDL particle, particularly under conditions of increased cholesteryl ester production (i.e. cholesterol-rich diets). However, the process by which cholesterol is transferred from the cell to HDL and from the HDL to other lipoproteins and tissues is still not totally understood (Eckardstein et al 1994).

LIPOPROTEIN(A) (LP(A))

Lipoprotein(a) was discovered nearly 20 years ago and since then it has become the subject of investigation as an indicator for heart disease (Ridker & Hennekens 1994). Cross-sectional and retrospective studies have suggested that high plasma levels of Lp(a) correlate with heart disease (Berg et al 1974, Kostner et al 1981, Sandkamp et al 1990) and may be an independent indicator (Sandkamp et al 1990).

Lipoprotein(a) is structurally related to LDL, though found in lower plasma concentrations (Schreiner et al 1994), and is catabolized in a similar way to LDL (Krempler et al 1983). Lipoprotein(a) is composed of two distinct apos, apo B_{100}, identical to the B_{100} of LDL, and apo (a), which is unique to Lp(a) (Schreiner et al 1994) and is similar in structure to plasminogen, a substance involved in fibrinolysis (anticoagulation) (Utermann 1989). The apo B_{100} of Lp(a) carries cholesterol and cholesteryl esters as it does in LDL, which may contribute towards Lp(a)'s thrombogenic capacity. The similarity of the apo (a) to plasminogen may cause it to compete with plasminogen for fibrin binding, potentially inhibiting tissue plasminogen activator activity (Albers et al 1990, Schreiner et al 1994) and intrinsic fibrinolysis (Ridker & Hennekens 1994), thus increasing the potential for the development of thrombi. Lp(a) is synthesized independently of other cholesterol ester-rich

apo B_{100} containing lipoproteins and its rate of synthesis is the determinant of plasma Lp(a) concentration (Krempler et al 1983), which varies between individuals (0.02–3.87 mmol/l (~<1–>150 mg/dl)) and is thought to be genetically determined.

The exact biological function of Lp(a) is unknown and there are no indications that individuals with very low concentrations of Lp(a) or who lack Lp(a) suffer from any metabolic disease. It is postulated that Lp(a) may be secreted by the liver and that it is not derived from TG-rich precursors, in contrast to LDL. This may explain why Lp(a) concentrations have been found to remain stable for months or even years and are hardly influenced by low-fat and calorie-restricted diets (Hoefler et al 1988).

INTRAVASCULAR LIPID METABOLISM

The process of lipid metabolism is complex and in constant flux, and in order to provide an understandable explanation of this process a simplified pathway of the events from the ingestion of dietary fats is provided.

Dietary lipids transported by chylomicrons, via lymph into the plasma, are degraded to remnants (IDL) by extrahepatic LPL, which is activated by apo C-II on the chylomicron surface. Chylomicron remnants (IDL) are then taken up by hepatic receptors, which recognize the apo E on their surface. Very low-density lipoprotein delivered into plasma from the liver carries endogenously synthesized TGs; like chylomicrons they too undergo partial degradation to IDL. The IDL remnant is then either taken up by the LDL receptor, which recognizes both the apo E and apo B_{100} on the remnant surface (the B_{100} on the IDL remnant surface is distinct from the smaller B_{48} present in chylomicrons), or is further degraded to LDL, which contains apo B_{100} but not apo E (hepatic lipase may be involved in this process). Low-density lipoprotein in turn undergoes catabolism, partly mediated by the LDL receptors. The lipid of HDL is derived from free cholesterol and phospholipid released during lipolysis of chylomicrons and VLDL, as well as free cholesterol efflux from peripheral cells, and its major apo, apo A-I, is synthesized from both the liver and small intestine. The newly formed HDL particles initially form HDL_3 in plasma, which eventually become converted to the larger HDL_2 particles by the action of LCAT, which is activated by apo A-I; they are then transported back to the liver where the HDL_2 is converted back to HDL_3 (Fig. 3.3).

AETIOLOGY

Hyperlipidaemia may be caused through genetic disorders, often termed familial or primary hyperlipidaemia, and/or as a result of a fault in lipid metabolism in conjunction with a metabolic or organic disease. High intake of dietary carbohydrate and/or fat is also a contributing factor and is the most modifiable of all the causes of hyperlipidaemia (Assmann 1982).

FAMILIAL HYPERLIPIDAEMIA

The causes of familial hyperlipidaemias are hereditary and may be the result of defects in the metabolism of lipoproteins, which can be in the form of (i) defects in the biosynthesis, composition or a section of the lipoproteins, (ii) faults in apo structure, (iii) problems with enzymes such as LPL and/or LCAT and/or (iv) defects in the recognition, uptake or degradation of lipoproteins by the cells (Assmann 1982).

Impaired LDL receptor function is one of the main physiological defects, and the outcome of this is an accumulation of LDL in the plasma, which ultimately leads to atherosclerosis (Assmann 1982, Brown & Goldstein 1986). Although underlying genetic or biochemical abnormalities for some of the familial hyperlipidaemias are understood, many have still not been fully determined. Since there are several different types of familial hyperlipidaemias and dyslipidaemias, an explanation for all these goes beyond the scope of this text; a fuller description is provided in Assmann (1982) and Thompson (1989).

SECONDARY HYPERLIPIDAEMIA

Secondary hyperlipidaemia is a disorder of lipid metabolism generally found in conjunction with a metabolic or organic disease, such as diabetes mellitus, thyroid disorders, liver and kidney disease. Secondary hyperlipidaemia may also be caused by a high intake of carbohydrate and/or fat, by alcohol abuse and/or by certain medications. Secondary hyperlipidaemia appears in about 3–5% of the adult population and it is estimated that around 40% of all hyperlipidaemias are of secondary origin. The majority of cases are due to impaired catabolism of lipoproteins. Secondary hyperlipidaemias are often treatable, by correcting or optimal management of the primary disease, and/or change in lifestyle (Assmann 1982). Plasma lipid and lipoprotein levels are also markedly influenced by intrinsic characteristics such as age, gender and genetic factors, as well as modifiable factors such as diet, body weight and physical activity. It is therefore often difficult to clearly determine the individual effect of these factors; for example, increasing age is often accompanied by an increase in body weight and a reduction in physical activity (Thompson 1989).

Body weight

Overweight and particularly obesity have been associated with hyperlipidaemia (Ortlepp et al 2003, Residori et al 2003), and several studies have shown a strong positive correlation between the degree of adiposity and fasting TGs when corrected for other variables (Phillips et al 1981, Connor et al 1982). Furthermore, a study carried out on 5220 men and 5869 women found a dose–response relationship between serum lipids and body mass index (BMI) (Thune et al 1998). High-density lipoprotein cholesterol has also been found to correlate inversely with body weight (Thompson 1989), and in the Lipid Research Clinic's Program Prevalence Study weight was the strongest independent correlate of TG levels in both men and women (Cowan et al 1985), which may reflect the observed association of body weight and increased VLDL synthesis (Phillips et al 1981). Additionally, the positive correlation with plasma cholesterol and BMI also probably reflects an increase in VLDL-C rather than LDL-C (Thompson 1989).

Diet

There is a wealth of research into the effect of diet upon BLP. Kilocalories consumed, carbohydrates, fat, cholesterol, protein, fibre, alcohol and coffee, as well as tobacco smoking may all have an effect upon BLP and are outlined below.

Kilocalories

Consumption of excessive calories sufficient to cause obesity is the most common cause of fasting hypertriglyceridaemia and is manifested by an increase in VLDL. One possible mechanism is that expanded adipocytes are relatively insulin-resistant and that this results in reactive hyperinsulinaemia, which leads to stimulation of hepatic TG synthesis and thus to increased rate of secretion of VLDL. Alternatively, TG clearance may be defective, resulting in a reduced rate of catabolism of VLDL in peripheral tissue (Groer & Shekleton 1989). Regardless of the mechanism regarding reduction in body weight to desirable levels, restriction of calorific intake often brings serum TG levels to within normal range. Indeed calorific restriction that is sufficient to induce weight reduction causes a rise in HDL-C in obese individuals, whose HDL-C levels tend to be lower than normal (Thompson 1989).

Carbohydrate

Healthy individuals show an increase in serum TG when fed a carbohydrate-rich diet, particularly if it contains considerable amounts of sucrose, but this rise is transient if the diet is isocaloric. For those with existing hypertriglyceridaemia, this type of diet may result in impaired TG clearance, which may be accompanied by increases in plasma insulin levels. Since the activity of LPL, which mediates TG clearance, is markedly influenced by insulin, this has led to the suggestion that carbohydrate-induced hypertriglyceridaemia results from defective lipolysis of VLDL, secondary to insulin resistance at the adipocyte level, rather than from an increase in hepatic TG synthesis. Additionally, HDL-C levels also tend to decrease when the diet is rich in carbohydrate (Thompson 1989).

Fat

Generally dietary saturated fats increase serum cholesterol, and polyunsaturated fats cause it to decrease, and similar changes occur in fasting serum TG. A diet containing 40% of its calories from monounsaturated fat lowers LDL-C to a similar extent as a diet containing 40% polyunsaturated fat, and does so without the undesirable reduction in HDL-C. Furthermore, this type of diet does not appear to show increases in serum TG as has been observed when low-fat diets are undertaken (Grundy 1986). This might explain the relatively low serum lipids in populations living in the Mediterranean, whose consumption of olive oil is considerable (Thompson 1989).

Changes in serum cholesterol, induced by dietary fat, are predominantly due to changes in concentration of LDL-C. Research has suggested that when polyunsaturated fat is substituted for saturated fat, LDL synthesis is reduced and catabolism is enhanced, contributing to a reduction in the size of the intravascular pool of LDL (Muesing et al 1995). These changes are accompanied by alterations in the fatty acid composition of the lipid constituents of VLDL and LDL (Thompson 1989).

Cholesterol

Increasing the intake of dietary cholesterol may result in increases in LDL-C, although cholesterol from ingestion of shellfish has a relatively small effect on serum cholesterol in normal subjects (Connor & Lin 1982). The main difficulty in assessing the importance of dietary cholesterol, apart from the source of this cholesterol, is the considerable inter-individual variation in response (Thompson 1989).

Protein

The substitution of dietary soya bean protein in place of animal protein has been shown to cause a reduction in cholesterol, despite the fat and cholesterol content being similar. However, the mechanism for this is unclear. Vegetarians also tend to have lower serum lipid levels than non-vegetarians, which is only partly attributable to the source of protein. Although HDL-C levels tend to be lower in vegetarians than in those on diets that include meat (D'Amico et al 1992), their ratio of HDL:total cholesterol tends to be higher (Thompson 1989).

Fibre

A study investigating the dietary habits of hyperlipidaemic subjects found dietary fibre intake to be inadequate (Kralikova et al 1996). Additionally, dietary intervention studies have found that a fibre-rich diet is effective in reducing blood LDL-C and TG levels (Rivellese et al 1994) in hyperlipidaemic subjects; and water-soluble dietary fibre, such as pectin, was found to decrease serum cholesterol levels (Veldman et al 1997).

Alcohol

In the animal model, chronic moderate alcohol consumption appears to reduce fasted blood lipids, and lowers postprandial chylomicrons and TG levels (Daher et al 2003). In human studies, regular consumption of small amounts of alcohol has been shown to increase levels of HDL-C (Hannuksela et al 2002). For instance, drinking two units of alcohol per day (approximately one glass of wine) has been shown to significantly increase HDL-C by around 0.33 mmol/l (12.8 mg/dl) compared to non-drinkers (Castelli et al 1977); and drinking around 40.2 g of alcohol per day has shown modest but statistically significant increases in HDL-C of around 0.08 mmol/l (3.1 mg/dl) (Samanek et al 2002). Increases in both HDL_2 and HDL_3 cholesterol have been found, which may be due to induced increases in LPL (Phillips et al 1981). The cardioprotective effect of alcohol consumption may be, in part, due to its enhancement of the cholesterol esterification rate in the HDL particle (Perret et al 2002). In contrast, hyperlipidaemia (mainly hypertriglyceridaemia) is found in more than 80% of cases of alcoholism. This has been attributed to an increase in hepatic synthesis of VLDL as a result of liver disease, and extreme hyperlipidaemia may be found in those with clinically manifest alcohol-induced pancreatitis. Around 60% of alcoholics suffer myocardial infarction, regardless of the observed increase in HDL-C with moderate alcohol intake. Therefore, alcohol intake cannot be recommended as a prophylaxis for atherosclerosis, due to its probable association with organ damage, most notably cirrhosis of the liver and/or cardiomyopathy (Assmann 1982).

Coffee

The ingestion of large quantities of coffee, particularly boiled coffee, has been found to increase serum cholesterol, which has not been found with equivalent quantities of tea or instant coffee. Therefore this rise in serum cholesterol is unlikely to be due to caffeine (Thelle et al 1987, Pirich et al 1993).

Tobacco

Cigarette smokers generally tend to show lower levels of HDL-C compared to non-smokers. However, HDL-C has been shown to improve after about 8 weeks of smoking cessation (Eliasson et al 2001). It appears that cigarette smoking stimulates oxidation of LDL particles, producing significant decrease of TGs and HDL-C (Lepsanovic et al 2001), and impairs lipolysis, which prevents the postprandial increase in HDL_2 normally found in non-smokers after a fatty meal (Thompson 1989, AHA 2004).

Illness and disease

Illnesses such as an acute myocardial infarction or viral infection have been found to affect serum lipids. For instance, after a myocardial infarction total cholesterol tends to fall, which reflects a decrease in LDL that is accompanied by a rise in plasma TG and fall in HDL-C, the cause in part being due to a rise in catecholamines and other hormones. These changes do not generally occur until around 24 hours post-event and may take several weeks to settle down to pre-event values. Similar changes have been observed after surgical operations and/or febrile illnesses (Thompson 1989).

Liver disease

Acute hepatitis, chronic hepatitis, liver cirrhosis and obstructive liver disease all show considerable variation with regard to secondary hyperlipidaemia. Non-alcoholic fatty liver disease comprises a wide spectrum of liver damage and although the prevalence of this disease is unknown, it is estimated to affect 10–24% of the general population of various countries. The natural history of this disease still remains to be defined but is often associated with hyperlipidaemia (Allard 2002, Alba & Lindor 2003).

Kidney disease

Hyperlipidaemia is frequently observed in patients with kidney disease who undergo dialysis as well as post-kidney transplantation and is an inevitable result of nephritic syndrome (a group of urinary tract disorders). Lipoprotein biosynthesis is increased in nephritic syndrome as a consequence of proteinuria (Gretz et al 1996) and elevations in HDL-C, apo A-I and A-II levels are commonly observed (Assmann 1982).

Diabetes

Hyperlipidaemia is seen in approximately 40% of all diabetics and more than 80% suffer from hypertriglyceridaemia (Assmann 1982), which is associated with insulin resistance (Saltiel & Kahn 2001). The increase in VLDL and reduced LPL activity contribute toward the pathogenesis of hypertriglyceridaemia. However, it is often difficult to determine if this is due to primary or secondary causes. If hyperlipidaemia persists after optimal regulation of the diabetes then it is considered to be of primary cause. The combination of hypertriglyceridaemia and low HDL-C results in cardiovascular disease complications and around 50% of diabetics suffer myocardial infarction. Serum lipids often normalize with appropriate weight reduction, restriction of rapidly absorbed carbohydrates, alcohol avoidance and/or medical intervention (Assmann 1982) (see Ch.4).

Thyroid disorders

Generally, hypothyroidism tends to be accompanied by hypercholesterolaemia due to the reduction in LDL catabolism; and females with hypothyroidism (defined as thyroid-stimulating hormone >3.75 mU/l) have been found to have serum cholesterol levels >7 mmol/l (271 mg/dl). It is speculated that hypothyroidism also causes a decrease in the enzyme activity responsible for the degradation and excretion of plasma cholesterol (Kobayashi et al 1997), resulting in increased levels of circulating lipids. Conversely, hyperthyroidism is associated with hypocholesterolaemia, as a result of increased LDL catabolism. Secondary dyslipidaemias are generally resolved with treatment of the underlying problems (Assmann 1982).

Age

During the first 6 months of life there is a rapid rise in serum cholesterol; thereafter there is little change until puberty, after which there is a rise in TG and LDL cholesterol in both sexes. There is also a fall in HDL for boys but not for girls. During adult life, plasma lipid levels continue to rise in both sexes, especially in the elderly (Saito 2001). The concentration of cholesterol tends to be higher in men up to the age of 55, but higher in women thereafter (Table 3.4). Triglyceride levels remain higher in men until the age of 65, when they become similar in both sexes (Heiss et al 1980). The increase in total cholesterol mainly reflects an increase in LDL-C. HDL-C levels, however, are higher in women than in men at all ages from puberty onwards and do not decrease after the menopause. Studies have shown that cholesterol, TG and LDL-C are correlated with age even when body weight is taken into account (Connor et al 1982). The rise in LDL-C observed in women as they increase in age is associated with the effect of hormonal changes on the breakdown of LDL (Thompson 1989).

Gender

From puberty up until women reach the menopause, females tend to have lower TG, LDL-C and VLDL-C levels and higher HDL-C levels than males. Once women reach the menopause, however, their LDL-C levels generally tend to become higher than those of men of a similar age, unless they are on hormone replacement therapy. Women who are on oestrogen and/or progesterone therapy tend to have higher TG levels with lower levels of LDL-C than women not on hormone replacement treatment (Heiss et al 1980). The higher HDL-C of females reflects a higher concentration of HDL$_2$ whereas the concentration of HDL$_3$ has been found to be similar in both sexes. Differences in endogenous sex hormones account for much of the gender differences. Oestrogen, for instance, tends to lower LDL-C, raise HDL-C (Levy 1981, Bush & Barrett-Connor 1985) and cause elevations in coagulation factors (Levy 1981), whereas androgens tend to have the opposite effect (Thompson 1989).

For premenopausal women, levels of the sex hormones oestrogen and progesterone vary throughout the menstrual cycle, and generally cholesterol and TG levels are higher and HDL-C is lower during the follicular phase compared to the luteal phase. It is strongly suggested that these changes are linked to oestrogen levels, which peak prior to ovulation. These factors should be a consideration for the exercise practitioner when determining a client/patient's blood lipid profile.

At any given serum cholesterol level the risk of CHD in men is roughly three times that of women of comparable age (AHA 1973). Women tend to get CHD at higher cholesterol levels than men, which may be due to women having a greater proportion of their serum cholesterol in the form of HDL, accompanied by lower TG, VLDL (Kannel 1987) and possibly Lp(a) levels (Barletta et al 1993). However, after the onset of menopause, when LDL-C levels tend to resemble those of men, the risk of CHD for women is increased.

Genetic factors relating to LDL receptors (Bush et al 1988) and Lp(a) (Howard et al 1994) do not appear to be gender-linked. However, there is some evidence to suggest that concentrations of HDL are influenced by genetic factors for both men and women, and several twin studies have found levels of HDL and apos A-I and A-II to be genetically determined (Mjos et al 1977, Dahlen et al 1983).

Race

Although it is difficult to determine the influence of factors such as diet and physical activity on blood lipids with regard to race, the Lipid Research Clinics Prevalence Study showed that black American males have higher HDL:total cholesterol ratios than their white counterparts (Green et al 1985), and a similar tendency has been reported in international comparisons between African and European countries. Hence there may be a genuine racial trait in those of African origin (Green et al 1985, Thompson 1989). Levels of Lp(a) too may be influenced by race (Howard et al 1994).

Seasonal and day-to-day variation

The variation in blood lipids found within an individual can be the result of measurement imprecision and biological variability. In healthy individuals variations in fasting serum lipids over the course of a year range from 4 to 11% for total cholesterol, 13 to 41% for TG and 4 to 12% for HDL-C. Over 60% of these variations have been attributed to biological fluctuation and the remainder to analytical variability (Demacker et al 1982). Part of the biological fluctuations have been attributed to seasonal changes, which are most marked in parts of the world where summer and winter have the greatest differential; pre-menopausal women also experience the additional effect of the menstrual cycle upon their serum lipids (Thompson 1989).

MEDICATIONS AND SECONDARY HYPERLIPIDAEMIA

Certain medications has been shown to produce hyperlipidaemia as a side effect, and this is something to be considered when prescribing PA/exercise. However, medications prescribed to treat hyperlipidaemia may have side effects that could influence PA/exercise prescription (Ch. 14).

Beta-adrenergic receptor blockers (beta-blockers)

Beta-adrenergic receptor blockers (beta-blockers) are often prescribed to patients with heart and vascular disease as a means of reducing cardiac work and lowering blood pressure. Furthermore, the nature of cardiovascular diseases is related to the fact that these individuals often have hyperlipidaemia. However, beta-blockers have been reported to result in increases in blood TG levels (Passotti et al 1986, Szollar et al 1990) whilst showing no significant change in total blood cholesterol (Passotti et al 1986). Though the underlying mechanisms are still not fully understood, the elevation in TGs has been attributed to an increase in VLDL TGs, while the lack of change in cholesterol levels has been speculated to be due to reductions in HDL-C, although some studies have found no significant change in HDL-C (Szollar et al 1990). One proposed mechanism for these changes in blood lipids, as a result of taking beta-blockers, is the possibly augmented resynthesis of TGs in the liver from the increased supply of FFA. This increase in FFA is due to pronounced lipolysis as a result of increased LPL activity (Lehtonen 1985), which becomes active in response to the inhibition of catecholamine-induced lipolysis. However, research findings have been contradictory and the greatest increases in TGs have been observed in those patients who also gain weight. The use of different beta-blockers, varying doses, experimental conditions and subject weight fluctuation make it difficult to clearly determine the effect of beta-blockers on blood lipids (Assmann 1982).

Diuretics

Diuretics are often employed as a means of lowering blood pressure, and have been found to cause elevations in total cholesterol, LDL-C and VLDL TGs (Middeke et al 1997, Van der Heijden et al 1998) and reductions in HDL-C (Middeke et al 1997) and apos A-I and B (Marquest-Vidal et al 2000). The underlying cause for the increase in LDL, however, remains unclear. Diuretics can also increase sympathetic activity, which induces lipolysis and thus circulating FFAs, and possibly may be the impetus for an increase in VLDL synthesis by the liver. Nonetheless, the research findings have been conflicting, for similar reasons to those mentioned for beta-blockers.

Oral hypoglycaemic agents

Oral hypoglycaemic agents, often prescribed to diabetics whose blood glucose is not well controlled (Pan et al 2002), have been shown to reduce TG and LDL-C as well (Derosa et al 2003).

Thyroid treatments

Treatments prescribed to those with an underactive thyroid (hypothyroidism) have been found to increase hepatic LDL–receptor activity, thereby lowering total cholesterol and LDL-C levels (Caraccio et al 2002).

Sex hormones

The effects of sex hormones upon blood lipids (p. 44) vary according to the drug, dose and route of administration (Donahoo et al 1998).

TREATMENT

There are numerous pharmacological interventions that can be given to try and control hyperlipidaemia, and the major non-pharmacological intervention would be through appropriate PA/exercise intervention.

PHARMACOLOGICAL

The most commonly prescribed drugs for the control of hyperlipidaemia are bile-acid binders, fibrates and statins.

Bile–acid binders

Bile-acid binders work by reducing LDL-C. They are ion-exchanging resins that act by binding bile acids, preventing their absorption, which promotes hepatic conversion of cholesterol into bile acids. This results in an increase in LDL-receptor activity of the liver cells and increases the clearance of LDL-C. However, they can raise TG and can cause gastrointestinal problems (BMA, RPS GB 2005).

Fibrates

Fibrates generally act by decreasing serum TG. They tend to have variable effects on LDL-C and may reduce risk of CHD events in those with low HDL-C or raised TG levels. However, if combined with a statin they can increase the risk of effects on the muscles. Fibrates may also cause gallstones, rash and gastrointestinal upset (BMA, RPS GB 2005).

Statins

Statins are extremely effective at reducing LDL-C levels. Statins inhibit HMG CoA reductase, the enzyme involved in cholesterol synthesis, particularly in the liver. Thus, they are more effective than other types of drugs in lowering LDL-C, but are less effective than fibrates in reducing TG levels. They can, however, have a mild lowering effect on TG and cause a slight increase in HDL-C (BMA, RPS GB 2005).

REGULAR PHYSICAL ACTIVITY AND EXERCISE

A review of intervention studies on the effect of PA/exercise upon blood lipids found that although not all studies reported favourable changes in TG and HDL-C, the majority of studies did (Wilmore 2001). Numerous studies have investigated the effect of regular PA/exercise upon blood lipid profile and have found increases in the concentration of HDL-C (Huttunen et al 1979, Seip et al 1993), HDL_2-C (Ballantyne et al 1982), HDL_2 (Wood et al 1983 & 1984), proportion of HDL-C/LDL-C (Seip et al 1993), HDL-C/total cholesterol (Rauramaa et al 1995), as well as decreases in total cholesterol, TG, VLDL-C and apo B (Hughes et al 1990a & 1990b, Seip et al 1993). However, consistent reductions in LDL-C have not been convincingly demonstrated (Goldberg & Elliot 1987) and though reductions in serum total cholesterol have been observed as a result of habitual PA/exercise they appear to be greatest in those who exercise at higher intensities. For example, although Savage et al (1986) found reductions in total cholesterol from two groups, one working at 75% $\dot{V}O_2max$ and the other at 45% $\dot{V}O_2max$, the reductions in total cholesterol were greatest in the group that exercised at the higher intensity, suggesting a dose response.

However, not all studies have observed changes in blood lipids as a result of PA/exercise intervention (Brownell et al 1982, Wood et al 1991, Houmard et al 1993), and changes appear to be related to the baseline blood lipid profile, in that the poorer the baseline lipid profile the greater the potential for change from PA/exercise intervention (Woolf-May 1998). But despite relatively poor baseline HDL-C values (1.26 mmol/l, 48.8 mg/dl), Suter et al (1994) failed to find significant increases in HDL-C after exercise intervention, indicating that other factors are probably involved in PA/exercise-induced changes in blood lipids.

Mechanism

The mechanisms responsible for changes in BLP, as a response to PA/exercise intervention, still remain to be fully determined; and other factors, such as lipid-lowering medications, may also have an influence upon these changes. However, the lower TG and VLDL-C concentrations often observed in healthy, physically active individuals have been attributed to the enhanced rate of removal, due to the increase in LPL in trained muscle (Nikkila 1978, Mowri et al 1994) and adipose tissue (Wood & Stefanick 1990). Lipolysis of TG and VLDL-C results in surface components being released into plasma, including free cholesterol, which is taken up by HDL_3, due to the action of

LCAT, and is then transformed to HDL_2 (Fig. 3.3). This process is assisted not only by an increase in LPL but also by a reduction in levels of hepatic lipase, the function of which is to promote the conversion of HDL_2 back to HDL_3. Consequently, TG-rich lipoprotein particles are reduced in number and size, and HDL particles are increased in size and cholesterol content (Lampman et al 1977). Physical activity intervention has been found to show increases in levels of the LCAT enzyme (Hostmark 1982, Marniemi et al 1982, Lehmann et al 2001) and physically active individuals have been shown to have increased activity levels of LCAT and CETP (Gupta et al 1993), which also promote reverse cholesterol transport and the ability of HDL to continue in this process, respectively.

The extent of change in lipids and lipoproteins with PA/exercise intervention is dependent upon several factors, such as PA/exercise intensity, duration and frequency, diet, medications, gender and pre-intervention BLP. However, this would pertain to those whose dyslipidaemia is alterable. For those individuals whose dyslipidaemia is of genetic origin, PA/exercise intervention may have little or no effect. Individuals with LPL deficiency, for instance, will not benefit from the PA/exercise training response of increased LPL activity, nor will the HDL particles increase in individuals with Tangier disease, since it is characterized by the virtual absence of circulating plasma HDL (Ordovas 2000). However, it is important to consider the other potential health benefits of regular PA/exercise for dyslipidaemic individuals.

Energy expenditure

For those individuals who do not possess any genetic dyslipidaemia, it appears that for changes to HDL-C concentration around a 1000 kcal per week is necessary, which is roughly equivalent to walking/running 1.5 miles a day. However, for increases in HDL_2-C, energy expenditure of more than 1500 kcal per week may be required (Haskell 1986, Superko 1991). Above this level, a dose–response relationship exists, with greater changes occurring up to energy expenditures of 4500 kcal per week (Haskell 1986). For those with existing atherosclerosis, not taking lipid-lowering medication, research suggests that a weekly energy expenditure of 2200 kcal is required to show a regression in atherosclerotic plaques (Hambrecht et al 1993), which in part may be related to blood lipid levels.

Intensity

It appears that regular PA/exercise intensity has an effect upon blood lipids (for those individuals without genetic dyslipidaemia), and Savage et al (1986) observed from a group of prepubescent boys and adult males that significant increases in HDL-C levels occurred when the subjects trained at 74% but not at 40% $\dot{V}O_2$max. Similarly, Stein et al (1990) found that a minimum of 75% $\dot{V}O_2$max (over a period

of 12 weeks, 3 times a week for 30 minutes each session) was needed for increases in HDL-C. Additionally, a study on a group of male myocardial patients (aged 63.5 ± 6.5 years) taking lipid-lowering medication, who carried out PA/exercise of varying types (excluding swimming), within the boundaries of moderate intensity (40–60% $\dot{V}O_2$max), showed that those subjects who worked at a higher PA/exercise intensity had lower TG levels (Woolf-May et al 2003).

Duration

The effect of PA/exercise duration upon blood lipids may have more to do with total energy expenditure than the duration of the exercise sessions per se. For instance, it has been suggested that if the duration of the exercise is long enough, changes in HDL-C (Tran et al 1983) and other blood lipids (Haskell 1986) will occur. Hence, energy expenditure may be one of the possible underlying mechanisms for favourable changes in blood lipids (Wood et al 1984, Haskell 1986, Hardman et al 1989).

Frequency

Government guidelines from the USA, which have been adopted by the UK, recommend that in order to reduce risk of all-cause and cardiovascular mortality by around 20–30%, on at least 5 days of the week adults should accumulate around 30 minutes of physical activity per day (Pate et al 1995). However, intervention studies into the effect on blood lipids of accumulative bouts versus continuous bouts of PA/exercise of similar volume and intensity have been mixed. For instance, some studies have found that exercise regimens consisting of repetitive short bouts of PA/exercise are less effective at improving blood lipids (Savage et al 1986, Woolf-May 1998), whereas others suggest that they are more effective (Ebisu 1985). However, there is still much work to be carried out in this area, especially employing interventions of moderate-intensity PA/exercise.

Age

A review of various studies has shown that while factors such as gender and health status may influence the extent of change in blood lipids, as a result of PA/exercise intervention, when direct comparisons were made across age groups, age did not appear to affect response (Wilmore 2001).

Gender

A review of studies found no consistent differentiating response in blood lipids between males and females as a result of PA/exercise. Nonetheless, some studies reported greater increases in HDL-C for males when compared to females (Wilmore 2001). The gender divide may be explained by the fact that males tend to have poorer BLPs than females. Therefore men tend to possess the greater potential for change as a result of PA/exercise intervention (Woolf-May et al 1998, Wilmore 2001). Furthermore, weight loss is an important factor in change in blood lipids and men tend to lose weight more easily through PA/exercise than women (Despres et al 1984, Bjorntorp 1989), probably due to the fact that the gluteofemoral fat, the major fat storage area in females, compared to the abdominal area in males, is known to be less lipolytically active than other fat (Bjorntorp 1989). This might explain the observed gender differences and is a factor that needs considering when looking for alterations in blood lipids in response to PA/exercise intervention.

SINGLE BOUT OF PHYSICAL ACTIVITY EXERCISE

An acute bout of PA/exercise may induce short-term transient changes in plasma lipids and lipoproteins, and although the exercise practitioner is generally aiming to induce longer-term improvements to their client/patient's BLP, understanding the potential influence of transient changes is essential.

Observed acute changes in blood lipids after PA/exercise may be dependent upon the intensity and duration of the PA/exercise undergone; and it appears that short-term transient changes in blood lipids tend to last for around 48 hours after an intense bout of PA/exercise and generally return to baseline values within 24 hours after less intense activities (Pronk 1993). Therefore, it is important when reviewing an individual's BLP that any blood lipids are taken at least 24 hours after moderate-intensity PA/exercise and 48 hours after more intense activities.

Intensity

The intensity of an acute bout of PA/exercise may affect the extent of the transient change in blood lipids. For example, a study carried out by Tsetsonis & Hardman (1995) observed (from a group of 5 males and 7 females, mean age of 25 years) that there were greater decreases in TG after 90 minutes of treadmill walking at 60% $\dot{V}O_2$max compared to 90 minutes of treadmill walking at 32% $\dot{V}O_2$max, yet found no significant fluctuations in HDL-C between the two intensities. Nonetheless, Angelopoulos & Robertson (1993) found no significant change in TG levels, in a group of 7 sedentary men, after treadmill running at 65% $\dot{V}O_2$max for 30 minutes, but did find significant changes in HDL-C 5 minutes post-exercise, which returned to baseline level 24 hours post-exercise; in another study Angelopoulos et al (1993) also found elevated levels of HDL$_3$-C 24 hours post-exercise after 30 minutes of treadmill exercise at 65% $\dot{V}O_2$max. Additionally, Gordon et al (1994) observed an increase in HDL$_3$-C 24 hours post-exercise when subjects ran to an energy expenditure of 800 kcal at 75% $\dot{V}O_2$max, but not when, on a separate

occasion, these same subjects ran at 65% $\dot{V}O_2$max. Similarly Hicks et al (1987) found greater increases in both HDL-C and apo A when their subjects exercised at 90% as opposed to 60% $\dot{V}O_2$max. Thus, these studies indicate that exercise intensity may be an important factor for transient elevations in the HDL-C.

Interestingly, anaerobic activities appear to result in a poorer BLP than aerobic activities. For example, a study carried out by Bubnova et al (2003) found that when cardiac patients and healthy individuals worked at high-intensity dynamic exercise (80–100% of peak aerobic capacity) there were increases in total cholesterol and LDL-C, TG, apo B and ratio of apo B/apo A-I, but found that after moderate-intensity exercise (60% of peak aerobic capacity) there were reductions in apo B and increases in apo A-I. Another study looking into the effect of static leg exercise on both healthy and cardiac patients found that following exercise there were elevations in TG, apo B and ratio of apo B/A, an increase in LDL-C in cardiac patients only and no changes in HDL-C for either group (Aronov et al 2003). Thus, these findings suggest that post-exercise anaerobic activities produce unfavourable changes in BLP.

Duration

The duration of an acute bout of PA/exercise has been shown to affect transient changes in blood lipids, and an extreme example of this can be seen from a study carried out by Foger et al (1994) who looked at the effect of cycling racing over 250 km (~156 miles). They found that after the race, total cholesterol, TG, LDL-C and apo B were all significantly reduced and HDL-C and HDL$_2$-C were significantly increased, whilst HDL$_3$-C was slightly decreased (probably at the expense of HDL$_2$-C). Interestingly, even 8 days post-race apos A-I and A-II were still significantly elevated. Although, it is unlikely that one would prescribe this duration of PA/exercise to any patient/client, it does highlight how duration of a PA/exercise bout can influence blood lipids and a review of various studies suggested that the more exhaustive the exercise the more prolonged the response (Pronk 1993).

Training status

The baseline training status of an individual may very well determine the degree of response in blood lipids to an acute bout of PA/exercise. For example, Kantor et al (1987) found that 48 hours after cycling on an ergometer, at around 80% of maximum heart rate (HRmax) (~75% $\dot{V}O_2$max), trained individuals showed greater increases in HDL$_2$-C than untrained individuals who only showed increases in HDL$_3$-C. This may be related to the increases in LPL (Nikkila 1978, Mowri et al 1994) found in trained muscle and decreased hepatic lipase activity (Lampman et al 1977).

Gender

There is evidence to suggest that women do not respond to the same extent as men to an acute bout of PA/exercise. However, research has been conflicting and the differences have mainly been between pre- and postmenopausal women (Pronk 1993) and men having poorer baseline levels than women. Hence, the gender variability may be subject to similar influences as for those discussed for chronic PA/exercise.

Prior physical activity

A single session of PA/exercise several hours before a high-fat meal reduces the extent of the usual post-meal rise in blood TGs, namely postprandial lipaemia (Malkova et al 1999), possibly by altering muscle LPL activity (Herd et al 2001). A review of studies suggests that the energy expenditure of prior exercise may also play a role in the magnitude of this effect, and that there appears to be no significant effect of gender, age, type of meal ingested, exercise intensity, exercise duration or timing of exercise on the postprandial response between the studies (Petitt & Cureton 2003).

PRE-EXERCISE PRESCRIPTION

As for all individuals undertaking PA/exercise intervention, those with dyslipidaemia should undergo a thorough screening process in order to detect associated risk factors and other co-morbidities. This should involve the completion of medical and pre-PA/exercise activity screening questionnaires, and where applicable appropriate assessments should be carried out (Appendix A). In addition to the dyslipidaemia any co-morbidities also require careful consideration prior to PA/exercise prescription.

REGULAR PHYSICAL ACTIVITY AND EXERCISE PRESCRIPTION

It is unlikely that anyone with longstanding hyperlipidaemia will be without at least some of the related co-morbidities, such as high blood pressure, overweight and heart and vascular disease. Hence, these factors should be considered in addition to other non-related co-morbidities. The aim therefore is to consider these factors and improve BLP. Hence, if the client/patient is overweight, then weight loss would undoubtedly help to improve BLP and dietary changes may also need to be suggested. Furthermore, some of the hyperlipidaemias may be of genetic (primary) origin (p. 42) and PA/exercise may have little influence upon these individuals' BLP. Nonetheless, appropriate habitual PA/exercise is known to produce physiological and psychological benefits other than those relating to blood lipids, which are likely to be of advantage to the person's health.

PHYSICAL ACTIVITY/EXERCISE INTENSITY

Generally it appears that higher PA/exercise intensity levels produce lower TG levels, and an intensity of around 75% $\dot{V}O_2$max is required to produce favourable changes in levels of HDL-C. However, this may be too high for those individuals just beginning a programme and initially the intensity should be at around 40–60% of $\dot{V}O_2$max, though this too will depend upon the individual's health status.

ENERGY EXPENDITURE

Total energy expenditure through PA/exercise may be an important factor in producing favourable changes in BLP, and it appears that around a minimum of 1000 kcal per week is required to induce improvements in HDL-C. Weekly energy expenditure through PA/exercise of around 1533 and 2200 kcal per week, in those with heart disease, may also be required to halt progression and show some regression in atherosclerotic plaques, respectively, in those not taking any lipid-lowering medication (Hambrecht et al 1993), which may in part be related to an improved BLP. Therefore, for dyslipidaemic individuals and those with a poor BLP a programme that progressively builds up energy expenditure through PA/exercise would be recommended, and may initially commence at a low exercise intensity level of longer duration. Nonetheless, this will ultimately depend upon the health status of each individual patient/client.

LOW-DENSITY LIPOPROTEIN CHOLESTEROL

Usually PA/exercise intervention does not appear to affect LDL-C levels, unless accompanied by weight loss (Durstine et al 2002) and/or if pre-intervention baseline levels are relatively high, thus increasing the potential for change.

AEROBIC ACTIVITIES

The majority of studies investigating the effect of PA/exercise upon blood lipids have employed aerobic activities; and a study comparing 16 weeks of aerobic training, resistance training and cross-training, in a group of 48 sedentary healthy women (aged 20.4 ± 1 years), found that whilst aerobic training resulted in significant reductions in blood TG and increases in blood HDL-C, resistance and cross-training caused no significant change in these parameters, but improvements in muscular strength were observed. Moreover, the rise in HDL-C, as a result of aerobic training, was partly explained by the

13% reduction in body fat; however, post-training blood lipid changes returned to baseline levels after 6 weeks of detraining (LeMura et al 2000). These findings therefore highlight the importance of aerobic PA/exercise in reducing TG levels and associated weight loss that lead to enhanced HDL-C. Furthermore, whilst the majority of studies have been carried out on healthy sedentary individuals, similar findings have also been seen in less healthy individuals. For instance, research carried out on a group of coronary artery disease (CAD) patients, where 14 patients participated in 8 months of supervised training, composed of two strength sessions (60% of 1 repetition maximum) and two aerobic training sessions (at 60–80% of HRmax) per week, found favourable changes in total cholesterol, TG, HDL-C and apo A-I levels, which returned to near baseline levels after 3 months of detraining: similar findings were also observed in muscular strength (Tokmakidis & Volaklis 2003). This indicates that for both healthy sedentary individuals and those with CAD, in order to retain a more healthy BLP it is important for PA/exercise to be current and regular. Furthermore, a study carried out on a group of 11 male overweight subjects (aged 25.6 ± 1.4 years) with a BMI of 27.7 ± 0.2 found that after 4 months of moderate-intensity aerobic exercise, carried out 5 days a week, plasma non-esterified fatty acid levels, both at rest and during exercise, were significantly lower, lipolysis of subcutaneous adipose tissue was also significantly higher and the anti-lipolytic effect observed in subcutaneous adipose tissue prior to the exercise intervention was no longer apparent. Furthermore, the percentage of lipid oxidation was also higher after training, during both rest and exercise. Hence aerobic exercise intervention in overweight men appeared to improve lipid mobilization through a decrease in the anti-lipolytic effect upon subcutaneous adipose tissue and enhanced lipid oxidation during moderate exercise (de Glisezinski et al 2003).

RESISTANCE CIRCUIT TRAINING AND WEIGHT TRAINING

Studies investigating the effect of resistance training upon blood lipids have produced variable findings. For instance, 12 weeks of resistance training, in a group of men and women aged 54 to 71 years, revealed that whilst the men showed mean increases in levels of HDL-C, the women actually showed mean decreases, which were not related to changes in body weight (Joseph et al 1999). Furthermore, LeMura et al (2000) found that after comparing resistance training with aerobic and cross-training, only aerobic training showed any significant improvement in BLP. Additionally, in a group of 5 paraplegic men who carried out circuit-based upper body resistance training three times per week, there were reductions in LDL-C and increases in HDL-C (Nash et al

2001). However, 8 weeks of supervised low-intensity resistance training (80% of 10 repetition maximum) in a group of sedentary postmenopausal women (aged 49–62 years) found significant improvements in muscular strength but no significant changes in blood lipids or body composition (Elliott et al 2002). Hence the effect of resistance training on blood lipids may be dependent upon the particular subject group, and is an important consideration for the exercise practitioner when prescribing PA/exercise.

INTERVAL TRAINING

Changes in blood lipids in response to PA/exercise training have been discussed above (p. 46) and it appears that, although interval training tends to enhance $\dot{V}O_2max$ to a greater extent than other forms of PA/exercise, in terms of blood lipids results tend to be similar to those found in continuous forms of PA/exercise (Thomas et al 1984). For instance, 59 untrained men and women (aged 18–32 years) were randomly assigned to one of four groups: a control group, a group who ran 4 miles continuously at 75% HRmax (~500 kcal per session), a group who ran 2 miles continuously at 75% HRmax (~250 kcal per session), and a group who did interval running for one minute at 90% HRmax, followed by 3 minutes walking for 8 sets (~500 kcal per session), 3 times per week for 12 weeks. It was found that whilst interval training showed the greatest improvement in $\dot{V}O_2max$, percentage fat loss and changes in TG, total cholesterol and HDL-C were similar between the exercising groups. Additionally, 9 weeks of interval training, consisting of hospital-based cycle ergometry of two times 30-minute daily sessions, resulted in decreased levels of plasma TG and LDL-C but no change in HDL-C or apos A-I and B, which significantly reverted 3 weeks after training ceased (Stubbe et al 1983).

CONSIDERATIONS AND CONTRAINDICATIONS

When planning a PA/exercise intervention the exercise practitioner needs to consider the aim of the PA/exercise intervention in conjunction with the patient's health status and medications (Ch. 14), which will therefore affect the exercise prescription. Hence, considerations and contraindications will be as they are for these and other co-morbidities, some of which are stated elsewhere.

MEDICATIONS

Various lipid-lowering medications may have an influence upon individuals' PA/exercise ability and will therefore require careful consideration (Ch. 14).

ABSOLUTE CONTRAINDICATIONS FOR EXERCISE

Depending on any other co-morbidities absolute contraindications for exercise will be as for those cited for other individuals (Appendix A, Table A.1)

SUMMARY

- Hyperlipidaemia is characterized by increased levels of serum TGs, cholesterol and fatty acids, and is a primary risk factor for heart and vascular disease.
- CHD rises appreciably when serum cholesterol is >6.5 mmol/l (250 mg/dl), and more so when >7.8 mmol/l (300 mg/dl). Lowest rates occur in men with serum cholesterol ≤5.2 mmol/l (200 mg/dl).
- LDL-C >3.36 mmol/l (130 mg/dl) is a risk to health and generally deposits some cholesterol into arterial walls.
- Compared to premenopausal women, men tend to have a poorer BLP. After menopause the gender difference tends to diminish.
- Regular PA/exercise reduces TG and increases HDL-C levels. Changes appear dependent on PA/exercise intensity, duration and total energy expenditure, and baseline blood lipid levels.
- Regular energy expenditure through physical activity of around 1000 kcal per week is required to induce improvements in HDL-C.
- Habitual aerobic PA/exercise appears more effective than strength or cross training in producing favourable changes in BLP in healthy, previously sedentary adults.
- Regular resistance training has been shown to produce improvements in BLP.
- Transient changes in TG, HDL and apo A can result from a single bout of PA/exercise, through the action of LPL. The magnitude appears dependent on training status, duration, intensity and energy expenditure of the PA/exercise bout.
- Individuals with familial dyslipidaemia/s may not respond to PA/exercise intervention in the same way as individuals suffering from secondary dyslipidaemia. However, other potential health benefits may be gained.
- The PA/exercise-induced changes in BLP tend to diminish within several weeks from the cessation of training.
- Medications prescribed for dyslipidaemic and hyperlipidaemic individuals may affect PA/exercise capacity.

Suggested readings, references and bibliography

Suggested reading

Assmann G 1982 Lipid metabolism and atherosclerosis. Schattauer Verlag, Stuttgart. (In-depth description of the various hyperlipidaemias and dyslipidaemias.)

Miller N E, Miller G J 1984 Clinical and metabolic aspects of high-density lipoproteins. Elsevier, Amsterdam

Thompson G R 1989 A handbook of hyperlipidaemia. Current Science, London. (In-depth description of the various hyper- and dyslipidaemias.)

References and bibliography

AHA (American Heart Association) 1973 Estimating risk of coronary heart disease in daily practice. Coronary risk hand book. AHA, New York, p 1–50

AHA 1990 A summary of the evidence relating dietary fats, serum cholesterol and coronary heart disease. Circulation 8:1721–1732

AHA 2004 What are healthy levels of cholesterol? Online. Available: http://www.americanheart.org January 2004

Alba L M, Lindor K 2003 Non-alcoholic fatty liver disease. Alimentary Pharmacology and Therapeutics 17(8):977–986

Albers J J, Marcovina S M, Lodge M S 1990 The unique lipoprotein(a): properties and immunochemical measurement. Clinical Chemistry 36(12):2019–2026

Allard J P 2002 Other disease associations with non-alcoholic fatty liver disease (NAFLD). Best Practice and Research in Clinical Gastroenterology 16(5):783–795

Anderson D M, Keith J, Novak P D et al (eds) 2002 Mosby's medical, nursing and allied health dictionary, 6th edn. Mosby, St Louis

Angelopoulos T J, Robertson R J 1993 Effect of a single exercise bout on serum triglyceride in untrained men. Journal of Sports Medicine and Physical Fitness 33:264–267

Angelopoulos T J, Robertson R J, Goss F L et al 1993 Effect of repeated exercise bouts on high density lipoprotein-cholesterol and its subfractions HDL$_2$-C and HDL$_3$-C. International Journal of Sports Medicine 14(4):196–201

Aronov D M, Bubnova M G, Perova N V et al 2003 Physical exercise and atherosclerosis: proatherogenic effects of high and moderate intensity static exercise on blood lipid transport. Kardiologiia 43(2):35–39

Assmann G 1982 Lipid metabolism and atherosclerosis. Schattauer Verlag, Stuttgart

Ballantyne F C, Clark R S, Simpson H S et al 1982 The effect of moderate physical exercise on the plasma lipoprotein subfractions in male survivors of myocardial infarction. Circulation 65:913–918

Barletta C, Coiloi I, Barlolomei D I et al 1993 Influence of aerobic physical activity on blood lipids in relation to sex and training. Medicine and Science in Sports and Exercise 46:397–402

Berg K, Dahlen G, Frick M H 1974 Lp(a) lipoprotein and pre-beta$_1$-lipoprotein in patients with coronary heart disease. Clinical Genetics 6:230–235

Bjorntorp P A 1989 Sex differences in the regulation of energy balance with exercise. American Journal of Clinical Nutrition 17:55–65

BMA, RPS GB (British Medical Association, Royal Pharmaceutical Society of Great Britain) 2005 British National Formulary. Pharmaceutical Press, London

Brown M S, Goldstein J L 1984 How LDL receptors influence cholesterol and atherosclerosis. Science America Nov: 58–66

Brown M S, Goldstein J L 1986 A receptor-mediated pathway for cholesterol homeostasis. Science 232(4):34–47

Brownell K D, Bachorik P S, Auerle R S 1982 Changes in plasma lipid and lipoprotein levels in men and women after a program of moderate exercise. Circulation 65(3):477–484

Bubnova M G, Aronov D M, Perova N V et al 2003 Physical exercise and atherosclerosis: dynamic high intensity exercise as a factor inducing exogenous dyslipidemia. Kardiologiia 43(3):43–9

Bush T L, Barrett-Connor E 1985 Cholesterol, lipoproteins and coronary heart disease. Epidemiological Review 7:80–104

Bush T L, Fried L P, Barret-Connor E 1988 Cholesterol, lipoproteins and coronary heart disease in women. Clinical Chemistry 34(8B):B60–B70

Caraccio N, Ferrannini E, Monzani F 2002 Lipoprotein profile in subclinical hypothyroidism: response to levothyroxine replacement, a randomised placebo-controlled study. Journal of Clinical Endocrinology and Metabolism 87(4):1533–1538

Castelli W P, Doyle J T, Gordon T et al 1977 Alcohol and blood lipids. The cooperative lipoprotein phenotyping study, Lancet 2(8030):153–155

Castelli W P, Garrison R J, Wilson P W F 1986 Incidence of coronary heart disease and lipoprotein cholesterol levels. The Framingham Study. Journal of the American Medical Association 256:2835–2838

Connor S L, Connor W E, Sexton G et al 1982 The effects of age, body weight and family relationships on plasma lipoproteins and lipids in men, women and children of randomly selected families. Circulation 65:1290–1298

Connor W E, Lin D S 1982 The effect of shellfish in the diet upon the plasma lipid level in human. Metabolism 31:1046–1051

Cowan L D, Wilcosky T, Criqui M H et al 1985 Demographic, behavioural, biochemical and dietary correlates of plasma triglycerides. Lipid Research Clinics Program Prevalence Study. Atherosclerosis 5:466–480

Daher C F, Berberi R N, Baroody G M 2003 Effect of acute and chronic moderate alcohol consumption on fasted and postprandial lipemia in the rat. Food and Chemical Toxicology 41(11):1551–1559

Dahlen G H, Encson C, de Garie U et al 1983 Genetic and environmental determinants of cholesterol and HDL-cholesterol in concentrations in blood. International Journal of Epidemiology 12:32–35

D'Amico G, Gentile M G, Manna G et al 1992 Effect of vegetarian soy diet on hyperlipidaemia in nephritic syndrome. Lancet 339(8802):1131–1134

de Glisezinski I, Moro C, Pillard F et al 2003 Aerobic training improves exercise-induced lipolysis in SCAT and lipid utilization in overweight men. American Journal of Physiology – Endocrinology and Metabolism 285(5):E984–E990

Demacker P N M, Schade R W B, Jansen R T P et al 1982 Intra-individual variation of serum cholesterol, triglycerides and high density lipoprotein cholesterol in normal humans. Atherosclerosis 45:259–266

Derosa G, Mugellini A, Ciccarelli L et al 2003 Comparison of glycaemic control and cardiovascular risk profile in patients with type 2 diabetes during treatment with either repaglinide or metformin. Diabetes Research and Clinical Practice 60(3):161–169

Despres J P, Bouchard C, Savard et al 1984 The effect of a 20-week endurance training program on adipose tissue morphology and lipolysis in men and women. Metabolism 33:235–239

Donahoo W T, Kosmiski L A, Eckel R H 1998 Drugs causing dyslipoproteinemia. Endocrinology and Metabolism Clinics of North America 27(3):677–697

Drexel H, Franz W, Amann W et al 1992 Relation of the level of high-density lipoprotein subtractions to the presence and extent of coronary artery disease. American Journal of Cardiology 70:436–440

Durstine J L, Grandjean P W, Cox C A et al 2002 Lipids, lipoproteins, and exercise. Journal of Cardiopulmonary Physiology 22:385–398

Ebisu T I 1985 Splitting the distance of endurance running: on cardiovascular endurance and blood lipids. Japanese Journal of Physical Education 30–31:37–43

Eckardstein A V, Huang Y, Assmann G 1994 Physiological role and clinical relevance of high-density lipoprotein subclasses. Current Opinion in Lipidology 5:404–416

Eliasson B, Hjalmarson A, Kruse E et al 2001 Effect of smoking reduction and cessation on cardiovascular risk factors. Nicotine and Tobacco Research 3(3):249–255

Elliott K J, Sale C, Cable N T 2002 Effects of resistance training and detraining on muscular strength and blood lipids profiles in postmenopausal women. British Journal of Sports Medicine 36(5):340–344

Fielding P E, Fielding C J 1984 A cholesteryl ester transfer complex in human plasma. In: Miller N E, Miller G J (eds) Clinical and metabolic aspects of high density lipoproteins. Elsevier, Amsterdam

Foger B, Wohlfarter T, Ritsch A 1994 Kinetics of lipids. Apolipoproteins and cholesteryl ester transfer protein in plasma after bicycle marathon. Metabolism 43(5):633–639

Fruchart J C, Ailhaud G 1991 Recent progress in the study of apo A containing lipoprotein particles. Progress in Lipid Research 30(2/3):145–150

Glomset J A 1968 The plasma lecithin:cholesterol acyltransferase reaction. Journal of Lipid Research 9:155–167

Goldberg L, Elliot D L 1987 The effect of exercise on lipid metabolism in men and women. Sports Medicine 4(5):307–321

Gordon P M, Goss F L, Visich P S et al 1994 The acute effects of exercise intensity on high density lipoprotein-cholesterol metabolism. Medicine and Science in Sports and Exercise 26(6):671–677

Green M S, Heiss G, Rifkind B M et al 1985 The ratio of plasma high density lipoprotein cholesterol to total and low density lipoprotein cholesterol: age-related changes and race and sex differences in selected North American populations: the Lipid Research Clinic Program Prevalence Study. Circulation 72:93–104

Gretz N, Kranzlin B, Pey R et al 1996 Rat models of autosomal dominant polycystic kidney disease. Nephrology Dialysis Transplantation 11(Suppl 6):46–51

Groer M W, Shekleton M E 1989 Basic pathophysiology: a holistic approach, 3rd edn. Mosby, St Louis

Grundy J M 1984 Hyperlipoproteinemia: metabolic basis and rationale for therapy. American Journal of Cardiology 54:20C–26C

Grundy S M 1986 Comparison of monounsaturated fatty acids and carbohydrates for lowering plasma cholesterol. New England Journal of Medicine 314:745–748

Gupta A K, Ross E A, Myers J N et al 1993 Increased reverse cholesterol transport in athletes. Metabolism: Clinical and Experimental 42(6):684–690

Hambrecht R, Niebauer J, Marburger C et al 1993 Various intensities of leisure time physical activity in patients with coronary artery disease: effects on cardiorespiratory fitness and progression of coronary atherosclerotic lesions. Journal of the American College of Cardiology 22:468–477

Hannuksela M L, Liisanantt M K, Savolainen M J 2002 Effect of alcohol on lipids and lipoproteins in relation to atherosclerosis. Critical Reviews in Clinical Laboratory Sciences 39(3):225–283

Hardman A E, Hudson A, Jones P M R et al 1989 Brisk walking and plasma high density lipoprotein cholesterol concentration in previously sedentary women. British Medical Journal 229:1204–1205

Hartmann G, Stahelin H B 1981 Hyperlipidamie und atherosklerose in der schweis: ergebnisse aus der Basler Studie. Therapeutische Umschau 37:980

Haskell W L 1986 The influence of exercise training on plasma lipids and lipoproteins in health and disease. Acta Medica Scandinavica Supplement 711:25–37

Heiss G, Tamir I, Davis C E et al 1980 Lipoprotein cholesterol distribution in selected North American populations: the Lipid Research Clinics Program Prevalence Study. Circulation 61:302–315

Herd S L, Kiens B, Boobis L H et al 2001 Moderate exercise, postprandial lipemia, and skeletal muscle lipoprotein lipase activity. Metabolism: Clinical and Experimental 50(7):756–762

Hicks A L, MacDougall J D, Muckle T J 1987 Acute changes in high density lipoprotein cholesterol with exercise of different intensities. Journal of Applied Physiology 63(5):1956–1960

Hoefler G, Harnoncour F, Paschke E et al 1988 Lipoprotein Lp(a): a risk factor for myocardial infarction. Atherosclerosis 8:398–401

Hostmark A T 1982 Physical activity and plasma lipids. Scandinavian Journal of Social Medicine Supplementation 29:83–91

Houmard J A, Bruno N J, Bruner R K et al 1993 Effects of exercise training on the chemical composition of plasma LDL. Atherosclerosis and Thrombosis 14:325–330

Howard B V, Ngoc-Anh L, Belcher J D et al 1994 Concentrations of Lp(a) in black and white young adults: relations to risk factors for cardiovascular disease. Annals of Epidemiology 4:341–350

Huang T, Von Eckardstein A, Wu S et al 1995 Cholesterol efflux, cholesterol etherification and cholesteryl ester transfer by Lp A-I and Lp A-I/A-II in native plasma. Atherosclerosis, Thrombosis and Vascular Biology 15(9):1412–1418

Hughes R A, Thorland W G, Eyford T et al 1990a The acute effects of physical exercise duration on serum lipoprotein metabolism. Journal of Sports Medicine and Physical Fitness 30:37–44

Hughes R A, Thorland W G, Housh T J et al 1990b The effect of exercise intensity on serum lipoprotein response. Journal of Sports Medicine and Physical Fitness 30:254–260

Huttunen J K, Lansimies E, Voutilainen E et al 1979 Effect of moderate physical exercise on serum lipoproteins: a controlled clinical trial with special reference to serum HDL. Circulation 60:1220–1229

Jackson R L, Gotto A M 1974 Phospholipids in biology and medicine. New England Journal of Medicine 290:24–29, 87–93

Jackson R L, Morrisett J D, Gotto A M 1976 Lipoprotein structure and metabolism. Physiological Review 56(2):259–303

James R W, Pometta D 1994 Postprandial lipemia differentially influence high density lipoprotein subpopulations LpAI and LpAI, AII. Journal of Lipid Research 35:1583–1591

Johnson C L, Rifkind B M, Sempos C T et al 1993 Decline in serum total cholesterol levels among US adults: the national health and nutrition examination surveys. Journal of the American Medical Association 269(23):3002–3008

Joseph L J, Davey S L, Evans W J et al 1999 Differential effect of resistance training on the body composition and lipoprotein-lipid profile in older men and women. Metabolism: Clinical and Experimental 48(11):1474–1480

Kannel W B 1987 Metabolic risk factors for CHD in women: perspective from the Framingham study. American Heart Journal 114:413–419

Kantor M A, Cullinane, E M, Sady S P et al 1987 Exercise, acutely increased high density lipoprotein-cholesterol and lipoprotein lipase activity in trained and untrained men. Metabolism 36(2):188–192

Kobayashi J, Yamazaki K, Tashiro J et al 1997 Type III hyperlipidaemia with primary hypothyroidism: a unique clinical course of hyperlipidaemia during replacement therapy of thyroid hormone. Clinical Endocrinology 46(5):627–630

Kostner G M, Avogaro P, Cazzolato G et al 1981 Lipoprotein Lp(a) and the risk of myocardial infarction. Atherosclerosis 38:51–61

Kralikova E, Sobra J, Ceska R et al 1996 Analysis of nutritional habits in patients with familial combined hyperlipidemia. Casopis Lekaru Keskych 135(7):220–224

Krempler F, Kostner G M, Roscher A et al 1983 Studies on the role of specific cell surface receptors on the removal of Lp(a) in man. Journal of Clinical Investigation 71:1431–1441

Kuhar M B 2002 Update on managing hypercholesterolemia. The new NCEP guidelines. AAOHN Journal 50(8):360–364

Lagrost L, Dengremont C, Athias A et al 1995 Modulation of cholesterol efflux from FuSAH hepatoma cells by the apolipoprotein content of high density lipoprotein particles. Particles containing various proportions of apolipoprotein A-I and A-II. Journal of Biological Chemistry 270(22):13004–13009

Lampman R M, Wood P D, Giotas C et al 1977 Comparative effects of physical training and diet in normalising serum lipids in men with type IV hyperlipoproteinemia. Circulation 55:652–659

Lehmann R, Engler H, Honegger R et al 2001 Alterations of lipolytic enzymes and high-density lipoprotein subfractions induced by physical activity in type 2 diabetes mellitus. European Journal of Clinical Investigation 31(1):37–44

Lehtonen A 1985 Effect of beta blockers on blood lipid profile. American Heart Journal 109(5 Pt 2):1192–1196

LeMura L M, von Duvillard S P, Andreacci J et al 2000 Lipid and lipoprotein profiles, cardiovascular fitness, body composition, and diet during and after resistance, aerobic and combination training in young women. European Journal of Applied Physiology 82(5–6):451–458

Lepsanovic L, Brkljac O, Lepsanovic L 2001 Effect of smoking on lipoprotein metabolism. Medicinski Pregled 54(9–10):453–458

Levy R I 1981 Cholesterol, lipoproteins, apolipoproteins and heart disease: present status and future prospects. Clinical Chemistry 27(5):653–662

Lewis B 1976 Disorders in lipid transport. In: The hyperglycaemias: clinical and laboratory practice. Blackwell Scientific, Oxford, p 9.58–9.70

Lippel K, Tyroller H, Eder H et al 1981 Relationship of hypertriglyceridemia to atherosclerosis. Arteriosclerosis 1:406–417

Lithell H, Vessby J B, Karlsson J 1982 Decrease of LPL activity in skeletal muscle in man during short term carbohydrate rich dietary regime. Metabolism 31:994–998

Mahlberg F H, Glick J M, Lund-Katz S et al 1991 Influences of apolipoproteins A-I, A-II and C on the metabolism of membrane and lysosomal cholesterol in macrophages. Journal of Biological Chemistry 266(30):19930–19937

Malkova D, Hardman A E, Bowness R J et al 1999 The reduction in postprandial lipemia after exercise is independent of the relative contributions of fat and carbohydrate to energy metabolism during exercise. Metabolism: Clinical and Experimental 48(2):245–251

Malloy M J, Kane J P 2001 A risk factor for atherosclerosis: triglyceride-rich lipoproteins. Advances in Internal Medicine 47:111–136

Marckmann P, Sandstrom B, Jespersen J 1992 Fasting blood coagulation and fibrinolysis of young adults unchanged by reduction in dietary fat content. Atherosclerosis and Thrombosis 12:201–205

Marniemi J, Dahlstrom S, Kvist M et al 1982 Dependence of serum lipid and lecithin: cholesterol acyltransferase levels on physical training in young men. European Journal of Applied Physiology and Occupational Physiology 49(1):25–35

Marquest-Vidal P, Montaye M, Haas B et al 2000 Association of hypertensive status and its drug treatment with lipid and haemostatic factors in middle-aged men: the PRIME study. Journal of Human Hypertension 14(8):511–518

Martin M J, Hulley S B, Browner W S et al 1986 Serum cholesterol, blood pressure and mortality: implications from a cohort of 361 662 men. Lancet 2(8513):933–936

Medline plus 2004 Familial combined hyperlipidemia. Online. Available: http://www.nih.bov/medlineplus/ency/artricle/000396.htm January 2004

Middeke M, Richter W O, Schwandt P et al 1997 The effects of antihypertensive combination therapy on lipid and glucose metabolism: hydrochlorothiazide plus sotalol vs. hydrochlorothiazide plus captopril. International Journal of Clinical Pharmacology and Therapeutics 35(6):231–234

Miller N E 1984 Clinical and metabolic aspects of high-density lipoproteins. Elsevier, Amsterdam

Mjos O D, Thelle D S, Forde O H et al 1977 Family study of HDL-cholesterol and relation to age and sex. Acta Medica Scandinavica 201:323–329

Mowri H, Patsch J R, Ritsch A et al 1994 High density lipoproteins with differing apolipoproteins: relationships to postprandial lipemia, cholesteryl ester transfer protein, and activities of lipoprotein lipase, hepatic lipase and lecithin:cholesterol acyltransferase. Journal of Lipid Research 35:291–300

Muesing R A, Griffin P M, Mitchell P 1995 Corn oil and beef tallow elicit different postprandial responses in triglycerides and cholesterols, but similar changes in constituents of high-density lipoprotein. Journal of the American College of Nutrition 14(1):53–60

Nash M S, Jacobs P L, Mendez A J et al 2001 Circuit resistance training improves the atherogenic lipid profiles of persons with chronic paraplegia. Journal of Spinal Cord Medicine 24(1):2–9

NCEP (National Cholesterol Education Program) 1988 Public screening strategies for measuring blood cholesterol in adults – issues for special concern. NCEP, USA

NCEP Executive Summary of the Third Report 2001 Expert panel on detection, evaluation, and treatment of high blood cholesterol in adults. Journal of the American Medical Association 285:2486–2497.

NHANES (National Health and Nutrition Examination Survey) III 1988–1994. Centers for Disease Control/National Center for Health Statistics, Atlanta, GA

Nikkila E A 1978 Metabolic and endocrine control of plasma high density lipoprotein concentration. Relation to catabolism of triglyceride-rich lipoproteins. In: Gotto Jr A M, Miller N E, Oliver M F (eds) High density lipoproteins and atherosclerosis. Elsevier, New York

Ordovas J M 2000 ABC1: the gene for Tangier disease and beyond. Nutrition Reviews 58(3 Pt 1):76–79

Ortlepp J R, Metrikat J, Albrecht M et al 2003 Relation of body mass index, physical fitness and cardiovascular risk profile in 3127 young normal weight men with an apparently optimal lifestyle. International Journal of Obesity and Related Metabolic Disorders: Journal of the International Association for the Study of Obesity 27(8):979–982

Pan J, Lin M, Kesala R L et al 2002 Niacin treatment of the atherogenic lipid profile and Lp(a) in diabetes. Diabetes, Obesity and Metabolism 4(4):255–261

Passotti C, Zoppi A, Capra A et al 1986 Effect of beta-blockers on plasma lipids. International Journal of Clinical Pharmacology, Therapy and Toxicology 24(8):448–452

Pate R P, Pratt M, Blair S N et al 1995 Physical activity and public health. A recommendation from the Centers for Disease Control and Prevention and the American College of Sports Medicine. Journal of the American Medical Association 273:402–407

Perret B, Ruidavets J B, Vieu C et al 2002 Alcohol consumption is associated with enrichment of high-density particles in polyunsaturated lipids and increased cholesterol esterification rate. Alcoholism, Clinical and Experimental Research 26(8):1134–1140

Petitt D S, Cureton K J 2003 Effects of prior exercise on postprandial lipemia: a quantitative review. Metabolism: Clinical and Experimental 52(4):418–424

Phillips N R, Havel R J, Kane J R 1981 Levels and interrelationships of serum and lipoprotein cholesterol and triglycerides. Association with adiposity and the consumption of ethanol, tobacco and beverages containing caffeine. Atherosclerosis 1:13–24

Pirich C, O'Grady J, Sinzinger H 1993 Coffee, lipoproteins and cardiovascular disease. Wiener Klinische Wochenschrift 105(1):306

Pronk N P 1993 Short term effect of exercise on plasma lipids and lipoproteins in humans. Sports Medicine 16(6):431–448

Rauramaa R, Vaisanen S B, Rankinen T et al 1995 Inverse relation of physical activity and apolipoprotein A-I to blood pressure in elderly women. Medicine and Science in Sport and Exercise 27(2):164–169

Residori L, Garcia-Lorda P, Flancbaum L et al 2003 Prevalence of co-morbidities in obese patients before bariatric surgery: effect of race. Obesity Surgery 13(3):333–340

Ridker P N, Hennekens M D 1994 Lipoprotein(a) and risks of cardiovascular disease: commentary. Annals of Epidemiology 4:360–362

Rivellese A A, Aulteea P, Marotta G et al 1994 Long term metabolic effects of two dietary methods of treating hyperlipidaemia. British Medical Journal 308(6923):227–231

Rothblat G H, Bamberger M, Phillips M C 1986 Reverse cholesterol transport. Methods of Enzymology 129:628–644

Rothblat G H, Mahlberg F H, Johnson W J et al 1992 Apolipoprotein membrane cholesterol domains and regulation of cholesterol efflux. Journal of Lipid Research 33:1091–1097

Saito Y 2001 Plasma lipid level in the elderly. Japanese Journal of Clinical Pathology 49(5):438–441

Saltiel A R, Kahn C R 2001 Insulin signalling and the regulation of glucose and lipid metabolism. Nature 414(6865):799–806

Samanek M, Dobiasova M, Urbanova Z et al 2002 Consumption of white wine retards development of atherosclerosis and affects anticoagulation. Casopis Lekaru Ceskych 141(8):251–254

Sandkamp M, Funke H, Schult H 1990 Lipoprotein(a) is an independent risk factor for myocardial infarction at a young age. Clinical Chemistry 36:20–23

Savage M P, Petratis M M, Thompson W H et al 1986 Exercise training effects on serum lipid of prepubescent boys and adult men. Medicine and Science in Sports and Exercise 18(2):197–204

Scanu A M, Edelstein C, Gordon J I 1984 Apolipoproteins of human plasma high density lipoprotein. Clinical Physiology Biochemistry 2:111–122

Schreiner P J, Chambless L E, Brown S A 1994 Lipoprotein(a) as a correlate of stroke and transient ischaemic attach prevalence in a biracial cohort: the ARIC study. Annals of Epidemiology 4:531–539

Seip R L, Moulin P, Cocke T et al 1993 Exercise training decreased plasma cholesteryl ester transfer protein. Arteriosclerosis and Thrombosis 13:1359–1367

Shaper A G, Pocock S J, Walker M et al 1985 Risk factors for ischaemic heart disease: the prospective phase of the British Heart Study. Journal of Epidemiology Community Health 39:197–209

South African Medical Association and Lipid and Atherosclerosis Society of South African Working Group 2000 Diagnosis, management and prevention of the common dyslipidaemias in South Africa – clinical guidelines. South African Medical Journal 90(2 Pt 2):164–174, 176–178

Spector A A 1984 Plasma lipid transport. Clinical Physiology and Biochemistry 2:123–134

Stein R A, Donald M D, Michielli D W et al 1990 Effects of different exercise training intensities on lipoprotein cholesterol fractions in healthy middle-aged men. American Heart Journal 119:277–283

Stubbe I, Gustafson A, Nilsson-Ehle P et al 1983 In-hospital exercise therapy in patients with severe angina pectoris. Archive of Physical Medicine & Rehabilitation 64(9):396–401

Superko H R 1991 Exercise training, serum lipids, and lipoprotein particles: is there a change threshold? Medicine and Science in Sports and Exercise 23(6):677–685

Suter E, Marti B, Gutzwiller F et al 1994 Jogging or walking – comparison of health effects. Annals of Epidemiology 4:375–381

Szollar L G, Meszaros I, Tornoci L et al 1990 Effect of metoprolol and pindolol monotherapy on plasma lipid- and lipoprotein-cholesterol levels (including the HDL subclasses) in mild hypertensive males and females. Journal of Cardiovascular Pharmacology 15(6):911–917

Thelle D S, Heyden S, Fodor J G 1987 Coffee and cholesterol in epidemiological and experimental studies. Atherosclerosis 67: 97–103

Thomas T R, Adeniran S B, Etheridge G L 1984 Effects of different running programs on $\dot{V}O_2max$, percentage fat, and plasma lipids. Canadian Journal of Applied Sport Science 9(2):55–62

Thompson G R 1989 A handbook of hyperlipidaemia. Current Science, London

Thune I, Njolstad I, Lochen M et al 1998 Physical activity improved the metabolic risk profiles of men and women: The Tromso study. Archives of International Medicine 158(15):1633–1640

Tokmakidis S P, Volaklis K A 2003 Training and detraining effects of a combined-strength and aerobic exercise program on blood lipids in patients with coronary artery disease. Journal of Cardiopulmonary Rehabilitation 23(3):193–200

Tran V Z, Weltman A, Glass G V et al 1983 The effects of exercise on blood lipids and lipoproteins: a meta-analysis of studies. Medicine and Science in Sports and Exercise 15(2):393–402

Tsetsonis N V, Hardman A E 1995 The influence of the intensity of treadmill walking upon changes in lipid and lipoprotein variables in healthy adults. European Journal of Applied Physiology 70:329–336

Utermann G 1989 The mysteries of lipoprotein(a). Science 246:904–910

Vander A J, Sherman J H, Luciano D S 1990 Human physiology. McGraw-Hill, New York

Van der Heijden M, Donders S H, Cleophas T J et al 1998 A randomised. Placebo-controlled study of loop diuretics in patients with essential hypertension: the bumetanide and furosemide on lipid profile (BUFUL) clinical study report. Journal of Clinical Pharmacology 38(7):630–635

Veldman F J, Nair C H, Vorster H H et al 1997 Dietary pectin influences fibrin network structure in hypercholesterolaemic subjects. Thrombosis Research 86(3):183–196

Wallace R B, Anderson R A 1987 Blood lipids, lipid-related measures, and the risk of atherosclerotic cardiovascular disease. Epidemiological Reviews 9:95–119

Wilmore J H 2001 Dose-response: variation with age, sex, and health status. Medicine and Science in Sports and Exercise 33(6):S622–S627

Wood P D, Stefanick M L 1990 Exercise fitness and atherosclerosis, In: Bourchard C, Shephard T, Sutton J R et al (eds) 1993 Exercise, fitness and health: a consensus of current knowledge. Human Kinetics, Champaign, IL

Wood P D, Haskell W L, Blair S N et al 1983 Increased exercise level and plasma lipoprotein concentrations: a one year randomised, controlled study in sedentary middle aged men. Metabolism 32:31–39

Wood P D, Williams P T, Haskell W L 1984 Physical activity and high density lipoproteins. In: Miller N E, Miller G J (eds) Clinical and metabolic aspects of high density lipoproteins. Elsevier, Amsterdam, p 135–165

Wood P D, Stefanick M L, Williams P T et al 1991 The effects on plasma lipoproteins of prudent weight-reducing diet, with or without exercise in overweight men and women. New England Journal of Medicine 325:461–466

Woolf-May K 1998 The effect of single versus repetitive bouts of brisk walking upon cardiovascular risk factors and left ventricular function in sedentary/low active adults, appendix D, PhD Thesis, CCCUC

Woolf-May K, Kearney E M, Jones W et al 1998 The effect of two different 18-week walking programmes on aerobic fitness, selected blood lipids and factor XIIa. Journal of Sport Sciences 16(8):701–710

Woolf-May K, Owen A, Jones D W et al 2003 The effect of phase IV cardiac rehabilitation upon cardiac function, factor XIIa, blood lipid profile and catecholamines. Research Findings Register

Chapter 4

Diabetes and insulin resistance/insensitivity

CHAPTER CONTENTS

Introduction 58
Prevalence 58
Metabolic syndrome 58
Aetiology 58
   Type I diabetes/insulin-dependent diabetes
      mellitus (IDDM) 58
   Type II diabetes/non-insulin-dependent diabetes mellitus
      (NIDDM) 58
      Type II, obese 59
      Type II, non-obese 59
   Gestational diabetes mellitus 59
   Impaired glucose homeostasis 59
   Other identifiable causes 59
The pancreas 59
Normal regulation of blood glucose 60
Glucagon 60
Insulin 60
   Carbohydrate metabolism 60
      Storage of glucose 60
   Lipid metabolism 61
      Promotion of fatty acid synthesis within the liver 61
      Inhibition of breakdown of fat 61
      Fat sparing 61
   Protein and minerals 61
   Insulin absence and/or resistance 61
   Receptor and mechanism of action 61
      Entry of glucose into muscle, adipose and other
        tissues 62
Pathology of diabetes 63
Microvascular and macrovascular complications 63
   Microvascular complications 63
      Retinopathy 63
      Nephropathy 63
      Neuropathy 63
      Peripheral vascular disease and diabetic foot 64
   Macrovascular complications 64
      Hyperinsulinaemia 64

Atherosclerosis and cardiovascular complications 64
   Hypertension 64
   Obesity 65
   Hyperlipidaemia 65
   Hypercoagulation 65
   Cancer 65
Ketoacidosis 65
   Hyperosmolar non-ketotic coma 66
   Lactic acidosis 66
Hypoglycaemia 66
Hyperglycaemia 67
   Glycosylated haemoglobin 67
Diuresis 67
Sympathetic nervous system 68
Treatment 68
   Glycaemic control 68
   Type I diabetic 68
   Type II diabetic 68
Physical activity/exercise 69
   Energy expenditure 69
   Physical activity/exercise intensity 69
   Physical activity/exercise and insulin resistance 69
   Mechanism 70
   Acute bouts of physical activity/exercise 70
   Regular aerobic physical activity/exercise 70
Pre-exercise prescription 71
Physical activity/exercise prescription 71
Physical activity/exercise considerations 71
   Blood glucose levels and physical activity/exercise 72
   Hypoglycaemia and physical activity/exercise 72
      Pre-physical activity/exercise blood glucose levels 72
      Insulin-treated diabetics 72
      Non-insulin-dependent diabetics 73
      Ingestion of carbohydrate and meals 73
      Post-physical activity/exercise or delayed
        hypoglycaemia 74
      Time of day 74
      Masking of hypoglycaemia 74
   Hyperglycaemia and physical activity/exercise 74

The diabetic cardiac patient 75
Ketoacidosis 75
Nephropathy 75
Retinopathy 76
Neuropathy 76
   Autonomic neuropathy 76
   Peripheral neuropathy 76
Warming up and cooling down 76
Contraindications for physical activity/exercise 76
Medications 76
Summary 77
Suggested Readings, references and bibliography 77

INTRODUCTION

There are numerous challenges when prescribing physical activity (PA)/exercise to the diabetic individual, and most of these are primarily based around when it is appropriate for these individuals to perform PA/exercise. The aim of this chapter therefore is not only to assist the exercise practitioner in understanding the physiological background to diabetes and insulin resistance, but also to look at the ways in which the diabetic condition may influence and be influenced by PA/exercise. The current PA/exercise guidelines for those with diabetes and insulin resistance will also be looked into and discussed in relation to the problems of prescribing PA/exercise to these individuals.

PREVALENCE

Diabetes is characterized by the excessive excretion of urine. This excess excretion may be caused by a deficiency of antidiuretic hormone, as in diabetes insipidus, or by the hyperglycaemia that occurs in diabetes mellitus (Anderson et al 2002); this chapter will be chiefly concerned with the latter. Diabetes is a syndrome of disordered metabolism with inappropriate hyperglycaemia, which is primarily the result of deficient or complete lack of insulin secretion by the beta cells of the pancreas, and/or resistance to insulin. There are two main types of diabetes. Diabetes mellitus is a chronic disease and has no known cure. Figures from Diabetes UK (2000) indicate that diabetes affects around 1.4 million individuals (~3 in 100 people) and another million are unaware that they have the disorder. Diabetes is also a major cause of blindness (p. 63) and amputation (p. 64) as well as kidney diseases (p. 63). In the USA, diabetes is the seventh leading cause of death, where around 5.9% of the population suffer from diabetes (~15.7 million people), costing the US government approximately $98 billion per annum (Diabetes 2001), and

in Canada it affects around 5% of the population, costing around $1 billion a year (Bonen 1995).

METABOLIC SYNDROME

Type II diabetes may be precipitated by a cluster of conditions termed metabolic syndrome or syndrome X (AHA 2003). Metabolic syndrome is characterized by insulin resistance in the presence of obesity and high levels of abdominal fat, blood glucose, cholesterol and triglyceride and high blood pressure. It is now extremely common in Western societies and findings from the third NHANES Survey (2002) estimate that in the USA around 47 million Americans may exhibit this syndrome. More research is required, however, to fully determine the underlying cause of this syndrome, and whether interventions such as PA/exercise have any beneficial effect has still to be determined. It is nonetheless important to recognize the signs associated with this syndrome, as these individuals may be at risk of developing diabetes.

AETIOLOGY

There are two major types of diabetes, type I and type II, and both are characterized by an internal starvation of glucose despite sufficient blood glucose being available.

TYPE I DIABETES/INSULIN–DEPENDENT DIABETES MELLITUS (IDDM)

Type I diabetes occurs in about 5–10% of diabetics. It results in inadequate functioning of the pancreatic cells (islets of Langerhans) in producing the peptide solution insulin. This type of diabetes appears most often in children and young adults, who require daily insulin injections. It occurs in two forms, one being immune-mediated diabetes, where there is cell-mediated autoimmune destruction of the pancreatic beta cells, the other being idiopathic diabetes (diabetes of no known aetiology) (IDF 2003). Those at risk of type I diabetes are siblings of individuals with type I diabetes, and children of parents with type I diabetes. Therefore, appropriate screening prior to PA/exercise should identify individuals at risk. The symptoms of type I diabetes are shown in Table 4.1.

TYPE II DIABETES/NON–INSULIN–DEPENDENT DIABETES MELLITUS (NIDDM)

Until recently type II diabetes was seen predominantly as an adult disorder. However, with the rise in childhood obesity, levels of type II diabetes have also risen in children. There are two main types of type II diabetes (outlined below). Those at risk of developing type II diabetes are listed in Table 4.2.

Table 4.1 Commonly seen symptoms for type I and type II diabetes

Type I	Type II
Frequent urination	Any of the type I symptoms
Unusual thirst	Frequent infections
Extreme hunger	Blurred vision
Unusual weight loss	Cuts/bruises that are slow to heal
Extreme fatigue	Tingling/numbness in the hands or feet
Irritability	Recurring skin, gum or bladder infections
	Often there are no symptoms

Table 4.2 Factors that may predispose an individual to type II diabetes

Aged between 45 and 75 years
Family history of diabetes
Obese and overweight
Physically inactive
Low blood levels of high-density lipoprotein cholesterol
High blood levels of triglyceride
Previous gestational diabetes
Certain ethnic groups

Type II, obese

There is a linear relationship between being overweight and the risk of developing type II diabetes, and over 80% of those with type II diabetes are overweight (IDF 2003). Analogous to type I diabetes, type II is a metabolic disorder characterized by the inability of the pancreas to produce insulin and/or reduced sensitivity to insulin, and is probably the result of receptor and post-receptor defects. The beta cells of the pancreas often show hypertrophy and dysregulation and become insensitive to glucose, resulting in hyperglycaemia and hyperinsulinaemia (Kopp 2003).

Type II, non-obese

Non-obese type II diabetes occurs in around 20% of type II diabetics, where there is a strong genetic link. It is often associated with mutations in insulin receptor and/or signal transduction molecules (IDF 2003).

GESTATIONAL DIABETES MELLITUS

Some pregnant women are prone to what is termed gestational diabetes. Gestational diabetes develops in around 3–6% of all pregnancies, which is alleviated postpartum, and is partly the result of a deficiency in insulin, possibly as a result of placental destruction of insulin. Additionally, however, these women are at greater risk of type II diabetes in later life (IDF 2003).

IMPAIRED GLUCOSE HOMEOSTASIS

Impaired glucose homeostasis is an intermediate stage between normal function and diabetes, and is considered a risk factor for cardiovascular disease (Ch. 2). Impaired glucose tolerance is diagnosed by fasting plasma glucose higher than normal ($\geq$6.1 mmol/l, ~110 mg/dl) and less than that diagnostic for diabetes ($\geq$7.0 mmol/l, ~126 mg/dl), or by an impaired glucose tolerance test, where plasma glucose is higher than normal following the administration of 75 grams of ingested glucose ($\geq$7.8 mmol/l, ~140 mg/dl and $\leq$11.1 mmol/l, ~200 mg/dl) (Diabetes Monitor 2001). However, these definitional values do vary between countries, organizations and over time (Harris et al 2000). Therefore, it is important for the exercise practitioner to be aware of current regional guidelines.

OTHER IDENTIFIABLE CAUSES

Other identifiable causes of diabetes are genetic defects in pancreatic beta cells or in insulin action, disease of the exocrine pancreas, such as cancer of the pancreas; cystic fibrosis and pancreatitis; endocrinopathies such as Cushing's disease; drug or chemically induced, by steroids, for example; infection such as rubella; uncommon forms of immune-related diabetes and other genetic syndromes (IDF 2003).

THE PANCREAS

The pancreas is a gland in the abdomen situated near the stomach and is connected to the small intestine by a duct (Fig. 4.1). The pancreas has many diverse functions involving endocrine gland cells, which secrete the hormones insulin and glucagon into systemic circulation, and exocrine gland cells, which secrete digestive enzymes and bicarbonate into the intestines to aid with digestion and neutralize acids, respectively (Vander et al 1990). The secretion of the hormones insulin and glucagon is integral in the control of blood glucose levels and any imbalance in these hormones can result in either hyper- or hypoglycaemia.

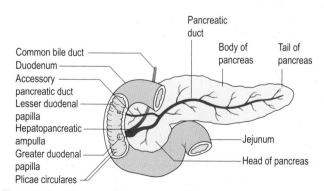

Figure 4.1 Diagram of the pancreas. (From Anderson et al 2002, p. 1268, with permission of Mosby.)

NORMAL REGULATION OF BLOOD GLUCOSE

In the non-diabetic, the control of blood glucose is normally maintained within a narrow range of around 3.3–5.6 mmol/l (though postprandial values can be higher and yet still be considered within the normal range (Table 4.3)) by the hormones insulin and glucagon (Fig. 4.2). These hormones are both secreted by the pancreas and are referred to as pancreatic hormones. The pancreas is involved in food digestion, and within the pancreas are the islet cells, which secrete both insulin and glucagon in response to the levels of blood glucose. Insulin is secreted from the beta cells when levels of blood glucose are high, though there is always a low level of insulin secretion by the pancreas and glucagon is secreted when blood glucose levels are low. It is not, however, the level of insulin per se that affects blood glucose levels; it is the ratio of insulin/glucagon (Endocrineweb 1998).

The untreated and poorly controlled diabetic is prone to both hyperglycaemia and hypoglycaemia. Hyperglycaemia

Table 4.3 Reference values for fasting plasma glucose (mmol/l) (adapted from BDA 1993[a] and ADA 2000)

Stage	mmol/l
Good[a]	4.4 (78 mg/dl) to 6.7 (120 mg/dl)
Normal	<6.1 (109 mg/dl)
Impaired glucose homeostasis	6.1 (109 mg/dl) to 7.0 (125 mg/dl)
Diabetes	≥7.0 (125 mg/dl)

[a]Inclusive of postprandial levels.

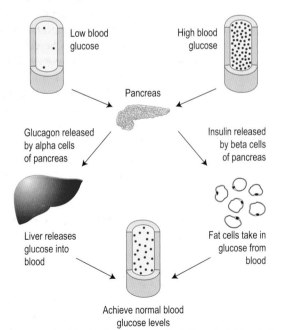

Figure 4.2 Negative feedback regulation of normal blood glucose by the hormones insulin and glucagon. (Reproduced with permission from EndocrineWeb and the Norman Endocrine Surgery Clinic, copyright © 1997–2002.)

occurs primarily as a result of large increases in postprandial blood glucose as the excess glucose is not able to be taken up by the cells and stored. Hypoglycaemia, on the other hand, is a result of the body having no stores to top up blood glucose when levels fall below normal.

GLUCAGON

The alpha cells of the pancreatic islets, in response to low blood glucose levels, secrete glucagon. When blood glucose is high, glucagon is not secreted. When blood glucose is low, however, after exercise or between meals, for example, more glucagon is secreted. Glucagon has an effect on many cells of the body, most notably the liver. The effect of glucagon is to cause the liver to release glucose, which is stored as a polymer in the form of glycogen, into the blood circulation, thus causing a rise in blood glucose levels. Glucagon also induces the liver and muscle cells to make glucose out of other nutrients, such as protein, a process termed gluconeogenesis (Endocrineweb 1998).

INSULIN

Insulin is a key player in the control of intermediary metabolism. It has a profound effect on both carbohydrate and lipid metabolism, and has a significant influence on both protein and mineral metabolism (Table 4.4). Consequently disturbances in insulin production and sensitivity have a widespread and devastating effect on many organs and tissues (NIH 2000).

CARBOHYDRATE METABOLISM

Glucose released from dietary carbohydrate within the small intestine is absorbed into the blood, where elevated blood glucose levels stimulate the release of insulin. Insulin acts on cells throughout the body to stimulate the uptake, utilization and storage of glucose, and the effects of insulin on glucose metabolism vary depending on the target tissue. Insulin has two important effects, one being the facilitation of the entry of glucose into the muscle, adipose and other tissues, and the other being the stimulatory effect upon the liver to store glucose in the form of glycogen (NIH 2000). Therefore, a lack of, or a reduction in, sensitivity to insulin can have widespread effects.

Storage of glucose

A large proportion of glucose absorbed from the small intestine is taken up by the hepatocytes of the liver where it is converted into glycogen and stored. Insulin has several effects upon the liver, one of which is to stimulate glycogen synthesis. Insulin activates the enzyme hexokinase, which phosphorylates glucose, trapping it within the cell. Insulin also inhibits the activity of glucose-6-phosphatase, thereby

Table 4.4 Effects of insulin

Muscle	Adipose tissue	Liver
↑ glucose entry	↑ glucose entry	↑ protein synthesis
↑ glycogen synthesis	↑ fatty acid synthesis	↑ lipid synthesis
↑ amino acid uptake	↑ glycerol phosphate synthesis	↓ glucose uptake (↑ glycogen synthesis)
↑ protein synthesis	↑ triglyceride deposition	
↓ protein catabolism	Stimulation of lipoprotein lipase	
↓ release of gluconeogenic amino acids	Inhibition of hormone sensitive lipase	
↑ ketone uptake		

inhibiting glucose metabolism. Insulin also activates several other enzymes that are directly involved in glycogen synthesis, including phosphofructokinase and glycogen synthase. The net effects of the activation of these enzymes are to instruct the liver, when there is an abundance of glucose, to store as much glucose as possible for later use (NIH 2000).

LIPID METABOLISM

The metabolic pathways involved in the utilization of fats and carbohydrates are entwined. Given that insulin enhances glucose uptake and utilization, lack of insulin and/or insulin resistance will enhance fatty acid use and therefore affects lipid metabolism (NIH 2000).

The rate of catabolism of these triglyceride-rich lipoproteins appears to be regulated by the activity of the enzyme lipoprotein lipase (LPL) (Lewis 1976, Spector 1984, Thompson 1989), whose action in adipose tissue increases in the fed state and is promoted by insulin (Ch. 2, p. 36).

Promotion of fatty acid synthesis within the liver

The stimulatory effect of insulin to enhance glycogen synthesis also has an effect upon synthesis of fatty acids. As the liver becomes saturated with glycogen, which is around 5% of liver mass, further synthesis is suppressed. Any additional glucose taken up by the hepatocytes is shunted into pathways that lead to synthesis of fatty acids. These fatty acids are then exported from the liver, as lipoproteins, into the circulating blood (p. 35), where in the healthy individual, they are taken up by other tissues, such as adipocytes, which use them for synthesis of triglyceride (NIH 2000).

Inhibition of breakdown of fat

Insulin causes an inhibition of the intracellular lipase that hydrolyzes triglycerides to release fatty acids, but facilitates entry of glucose into adipocytes, and within those cells, glucose can be used to synthesize glycerol. These glycerols, along with the fatty acids delivered from the liver, are used to synthesize triglycerides within the adipocyte. By these mechanisms, insulin is involved in further accumulation of triglyceride in fat cells (NIH 2000).

Fat sparing

Insulin drives most cells to preferentially oxidize carbohydrates instead of fatty acids for energy, thereby indirectly stimulating accumulation of fat in adipose tissue (NIH 2000).

PROTEIN AND MINERALS

In addition to the effect that insulin has upon certain cells to take up glucose, insulin also stimulates the uptake of amino acids. When there is lack of and/or resistance to insulin, the balance is placed toward intracellular protein degradation.

Insulin also increases permeability of certain cells to potassium, magnesium and phosphate ions, and activates sodium-potassium ATPase (NIH 2000).

INSULIN ABSENCE AND/OR RESISTANCE

The main effect of insulin is to decrease the blood concentration of glucose, and when blood glucose concentrations fall so does the secretion of insulin. In the absence of and/or resistance to insulin, the bulk of the cells within the body become unable to take up glucose and therefore switch to using alternative fuels, such as fatty acids, for energy. Neurons require a constant supply of glucose and in the short term use stored glycogen for energy. Insulin absence and/or resistance will also cause the liver to cease glycogen synthesis and cause enzymes responsible for the breakdown of glycogen to become active (NIH 2000). In addition, glycogen breakdown is stimulated not only by the insulin absence and/or resistance but by the presence of glucagon (p. 60), which is secreted when blood glucose levels fall below the normal range (normal range 3.3–5.6 mmol/l) (Fig. 4.2).

RECEPTOR AND MECHANISM OF ACTION

The receptor for insulin is embedded for instance in the plasma membrane of adipose and muscle tissue. The insulin receptor is composed of two alpha subunits and two beta subunits linked by bonds. The alpha chains are entirely extracellular and house insulin-binding domains, while the linked beta chains penetrate through the plasma

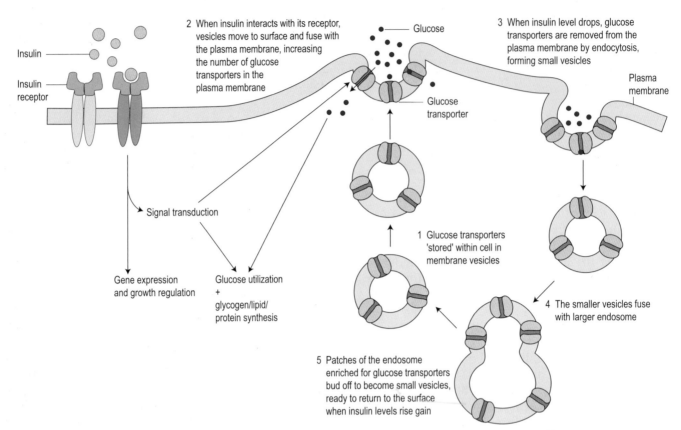

Figure 4.3 Glucose transport (adapted from http://www.betacell.org/content/articles/print.php?aid=1 and http://www.health.on-topic.net/health/insulin-resistance).

membrane. Binding of insulin to the alpha subunits causes the beta subunits to phosphorylate themselves, thus activating the catalytic activity of the receptor. The activated receptor then phosphorylates a number of intracellular proteins, which in turn alters their activity, thereby generating a biological response. Several intracellular proteins have been identified as phosphorylation substrates for the insulin receptor, the most commonly studied being insulin receptor substrate 1 (IRS-1), which when activated results in many physiological processes (NIH 2000), most notably the uptake of glucose by the cell.

Entry of glucose into muscle, adipose and other tissues

The only mechanism by which cells can take up glucose is by facilitated diffusion through a group of transporters. In many tissues, particularly muscle, the major transporter used for uptake of glucose is GLUT 4, which is made available in the plasma membrane through the action of insulin (p. 60). In the absence of, or if there is resistance to, insulin, GLUT 4 glucose transporters present in the cytoplasmic vesicles are unable to transport glucose across the plasma membrane. The binding of insulin to receptors on such cells leads rapidly to fusion of those

vesicles with the plasma membrane and insertion of the glucose transporters, thereby giving the cell the ability to take up glucose efficiently. When blood levels of insulin decrease and insulin receptors are no longer occupied, the glucose transporters are recycled back into the cytoplasm (Fig. 4.3). There are, however, some tissues that do not require insulin for efficient uptake of glucose, such as those of the brain and liver, and these tissues import glucose into their tissue by means of GLUT 1 and GLUT 2 transporters, respectively. (NIH 2000, Dorsch 2000). It was hypothesized that there may be a reduction in the number of GLUT 4 glucose transporters in diabetic individuals. It has been reported, though, that GLUT 4 transport molecules are the same in both normal and diabetic individuals, therefore ruling this out (Ryder et al 2001). However, the speculated reduction in the number of GLUT 4 transporters may be related to a reduction in the translocation of GLUT 4, rather than a reduction in GLUT 4 per se. For instance, compared to non-diabetic muscle following insulin stimulation, GLUT 4 distribution in diabetic skeletal muscle was reduced by around 40%, and GLUT 4 translocation by around 71%. This suggests that insulin resistance in skeletal muscle is a result of defective GLUT 4 trafficking and translocation (Lund et al 1997).

PATHOLOGY OF DIABETES

There are numerous pathophysiological manifestations of diabetes, and the development of these long-term chronic pathological changes are generally more prevalent in those type I diabetics who have absolute loss of insulin production. These individuals are also most susceptible to complications such as retinopathy, neuropathy, peripheral vascular disease, atherosclerosis and nephropathy, but these may be exhibited in all diabetics. Hyperinsulinaemia has a considerable pathophysiological effect (p. 64), contributing to various diseases, and is seen in type II diabetics. To a large degree these conditions can, in part or fully, be explained by changes to the small and larger blood vessels, namely *microvascular* or *macrovascular* complications, respectively. The basic aetiology of these complications has still to be fully determined. Nonetheless, these vascular changes account for most of the morbidity and mortality directly caused by diabetes (Groer & Shekleton 1989).

MICROVASCULAR AND MACROVASCULAR COMPLICATIONS

The nature of diabetes predisposes the diabetic individual to complications, which need to be determined prior to any PA/exercise prescription. These complications are categorized into microvascular and macrovascular complications and have implications for PA/exercise prescription.

MICROVASCULAR COMPLICATIONS

Microvascular complications are thought to be the result of thickening of the capillary base membrane and changes to the glucoprotein composition of the vascular structure. Damage to these vessels and the base membrane impairs the delivery of nutrients and hormones to the tissues, which results in further damage to the tissues, leading to hypoxia and ischaemia of various organs. The precise mechanisms concerned in the development of these microvascular complications are complex and still remain to be fully determined. It is possible, however, that the base membrane may be faulty in the diabetic individual and that some metabolic dysfunction is responsible for these changes. Furthermore, it is thought that chronic hyperglycaemia may downregulate the GLUT 4 transporters (p. 61), inhibiting glucose uptake, in addition to glucose toxicity and the accumulation of advanced glycated end products (Duckworth 2001). The main affected areas are the retina, the renal glomerulus and nerve sheath, leading to retinopathy, nephropathy and peripheral neuropathy, respectively (Groer & Shekleton 1989, Patel 1999).

Retinopathy

Diabetes is the leading cause of new cases of blindness in people aged 20 to 74 years. Microvascular damage to the retina tends to develop over a number of years, although in some type I patients it can develop quite rapidly, resulting in blindness at adolescence. Aneurysms may also develop and it is therefore important that the diabetic individual has regular eye checks. However, vision is not affected by all retinopathies, though diabetic control is required in order to maintain vision (Groer & Shekleton 1989, Patel 1999).

Nephropathy

Around 30% of type I diabetics develop nephropathy. Diabetic nephropathy is characterized by distinctive lesions in the kidney, which may develop prior to the overt manifestation of diabetes. Both kidneys are generally hypertrophied and there is usually a round clear mass in the glomerulus, with ischaemic changes to the kidney's vessels as a result of thickening of the basement membrane of the capillaries. The process is termed 'diffuse intercapillary glomerulosclerosis'. The manifestation of nephropathy appears when protein is found in the urine, termed proteinuria or albuminuria, since the protein albumin can be found in the urine. An albumin excretion rate of >30 mg per day (or >20 µg/min) is characteristic of albuminuria (Table 4.5). Hypertension is usually present and needs to be treated since increased arterial blood pressure can cause additional kidney damage. Oedema may also be present, as well as retinopathy, dyslipidaemia and atherosclerotic complications. With further decline in the glomerular filtration rate there may be a need for renal dialysis or kidney transplantation (Groer & Shekleton 1989, Patel 1999).

Neuropathy

Around 60–70% of those with diabetes have mild to extreme kinds of diabetic nerve damage, which in its severe form can lead to lower limb amputations. Diabetes is therefore one of the most common causes of non-traumatic lower amputation (Patel 1999). Oxidative stress, due to damaged vessels not supplying sufficient nutrients to the

---

Table 4.5 Normal renal function reference values (adapted from Viberti 1997, Patel 1999)

Factors	Reference values
Albumin in urine	<200 mg/l
Albumin excretion rate	<20 µg/min

Transient increase in urinary albumin excretion can be found in urinary tract infections, cardiac failure, acute illness and heavy exercise.

nerves, results in ischaemia. This is manifested in reduced nerve blood flow and conduction deficits, impaired neurotrophic support, changes in signal transduction and metabolism (Obrosova 2002) and morphological abnormalities (Kamiya et al 2003). These are all characteristic of peripheral diabetic neuropathy, and hyperglycaemia appears to play a key role in this process (p. 67) (Obrosova 2002).

Although there are varying symptoms for neuropathy, common signs are unusual sensations felt in the upper and lower extremities, as well as muscular weakness and motor impairment. Other signs are postural hypotension, gastrointestinal and bladder problems and muscular paralysis (Groer & Shekleton 1989, Patel 1999).

Autonomic neuropathy predisposes the individual to a greater risk of an adverse cardiac event especially during PA/exercise. Signs such as weakness and breathlessness are indicative of cardiovascular complications. However, these symptoms may also occur with hyperglycaemia and therefore may make it difficult to clearly determine an individual's physical state. If cardiovascular complications are suspected, the exercise practitioner should refer the individual back to their general practitioner for medical assessment (White & Sherman 1999).

Peripheral vascular disease and diabetic foot

Owing to diabetic neuropathy and vascular damage (p. 63), circulation is often impaired in the diabetic individual, particularly to the extremities. This may result in ulceration, infection and untreated gangrene, and where necrosis has occurred amputation may be required. Diabetics often have what is termed 'diabetic foot'. Peripheral neuropathy can cause sensory loss in the feet and legs, thus resulting in loss of the protective sensation in the feet. This in combination with diminished blood flow, as a result of vascular impairment, can cause small lesions or ulcers to develop from dry skin, and since the diabetic has impaired sensation, these may go unnoticed until an infection or gangrene is present (Groer & Shekleton 1989, Patel 1999). Other signs are intermediate claudication, cold feet, decreased or absent pulses, atrophy of subcutaneous tissues and hair loss (ADA 2000).

MACROVASCULAR COMPLICATIONS

Macrovascular complications are usually related to the cardiovascular complications found in the type II diabetic. These are generally the result of insulin resistance, hyperinsulinaemia, hyperglycaemia, central obesity, dyslipidaemia, hypercoagulation and hypertension (Patel 1999).

Hyperinsulinaemia

The nature of type II diabetes dictates that there is a degree of insulin resistance (cells becoming resistant to insulin) and/or insufficient production from the beta cells of the pancreas. Insulin resistance has a profound effect upon the body, especially if insulin is being produced, and if left untreated results in hyperinsulinaemia. Hyperinsulinaemia is defined as excessively high levels of blood insulin, where normal finding of insulin assay in adults is around 5–24 μmU/ml (Anderson et al 2002). Uncontrolled hyperinsulinaemia can have a devastating effect upon the body; the acute state (generally as a result of an overdose of insulin) can result in insulin shock, and in the longer term contribute toward various diseases and disorders, some of which are outlined below.

Atherosclerosis and cardiovascular complications

Damage to the vasculature (p. 11) allows for the development of atherosclerosis, which can lead to cardiovascular complications. Multiple factors contribute toward the development of cardiovascular disease, and high levels of circulating insulin are known to contribute to the acceleration of atherosclerosis and vascular damage (Preuss 1997). Consistently high levels of circulating insulin stimulate arterial vascular smooth muscle hypertrophy (Kopp 2003), which as a consequence alters membrane ion transport. This leads to an increase in intracellular calcium and augmentation of vascular tone and blood pressure. Additionally, insulin enhances proliferation of growth hormone (Ledet 1976), smooth muscle cells (Stout 1985) and possibly synthesis of collagen (DeFronzo & Ferrannini 1991), and increases the production of von Willebrand factor (which facilitates adherence of platelets) from the walls of the damaged vasculature (Meyer & Baumgartner 1983). Other factors that are outlined in Chapter 2 (p. 9) also contribute toward the development of cardiovascular disease.

Hypertension

Hyperinsulinaemia is a contributing factor in primary hypertension (of a known cause) (Ch. 5, p. 84), which in turn contributes toward cardiovascular disease, and although the hypertensive mechanisms of insulin are not yet fully known, reductions in blood pressure have been observed in association with a fall in blood glucose levels (i.e. enhanced insulin sensitivity) (Jaber et al 1992).

High circulating levels of plasma insulin lead to an augmentation in sympathetic nervous system (SNS) activity (Facchini et al 1996), which results in a release of catecholamines (noradrenaline and adrenaline). Catecholamines cause an increase in sympathetic tone, which contributes towards the stimulation of the renin–angiotensin–aldosterone system (Esler et al 2001) resulting in vasoconstriction and aldosterone-led renal sodium reabsorption by the kidney tubules, and an increase in intravascular volume and blood pressure. Over a period of time high blood pressure will also affect the vasculature, resulting in impaired vasodilation, which contributes toward cardiovascular disease (Ch. 2).

Secondary hypertension (of a known origin) is not known to be associated with insulin insensitivity (Sharma & Haldiya 2002, Voiculescu et al 2003).

Obesity

There is a relationship between hypertension, hyper-insulinaemia and obesity (Pouliot et al 1994, Esler et al 2001) and those who possess high levels of abdominal fat are at particular risk of diabetes (Ramachandran et al 2000, Idzior-Walus et al 2001) and cardiovascular disease. The mechanisms linking obesity and hyperinsulinaemia are complex and still to be determined. However, one possible mechanism may be related to the fact that expanded adipocytes of the obese are relatively insulin-resistant, resulting in reactive hyperinsulinaemia (Frayn 2001). Furthermore, obese individuals often possess hypertrophied pancreatic beta cells (Kopp 2003) and show diminished insulin clearance (Lewis et al 2002), thus contributing toward hyperglycaemia and a predisposition to diabetes. Nonetheless, hyperinsulinaemia and insulin resistance may result from abnormal insulin cell membrane receptors (Shafrir & Ziv 1998), and/or response of the tissues to constant exposure to high levels of insulin. The tissues become more tolerant to insulin, and/or the pancreas compensates for primary insulin resistance by increasing insulin output, leading to hyperinsulinaemia. It is also thought that hyperinsulinaemia may be the primary defect that causes obesity, although others consider it to be a response (Groer & Shekleton 1989).

Hyperlipidaemia

Hyperlipidaemia is seen in approximately 40% of all diabetics and more than 80% suffer from hypertriglyceridaemia (Assmann 1982) (Ch. 3), which is associated with insulin resistance (Saltiel & Kahn 2001). The increase in very low-density lipoproteins and reduced LPL activity contribute toward the pathogenesis of hypertriglyceridaemia. However, it is often difficult to determine if this is a primary or secondary cause. If hyperlipidaemia persists after optimal regulation of the diabetes then the cause is considered to be primary.

The combination of hypertriglyceridaemia and a low level of high-density lipoprotein cholesterol results in cardiovascular disease complications, and myocardial infarction occurs in around 50% of diabetics. However, serum lipids often normalize with appropriate weight reduction, restriction of rapidly absorbed carbohydrates, alcohol avoidance and/or medical intervention (Assmann 1982).

The normal role of insulin in lipid metabolism is to promote lipogenesis and fat storage. Thus if insulin resistance is present, there may be an increased production of triglycerides, which in insulin-resistant individuals cannot then be taken up normally by the liver, adipose tissue and muscle. The normal stimulatory effect of insulin on LPL activity is also depressed in obesity (Ljung et al 2002). Therefore, insulin resistance may actually cause the hyperlipidaemia in obese individuals. Additionally, carbohydrates are insulinogenic. Thus high carbohydrate diets tend to aggravate this situation, especially since obese individuals appear to make more lipids from ingested carbohydrate, though physical exercise and weight reduction appear to improve the situation (Groer & Shekleton 1989).

Hypercoagulation

Hypercoagulation can be characteristic of ketosis (Alakhverdian & Koev 1987, Golubiatnikova et al 1987) and complications such as hypertension, arteriosclerosis and smoking tend to influence blood fluidity and contribute toward the development of microcirculatory blood flow disorders, which can cause platelet hyperactivity and hypercoagulation. Hypercoagulation is common in diabetics who display deterioration of blood flow, and these individuals tend to show raised fibrinogen levels, which have been linked with increased plasma viscosity and erythrocyte aggregation (Volger 1986). Additionally, hypertriglyceridaemia is often found in hyperinsulinaemic individuals and given that triglyceride-rich lipoproteins have been found to stimulate blood coagulation (Mitropoulos et al 1989, Kelleher et al 1992) this may further increase their risk of thrombosis. Physical activity/exercise also affects coagulation and fibrinolysis, and in certain individuals will favour coagulation. Therefore, it is important to be aware of any additional PA/exercise complications (Ch. 7).

Cancer

Insulin resistance and elevated levels of insulin-like growth factor have been associated with cancer (Ballard-Barbash et al 1997, Hu et al 1999b). Indeed, serum insulin levels have been found to be elevated in individuals with cancer, without disease-related hyperinsulinaemia (Del Giudice et al 1998). Hence individuals with insulin resistance and those with NIDDM are potentially at risk (Westerlind 2003).

KETOACIDOSIS

Ketoacidosis is found in uncontrolled type I diabetics, the most common cause of which is the omission of insulin. Absolute insulin deficiency leads to an increase in glucose output by the liver and decreased glucose uptake by the peripheral tissues. This results in hyperglycaemia (p. 67) with glucosuria (glucose in the urine), which leads to a depletion of fluid and electrolytes and a fall in the rate of renal perfusion. This condition, however, also resembles that of the fasted state, where the diabetic relies on fatty acid metabolism for energy since insulin-dependent cells, such as muscle, cannot take up glucose. Ketones develop when there is an excessive breakdown of fatty acids, via acetyl-CoA in the liver, and are converted to ketone bodies (acetone acetate, acetone and beta-hydroxybutyrate). The increase in these ketone bodies causes elevated levels of blood beta-hydroxybutyric acid, which causes a drop in blood pH. A drop in blood pH less than the neutral value of 7.0 may cause acidosis. This may also cause a reduction in the effectiveness of pH-dependent enzyme systems, further contributing to metabolic disturbances. Ketoacidosis is life-threatening and requires immediate medical attention. Non-acidotic ketosis can usually be treated outside of hospital and is differentiated from metabolic acidosis by blood pH levels over 7.3 and bicarbonate levels over 15 mEq/l. Appropriate insulin administration and rehydration with electrolytes generally tends to correct the acidosis, if renal function is not impaired (Groer & Shekleton 1989, Patel 1999). If ketosis does occur or is present, it is important for the client/patient to seek medical assistance.

The biochemical markers for ketoacidosis are hyperglycaemia and ketonaemia (ketones in the blood). Other common signs include ketonuria (ketones in the urine), dehydration due to diuresis (increased passing of urine) (p. 67), dry skin, acetone odour on the breath (sweet sickly smell), tachycardia, hypotension, central nervous system depression and laboured breathing, as well as abdominal pain, anorexia, nausea and vomiting (Groer & Shekleton 1989, Patel 1999).

HYPEROSMOLAR NON-KETOTIC COMA

Non-ketotic coma is characteristic of type II diabetes and develops in those with sufficient insulin production to depress excessive fatty acid breakdown but not enough to permit glucose use and transport across the cell membranes. Thus, blood and urine tests for ketone are often close to normal. However, insufficient endogenous insulin leads to ketogenesis (Patel 1999) with similar results to those described above. The associated hyperglycaemia induces osmotic diuresis (p. 67) leading to thirst. If subsequent ingestion of high sugar drinks occurs, plasma osmolarity will increase, leading to changes in the sensorium and a condition of increased fluid intake, thus further aggravating the hyperosmolarity and hyperglycaemia. With hyperosmolarity the glomerular filtration rate decreases, leading to excessive amounts of nitrogenous compound in the blood, caused by failure of the kidneys to remove urea from the blood; further increases in blood glucose result. In contrast to ketoacidosis, this condition develops quite slowly. The treatment is rehydration, administration of small spaced doses of insulin

and replacement of potassium, as low potassium levels are a problem in these individuals, which tends to diminish with restored glucose metabolism (Groer & Shekleton 1989, Lulsegged & Sharma 2001).

LACTIC ACIDOSIS

Lactic acidosis is a metabolic acidosis due to excess lactic acid in the blood and is produced by conditions that impair cellular respiration (Patel 1999). During lactic acidosis blood glucose levels may be normal, but blood keto-acids are increased. Dehydration, hypotension and hyperventilation are often present. Lactic acid is produced normally in adults and utilized by other organs as a substrate, such as the heart. Generation of excess lactic acid is an effect of cellular hypoxia and/or anaerobic PA/exercise. Diabetics often have associated chronic diseases that predispose them to cellular hypoxia and ischaemia (Groer & Shekleton 1989), which predisposes these individuals to lactic acidosis during PA/exercise.

HYPOGLYCAEMIA

Hypoglycaemia is defined as subnormal blood glucose levels, and although there are no agreed values that define hypoglycaemia, the potential effects of low blood glucose levels are outlined in Table 4.6. Symptoms of low blood glucose tend to present as a result of either the release of catecholamines, via activation of the sympathetic nervous activity, or defective nervous systems, through stimulation of the central nervous system (Table 4.7).

Table 4.6 Hypoglycaemia and presence of symptoms (adapted from Patel 1999)

Blood glucose levels	Presence of symptoms
<2.8 mmol/l (50 mg/dl)	Symptoms may or may not be present
<2.2 mmol/l (<40 mg/dl)	Symptoms are usually present
<1.1 mmol/l (<20 mg/dl)	Seizures and coma usually occur

Table 4.7 Common signs and symptoms of hypoglycaemia

Signs and symptoms	Activation
Anxiety, sweating, tremor, palpitations, hunger, tachycardia, irritability, pallor, perspiration	Sympathetic nervous system
Headache, blurred vision, fatigue, numbness of lips and tongue, emotional changes, confusion	Central nervous system
Severe – convulsions, coma	

Hypoglycaemia is most common before meals and at night. Hypoglycaemia may be caused by a variety of factors, and under resting conditions usually occurs in those with uncontrolled diabetes or when too much insulin has been administered. Individuals will vary in the amount of injected insulin required and in their peak responses. Physical activity/exercise may also require adjustment to the amount of insulin required, since exercise increases insulin sensitivity (p. 70) and glucose uptake irrespective of the presence of insulin, thereby predisposing the individual to hypoglycaemia. Additionally, since during PA/exercise, the working muscles become more insulin sensitive, the diabetic will need to adjust the site of injection to a 'non-working' area, such as the abdomen, to avoid hypoglycaemia (for more details refer to Patel 1999 and Burr & Dinesh 1999).

If hypoglycaemia does occur under non-PA/exercise conditions, ingestion of fast-acting carbohydrates such as fruit juice is required. This results in hyperglycaemia. Approximately 10 to 20 g of carbohydrate is generally recommended, which is around two teaspoonfuls of sugar. If after 15 minutes, however, blood glucose levels remain low, a further 10 to 20 g of fast-acting carbohydrate should be ingested (for more details refer to Patel 1999).

HYPERGLYCAEMIA

Hyperglycaemia is as much of a problem to the diabetic as is hypoglycaemia. Hyperglycaemia is defined as a fasting blood glucose level greater than 6.1 mmol/l (109 mg/dl). Blood glucose levels of around 10 mmol/l (178 mg/dl) result in a change in the osmolarity of the blood (Table 4.8), causing glucose to be excreted in the urine, which can lead to diabetic diuresis. Diuresis can result in dehydration and loss of potassium and sodium,

Table 4.8 Possible consequences of acute hyperglycaemia (blood glucose levels greater than 10 mmol/l (~178 mg/dl))

↑ blood osmolarity
↑ urination
Dehydration
Increased thirst
↓ potassium and sodium levels
↓ blood volume
↑ blood viscosity
↑ platelet reactivity
↓ endothelium function
↓ muscle blood flow
Hypotension
Exhaustion
Leads to diuresis
Leads to ketoacidosis

and left untreated can contribute toward ketoacidosis (p. 65). Diuresis and subsequent dehydration can cause a reduction in blood volume, leading to thickening of the blood. The increase in blood osmolarity is also associated with enhanced platelet reactivity (Keating et al 2003), which may contribute toward risk of thrombosis.

Hyperglycaemia is a contributing factor in vascular and cell damage, commonly seen in diabetic patients. In early nephropathy (p. 63) the animal model shows how hyperglycaemia can cause cell cycle arrest and hypertrophy of the mesangial cells (the cellular network of the renal glomerulus) (Wolf et al 1998). Hyperglycaemia is also associated with impaired wound healing, partly due to decreased oxygenation and perfusion (Terranova 1991), as a result of ischaemia.

Although it is chronic hyperglycaemia that is generally associated with microvascular disease, acute hyperglycaemia has been found to cause attenuation of endothelial function (Du et al 2001), leading to significant reductions in muscle blood flow (Kim et al 2003b). In the animal model the onset of hyperglycaemia has also been found to increase the production of superoxides (Kim et al 2003a), which are known to attack lipids, proteins and nucleic acids, and is probably part of the mechanism that contributes toward hyperglycaemic vascular damage.

Hyperglycaemia is commonly seen in conjunction with hyperlipidaemia. Since absolute insulin deficiency leads to an increase in hepatic glucose output and there is a decrease in glucose uptake, there is an increase in the breakdown and mobilization of fatty acids from the adipose tissue to the liver. These fatty acids are then delivered into the blood in the form of lipoproteins (very low-density lipoproteins), which cannot be taken up, as the action of LPL is inhibited (Assmann 1982).

GLYCOSYLATED HAEMOGLOBIN

Glycosylated haemoglobin is a haemoglobin (Hb) A molecule with a glucose group attached. This reaction occurs more readily when blood glucose rises above normal. Glycosylated Hb blood concentration represents the average blood glucose level over a period of several weeks, and glycated Hb tests measure the amount of Hb that is irreversibly bound to glucose (usually HbA_{1c}). Although these values may vary between different laboratories (Patel 1999), in controlled diabetes this should stay within the normal range of around 5.0–7.5% for HbA_1 and 4.0–6.0% HbA_{1c} for the total glycated Hb (BDA 1993).

DIURESIS

When blood glucose is elevated to levels that exceed the capacity of the kidney to reabsorb the glucose, which is around 10 mmol/l, glucose will remain in the tubular filtrate of the kidney, which is then excreted in the urine.

Therefore, glucose will appear in the urine, and is a good indicator of blood hyperosmolarity. In order to reach an isosmotic concentration, excess glucose molecules in the tubular filtrate cause water to osmose from the spaces between the cells, and through the tubular cells. Electrolytes are also present and retained in the tubular filtrate. The increase in water drawn to the tubular filtrate dilutes sodium ions and causes the reabsorption of sodium to be diminished. The loss of water and electrolytes causes an increase in extracellular osmolarity and cellular dehydration. Consequently, this causes the individual to feel extremely thirsty, so that they will replace the fluid being lost (Groer & Shekleton 1989). However, the individual should not rehydrate with carbohydrate drinks.

SYMPATHETIC NERVOUS SYSTEM

During PA/exercise the build up of local metabolites activate afferent nerves to stimulate the sympathetic nervous system. The sympathetic nervous system has numerous effects, which are mainly the result of catecholamines noradrenaline (norepinephrine) and adrenaline (epinephrine). Noradrenaline is released from the nerve terminals in the beta-cell islets and adrenaline from the adrenal medulla. Their effect is to speed up heart rate by acting on special beta-adrenergic-1 receptors (beta$_1$ receptors) and to cause vasoconstriction by acting on beta$_1$ receptors of the smooth vascular muscle, thereby increasing total peripheral resistance and blood pressure. Catecholamines also affect blood pressure, through the stimulation of the renin–angiotensin–aldosterone system (Esler et al 2001), resulting in vasoconstriction and aldosterone-led renal sodium reabsorption by the kidney tubules, and an increase in intravascular volume. In addition, catecholamines increase hepatic glucose output in response to a drop in blood glucose levels and inhibit insulin section via the alpha-adrenoceptors on the beta cell. This inhibitory effect is important when there is a need for elevated blood glucose, such as at times of stress or during PA/exercise, and in the healthy individual is part of the blood glucose balance.

TREATMENT

Whether the diabetic has type I or type II diabetes some sort of day-to-day management will be required (Table 4.9). It is important that diabetic individuals have a good concept as to how to manage their treatment before they embark upon any type of unsupervised PA/exercise. Therefore, initially coordination between the client/patient, the diabetic team and the exercise practitioner may be required in order for this to be achieved.

Table 4.9 Basic management for diabetic individuals

Type of diabetes	Type of management
Type I	Insulin injections Healthy diet (with low glycaemic carbohydrates)
Type II obese	Energy-restricted healthy diet and regular PA/exercise If ineffective, additional oral medication If insulin output is reduced and oral medication ineffective, inclusion of insulin injections
Type II non-obese	Healthy diet with oral medication/s, with regular PA/exercise If insulin output is reduced and oral medication ineffective, inclusion of insulin injections

GLYCAEMIC CONTROL

Maintaining glycaemic control (blood glucose levels <6.0 mmol/l) can substantially reduce microvascular and macrovascular complications (Zimmerman 1994, UKPDS 1998). Ideally blood glucose should be within the normal range (Table 4.3) with fasting levels of between 4.4 and 6.7 mmol/l and postprandial values of <10 mmol/l (Patel 1999).

TYPE I DIABETIC

Given that the type I diabetic does not produce insulin, at present the only source of treatment is regular insulin injections. These are required to enable the uptake of blood glucose and the dose of insulin and site of injection may vary according to types and levels of PA/exercise. The type I diabetic's diet should also be monitored, avoiding high glycaemic foods, such as simple carbohydrates.

TYPE II DIABETIC

Type II diabetes can be controlled by a lifestyle change which incorporates appropriate diet and increased PA/exercise (p. 69) in order to reduce body weight and blood lipid levels. This type of intervention is generally the one initially employed for obese type II diabetics. Nonetheless, even this lifestyle change does not always regulate blood glucose levels, and medication may therefore be required, usually in the form of tablets, which are usually prescribed for the non-obese type II diabetic. If, however, insulin output is also reduced, and oral medication is ineffective, insulin injections may be required (Patel 1999).

New medications are always being developed but at present the most common types of oral medication for the type II diabetic are sulphonylureas, which increase insulin secretion (there are short- and longer-acting types); biguanides (metformin), which increase intracellular glu-

Table 4.10   Medications commonly prescribed to diabetic individuals

	Medication	Effect
Type I diabetic	Insulin injection	↑ glucose uptake
Type II diabetic	Sulphonylureas	↑ insulin secretion
	Biguanides (metformin)	↑ intracellular glucose metabolism and ↓ hepatic glucose output
	Thiazolidinediones	↑ insulin action
	Alpha-glucosidase (acarbose)	↓ postprandial hyperglycaemia by ↓ digestion of carbohydrate
	May also require insulin	

cose metabolism and decrease hepatic glucose output; thiazolidinediones, which enhance insulin action by promoting glucose uptake in the peripheral tissues, and alpha-glucosidase inhibitors (acarbose), which reduce postprandial hyperglycaemia by slowing down the digestion of carbohydrate, thereby reducing the glycaemic effect (Patel 1999, BMA, RPS GB 2004) (Table 4.10). These types of drugs do have side effects and may be prescribed in combination. It is therefore important for the exercise practitioner to be aware of the potential effects of these drugs (see BMA, RPS GB 2004). For more details on diabetic drug therapies refer to Patel (1999) and Bailey & Feher (2004).

PHYSICAL ACTIVITY/EXERCISE

Regular PA/exercise is known to have a protective effect against type II diabetes (Manson et al 1992). Whilst the optimal amount of PA/exercise for reducing the occurrence of type II diabetes has yet to be determined, epidemiological evidence indicates that increased levels of leisure time energy expenditure and exercise intensity reduce one's risk of developing this disease.

ENERGY EXPENDITURE

Epidemiological evidence from a prospective study, carried out on 5900 males from the alumni of the University of Pennsylvania, showed that the incidence of non-insulin-dependent diabetes declined with an increase in leisure time energy expenditure. Energy expenditure was measured in 500 kcal per week increments, and for each incremental increase diabetes was reduced by around 6%. The protective effect of the physical activity was strongest in those individuals with the highest risk of diabetes, notably those with high body mass index, a history of hypertension or parental history of diabetes (Helmrich et al 1991). Similarly, another study found that the greater the energy expenditure through PA/exercise, including low-intensity activities such as gardening and walking, the lower the risk of developing type II diabetes (Hu et al 1999a), providing support for the role of PA/exercise in reducing incidence of type II diabetes.

PHYSICAL ACTIVITY/EXERCISE INTENSITY

The exact intensity of PA/exercise required to reduce the risk of type II diabetes has not yet been established, and although Hu et al (1999a) found even low level PA/exercise to reduce risk of type II diabetes, Manson et al (1991) did not. Manson et al (1991) followed a group of 87253 female nurses for a period of 8 years. The findings of the study revealed that those nurses who carried out vigorous exercise at least once a week had a 67% reduced risk of developing type II diabetes when compared to their sedentary counterparts. Interestingly, frequency and duration of PA/exercise did not appear to influence this outcome.

PHYSICAL ACTIVITY/EXERCISE AND INSULIN RESISTANCE

Skeletal muscle insulin resistance entails the dysregulation of both glucose and fatty acid metabolism. The effect of physical activity on glucose intolerance and insulin resistance in relation to obesity has been reviewed, and has shown that physical activity has a favourable effect on reducing insulin resistance in obesity and among type II diabetics. The probable mechanisms for this are outlined on page 70. The effect of PA/exercise on glucose tolerance, however, has been less consistently observed, and appears to be related to variations in PA/exercise intensity between the different studies, changes in adiposity, the interval between PA/exercise, testing of glucose tolerance and baseline severity of glucose intolerance (Kelley & Goodpaster 1999).

Although PA/exercise alone has been reported to be effective in the enhancement of insulin sensitivity (p. 70), many interventions looking at insulin resistance in obese individuals employ interventions of PA/exercise with diet control. For example, a study carried out on 9 obese men and 16 obese women (age 39±4 years), who underwent 16 weeks of moderate-intensity physical activity with a calorie-reduced diet, found that rates of resting fat oxidation were enhanced, with greater proportions of resting energy being derived from fat, which was also found to be the strongest predictor of improved insulin sensitivity (Goodpaster et al 2003). This indicates the effectiveness of PA/exercise and diet combined in enhancing insulin sensitivity.

MECHANISM

Whilst regular PA/exercise is now seen as an essential part of the treatment for type II diabetes, it does not assist in the control of type I diabetes. Furthermore, despite regular PA/exercise being associated with enhanced insulin sensitivity, the exact mechanism by which PA/exercise assists individuals with type II diabetes is still under investigation. Nonetheless, PA/exercise is known to assist through its effect on glucose uptake, enhanced insulin sensitivity and the downregulated secretion from the pancreatic beta cell (Zonderland et al 2000).

The rate-limiting step in glucose metabolism is glucose transport, which in skeletal muscle is mediated by the translocation of glucose transported GLUT 4 (p. 62). In simplified terms, within the cell there are compartments that store the GLUT 4 transporters. These GLUT 4 transporters are required for the uptake of glucose into the cell, and in order for this to be achieved these need to translocate to the cell membrane (p. 62). In skeletal muscle two distinct and separate signalling pathways activate translocation of GLUT 4. Insulin activates one pathway (p. 61), and muscle contraction activates the other (Ryder et al 2001). Although the mechanisms behind PA/exercise-induced activation of glucose transport still remain to be fully determined, the stimulatory effect of muscle contraction upon the activation of adenosine monophosphate (AMP)-activated protein kinase (Gautier & Mauvais-Jarvis 2001), nitric oxide synthase and release of calcium may be involved (Ryder et al 2001). AMP-activated protein kinase appears to stimulate the translocation of GLUT 4 to the cell membrane, thus allowing for the uptake of glucose into the cell (Gautier & Mauvais-Jarvis 2001) (Fig. 4.3) and improvement of whole-body glucose homeostasis in insulin resistant individuals (Ryder et al 2001). The resultant effect of this can be illustrated through the acute effect of PA/exercise. Interestingly, slow twitch muscle fibres possess larger quantities of GLUT 4 transporters than do fast twitch fibres, suggesting that aerobic activities provide greater glucose uptake than anaerobic activities. This does not appear to play a part in the pathogenesis of diabetes, since type II diabetics and non-diabetics appear to be similar in muscle fibre composition. There is, however, good evidence that PA/exercise training impacts upon insulin sensitivity in healthy individuals as well as in type II diabetics by increasing skeletal muscle GLUT 4 expression, which may partly explain the beneficial effect of regular PA/exercise (Daugaard & Richter 2001).

ACUTE BOUTS OF PHYSICAL ACTIVITY/EXERCISE

During a bout of PA/exercise glucose uptake in the working muscle may increase to around 7 to 20 times that of resting levels, the extent of the increase being dependent upon the intensity of the PA/exercise (Jeng et al 2003). Therefore, in order to meet this demand, transport of glucose into the working skeletal muscle needs to increase, and this demand is the same for diabetics and non-diabetics alike.

A single bout of PA/exercise brings about a transient effect that enhances insulin sensitivity and glucose transport into muscles (Lutoslawska 2000). For example, a study carried out on 10 untrained healthy young adults, who exercised for 60 minutes on a cycle ergometer at a mean of 73% peak oxygen uptake, found a post-exercise upregulation of skeletal muscle GLUT 4 transporters (Kraniou et al 2000). Furthermore, research on young healthy subjects, looking at the effect of 60 minutes of one-legged exercise, found that, in the exercised leg, insulin increased glucose uptake and glycogen synthase activity (an enzyme that increases the storage of glucose as muscle glycogen) by around two to four times (Wojtaszewski et al 2000). This PA/exercise-induced increase in glucose transport is also observed in insulin-resistant individuals and diabetics. Research carried out on diabetic rats, for instance, has shown muscle contraction to stimulate glucose transport despite severe insulin-induced insulin resistance (Wallberg-Henriksson & Holloszy 1984). Crucially, these effects have also been observed in human diabetics, since 45 to 60 minutes of cycling was also found to stimulate translocation of GLUT 4 in skeletal muscle of both healthy and type II diabetic subjects. This was regardless of there being around a 30% reduction in GLUT 4 in the diabetic subjects, compared to the non-diabetics, both prior to and after the exercise (Kennedy et al 1999), thus indicating the potential importance of acute PA/exercise in glucose homeostasis in type II diabetics. However, the intensity required to induce these effects may be at a level that some individuals are not able to tolerate (DoH 2004).

REGULAR AEROBIC PHYSICAL ACTIVITY/EXERCISE

In addition to the beneficial effect of acute PA/exercise upon glucose uptake, habitual PA/exercise has been shown to enhance whole-body glucose homeostasis, insulin-stimulated glucose transport (Houmard et al 1993) and insulin sensitivity, and to reduce insulin resistance (Rodgers et al 1988), although research has only found at most modest improvements in glycated Hb (DoH 2004). The mechanism by which regular PA/exercise enhances glucose uptake may, in part, be related to an increase in the expression and/or activity of key proteins, such as GLUT 4, hexokinase II and glycogen synthase. All of these are involved in the regulation of glucose uptake and metabolism in skeletal muscle, and are found to upregulate with exercise training. Although the role of GLUT 4 is clear, the roles of hexokinase II and glycogen synthase are less so. Initially hexokinase II was reported to enhance insulin-stimulated glucose transport, indicating that hexokinase activity may be the rate-limiting step for glucose uptake. However, reports have been conflicting, with some showing no improvement in glucose uptake with over-expression of hexokinase II. Additionally, even though glycogen synthase dramatically increased the storage of glucose as muscle glycogen, over-expression does not appear to enhance glucose transport capacity in skeletal muscle. Insulin signal transduction may be another process by which glucose homeostasis is improved through PA/exercise training (Ryder et al 2001). For instance, important signalling proteins have been found to upregulate within 5 days of swim training in rats (Chibalin et al 2000); and in humans, after 7 days of exercise training (Houmard et al 1999).

The beneficial effect of exercise training in reducing body mass and blood pressure is also linked to reduced insulin resistance (Esler et al 2001). Reductions in blood pressure are also paralleled by changes in insulin resistance, and favourable changes in insulin have been found to correlate with improved baroreflex function and a decrease in heart rate. Moreover, corrections in sympathetic nervous system activity have been associated with the amelioration of hyperinsulinaemia, suggesting improvement in neuro-metabolic factors (Kohno et al 2000).

PRE-EXERCISE PRESCRIPTION

Even though the majority of diabetics will be referred for PA/exercise prescription via other health professionals, they still require thorough screening in order to determine other related co-morbidities, such as cardiovascular complications, neuropathy, retinopathy and nephropathy (Table 4.11), which will significantly affect the PA/exercise prescription. If insulin resistance or diabetes (usually type II) is suspected in an individual who has not previously been considered at risk for insulin resistance or diabetes, it would be unwise to prescribe PA/exercise before further evaluation has been carried out. It would, however, be essential to refer the individual back to their general practitioner for further medical evaluation.

PHYSICAL ACTIVITY/EXERCISE PRESCRIPTION

Generally it is recommended that PA/exercise should not be prescribed until adequate diet, metabolic control and blood glucose levels are achieved. Prescribing PA/exercise to the diabetic individual is indeed a challenge to the exercise practitioner. There are numerous factors that need to be considered not only when prescribing a programme, but also immediately prior to and following a bout of PA/exercise. The nature of diabetes suggests that the diabetic individual will have or will be highly predisposed to micro and macro

Table 4.11 Risk factors, signs and symptoms for diabetic complications (adapted from ADA 2000)

Complication	Risk factors, signs and symptoms
Cardiovascular	>35 years Type II diabetes for >10 years Type I diabetes >15 years Coronary heart disease risk factors Microvascular disease Macrovascular disease Peripheral vascular disease Autonomic neuropathy
Peripheral vascular disease	Intermittent claudication Cold feet Decreased or absent pulses Atrophy of subcutaneous tissues Hair loss
Retinopathy	Blurred vision
Nephropathy	Microalbuminuria: Incipient – 30 –300mg/day albumin excretion rate Overt – >300 mg/day albumin excretion rate
Peripheral neuropathy	Insensitive feet Ulcerations Fractures
Autonomic neuropathy	Resting tachycardia Orthostatic hypotension Skin – tingling/numbness Gastrointestinal Thermo-dysregulation

complications (p. 63), and an attempt will be made below to simplify these complex issues.

Notwithstanding this, and taking into account any considerations and contraindications (p. 76), generally the type of PA/exercise prescribed for type II diabetics would be low-intensity aerobic PA/exercise of longer duration (around 40 to 60 minutes). This type of activity will maximize a reduction in any risk factors associated with macro complications (p. 63), and minimize any further micro complications (p. 64), though resistance training may be prescribed for certain diabetic individuals (p. 76 and Table 4.14). Similar types of PA/exercise may also be prescribed for type I diabetics, but maintaining metabolic control may be more of a problem.

PHYSICAL ACTIVITY/EXERCISE CONSIDERATIONS

The type, frequency, duration and intensity of PA/exercise suitable for the diabetic individual will depend upon glycaemic control, micro and/or macro complications, and any other co-morbidity. The individual's fitness status will also determine the type of PA/exercise prescription. For instance, despite the fact that the majority of diabetics requiring PA/exercise prescription will be physically unfit, there are many extremely physically fit diabetics who participate in competitive sports, and the type of prescription they require will be very different, despite the commonality of diabetes. This therefore highlights the vast range of variation between individuals, and challenges the skills of the exercise practitioner in determining appropriate PA/exercise prescription. Nonetheless, the benefits of regular aerobic PA/exercise are most notable for those with type II diabetes, as it assists with the metabolic control of the disease, and where possible PA/exercise should be carried out on most days. Although PA/exercise may help in enhancing glucose uptake (thus there is the need to adjust injected insulin), generally for the type I diabetic PA/exercise does not help in metabolic control. However, if PA/exercise is carried out under controlled conditions it can help reduce the impact of certain associated complications. Most PA/exercise programmes that have shown beneficial effects have typically consisted of three bouts of walking or cycling per week, for around 40 minutes in each bout (DoH 2004). Furthermore, studies that have included higher PA/exercise intensity tend to show greater improvements in fitness, glycated Hb (clinically significant reduction being around 15%) and insulin sensitivity (McAuley et al 2002, Boule et at 2003).

PA/exercise programmes should employ an adaptive programme of aerobic and resistance activities in addition to mobility and flexibility components (Tokmakidis et al 2000). However, when designing a PA/exercise programme, the fact that aerobic activities provide greater glucose uptake than anaerobic activities should be considered (Daugaard & Ritcher 2001).

BLOOD GLUCOSE LEVELS AND PHYSICAL ACTIVITY /EXERCISE

It is important to determine when it is and is not appropriate for the diabetic to carry out PA/exercise. Therefore, for anything other than very light PA/exercise (exercise intensity <20% of maximum aerobic capacity ~ <10 ratings of perceived exertion (RPE), Appendix B, Table B.3), prior to PA/exercise the diabetic individuals should carry out a test of their current blood glucose levels. This can detect risk of hypoglycaemia (p. 66), or hyperglycaemia (p. 67) and the respective metabolic consequences.

HYPOGLYCAEMIA AND PHYSICAL ACTIVITY/EXERCISE

Although PA/exercise assists in the control of type II diabetes, it does not assist the type I diabetic, who is at risk of hypoglycaemia. Whilst both type I and type II diabetics can become hypoglycaemic as a result of PA/exercise, it is relatively uncommonly in type II diabetics not injecting with insulin.

Hypoglycaemia (blood glucose levels around 2.8 mmol/l, ~50 mg/dl, Table 4.6) rarely occurs in non-diabetic individuals, and in the non-diabetic individual the control of blood glucose during PA/exercise is mediated by the hormones insulin and glucagon (p. 60). During the early stages of PA/exercise an increase in the ratio of glucagon/insulin is required in order for the liver to release glucose into the systemic circulation, and this is also the case during prolonged PA/exercise, when muscle glycogen stores start to diminish. In type I diabetics, who are insulin deficient, and type II diabetics injecting insulin, these hormonal adaptations are essentially respectively lost or inadequate (ADA 2000). The problems of blood glucose control in physically active insulin-treated diabetics can be explained by imbalances between blood insulin levels and available blood glucose. During PA/exercise, insulin-treated diabetics may have higher blood insulin levels than non-diabetic individuals undertaking similar PA/exercise. This is because the non-diabetic will naturally adjust the level of blood insulin to the body's increased sensitivity to insulin and blood glucose uptake during PA/exercise. But whilst the insulin-treated diabetic's body will still become increasingly sensitive to insulin and blood glucose uptake, if the insulin injection stays as it is under resting conditions, essentially there will be too much circulating blood insulin. Concurrently, under this situation where normal amounts of insulin have *not* been adjusted, blood glucose will also be too low, because high insulin levels block hepatic glycogenolysis, thus causing a propensity toward hypoglycaemia (Grimm 1999). It is therefore important for the client/patient and exercise practitioner to understand the ways to avoid hypoglycaemia during and after PA/exercise (Table 4.12).

Pre-physical activity/exercise blood glucose levels

Prior to the commencement of any PA/exercise, other than that of very low intensity, it is vital for diabetics to become habituated to taking their blood glucose levels. If blood glucose levels are <4.0 mmol/l (~71 mg/dl) or <5.6 mmol/l (100 mg/dl) for vigorous PA/exercise, it is advisable not to carry out PA/exercise (White & Sherman 1999, Colberg & Swain 2000), ingest some fast-acting carbohydrate and wait for levels to come up to a suitable level, which may be around 5.6 mmol/l (100 mg/dl) and, for some top sports people as much as 20 mmol/l (~358 mg/dl). However, suitable pre-PA/exercise levels will vary according to the individual and it is important for the client/patient and the exercise practitioner to become familiar with an individual's responses.

Insulin-treated diabetics

The way to avoid hypoglycaemia in insulin-treated diabetics is to reduce the amount of injected insulin and/or adjust the amount of food ingested (Table 4.12). It has been

Table 4.12 Hypoglycaemia and physical activity/exercise

Insulin-dependent diabetics	
How to avoid hypoglycaemia	Do not carry out PA/exercise if blood glucose levels are <4.0 mmol/l (~71 mg/dl) or <5.6 mmol/l (100 mg/dl) for vigorous PA/exercise
	Pre-PA/exercise blood glucose levels should be between 5.6 (100 mg/dl) and 11.1 mmol/l (200 mg/dl)
	Carry out PA/exercise in the morning rather than the evening
	Reduce amount of injected insulin
	Do not inject insulin into the active muscles
	↓ insulin by ~30% and ingest fast acting carbohydrate at a rate of 40 g/h (~3–4 teaspoonfuls of sugar)
Non-insulin-dependent diabetics	
How to avoid hypoglycaemia	Individuals taking sulphonylureas and thiazolidinediones may need to adjust their dose of medication
	Be aware when treating hypoglycaemia that alpha glucosidases slow the ingestion of carbohydrates
Masking of hypoglycaemia (Table 4.7)	
	Individuals with autonomic dysfunction (i.e. cardiac patients) may not show signs of hypoglycaemia
	Individuals taking beta-blockers may not show signs of hypoglycaemia
	The effect of increased circulating catecholamines in response to PA/exercise may mask signs of hypoglycaemia
Post-PA/exercise hypoglycaemia	
	Be aware that PA/exercise-induced sensitivity to insulin may last for several hours post PA/exercise. Therefore, there is still a risk of hypoglycaemia. Hence carry out PA/exercise in the morning rather than the evening

suggested that the amount of injected insulin should be reduced by around 30–35% for intermediate-acting insulin, and 50–65% for short-acting insulin (Schneider et al 1988). However, this will vary between individuals. A reduction in exogenous insulin will reduce blood glucose uptake and lessen the risk of hypoglycaemia (Patel 1999) (p. 66).

Additionally, since working muscles cause an increase in insulin sensitivity (Koivisto & Felig 1978), injecting insulin into the working muscles will further increase risk of hypoglycaemia. Thus it is advised that insulin be injected into non-active areas (for more details refer to Patel 1999 and Burr & Dinesh 1999).

Balancing the amount of insulin required during PA/exercise is initially by trial and error, as each individual will respond slightly differently. Therefore, a pattern of response needs to be established prior to any unsupervised PA/exercise, and it is generally recommended that type I diabetics do not carry out anything other than mild PA/exercise. It is always advisable, where possible, to discuss these and any adjustments in medications with the individual's diabetic team.

Non-insulin-dependent diabetics

Although hypoglycaemia is unlikely to occur in non-insulin-dependent diabetics, certain medications, such as sulphonylureas and thiazolidinediones (Table 4.10), do increase the action of insulin and thereby, with the increase in insulin sensitivity during PA/exercise, may result in too great an uptake of blood glucose, and the potential for hypoglycaemia. Therefore, adjustment of the dose of these medications may be required, though the extent will be dependent upon the individual response (White & Sherman 1999). Type II diabetics taking biguanides (metformin) are unlikely to suffer from hypoglycaemia as a result of PA/exercise, but may need some food soon after (Diabetes UK 2000). Furthermore, since alpha-glucosidases slow the digestion of carbohydrate, they may inhibit oral treatment for hypoglycaemia (White & Sherman 1999).

As with insulin-dependent diabetics, any modifications to medications should be discussed with the individual's diabetic team.

Ingestion of carbohydrate and meals

In order to avoid hypoglycaemia some diabetics may need to ingest carbohydrate prior to embarking upon PA/exercise. It has been suggested that during prolonged exercise, in conjunction with around a 30% reduction in insulin, fast-acting carbohydrate should be ingested at a rate of around 40 grams per hour (3 to 4 teaspoonfuls of sugar) (Schneider et al 1988). However, the amount required will depend upon the individual's response, the volume and intensity of PA/exercise being carried out and medications being taken, and their adjustment. Therefore, discussion with the client/patient and their diabetic team is advisable in order to establish the best protocol for the individual, and over time a pattern of procedures and responses should develop. Supplemental carbohydrate is not generally needed for non-insulin-injecting diabetics. However, monitoring of blood glucose levels is essential in order to respond to low blood glucose levels and prevent the possibility of hypoglycaemia (White & Sherman 1999, Colberg & Swain 2000).

The timing of meals in relation to PA/exercise is also important and it has been suggested that a suitable time to carry out postprandial PA/exercise is around 1 to 2 hours after eating, or when insulin is not at its peak. Additionally, after prolonged PA/exercise it is essential to replenish muscle glycogen stores within 1 to 2 hours of the PA/exercise (White & Sherman 1999), which is when glycogen synthase activity is at its greatest (Ryder et al 2001).

Post–physical activity/exercise or delayed hypoglycaemia

The PA/exercise-induced increase in insulin may persist for anywhere between 6 (Nagasawa et al 1991) and 15 hours and possibly (MacDonald 1987, White & Sherman 1999) 28 hours after prolonged PA/exercise (Horton 1988, White & Sherman 1999). This is generally the result of the PA/exercise-induced increased glucose uptake (MacDonald 1987) and, after prolonged PA/exercise, hepatic synthesis of depleted glycogen stores (Bogardus et al 1983), which take longer to replenish (Horton 1988). Hence, there is still a risk of hypoglycaemia during this time. Thus, if carrying out PA/exercise late in the day, to avoid hypoglycaemia during the night (nocturnal hypoglycaemia) blood glucose levels should be checked and food taken to make sure that blood glucose levels are not too low. It is therefore recommended that most diabetics do not carry out PA/exercise in the evening (White & Sherman 1999).

Time of day

As explained above, it is better to exercise during the day rather than in the evening when there is a greater risk of nocturnal hypoglycaemia. Moreover, given that in the morning insulin levels are generally lower, and there are higher levels of the hormone cortisol, which also raises blood glucose levels, the morning is a good time for the insulin-treated diabetic to carry out PA/exercise.

Masking of hypoglycaemia

There are certain factors that can mask hypoglycaemia. For instance, catecholamines of the sympathetic nervous system increase during PA/exercise (Farrell et al 1987), and their effect can produce symptoms that are similar to those of hypoglycaemia (Table 4.7). Likewise, individuals who possess autonomic dysfunction, such as cardiac patients, may also exhibit symptoms that are comparable to those of hypoglycaemia and therefore may not be aware of its onset. Furthermore, since beta-blockers essentially block the action of the sympathetic nervous system, individuals taking beta-blockers may not display the effects of hypoglycaemia (Patel 1999).

HYPERGLYCAEMIA AND PHYSICAL ACTIVITY/EXERCISE

Whilst hypoglycaemia is a major consideration during PA/exercise, so is hyperglycaemia; the metabolic consequences can be just as deleterious and therefore blood glucose monitoring prior to PA/exercise is essential. Hyperglycaemia, when blood glucose levels exceed 10 mmol/l (178 mg/dl), is usually a problem in poorly controlled diabetics (p. 67). At this level the osmolarity of the blood increases, leading to a cascade of metabolic reactions (Table 4.8). However, pre-PA/exercise levels of 10 mmol/l (178 mg/dl) are acceptable, as enhanced exercise-induced glucose uptake should lower this value. Nonetheless, at blood glucose levels above 10 mmol/l (178 mg/dl), the individual will probably be dehydrated, which needs correcting prior to PA/exercise. During PA/exercise sweating may further exacerbate the situation. Therefore, adequate intake of fluids is essential. However, fluid intake should be free of carbohydrate in order to avoid further increases in blood glucose levels. Some drinks contain potassium and sodium, which will help with rehydration. It is therefore a good idea to find a drink that contains these electrolytes without high carbohydrate levels.

When values exceed 14 mmol/l (250 mg/dl), the likelihood of the body being able to control these blood glucose levels is reduced and care should be taken. It is difficult at these blood glucose levels to determine whether it is safe or not to exercise. If blood glucose values do exceed 14 mmol/l (250 mg/dl), then check for ketones in the urine. If these are absent then ketoacidosis is not currently present, and PA/exercise may be carried out after rehydration. However, it is important that PA/exercise levels remain at a low intensity. The rationale is that as PA/exercise intensity rises so do catecholamine levels (Farrell et al 1987), and one of their effects is to enhance hepatic glucose output; therefore, there could be an increase in blood glucose levels, which would be undesirable. Thus it is imperative that blood glucose levels are checked at regular intervals.

There are other consequences of high pre-PA/exercise blood glucose (Table 4.8), regardless of lack of ketoacidosis, and these may affect the PA/exercise ability of the individual. High acute levels of blood glucose have been found to reduce the function of the endothelium (Du et al 2001) and muscle blood flow (Kim et al 2003b), and to enhance lactic acidosis (p. 66) as a result of cellular hypoxia. This is in conjunction with an increase in blood viscosity and consequent propensity toward hypercoagulation (Keating et al 2003), in addition to hypotension as a result of dehydration (Groer & Shekleton 1989), affecting PA/exercise ability. Therefore, if the client/patient is carrying out PA/exercise with high pre-PA/exercise blood glucose levels, regular assessment of the their physical status should be taken. Furthermore, as the symptoms, such as breathlessness and fatigue, are similar in PA/exercise to those for these metabolic disturbances it

Table 4.13 Physical activity/exercise recommendations (above light intensity) for diabetics from pre-PA/exercise blood glucose levels (mmol/l)

Blood glucose levels	PA/exercise recommendations	Potential consequences
<4.0 (~71 mg/dl)	Advisable not to carry out PA/exercise	Risk of hypoglycaemia
<5.6 (100 mg/dl)	Advisable not to carry out vigorous PA/exercise	Risk of hypoglycaemia
8.4 (150 mg/dl)	Fine to carry out PA/exercise	
>10 (180 mg/dl)	Vigorous or prolonged PA/exercise	Insulin-treated individuals should check for ketones. If no ketosis, only for individuals that are physically fit and healthy enough to carry out PA/exercise at this level, then risk of worsening metabolic state reduced
>10 (180 mg/dl)	Low to moderate intensity, PA/exercise with caution	Insulin-treated individuals should check for ketones. If no ketosis, still risk of worsening metabolic state. May cause additional problems for those with cardiovascular disease
>14 (250 mg/dl)	Vigorous intensity or prolonged PA/exercise. Athletic individuals only	Insulin-treated individuals should check for ketones. If no ketosis, only for individuals who are physically fit and healthy enough to carry out PA/exercise at this level, then risk of worsening metabolic state reduced
>14 (250 mg/dl)	PA/exercise not recommended	Insulin-treated individuals should check for ketones. Even if there is no ketosis there is still risk of worsening metabolic state. Only very light intensity PA/exercise advisable
≥16.9 (300 mg/dl)	PA/exercise not recommended	Risk of worsening metabolic state

may be difficult to determine the physical status of these individuals. Therefore, great care should be taken when they undertake PA/exercise. Blood glucose levels above 17 mmol/l (300 mg/dl) are seen as contraindicating PA/exercise as the metabolic state will be worsened (Leutholtz & Ripoll 1999). Based on the metabolic consequences of different pre-PA/exercise blood glucose levels, recommendations whether or not to carry out PA/exercise are summarized in Table 4.13.

THE DIABETIC CARDIAC PATIENT

Diabetes is a known risk factor for cardiovascular disease and those cardiac patients who also suffer from diabetes have to be additionally cautious when exercising with high blood glucose levels. In addition to the factors mentioned above, these individuals are likely to have endothelial dysfunction (p. 15) and are prone to ischaemia and arrhythmias that will be further aggravated by the consequences of high blood glucose levels (Table 4.8). Therefore, threshold levels such as 14 mmol/l (250 mg/dl) for diabetics without cardiovascular disease and ketoacidosis should be lowered in the cardiac-diabetic to avoid the consequence of an adverse cardiac event. Notwithstanding this, a study carried out on 17 non-ketotic cardiac patients with type II diabetes, who regularly had blood glucose levels ≥12 mmol/l (214 mg/dl), found that 6 hours post-PA/exercise blood glucose levels were significantly lower than pre-PA/exercise levels, with no consistently elevated blood glucose levels 24 hours post-PA/exercise. However, hypoglycaemia (blood glucose ≤3.3 mmol/l, ~59 mg/dl) was found in some patients, but no other complications were reported (Badenhop et al

2001). This further illustrates the fact that individuals will react differently and finding acceptable levels will be by trial and error. Therefore, it is advisable that these individuals carry out PA/exercise in consultation with the cardiac and diabetic teams. Furthermore, although water-based PA/exercises are often recommended for diabetic individuals, especially those who cannot undertake weight-bearing activities, these may be problematic for the cardiac patient with diabetes (p. 15).

KETOACIDOSIS

If a patient with diabetes is referred for PA/exercise prescription and their diabetes is under control, ketoacidosis should not occur. Ketoacidosis usually occurs in undiagnosed individuals or from an inadequate dosage of exogenous insulin. However, ketosis can be triggered by stress, illness and/or infection (Patel 1999). If a client/patient presents with high blood glucose levels, ≥10 mmol/l (178 mg/dl), then check for ketones in the urine. If these are present, then do not allow the individual to carry out PA/exercise; if they are not present then PA/exercise may be undertaken with caution (Table 4.14).

NEPHROPATHY

Specified PA/exercise recommendations have not been set for those with incipient or overt nephropathy. However, those with overt nephropathy often have impaired functional capacity, which leads a limitation in their activity levels; thus any PA/exercise greater than 60% of their aerobic capacity should be discouraged. There

Table 4.14 Basic considerations for physical activity/exercise prescription in diabetics with complications

Complication	Physical activity/exercise considerations
Cardiovascular	Keep intensity below ischaemic threshold
Peripheral vascular disease	PA/exercise to pain then change to non-weight-bearing activity until pain subsides
Retinopathy	Avoid strenuous, anaerobic activities, jarring or Valsalva manoeuvres – may lead to haemorrhage or retinal detachment
Nephropathy	Avoid high intensity strenuous activity
Peripheral neuropathy	Possible diabetic foot. Shock absorptive and supportive shoes required and regular foot care. In severe cases avoid weight-bearing activities
Autonomic neuropathy	At risk of adverse cardiac event and impaired thermoregulation; ensure appropriate hydration. Similar consideration to cardiac patients (Ch. 2, p. 26)

is, however, no research to suggest that low to moderate PA/exercise (around 40–60% of aerobic capacity) is harmful and this can therefore be prescribed if suitable for a particular individual (ADA 2000, Colberg & Swain 2000) (Table 4.14).

RETINOPATHY

Vitreous haemorrhage can result from unstable proliferative retinopathy. Diabetics with retinopathy should avoid vigorous PA/exercise as this can hasten haemorrhage or retinal detachment. Activities that cause a sudden increase in blood pressure such as vigorous PA/exercise involving strain, jarring or the Valsalva manoeuvre (p. 90) should be avoided as they may exacerbate the situation (White & Sherman 1999, ADA 2000, Colberg & Swain 2000) (Table 4.14).

NEUROPATHY

Neuropathy can be divided into autonomic and peripheral neuropathy and diabetics can be subject to both types.

Autonomic neuropathy

Autonomic neuropathy predisposes the diabetic to greater risk of an adverse cardiac event during PA/exercise. These individuals will be prone to complications similar to those outlined for individuals with cardiovascular disease, and will require the same PA/exercise considerations (White & Sherman 1999) (Ch. 2, p. 26). Those with autonomic neuropathy will be prone to both post-

PA/exercise hypotension and hypertension. Thermoregulatory mechanisms may also be impaired. Therefore, measures should be taken to ensure sufficient hydration during PA/exercise (ADA 2000, Colberg & Swain 2000) (Table 4.14).

Peripheral neuropathy

Peripheral neuropathy predisposes the diabetic to 'diabetic foot' (p. 64). Therefore it is vital that appropriate footwear be worn (White & Sherman 1999) and that regular foot checks are undertaken. During PA/exercise use of silica gel or cushioned midsoles, with polyester or synthetic-blend socks, may help reduce blisters and prevent additional damage. Feet should also be kept dry (Colberg & Swain 2000). In severe cases non-weight-bearing PA/exercise is suggested, such as water-based PA/exercise. However, for those with cardiovascular and autonomic complications this may not be advisable (p. 25).

Individuals with peripheral neuropathy may also suffer from peripheral vascular disease (PVD). The signs include intermittent claudication – intermittent pain in the lower leg during physical exertion, caused by local ischaemia and consequent build-up of lactic acid and anaerobic metabolites. Those with PVD should carry out walking (if able to do weight-bearing activities) interspersed at the onset of pain with non-weight-bearing activities, such as cycling, to allow for build-up of aerobic capacity (Appendix B, Table B.2) (Table 4.14).

WARMING UP AND COOLING DOWN

Diabetics with autonomic dysfunction will require longer warm-up and cool-down periods. The reasons are comparable to those for cardiac patients who are prone to similar complications (p. 25).

CONTRAINDICATIONS FOR PHYSICAL ACTIVITY/EXERCISE

Unplanned weight training is contraindicated in those with proliferative retinopathy, hypertension and uncontrolled diabetes (Canabal 1992), and also in those with ketosis, hypo- or hyperglycaemia. Other contraindications for PA/exercise are as given in Appendix A, Table A.1.

MEDICATIONS

Certain medications are known to affect glucose regulation and interfere with blood glucose tests. It is important therefore for the exercise practitioner to be aware of these effects. Hence, during the client/patient screening process the effect of medications should be looked into prior to PA/exercise prescription and constant updates regarding changes in medication should be made. Additionally, the acute effect of medications such as aspirin and paracetamol may cause falsely low glucose readings when home monitoring from a fingerprick blood sample. Since these types of blood samples are taken prior to PA/exercise it is important to determine whether such medications have been taken prior to these measures. Additionally, vitamin C (ascorbic acid) and aspirin can cause a false positive urine test. Furthermore, other types of medication may have a counter-regulatory effect upon insulin. For example, beta$_2$ agonists, commonly prescribed to asthmatics to dilate the bronchial tubes, reduce insulin output. Additionally,

beta-blockers, particularly the non-selective types, given to lower blood pressure and myocardial work, block the pancreatic beta$_2$ receptors, which are associated with the release of insulin. These drugs have also been known to mask the effects of hypoglycaemia, as they decrease the sympathetic system warning signs (Patel 1999) (Table 4.7). For the potential side effects of these and other medications refer to an up-to-date *National Formulary*, and for more details on diabetic drug therapies refer to Bailey & Feher (2004).

SUMMARY

- Diabetes is a syndrome of disordered metabolism with inappropriate hyperglycaemia; it affects around 1.4 million people in the UK and is the seventh leading cause of death in the USA.
- Metabolic syndrome is a precursor for diabetes.
- There are two types of diabetes:

  Type I diabetes is the result of inadequate production of insulin and may be caused by autoimmune destruction of pancreatic beta cells or arise from unknown causes.

  Type II diabetes is generally related to lifestyle (poor diet and inactivity leading to obesity and related disorders).
- Appropriate habitual PA/exercise intervention generally results in:

  ↑ general physical fitness

  modification of CHD risk factors, diabetes and insulin resistance, obesity, blood lipids, blood pressure

  ↑ insulin sensitivity

  ↑ metabolic control in non-insulin–dependent diabetics.
- Medications may affect blood glucose monitoring tests, and mask signs of hypoglycaemia, as can catecholamines.
- Diabetics are susceptible to micro and macro complications, such as retinopathy, peripheral and autonomic neuropathy, hypertension, cardiovascular disease, hyperlipidaemia and hypercoagulation, all of which need to be addressed when prescribing PA/exercise.
- Additional complications which have to be considered during PA/exercise are hyperglycaemia, ketosis, lactic acidosis and hypoglycaemia.

Suggested readings, references and bibliography

Suggested reading

Burr B, Dinesh N (eds) 1999 Exercise and sport diabetes. John Wiley, Chichester

Patel A 1999 Diabetes in focus. Pharmaceutical Press, London

References and bibliography

ADA (American Diabetic Association) 2000 Diabetes mellitus and exercise. Diabetic care. Online. Available: http://www.findarticle.com/cf_0/m0CUH/1_23/59175328/print.jhtml October 2001

AHA (American Heart Association) 2003 Heart disease and stroke statistics – 2003 update. Online. Available: http://www.americanheart.org/downloadable/heart/10461207852142003hdsstatsbook.pdf. July 2003

Alakhverdian R, Koev D 1987 Fibrinogen-fibrin degradation products in diabetes mellitus. Vutreshni Bolesti 26(6):72–75

Anderson D M, Keith J, Novak P D et al (eds) 2002 Mosby's medical, nursing and allied health dictionary, 6th edn. Mosby, St Louis

Assmann G 1982 Lipid metabolism and atherosclerosis. Schattauer Verlag, Stuttgart

Badenhop D T, Dunn C B, Eldridge S et al 2001 Monitoring and management of cardiac rehabilitation patients with type II diabetes. Clinical Exercise Physiology 3(2):71–77

Bailey C J, Feher M D 2004 Therapies for diabetes. Sherborne Gibbs, Birmingham, UK

Ballard-Barbash R, Birt D F, Kestin M et al 1997 Perspectives on

integrating experimental and epidemiological research on diet, anthropometry and breast cancer. Journal of Nutrition 127(5 Suppl):S936–S939

BDA (British Diabetic Association) 1993 Recommendations for the management of diabetes in primary care. British Diabetic Association, Diabetic Services Advisory Committee

BMA, RPS GB (British Medical Association, Royal Pharmaceutical Society Great Britain) 2004 British National Formulary. Pharmaceutical Press, Oxford

Bogardus C, Thuillez P, Ravussin E et al 1983 Effect of muscle glycogen depletion on in vivo insulin action in man. Journal of Clinical Investigation 72(5):1605–1610

Bonen A 1995 Benefits of exercise for type II diabetics: convergence of epidemiologic, physiologic and molecular evidence. Canadian Journal of Applied Physiology 20(3):261–279

Boule N G, Kenny G P, Haddad E et al 2003 Meta-analysis of the effect of structured exercise training on cardiorespiratory fitness in type 2 diabetes mellitus. Diabetologia 46:1071–1081

Burr B, Dinesh N (eds) 1999 Exercise and sport diabetes. John Wiley, Chichester

Canabal T 1992 Exercise, physical activity and diabetes mellitus. Asociacion Medica de Puerto Rico 84(2):78–81

Chibalin A V, Yu M, Ryder J W et al 2000 Exercise-induced changes in expression and activity of proteins involved in insulin-signal-transduction in skeletal muscle: differential effects on IRS-1 and IRS-2. Proceedings of the National Academy of Science USA 97:38–43

Colberg S R, Swain D P 2000 Exercise and diabetes control. The Physician and Sportsmedicine 28(4):63–64, 69–72, 81

Daugaard J R, Richter E A 2001 Relationship between muscle fibres composition, glucose transporter protein 4 and exercise training: possible consequences in non-insulin-dependent diabetes mellitus. Acta Physiologica Scandinavica 171(3):267–276

DeFronzo R A, Ferrannini E 1991 Insulin resistance. A multifaceted syndrome responsible for NIDDM, obesity, hypertension, dyslipidemia and atherosclerotic cardiovascular disease. Diabetes Care 14(3):173–194

Del Giudice M E, Fantus I G, Ezzat S et al 1998 Insulin and related factors in premenopausal breast cancer risk. Breast Cancer Research and Treatment 47(2):111–120

Diabetes 2001 The impact of diabetes. Online. Available: http://www.diabetes.org July 2001

Diabetes Monitor 2001 Diagnosing diabetes. Online. Available: http://www.diabetesmonitor.com/dx-class.htm July 2001

Diabetes UK 2000 Who gets diabetes and what causes it? Online. Available: http://www.diabetes.org.uk/whatis/get.htm July 2001

DoH (Department of Health) 2004 Physical activity, health improvement and prevention. At least five a week. Department of Health, London

Dorsch T R 2000 Insulin resistance. Online. Available: http://www.curediabetes.org/insulin_resistance_1.htm July 2001

Du X L, Edelstein D, Dimmeler S et al 2001 Hyperglycemia inhibits endothelial nitric oxide synthase activity by posttranslational modification at the Akt site. Journal of Clinical Investigation 108(9):1341–1348

Duckworth W C 2001 Hyperglycemia and cardiovascular disease. Current Atherosclerosis Reports 3(5):383–391

EndocrineWeb 1998 Normal regulation of blood glucose. Online. Available: http://www.endocrineweb.com/insulin.html January 2006

Esler M, Rumantir M, Wiesner G et al 2001 Review: sympathetic nervous system and insulin resistance: from obesity to diabetes. American Journal of Hypertension 14(11 Pt 2):304S–309S

Facchini F S, Stoohs R A, Reaven G M 1996 Enhanced sympathetic nervous system activity: The linchpin between insulin resistance, hyperinsulinemia and heart rate. American Journal of Hypertension 9:1013–1017

Farrell P A, Gustafson A B, Morgan W P et al 1987 Enkephalins, catecholamines and psychological mood alterations: effects of prolonged exercise. Medicine and Science in Sports and Exercise 19(4):347–353

Frayn K N 2001 Adipose tissue and the insulin resistance syndrome. Proceedings of the Nutritional Society 60(3):375–380

Gautier J F, Mauvais-Jarvis F 2001 Physical exercise and insulin sensitivity. Diabetes and Metabolism 27(2 Pt 2)255–260

Golubiatnikova G A, Valid B, Starosel'tseva L K et al 1987 Hemostasis and microcirculation in patients with diabetic ketosis. Terapevticheskii Arkhiv 59(7):109–111

Goodpaster B H, Katsiaras A, Kelly D E 2003 Enhanced fat oxidation through physical activity is associated with improved insulin sensitivity in obesity. Diabetes 52(9):2101–2197

Grimm J-J 1999 Exercise in type I diabetes. In: Burr B, Dinesh N (eds) Exercise and sport diabetes. John Wiley, Chichester, Ch 2

Groer M W, Shekleton M E 1989 Basic pathophysiology: a holistic approach, 3rd edn. Mosby, St Louis

Harris T J, Cook D G, Wicks P D et al 2000 Impact of the new American Diabetes Association and World Health Organization diagnostic criteria for diabetes on subjects from three ethnic groups living in the UK. Nutrition and Metabolism in Cardiovascular Disease 10:305–309

Helmrich S P, Ragland D R, Leung R W et al 1991 Physical activity and reduced occurrence of non-insulin-dependent diabetes mellitus. New England Journal of Medicine 325(3):147–152

Horton E S 1988 Role and management of exercise in diabetes mellitus. Diabetes Care 11(2):201–211

Houmard J A, Shinebarger M H, Dolan P L et al 1993 Exercise training increases GLUT-4 protein concentration in previously sedentary middle-aged men. American Journal of Physiology, Endocrinology and Metabolism 264:E896–E901

Houmard J A, Shaw C D, Hickey M S et al 1999 Effect of short-term exercise training on insulin-stimulated PI 3-kinase activity in human skeletal muscle. American Journal of Physiology, Endocrinology and Metabolism 277:E1055–E1060

Hu F B, Sigal R J, Rich-Edwards J W et al 1999a Walking compared with vigorous physical activity and risk of type 2 diabetes in women. Journal of the American Medical Association 282:1433–1439

Hu F B, Manson J E, Liu S et al 1999b Prospective study of adult onset diabetes mellitus (type 2) and risk of colorectal cancer in women. Journal of the National Cancer Institute 91(6):542–547

IDF (International Diabetes Federation) 2003 International Diabetes Federation. Online. Available: http://www.idf.org/home/index May 2004

Idzior-Walus B, Mattock M B, Solnica B et al 2001 Factors associated with plasma lipids and lipoproteins in type I diabetes mellitus: the EURODIAB IDDM Complications Study. Diabetic Medicine 18(10):786–796

Jaber L A, Melchior W R, Rutledge D R 1992 Possible correlation between glycemia and blood pressure in black, diabetic, hypertensive patients. Annals of Phamacotherapy 26:882–886

Jeng C, Ku C T, Huang W H 2003 Establishment of a predictive model of serum glucose changes under different exercise intensities and durations among patients with type 2 diabetes mellitus. Journal of Nursing Research 11(4):287–294

Kamiya H, Nakamura J, Hamada Y et al 2003 Polyol pathway and protein kinase C activity of rat Schwannoma cells. Diabetes/Metabolism Research Reviews 19(2):131–139

Keating F K, Sobel B E, Schneider D J 2003 Effects of increased concentrations of glucose on platelet reactivity in healthy subjects and in patients with and without diabetes mellitus. American Journal of Cardiology 92(11):1362–1365

Kelleher C C, Mitropoulos K A, Imeson J et al 1992 Hageman factor and risk of myocardial infarction in middle-aged men. Atherosclerosis 97:67–73

Kelley D E, Goodpaster B H 1999 Effects of physical activity on insulin action and glucose tolerance in obesity. Medicine and Science in Sports and Exercise 31(11 Suppl):S619–S623

Kennedy J W, Hirshman M F, Gervino E V et al 1999 Acute exercise induces GLUT 4 translocation in skeletal muscle of normal human subjects and type 2 diabetics. Diabetes 48(5):1192–1197

Kim I J, Kim Y K, Son S M et al 2003a Enhanced vascular production of superoxide in OLETF rat after the onset of hyperglycaemia. Diabetes Research and Clinical Practice 60(1):11–18

Kim S H, Park K W, Kim T S et al 2003b Effects of acute hyperglycemia on endothelium-dependent vasodilation in patients with diabetes mellitus or impaired glucose metabolism. Endothelium 10(2):65–70

Kohno K, Matsuoka H, Takenaka K et al 2000 Depressor effect by exercise training is associated with the amelioration of hyperinsulinaemia and sympathetic overactivity. Internal Medicine 39(12):1013–1019

Koivisto V A, Felig P 1978 Effects of leg exercise on insulin absorption in diabetic patients. New England Journal of Medicine 298(2):79–83

Kopp W 2003 High-insulinogenic nutrition–an etiologic factor for obesity and the metabolic syndrome? Metabolism: Clinical and Experimental 52(7):840–844

Kraniou Y, Cameron-Smith D, Misso M et al 2000 Effects of exercise on GLUT-4 and glycogenin gene expression in human skeletal muscle. Journal of Applied Physiology 88(2):794–796

Ledet T 1976 Growth hormone stimulating the growth of arterial medial cells in vitro. Absence of effect of insulin. Diabetes 25(11):1011–1017

Leutholtz B C, Ripoll I 1999 Exercise and disease management. CRC Press, Boca Raton, FL

Lewis B 1976 Disorders in lipid transport. In: The hyperglycaemias: clinical and laboratory practice. Blackwell Scientific Publications, Oxford, p 9.58–9.70

Lewis G F, Carpentier A, Adeli K et al 2002 Disordered fat storage and mobilization in the pathogenesis of insulin resistance and type 2 diabetes. Endocrine Reviews 23(2):201–229

Ljung T, Ottosson M, Ahlberg A C et al 2002 Central and peripheral glucocorticoid receptor function in abdominal obesity. Journal of Endocrine Investigation 25(3):229–235

Lulsegged A, Sharma S 2001 Diabetic Ketosis. Online. Available: http://www.medibyte.com/cme/tutorial108/tutdia.htm April 2004

Lund S, Holman G D, Zierath J R et al 1997 Effect of insulin on GLUT 4 translocation and turnover rate in human skeletal muscle as measured by exofacial bismannose photolabeling technique. Diabetes 46:1965–1969

Lutoslawska G 2000 Review: the influence of physical exercise on glucose transport into the muscle. Medicina Sportiva 5(1):9–15

McAuley K A, Williams S M, Mann J I et al 2002 Intensive lifestyle changes are necessary to improve insulin sensitivity: a randomized controlled trial. Diabetes Care 25:445–452

MacDonald M J 1987 Postexercise late-onset hypoglycemia in insulin-dependent diabetic patients. Diabetes Care 10(5):584–588

Manson J E, Rimm E B, Stampfer M J et al 1991 Physical activity and incidence of NIDDM in women. Lancet 338(8770):774–778

Manson J E, Nathan D M, Krolewski A S et al 1992 A prospective study of exercise and incidence of diabetes among USA male physicians. Journal of the American Medical Association 268:63–67

Meyer D E, Baumgartner H R 1983 Role of von Willebrand factor in platelet adhesion to the subendothelium. British Journal of Haematology 54:1–9

Mitropoulos K A, Martin J C, Reeves B E A et al 1989 The activation of the contact phase of coagulation by physiological surfaces in plasma: the effect of large negatively charged lyposomal vesicles. Blood 73:1525

Nagasawa J, Sato Y, Ishiko T 1991 Time course of in vivo insulin sensitivity after a single bout of exercise in rats. International Journal of Sports Medicine 12(4):399–402

NHANES (National Health and Nutrition Examination Survey) 2002 National Health and Nutrition Examination Survey. Department of Health and Human Services, USA

NIH (National Institutes of Health) 2000 Physiological effects of insulin. Online. Available: http://arbl.cvmbs.colostate.edu/hbooks/pathphys/endocrine/pancreas/insulin_phys.html November 2001

Obrosova J G 2002 How does glucose generate oxidative stress in peripheral nerve? International Review of Neurobiology 50:3–35

Patel A 1999 Diabetes in focus. Pharmaceutical Press, London

Pouliot M C, Despres J P, Lemineux S et al 1994 Waist circumference and abdominal sagittal diameter: Best simple anthropometric indexes of abdominal visceral adipose tissue accumulation and related cardiovascular risk in men and women. American Journal of Cardiology 73:460–468

Preuss H G 1997 Effects of glucose/insulin perturbations on aging and chronic disorders of aging: the evidence. Journal of the American College of Nutrition 16:397–403

Ramachandran A, Snehalatha C, Satyayani K et al 2000 Cosegregation of obesity with familial aggregation of type 2 diabetes mellitus. Diabetes, Obesity and Metabolism 2(3):129–154

Rodgers M A, Yamamoto C, King D S et al 1988 Improved glucose tolerance after 1 wk of exercise in patients with mild NIDDM. Diabetes Care 11:613–618

Ryder J W, Gilber L, Zierath J R 2001 Skeletal muscle and insulin sensitivity: pathophysiological alterations. Frontiers in Bioscience 6:D154–163

Saltiel A R, Kahn C R 2001 Insulin signalling and the regulation of glucose and lipid metabolism. Nature 414(6865):799–806

Schneider S H, Kim H C, Khachadurian A K, Ruderman N B 1988 Impaired fibrinolytic response to exercise in type II diabetes: effects of exercise and physical training. Metabolism 37:924–929

Shafrir E, Ziv E 1998 Cellular mechanism of nutritionally induced insulin resistance: the desert rodent Psammomys obesus and other animals in which insulin resistance leads to detrimental outcome. Journal of Basic and Clinical Physiology and Pharmacology 9(2–4):347–385

Sharma A, Haldiya S S 2002 Insulin sensitivity in pre-eclampsia. Journal of the Association of Physicians of India 50:1022–1027

Spector A A 1984 Plasma lipid transport. Clinical Physiology and Biochemistry 2:123–134

Stout R W 1985 Hyperinsulinaemia – a possible risk factor for cardiovascular disease in diabetes mellitus. Hormone and Metabolic Research 15(Suppl):37–41

Terranova A 1991 The effects of diabetes mellitus on wound healing. Plastic Surgical Nursing 11(1):20–25

Thompson G R 1989 A hand book of hyperlipidaemia. Current Science, London

Tokmakidis S, Angelopoulos T, Mitrakou A et al 2000 The role of exercise in the prevention and management of diabetes mellitus. Exercise and Society Journal of Sport Science 24:9–29

UKPDS (UK Prospective Diabetes Study) Group 1998 Intensive blood-glucose control with sulphonylureas or insulin compared with conventional treatment and risk of complications in patients with type 2 diabetes. Lancet 352:837–853

Vander A J, Sherman J H, Luciano D S 1990 Human physiology, 5th edn. McGraw-Hill, New York

Viberti G 1997 Diabetic nephropathy. Medicine 25:32–35

Voiculescu A, Hollenbeck M, Kutkuhn B et al 2003 Successful treatment of renovascular hypertension has no effect on insulin sensitivity. European Journal of Clinical Investigation 33(10):848–854

Volger E 1986 Hemorheologic findings in diabetes and their clinical relevance. Wiener Medizinische Wochenschrift. Journal Suisse de Medecine 136:5–10

Wallberg-Henriksson H, Holloszy J O 1984 Contractile activity increases glucose uptake by muscle in severely diabetic rats. Journal of Applied Physiology 57:1045–1049

Westerlind K C 2003 Physical activity and cancer prevention – mechanisms. Medicine and Science in Sports and Exercise 35(11):1834–1840

White R D, Sherman C 1999 Exercise in diabetes management. The Physician and Sportsmedicine 4(27):63–64, 66, 71, 74, 76

Wojtaszewski J F, Hansen B F, Gade J et al 2000 Insulin signalling and insulin sensitivity after exercise in human skeletal muscle. Diabetes 49(3):325–331

Wolf G, Schroeder R, Thaiss F et al 1998 Glomerular expression of p27Kip 1 in diabetic db/db mouse: role of hyperglycemia. Kidney International 53(4):869–879

Zimmerman B R 1994 Glycaemia control in diabetes mellitus. Towards the normal profile? Drugs 47:611–621

Zonderland M L, Dubbeldam S, Erkelens D W et al 2000 Lower beta-cell secretion in physical activity first-degree relatives of type II diabetes patients. Metabolism: Clinical and Experimental 49(7):833–838

Chapter 5

Blood pressure and hypertension

CHAPTER CONTENTS

Prevalence of hypertension   81
Definition   82
Blood pressure   82
Mechanisms that control blood pressure   82
  Renin–angiotensin–aldosterone system and blood
    pressure control   83
Primary hypertension   83
  Risk factors for developing primary
    hypertension   83
    Smoking   83
    Obesity   83
    Insulin resistance   84
    Increasing age   84
    Excess sodium intake   84
    Low physical activity   84
Secondary hypertension   84
Orthostatic or postural hypotension   85
Pathophysiology of hypertension   85
  Diastolic dysfunction, LVH and CAD   85
  Systolic dysfunction   85
  Stroke and cerebrovascular accidents   85
  Aorta and peripheral vasculature   86
  Nephropathy (disease of the kidneys)   86
  Hypertensive retinopathy   86
Treatment   86
  Pharmacological   86
  Non-pharmacological   86
Physical activity and exercise   87
Single bout of physical activity/exercise   87
  Local metabolites   87
Regular aerobic exercise   87
  Mechanisms   87
  Sympathetic nervous system   88
  Renin–angiotensin–aldosterone system   88
  Insulin   88
  Structural   88

Types of aerobic physical activity/exercise   88
Resistance training   89
Physical activity/exercise prescription   89
  Category A and B and stage I   89
    Intensity   90
    Monitoring intensity   90
    Duration   90
  Category C and stages II and III   90
    Intensity   90
    Duration   90
  Resistance circuit training and weight training   90
Considerations and contraindications   91
Summary   91
Suggested readings, references and bibliography   91

PREVALENCE OF HYPERTENSION

Hypertension (HT) is endemic throughout the world and is considered to be a significant public health problem, especially in middle-aged and elderly individuals. It is estimated that nearly 50 million people in the USA have this disorder (Burt et al 1995) and figures from the Australian Bureau of Statistics (2002) state that around 16% of Australians over the age of 18 years are hypertensive. Although the incidence of HT has been reported to be declining in the West (WHO 1986–1995, National Center for Health Statistics 1994), in countries like Mexico (Secretaria de Salud 1996) and the Middle East (National Nutritional Survey 1998) it appears to be still rising; and yet despite this decrease in the West it has been estimated that more than half of the 10 million individuals over 65 years of age in the UK are hypertensive (Colhoun et al 1998).

DEFINITION

Hypertension is defined as an abnormally high blood pressure (BP) (>140–159 mmHg systolic or >89–99 mmHg diastolic, AMA 1998) and is a primary risk factor for coronary heart disease (CHD). However, it must be noted that the classifications for BP differ slightly between the USA (Jones & Hall 2004) and Europe. The main difference is that in the USA guideline BPs of 120–139 mmHg systolic and 80–89 mmHg diastolic are termed 'prehypertension' and in Europe they have retained the previous classification of pressures for 'high normal' (Table 5.1). Hypertension often displays no symptoms, and around a third of those estimated to be hypertensive are unaware of their condition. Moreover, HT is highly related to other disorders, such as non-lethal myocardial infarction (MI) (heart attack), stroke and permanent retina and kidney damage, and because of the lack of symptoms is aptly named 'the silent killer'. The risk to health is evident even for those with 'high normal' BP (130–139 mmHg systolic or 85–89 mmHg diastolic, Table 5.1), as there is a linear relationship between BP and the related diseases. Therefore, high BP left untreate will soon lead to health complications. In some individuals, HT remains asymptomatic until the occurrence of an acute cardiovascular event, such as MI. It is evident therefore that screening for HT is extremely important, especially as one increases in age.

Several factors have been associated with HT (p. 83); thus it is difficult to clearly pinpoint the exact cause. The majority of hypertensives have what is termed *essential* or *primary* HT where the cause of their condition is unknown. Hypertension with an attributable cause is termed *secondary* HT. Primary or essential (p. 83) HT can in most cases be treated but is difficult to cure, as the cause is unknown. However, secondary (p. 84) HT is often curable as the cause can often be determined.

BLOOD PRESSURE

Blood pressure is essential for the function of the human body as it maintains a constant flow of blood to the tissues and organs. Blood pressure tends to increase with age (p. 84) and is dependent upon body size. For example, normal weight children and adolescents have lower blood pressure than normal weight adults. Blood pressure also varies within an individual and can change very quickly as it is very sensitive to emotions, such as stress and anxiety. An example of this is known as the 'white coat syndrome'. For instance, a doctor can induce patient stress merely by taking the BP and thereby cause the patient's BP to rise. However, in a relaxed and familiar situation the patient's BP tends to normalize and a truer indication can be gained.

MECHANISMS THAT CONTROL BLOOD PRESSURE

There are three major systems that are responsible for BP control and these are the heart, the blood vessels and the kidneys. These systems are also sensitive to hormones and chemicals, such as catecholamines and angiotensin II, which influence cardiac contractility and vasoconstriction, respectively (p. 83).

Cardiac output ($\dot{Q}$) and the total peripheral resistance (TPR) within the blood vessels have a significant effect on BP and alterations in either or both will cause BP to change. Likewise, $\dot{Q}$ is also influenced by stroke volume (SV) and heart rate (HR) and changes in these will also have an effect. Furthermore, SV is affected by cardiac contractility and venous return (Starling's law, p. 87) to the heart. Hence any factor that influences SV, HR and TPR will have an effect on BP (Fig. 5.1).

Hypertension is often seen as a cardiovascular problem. However, if $\dot{Q}$ and TPR are high, renal excretion can decrease blood pressure to normal by reducing the intravascular volume. Renal participation can normalize BP

Table 5.1 Blood pressure classifications for adults over 18 years and follow-up recommendations (AMA 1998, and Primary Care Clinical Effectiveness Guidelines 2000)

Category	Systolic BP (mmHg)		Diastolic BP (mmHg)	Follow-up recommendations
Optimal	<120	And	<80	Recheck in 2 years
Normal	120–129	And	80–84	Recheck in 2 years
High normal	130–139	Or	85–89	Recheck in 1 year
Hypertension				
Stage/grade I hypertension (mild)	140–159	Or	90–99	Confirmation within 2 months
Stage/grade II hypertension (moderate)	160–179	Or	100–109	Evaluate within 1 month
Stage/grade III hypertension (severe)	180 or >	Or	110 or >	Evaluate immediately or within 1 week
Isolated systolic hypertension	>140	With	<90	Not stated

A diagnosis of hypertension is based upon two or more BP readings taken at separate visits.

> $BP = \dot{Q} \times TPR$; changes in $\dot{Q}$ and/or TPR will affect BP
> $\dot{Q} = SV \times HR$; SV = cardiac contractility and venous return to the heart

Figure 5.1   Factors that contribute toward blood pressure.

even though the problem may not be in the kidneys. However, the kidney can induce a volume-based HT by retaining excessive sodium and water (Deshmukh et al 1997).

RENIN–ANGIOTENSIN–ALDOSTERONE SYSTEM AND BLOOD PRESSURE CONTROL

The kidneys' contribution to the control of blood pressure is based around many factors that influence the secretion of an enzyme known as *renin*. Renin catalyzes the cleavage of *angiotensin I* from a larger plasma protein called *angiotensinogen*, which is then converted to *angiotensin II* by a converting enzyme (angiotensin-converting enzyme (ACE)). Angiotensin II is a powerful vasoconstrictor, acting on the arterioles. It is also the predominant regulator of aldosterone synthesis and secretion. Aldosterone is secreted by the adrenal cortex (as is the catecholamine adrenaline). It acts on the distal renal tubule and also on the gut to promote the reabsorption of sodium and the secretion of potassium and hydrogen ions. The absence of aldosterone can cause the excretion of around 15 g of sodium per day, whereas, the presence of aldosterone will cause virtually no sodium to be excreted. Hence, the presence of aldosterone can cause an increase in blood volume through the retention of sodium and water. Thus the renin–angiotensin–aldosterone system plays a central role in the regulation of arterial BP and in the maintenance of sodium and potassium homeostasis (Vander et al 1990, Cartledge & Lawson 2000).

Renin is released in response to various physiological factors, the most important being sodium depletion, decrease in blood volume and pressure, and beta-adrenergic stimulation. Whenever the systemic BP falls, the rate of renin release increases (due to activation of the renal baroreceptors' stimulation of the sympathetic nervous system (SNS)). The elevation of circulating renin leads to an increase in the rate of angiotensin II formation. This promotes arteriolar vasoconstriction and maintenance of BP, and via the action of aldosterone, the increased reabsorption of sodium by the kidneys. It should be noted, that the renin–angiotensin–aldosterone system also interacts with several systemic circulatory and local factors (Cartledge & Lawson 2000).

PRIMARY HYPERTENSION

It is estimated that 95% of a hypertensive patient's condition is not definable, and because of the strong relationship between HT and certain ethic groups, such as African Americans (AHA 1997), it is probable that there are different underlying defects in different populations. Primary HT is likely to result from a synergy of many BP regulatory defects and interaction with environmental stressors. These may be acquired or genetically determined and independent of each other. Genetic factors are important in primary HT, although the markers have yet to be identified. Nonetheless, it is thought that genetic abnormalities include sodium sensitivity (p. 84) and/or abnormally high autonomic nervous system response to external stressors.

Around 80% of those with primary HT have stage I HT (Table 5.1) and the remaining 20% have either moderate or severe degrees. Since the majority of hypertensives have primary as opposed to secondary HT, primary HT is responsible for greater morbidity and mortality.

From a review on the prevalence of high BP, it appears that the main risk factors for HT are heredity, low birth weight for gestational age, large increase in weight as a teenager, low physical activity and excessive alcohol consumption (Krzesinski 2002). Other contributing factors for primary hypertension are thought to be smoking, age, hyperinsulinaemia and sodium sensitivity and consumption.

RISK FACTORS FOR DEVELOPING PRIMARY HYPERTENSION

Smoking

Smoking has been identified as a risk factor for HT as it leads to changes in the vasculature (Ch. 2, p. 10) and has a temporary effect on the nervous system. Nicotine causes a transient vasoconstriction and an increase in HR leading to augmented peripheral resistance and cardiac output, respectively. Smoking a cigarette can raise BP by about 5–10 mmHg for around 30 minutes, and combined with caffeine the effect is even greater and lasts for longer. Despite this, epidemiological studies have found that smokers and non-smokers of the same weight tend to have similar BP (National Cancer Institute 1995).

Obesity

There is a relationship between HT, hyperinsulinaemia and obesity (Pouliot et al 1994). A review from the department of medicine at the University of Mississippi (Wofford et al 2002) stated that obesity is closely associated with HT, and is now recognized as an independent risk factor for cardiovascular disease. Indeed a study carried out by Jones (1996) found that when overweight individuals lost weight there were also reductions in their BP. It was further concluded that there could have been additional reductions in BP with the inclusion of hypertensive drug therapy. However, the mechanisms linking changes in weight with changes in BP are complex and still not fully understood. Nonetheless, the link between obesity and insulin sensitivity may be a contributing factor.

Insulin resistance

Hyperinsulinaemia is defined as excessively high levels of blood insulin (see Ch. 4, p. 64, and Ch. 6, p. 102) and can lead to an increase in BP. Although the hypertensive mechanisms of insulin are not yet fully known, reductions in BP have been observed in association with a fall in blood glucose levels (Jaber et al 1992). High levels of insulin are known to stimulate the SNS (Facchini et al 1996) to release catecholamines (noradrenaline and adrenaline). Catecholamines cause an increase in sympathetic tone, which contributes to the stimulation of the renin–angiotensin–aldosterone system (Esler et al 2001), resulting in vasoconstriction and aldosterone-led renal sodium reabsorption, and an increase in intravascular volume (p. 83). Catecholamines also increase HR and force of myocardial contractility leading to enhanced cardiac output, all of which contribute towards an increase in BP. The release of sympathetic neurotransmitters, principally the catecholamine noradrenaline and the hormone adrenaline (transported in the blood), cause the heart rate to speed up by acting on special beta-adrenergic$_1$ receptors (beta$_1$ receptors). However, the effect of these catecholamines on the beta$_1$ receptors of the smooth vascular muscle is vasoconstriction, thereby increasing TPR and BP.

High levels of circulating insulin are also associated with the acceleration of atherosclerosis and vascular damage (Preuss 1997). This is caused, in part, by consistently high levels of circulating insulin stimulating arterial vascular smooth muscle hypertrophy, which as a consequence alters membrane ion transport leading to an increase in intracellular calcium and augmentation of vascular tone and BP. It can therefore be seen that hyperinsulinaemia has a considerable pathophysiological effect contributing to various diseases.

Increasing age

Rates of HT tend to increase with age. Whether this is partly due to age-related diseases, such as coronary heart and vascular disease, or ageing per se is difficult to determine clearly. However, the vascular changes related to ageing do tend to result in an increase in BP.

In hypertensive individuals of less than 40 years it is cardiac output that is relatively high with normal peripheral resistance. However, over time and with increasing age the contribution from cardiac output tends to decline, while peripheral resistance increases as the heart and vessels adapt to prolonged stress. Hypertrophy of the vessels due to disease also causes a narrowing of the lumen, further contributing to an increase in BP (Lilly 1997, Copstead & Banasik 2000). The tension produced by the heart muscle after contraction (afterload) as a result of HT leads to an increase in left ventricular wall thickness (concentric hypertrophy), which causes a reduction in diastolic filling (Liebson et al 1993). This is also seen in healthy individuals where concentric remodelling of the left ventricle (LV) is the result of the age-related stiffening of the arterial tree (Ganau et al 1995). This stiffening causes a reduction in vessel compliance that leads to the often age-related elevation in systolic blood pressure (SBP) (Guyton & Hall 1996). All of these factors have an effect on BP whether as a result of disease or increasing age.

Excess sodium intake

Epidemiological studies indicate that excess sodium intake is associated with high BP (Krzesinski 2002). There is also evidence to suggest that only the blood pressure of individuals who have a genetic predisposition toward sodium sensitivity will be affected by its consumption (Saruta et al 1995). This is supported by the fact that those who are insensitive to sodium tend not to show a reduction in BP when sodium intake is reduced (Guyton & Hall 1996). Type II diabetics, obese and hypertensive individuals are often sodium sensitive and usually respond to a reduction in intake after about 2 to 5 weeks (Conlin et al 2000, Feldstein 2002). Although the mechanisms regarding sensitivity are not fully known there does appear to be an interaction between sodium intake and noradrenaline concentration, which is capable of influencing blood pressure (Rankin et al 1981). In a study on rats it was found that the ingestion of sodium was associated with an increase in plasma angiotensin II (Hodge et al 2002), a potent vasoconstrictor, the effect of which is to increase peripheral resistance (p.83). Sodium retention occurs in exchange for potassium. Therefore, it has been postulated that BP may be controlled by an increase in potassium intake (Geleijnse et al 1996).

Low physical activity

The contribution of physical activity to the control of hypertension is of prime concern to the exercise practitioner (p. 87).

SECONDARY HYPERTENSION

Secondary HT is relatively uncommon and affects approximately 5% of hypertensives. It is often curable; however, if left untreated it can lead to adaptive cardiovascular problems (Ch. 2). Secondary HT is not known to be associated with insulin insensitivity but there does appear to be a genetic link. The cause is usually structural or hormonal and is indicated when it develops in young individuals less than 20 years of age. Furthermore, it presents abruptly, with BP raised to stage III rather than stages I or II (Table 5.1) (Deshmukh et al 1997). The most common cause of secondary HT for both adults and children is renal disease (Sadowski & Falkner 1996). Endocrine, neurological and vascular disorders also contribute to secondary HT (Copstead & Banasik 2000), as do exogenous factors, such as the oral contraceptive pill and other medications. Occasionally pregnant women develop a condition known as gestational HT, which is an abnormal rise in BP that often returns to normal postpartum.

ORTHOSTATIC OR POSTURAL HYPOTENSION

Orthostatic or postural hypotension is common in individuals with low BP, cardiovascular disease and/or taking medication to lower BP. It is characterized by a lack of venous return to the heart as a result of low BP (hypotension). This can cause a reduction in cerebral blood flow causing an individual to feel dizzy, light-headed or syncopic. Postural hypotension generally occurs when an individual moves from a supine to an upright position. When an upright position is assumed blood volume transiently shifts to the lower limbs. The baroreceptors in the carotid arteries and aortic arch sense a fall in circulating volume and trigger mechanisms (renin–angiotensin–aldosterone system) that cause peripheral vasoconstriction and an increase in HR to restore arterial BP (Copstead & Banasik 2000). The normal postural response to moving from a supine to an upright position is an increase in HR of about 15% above rest, and a decrease of up to 15 mmHg SBP and change in diastolic blood pressure (DBP) of around 10 mmHg (Guyton & Hall 1996). Changes in SBP and/or DBP greater than these values will result in postural hypotension. The lack of fluid volume returning to the heart as a result of these changes in BP will prevent the prompt return to normal BP with the postural change and cause postural hypotension.

Individuals with cardiovascular disease may have impaired responses to postural changes as a result of cardiac and/or vascular damage. Impaired vasoconstriction and/or HR response will cause a lack of venous return and consequently postural hypotension will occur. Diabetics who have peripheral neuropathy (which may limit vasoconstriction) are also susceptible to postural hypotension, especially if they are on medications to reduce fluid volume and BP (Copstead & Banasik 2000).

It is therefore important that the exercise practitioner be aware of those who are prone to postural hypotension and modify the individual's programme appropriately by avoiding sudden changes in posture.

PATHOPHYSIOLOGY OF HYPERTENSION

If left untreated, HT can lead to left ventricular hypertrophy (LVH), diastolic dysfunction, systolic dysfunction, coronary artery disease (CAD), cerebrovascular accidents (such as stroke), structural alterations to the aorta and peripheral vasculature, nephropathy (nephrosclerosis) and hypertensive retinopathy (Deshmukh et al 1997).

DIASTOLIC DYSFUNCTION, LVH AND CAD

Hypertension places an abnormally high stress on the arteries and arterioles, especially if left untreated over a long period of time. This can lead to a reduction in arterial elasticity and compliance, hardening of the vessels and CAD. Hypertension requires the heart to use more energy to work against the greater peripheral resistance. More energy requires more oxygen and, for someone with CHD/CAD, hypertension may eventually lead to angina pectoris (Ch. 2). Over time, the LV of the heart adapts to consistently having to work against an abnormally high pressure. It becomes thickened and enlarged (concentric hypertrophy) and less powerful, leading to LVH. Left ventricular hypertrophy affects diastolic filling eventually causing diastolic dysfunction. The weight of an average heart is about 500 g but an enlarged heart can be less efficient and weigh as much as 800 g. In the Framingham study LVH was associated with 21–33% mortality within 5 years of diagnosis (Kannel 1991).

SYSTOLIC DYSFUNCTION

Systolic dysfunction will generally occur if HT is left untreated. Left ventricular hypertrophy is initially compensatory through an increase in LV mass. However, this may be insufficient to offset the high wall tension caused by the increase in the tension produced by the heart muscle after contraction (afterload). Over time, LV contractility decreases, which leads to a decrease in cardiac output leading to systolic dysfunction and eventually pulmonary congestion with the back up of fluid. This can often be detected by oscilloscope from crackles in the lungs and an extra heart sound, dyspnoea (breathlessness) and fatigue.

STROKE AND CEREBROVASCULAR ACCIDENTS

Stroke was given its name because it happens very suddenly and the effects are often physically striking. Cerebrovascular accidents such as stroke are closely linked to the magnitude of SBP. High SBP leading to stroke can be the result of either a haemorrhage from ruptured microaneurysms, thrombosis or embolism (Ch. 7) or general narrowing of the vessels causing a significant reduction in blood flow to the tissue of the brain.

Table 5.2   Recommended lifestyle modifications for those with hypertension (adapted Leutholtz & Ripoll 1999 and ACSM 2000 guidelines for exercise testing and prescription)

Reduce body weight	For every 2 lb (~1 kg) of weight loss there is around a 2 mmHg reduction in mean arterial BP
Limit alcohol consumption	No more than 30 ml and 15 ml of ethanol for men and women (or lightweight individuals), respectively, the latter being around 720 ml beer or 300 ml wine per day
Reduce sodium intake	<2.4–3.0 g per day
Maintain potassium intake	3.5 g per day (about one banana)
Stop smoking	Prevent further vascular damage
Reduce saturated fat intake and cholesterol intake	<300 mg cholesterol per day to reduce CHD risk
Increase physical activity	Reduces risk of HT and CHD

It is therefore imperative that those will high resting SBP do not exercise until it is under control (Table 5.2).

AORTA AND PERIPHERAL VASCULATURE

Hypertension can contribute to an increase in atherosclerosis, which results in plaque formation and narrowing of arterial vasculature contributing to increased peripheral resistance. Furthermore, the damage to the vessels can also affect the vasodilatory mechanisms, again contributing to an increased peripheral resistance. Over time, the increase in peripheral resistance can weaken the vessel walls, particularly in areas of high mechanical stress such as the aorta (particularly in the abdominal area), which can in some cases lead to aneurysms.

NEPHROPATHY (DISEASE OF THE KIDNEYS)

It is clear that HT can lead to smooth muscle hypertrophy, resulting in a thickening of the vessel walls. This is also true for the vasculature of the kidneys, which can lead to a reduction in the blood supply to the kidneys, producing ischaemic atrophy of tubules and glomeruli and resulting in renal failure. This compromises the kidneys' ability to regulate blood volume, further contributing to an increase in BP.

HYPERTENSIVE RETINOPATHY

A visual examination is often able to detect poorly controlled blood pressure. This is usually evident by small indentations of the retinal veins and is often an asymptomatic clinical marker of high blood pressure. In severe HT small retinal vessels may burst, causing haemorrhages and local infarction resulting in blurred vision. Another condition not generally seen in those with chronic HT is a swelling of the optic disc known as papilloedema. This is the result of very high BP causing high intracranial pressure.

TREATMENT

Reductions in BP have been associated with decreased rates of mortality and morbidity (Roman et al 2002, Zarnke et al 2002). Figures from the USA show that a reduction of 15 mmHg and 6 mmHg for SBP and DBP, respectively, can reduce the risk of stroke by around 4% and CHD by around 19% over 5 years (National Center for Health Statistics 1995). Primary HT is usually treated by the use of medications and non-pharmacological treatments, such as lifestyle changes (Table 5.2). For those with high normal or stage I BP (Table 5.1) without organ damage, lifestyle changes may be effective on their own. However, for those with stage II or III hypertension, a mixture of pharmacological and non-pharmacological interventions should be employed.

PHARMACOLOGICAL

Pharmacological treatments can significantly reduce HT and risk of complications and there are numerous hypertensive medications on the market. These range in type from diuretics, vasodilators, angiotensin-converting enzyme (ACE) inhibitors, angiotensin II receptor antagonists to sympatholyic agents such as beta-blockers (Ch. 2, p. 13).

NON-PHARMACOLOGICAL

Lifestyle modifications include weight reduction, dietary intervention, smoking cessation, relaxation therapy and an increase in physical activity (PA)/exercise (Table 5.2).

The connection between weight reduction and fall in BP, although not yet fully understood, is probably related to the relationship between body weight, high circulating levels of insulin (hyperinsulinaemia) and catecholamines. The link between alcohol consumption and high BP is again not fully known but reductions in consumption are associated with reduced SBP. Despite the epidemiological link between sodium reduction and decrease in BP, this treatment may only be effective for those who are sodium sensitive.

Caffeine and nicotine have a transient effect on BP and therefore need to be modified. Caffeine raises BP through the stimulation of the SNS, which increases vessel tone and stiffness (Mahmud & Feely 2001, Okuno et al 2002). Smoking cessation is also extremely important in the treatment of HT because of its links with atherosclerosis (Ch. 2) and its transient effect on the nervous system. Relaxation therapy is also a valuable tool in the reduction of BP, especially for those who have an abnormally high autonomic nervous system response to external stressors.

PHYSICAL ACTIVITY AND EXERCISE

Low levels of physical fitness have been associated with increased risk for all-cause mortality in normotensive and hypertensive men (Blair et al 1991). However, since fitness is highly dependent upon genetic factors, the relationship between energy expenditure and physical activity probably gives a better indication of the influence of PA/exercise upon BP. Evidence suggests that those who expend more than 2000 kcal per week through physical activity have a significantly lower risk of developing HT than those who expend less than this amount (Paffenbarger et al 1983). A review of various interventional studies has shown that regular aerobic exercise reduces BP in both normotensive and hypertensive adults (Fagard & Tipton 1994), and although the mechanisms of training-induced hypotension are not fully known, a more recent review estimated that in about 75% of hypertensive individuals systolic and diastolic BP decreased by an average of 11 mmHg and 8 mmHg, respectively (Hagberg et al 2000).

SINGLE BOUT OF PHYSICAL ACTIVITY/EXERCISE

During an acute bout of aerobic activity there is a gradual increase in SBP due to an increase in stroke volume and cardiac output (due to the influence of catecholamines). In healthy adults SBP will peak during exercise at around 180–210 mmHg. However, for normotensive men, elevated SBP during exercise recovery is a predictor of new-onset HT (Singh et al 1999 (Framingham study)), which is an indication of preclinical, pathophysiological cardiovascular changes (ACSM 2001). The acute effect of exercise on DBP tends to show either no change or a decrease (60–85 mmHg) (due to dilation in the peripheral vasculature from the effect of catecholamines on the beta$_2$ receptors); and in normotensive adults an enhanced diastolic response to exercise is also a predictor of new-onset HT (Singh et al 1999 (Framingham study)). It has also been demonstrated that during exercise men at high risk of HT also show blood pressures ≥230 mmHg systolic and 100 mmHg diastolic. This is thought to be the result of a blunting in

vasodilation causing an increase in peripheral resistance during exercise (Wilson et al 1990).

An acute bout of mild to moderate aerobic exercise has been shown to reduce BP post-exercise (exercise hypotension) for both normotensive and hypertensive individuals. For example, when stage I hypertensive adults underwent 30 minutes of treadmill exercise at 50% and at 75% $\dot{V}O_2$max there were significant mean post-exercise reductions in systolic and diastolic blood pressure of 4 and 9 mmHg and 5 and 7 mmHg, respectively. These reductions in BP remained for around 13 and 4 hours for SBP, and for 11 and 4 hours for DBP, from exercise at 50% and at 75% $\dot{V}O_2$max, respectively. These results suggest that the greater the intensity the longer the post-exercise effect (Quinn 2000). However, for hypertensives with organ damage and stage II or III BP, exercise greater than 50% $\dot{V}O_2$max would not be recommended.

The mechanism for exercise hypotension is mainly due to a reduction in peripheral resistance as a result of the vasodilatory effect of local metabolites and the catecholamine stimulation of the beta$_2$ receptors.

LOCAL METABOLITES

During acute activity local metabolites, such as lactic acid, nitric oxide, hydrogen ions, adenosine and prostaglandins, are thought to have a local vasodilatory effect on the working muscles, causing an increase in blood flow (Deshmukh et al 1997). This effect can persist for several minutes after exercise and contributes to post-exercise hypotension (Hussain et al 1996).

REGULAR AEROBIC EXERCISE

The long-term resting adaptations to regular aerobic exercise include a reduction in sympathetic tone (decrease in sympathetic catecholamines), resulting in a decrease in resting HR and increase in stroke volume. The latter is partly associated with an augmented venous return and diastolic filling, leading to an enhanced systolic emptying due to the combined effect of *Starling's law* and enhanced contractile state of the myocardium, resulting in a decrease in SBP. This reduction in SBP and HR also reduces the workload on the heart. A method used to calculate cardiac workload, both at rest and during exercise, is known as the *rate pressure product* (RPP) and is based upon SBP multiplied by HR divided by 100 (RPP = (SBP × HR)/100). It can be a useful tool for determining changes in cardiac workload as a result of exercise intervention (Fig. 5.2).

MECHANISMS

In normotensive subjects it was found that the hypotensive effect of chronic aerobic training was the result of a

$$RPP = \frac{SBP \times HR}{100}$$

Figure 5.2 Calculation for rate pressure product (RPP).

reduction in vascular resistance of about 12–22% despite an increase in cardiac output. However, the mechanisms for the hypotensive effect of exercise on hypertensive patients are difficult to determine (Meredith et al 1990, 1991). Hence the possible mechanisms contributing towards the reduction in blood pressure, as a result of chronic aerobic training (training), are currently based primarily on non-hypertensive individuals.

SYMPATHETIC NERVOUS SYSTEM

Physical training results in a reduction in sympathetic tone at rest as the parasympathetic nervous system (acetylecholine) predominates.

RENIN–ANGIOTENSIN–ALDOSTERONE SYSTEM

Endurance trained athletes have been found to have lower plasma renin activity at rest compared to those who are non-endurance trained (Meyer et al 1988). It has also been found that despite little change in BP, resting plasma renin activity and aldosterone concentration were reduced in a group of 18 ischaemic heart disease patients after training for 3 months, three times a week at 70–90% of their maximal capacity (Vanhees et al 1984). However, in a group of 38 healthy elderly men and women (aged 60–82 years) after 6 months of endurance training, three times a week for 30–45 minutes at 75–85% of maximal HR reserve, there were no changes in aldosterone, sodium, potassium and catecholamines. It was postulated that this was due to a possible resetting of plasma and blood volume receptors (Carroll et al 1995). Nonetheless, the influence of training on the renin–angiotensin–aldosterone system remains to be elucidated as it is complex and may respond differently in different populations.

INSULIN

Insulin resistance is associated with obesity and HT; hence those who are overweight or obese are prone to hyperinsulinaemia (Esler et al 2001). The high circulating levels of plasma insulin lead to an augmentation in SNS activity and sodium reabsorption by the kidney tubules, resulting in an increase in BP. Over a period of time, high BP will also impair the vasculature. A single bout of PA/exercise and physical training increases insulin sensitivity and glucose transport into muscles (Ch. 4, p. 70), which can assist in the control of insulin insensitivity and diabetes (Lutoslawska 2000). Furthermore, since regular aerobic training tends to result in a decrease in body mass, this also helps to reduce insulin resistance and BP (Esler et al 2001). A study on 30 HT patients (63 ± 7 years) looking into the effect of 6 months of aerobic training found an increase in insulin sensitivity. The study also found that the small change in SNS activity had a strong positive relationship with the change in mean arterial BP. It was suggested that the suppression in SNS activity might play a role in the reduction of mean arterial blood pressure in response to aerobic training (Brown et al 2002). Similarly 3 weeks of aerobic training in a group of 29 hypertensive patients, at an intensity of 75% of $\dot{V}O_2$max, showed reductions in BP with parallel changes in insulin resistance. These changes in insulin were correlated with improved baroreflex function and a decrease in HR. Furthermore, the correction in SNS activity was associated with the amelioration of hyperinsulinaemia. These findings suggest that the improvement of neuro-metabolic factors may be involved in the depressor effect caused by aerobic training (Kohno et al 2000).

STRUCTURAL

Aerobic training appears to have no effect on vessel wall thickness; however, the animal model has shown an increase in the lumen area, causing a reduction in peripheral resistance and BP (Amaral et al 2000).

TYPES OF AEROBIC PHYSICAL ACTIVITY/EXERCISE

It is clear that regular aerobic activity is beneficial to those with HT and from the findings of meta-analysis that moderate to low-level intensity is most effective. A meta-analysis of 48 training groups using isotonic endurance exercise, such as walking, jogging, running or cycling, ranging between 4 and 68 weeks (median 16 weeks) with an average of 3 weekly sessions of 15–90 minutes at around 50–85% $\dot{V}O_2$max, found a net average reduction in blood pressure of 5.3 mmHg and 4.8 mmHg for SBP and DBP respectively, with only one of the studies showing an increase in BP. The beneficial changes became apparent at around 2 to 7 weeks of regular training; however, the hypotensive effect did not persist after training ceased. Thus training needs to be current and regular. Furthermore, it appeared that the hypotensive effect of training is greatest in hypertensive individuals (Table 5.3) (Fagard & Tipton 1994). This is commonly seen in exercise physiology where those with initially poor baseline values tend to show a greater potential for change. Nonetheless, the parameters of duration and intensity of training have not yet been able to explain the variance in BP response to training in normotensive or hypertensive individuals. Nevertheless, slightly greater reductions in BP have been found with exercise seven versus three times per week and

Table 5.3 Mean reductions in blood pressure (mmHg) after aerobic training (adapted from Fagard & Tipton 1994)

Category	Systolic blood pressure	Diastolic blood pressure
Normal	3.2	3.1
Borderline hypertensive	6.2	6.8
Hypertensive	9.9	7.6

with moderate versus vigorous exercise, respectively (Fagard & Tipton 1994, Cleroux et al 1999). However, the exact mechanisms for this response are not fully understood, and although low to moderate-intensity aerobic exercise has been found to be the most effective, the optimal frequency, intensity, time and type (FITT) of PA/exercise for HT has still to be determined.

RESISTANCE TRAINING

Weight training, isometric or high anaerobic work is not recommended as the primary exercise therapy for those with hypertension or cardiovascular disease. Isometric and any static component tends to increase afterload (Leutholtz & Ripoll 1999). These types of exercises may also increase HR, BP and RPP and may lead to an ischaemic event. In the past resistance training was also avoided. However, within the past 15–20 years appropriately prescribed resistance training, consisting of low weights and high repetitions, has gained support as a means of improving upper and lower body strength and self-confidence to perform daily tasks that require moderate amounts of strength (Vescovi & Fernhall 2000). Indeed, this type of resistance exercise causes the HR to increase less than aerobic exercise with, in numerous cases, a lower RPP than aerobic training of the same metabolic demand (ACSM 2001). An increase in muscle strength may also reduce RPP, as a given amount of muscular work will be proportionally less of the maximal voluntary muscle

contraction. Hence, there will also be a corresponding reduction in peripheral resistance, SBP and RPP (Franklin 2002).

The majority of studies looking into the effect of resistance training on hypertensive populations have been carried out on only mildly hypertensive subjects. Nevertheless, a meta-analysis looking at 11 studies found an average of a 2% and 4% reduction in resting SBP and DBP, respectively (Kelly & Kelly 2000). Research investigating the combined effect of circuit training and aerobic exercise versus antihypertensive medication on mildly hypertensive men found similar reductions in SBP and DBP (Keleman et al 1990, Stewart et al 1990).

PHYSICAL ACTIVITY/EXERCISE PRESCRIPTION

There are no specific PA/exercise prescription guidelines for those with hypertension. However, the following guidelines are given taking into account the known pathophysiology and evidence-based research.

Prior to the prescription of PA/exercise, an individual must be suitably screened (Appendix A), which should include risk stratification (Table 5.4) and if appropriate undergo some pre-exercise tests (Appendix A). This will assist in determining the appropriate type of PA/exercise programme for each individual.

The demands of the various physical activities will differ physiologically, psychologically and sociologically. It is therefore important for the practitioner to consider all these factors when prescribing to the individual.

CATEGORY A AND B AND STAGE I

Individuals who fall into categories A and B (Table 5.4) and stage I (Table 5.1) HT are initially advised to undertake regular aerobic exercise using large muscle groups, which might later include some resistance circuit training. It is not advisable for these individuals to carry out weight training unless they are low risk and capable of doing so.

Table 5.4 Risk stratification and treatment recommendations for those with hypertension (adapted from ACSM 1993, 2001)

Category	Classification	Recommendation
A	No CHD risk factors, no target organ damage or clinical cardiovascular disease (CVD)	Initial lifestyle modifications (Table 5.2) including exercise for those with high normal BP and stage I HT (Table 5.1)
B	One main CHD risk factor not including diabetes, no target organ damage or CVD	Initial lifestyle modifications (Table 5.2) including exercise for those with high normal BP and stage I HT (Table 5.1)
C	Target organ damage, CVD and/or diabetes with or without other risk factors	Any level of HT or any risk group with stage II and III HT should begin drug therapy prior to PA/exercise intervention. They should also initiate the other lifestyle modifications (Table 5.2)

Intensity

The initial aerobic intensity should start off at around 40% $\dot{V}O_2$max for elderly patients/clients and around 50% $\dot{V}O_2$max for those who are more capable. This can slowly increase over time to a maximum of around 50% $\dot{V}O_2$max for elderly persons and 70% $\dot{V}O_2$max for the majority of hypertensives. Those younger low-risk individuals, when habituated to exercise, may exercise at up to around 85% $\dot{V}O_2$max (if symptom free during exercise), but only if they are capable of working predominantly at an aerobic level. However, the PA/exercise intensity will depend very much upon the capabilities of the individual.

Monitoring intensity

During a session SBP should not exceed 250 mmHg and DBP should not exceed 120 mmHg in order to avoid undue strain on the heart and vasculature. Ratings of perceived exertion (RPE) should also not be greater than 13 (*somewhat hard*) on the 6–20 scale (Nobel et al 1983) (Appendix B) for the same reason.

For those patients who are on medications to lower their BP, such as beta-blockers (Ch. 14) it is better to use RPE. Medications can alter the HR response to activity and should therefore not be relied on as an indicator of exercise intensity. Moreover, once an individual is habituated to PA/exercise and their condition is reasonably stable, for this population, RPE is the preferred method of determining PA/exercise intensity.

Duration

The PA/exercise duration of each session is still very much under debate for asymptomatic and symptomatic individuals. However, the initial session may start at around 10–15 minutes. It is not advisable to increase the duration by more than 10% per week. Exceeding this increment will not allow the individual time to adjust to the activity and may put them at an increased risk of injury. Once the individual can manage about 20 minutes of aerobic activity they may increase the intensity if appropriate. The activity may range between 15 and 90 minutes per session, with between 3 and 7 sessions per week.

CATEGORY C AND STAGES II AND III

Individuals who fall into category C (Table 5.4) or have greater than stage II (Table 5.1) HT should initially undergo pharmacological treatment to stabilize their BP.

It is inadvisable for patients in this category to carry out weight training, but they may incorporate resistance circuit training into their regimen after they have become accustomed to a programme of aerobic training.

Intensity

As with other individuals with BP, this category of hypertensive should carry out aerobic activities at an intensity of 40–50% $\dot{V}O_2$max. When able to exercise at 50% $\dot{V}O_2$max light circuit training may be introduced. These individuals should be encouraged to breathe normally throughout all movements, exhaling on the 'sticking point' and under no circumstances should they hold their breath and force against a closed glottis (Valsalva manoeuvre).

During aerobic activity RPE and target HR should be at a level below that of the individual's peak SBP. If possible it is advisable to find out the individual's maximum SBP. Then a target SBP can be determined using a modified version of the Karvonen equation (for example, a target SBP of 60% of peak may be prescribed, then the equation would be: Target SBP = 0.60 x (peak SBP - resting SBP) + rest SBP = target SBP). Furthermore, during activity BP should not rise above SBP 250 mmHg or DBP 120 mmHg, nor should activity intensity be above an RPE of 13 (*somewhat hard*) (Nobel et al 1983).

Duration

For this category of HT, the duration of aerobic activity may be similar to that for category A, B and stage I, but at a lower intensity, especially at durations longer than 20 minutes.

RESISTANCE CIRCUIT TRAINING AND WEIGHT TRAINING

After a few weeks of training and if deemed appropriate resistance circuit training may be included into the regimen, and once the individual is experienced and stable they can use either free weights or machines, but correct technique must be taught to avoid strain and injury. Breath holding during resistance training (Valsalva manoeuvre) can cause BP to rise to values in excess of 200 mmHg (Childs 1999), placing some individuals at risk of stroke (Narloch & Brandstater 1995). Hence, resistance weight training is not advisable for those in category C and/or whose resting BP is greater than SBP 160 mmHg or DBP 100 mmHg (greater than stage II HT, Table 5.1).

The Valsalva manoeuvre during resistance exercise usually occurs during isometric or heavy resistance exercise of prolonged strenuous effort. The glottis closes and intra-abdominal pressure increases by the forcible contraction of the respiratory muscles. This results in a decrease in venous return to the heart, causing cardiac output to decrease and a transient drop in BP. Baroreceptors of the carotid sinus and aortic arch stimulate the secretion of renin and SNS to maintain BP. However, when the individual exhales there is a rapid return of venous return to the heart, causing an additional increase in BP resulting in an abnormal mechanical load on the heart (Kisner & Colby 1990). Therefore the teaching of correct breathing technique is of great importance for those with hypertension.

CONSIDERATIONS AND CONTRAINDICATIONS

Resting BP values of SBP >200 mmHg or DBP >115 mmHg are considered a contraindication for exercise and attaining SBP >250 mmHg or DBP >120 mmHg during an exercise session would indicate that the exercise session should be terminated (Nobel et al 1983, ACSM 1993), as would a sudden drop in BP (indicating ischaemic threshold and/or ventricular dysfunction). Hypertensives with uncontrolled SBP >160 mmHg or DBP >100 mmHg (stage II hypertension) should avoid circuit and weight training. Contraindications for any circuit weight training would include congestive heart failure, uncontrolled arrhythmias, severe valvular disease, aerobic capacity <17 ml/kg per minute (5 METs, Appendix B).

Patients on vasodilators (Ch. 14, p. 223) will require longer cool-downs to prevent venous pooling following an abrupt cessation of activity. Also, any sudden change in posture that may cause postural hypotension, such as from the supine to the upright position, should be avoided, as should any floor-based exercise that may increase venous return to the heart and cause an increase in cardiac work by increasing SBP through the principle of Starling's law.

As intravascular volume has such an effect on BP, practitioners should make their patients/clients aware of factors that might affect their BP such as heat and humidity and advise them on sufficient fluid intake, especially those on diuretics. Additionally, beta-blockers also impair the ability of the body to regulate temperature. Therefore, patients/clients should be made aware of the potential to develop 'heat illness' when exercising (Ch. 14, p. 223).

SUMMARY

- HT is endemic throughout the world and is a significant public health problem, especially in middle-aged and elderly individuals.
- HT is defined as abnormally high BP (>140–159 mmHg systolic or >89–99 mmHg diastolic).
- HT is a primary risk factor for CHD.
- Ninety-five per cent of HT is essential, i.e. without a known cause. The other 5% has a known cause and is often curable.
- Rises in BP can occur as a result of the 'white coat syndrome'.
- Many organs and systems are involved in the control of BP.
- BP is: stroke volume × heart rate = cardiac output × total peripheral resistance.
- BP tends to increase with age.
- Untreated hypertension can result in:
  diastolic dysfunction of the heart, LVH and CAD
  nephropathy (kidney disease)
  increase in atherosclerosis.
- High SBP can lead to stroke and cerebrovascular accidents.
- Hypertension can be treated pharmacologically and/or through change in lifestyle (Table 5.2).
- Acute and chronic PA/exercise affect BP.
- The dose of PA/exercise for optimal reductions in BP has yet to be determined.
- Aerobic PA/exercise of a moderate intensity carried out between 3 and 7 times a week for around 15–90 minutes has been found to be beneficial for showing reductions in BP of around 5.3 mmHg SBP and 4.8 mmHg DBP.
- Weight training is only recommended for individuals whose BP is stable and within acceptable limits.
- Contraindications for PA/exercise are:
  resting SBP >200 mmHg or DBP >115 mmHg
  exercising SBP >250 mmHg and DBP > 120 mmHg
  sudden drop in BP.
- Longer cool-down is required due to possibility of orthostatic hypotension.

Suggested readings, references and bibliography

References and bibliography

ACSM (American College of Sports Medicine) 1993 ACSM position stand: physical activity, physical fitness, and hypertension. Medicine and Science in Sports and Exercise 25(10):i–x

ACSM 2000 ACSM's guidelines for exercise testing and prescription, 6th edn. Lippincott Williams & Wilkins, Philadelphia

ACSM 2001 ACSM's resource manual for guidelines for exercise testing and prescription, 4th edn. Lippincott Williams & Wilkins, Philadelphia

AHA (American Heart Association) 1997 Heart and stroke statistical update. AHA, Dallas

AMA (American Medical Association)1998 Blood pressure classifications. AMA, Chicago, IL

Amaral S L, Zorn T M, Michelini L C 2000 Exercise training normalizes wall-to-wall ratio of the gracilis muscle arterioles and reduces pressure in spontaneously hypertensive rats. Journal of Hypertension 18(11):1563–1672

Australian Bureau of Statistics 2002 Australian social trends 2002: health state summary tables. Online. Available: www.abs.gov.au/ausst

Blair S N, Kohn H W, Barlow C E et al 1991 Physical fitness and all-cause mortality in hypertensive men. Annals of Medicine 23(3):307–312

Brown M D, Dengel D R, Hogikyan R V et al 2002 Sympathetic activity and the heterogeneous blood pressure response to exercise training in hypertensives. Journal of Applied Physiology 92(4):1434–1442

Burt V L, Cutler J A, Higgins M et al 1995 Trends in the prevalence, awareness, treatment, and control of hypertension in the adult US population: data from the health examination surveys 1960–1991. Hypertension 26:60–69

Carroll J F, Convertino V A, Wood C E et al 1995 Effect of training on blood volume and plasma hormone concentrations in the elderly. Medicine and Science in Sports and Exercise 27(1):79–84

Cartledge S, Lawson N 2000 Aldosterone and renin measurements. Annuals of Clinical Biochemistry 37:262–278

Childs J D 1999 One to one: the impact of the Valsalva maneuver during resistance exercise. Strength and Conditioning Journal 21(2):54–55

Cleroux J, Feldman R D, Petrella R J 1999 Lifestyle modifications to prevent and control hypertension: recommendations on physical exercise training. Canadian Medical Association Journal 160 (9 suppl):S21–28

Colhoun W, Dong W, Poulter N 1998 Blood pressure screening, management, and control in England: result from the health survey for England 1994. Journal of Hypertension 16:747–752

Conlin P R, Chow D, Miller E R et al 2000 The effect of dietary patterns on blood pressure control in hypertensive patients: results from the dietary approaches to stop hypertension (DASH). American Journal of Hypertension 13(9):949–955

Copstead L C, Banasik J L 2000 Pathophysiology: biological and behavioural perspectives, 2nd edn. Saunders, Philadelphia

Deshmukh R, Smith A, Lilly L S 1997 Hypertension. In: Lilly L S The pathophysiology of heart disease, 2nd edn. Lippincott Williams & Wilkins, Philadelphia, p 267–301

Esler M, Rumantir M, Wiesner G et al 2001 Sympathetic nervous system and insulin resistance: from obesity to diabetes. American Journal of Hypertension 14(11 Pt 2):304S–309S

Facchini F S, Stoohs R A, Reaven G M 1996 Enhanced sympathetic nervous system activity: the linchpin between insulin resistance, hyperinsulinemia and heart rate. American Journal of Hypertension 9:1013–1017

Fagard R H, Tipton C M 1994 Physical activity, fitness and hypertension. In: Bouchard C, Shepherd R J, Stephens T (eds) Physical activity, fitness and health. Human Kinetics, Champaign, IL

Feldstein C A 2002 Salt intake, hypertension and diabetes mellitus. Journal of Human Hypertension 16(suppl 1):S48–S51

Franklin B 2002 Resistance training for persons with and without heart disease: rationale, safety and prescriptive guideline. BACR Newsletter 2(2)

Ganau A, Saba P S, Roman M J et al 1995 Ageing induced left ventricular concentric remodelling in normotensive subjects. Journal of Hypertension 13(12 Pt 2):1818–1822

Geleijnse J M, Witteman J C M, den Breeijen J H et al 1996 Dietary electrolyte intake and blood pressure in older subjects: the Rotterdam study. Journal of Hypertension 14:737–741

Guyton A C, Hall J E 1996 Textbook of medical physiology, 9th edn. Saunders, Philadelphia

Hagberg J M, Park J J, Brown M D 2000 The role of exercise training in the treatment of hypertension: an update. Sports Medicine 30(3):193–206

Hodge G, Ye V Z, Diggan K A 2002 Salt-sensitive hypertension resulting from nitric oxide synthase inhibition is associated with loss of regulation of angiotensin II in the rat. Experimental Physiology 87(1):1–8

Hussain S T, Smith R E, Medbak S et al 1996 Haemodynamic and metabolic responses of the lower limb after high intensity exercise in humans. Experimental Physiology 8(2):173–187

Jaber L A, Melchior W R, Rutledge D R 1992 Possible correlation between glycemia and blood pressure in black, diabetic, hypertensive patients. Annals of Phamacotherapy 26:882–886

Jones D W 1996 Body weight and blood pressure: effects of weight reduction on hypertension. American Journal of Hypertension 9(suppl 8):50S–54S

Jones D W, Hall J E 2004 Seventh report of the joint national committee on prevention, detection, evaluation and treatment of high blood pressure and evidence from new hypertension trails. Hypertension (43):1–3

Kannel W B 1991 Left ventricular hypertrophy as a risk factor: the Framingham experience. Journal of Hypertension suppl 9(2):3–9

Keleman M H, Effron M B, Valenti S A et al 1990 Exercise training combined with antihypertensive drug therapy: effects on lipids, blood pressure, and left ventricular mass. Journal of the American Medical Association 263:2766–2771

Kelly G A, Kelly K S 2000 Progressive resistance exercise and resting blood pressure: a meta-analysis of randomised controlled trials. Hypertension 35:838–843

Kisner C, Colby L 1990 Therapeutic exercise: foundations and techniques. Davis, Philadelphia

Kohno K, Matsuoka H, Takenaka K et al 2000 Depressor effect by exercise training is associated with the amelioration of hyperinsulinaemia and sympathetic overactivity. Internal Medicine 39(12):1013–1019

Krzesinski J M 2002 Epidemiology of arterial hypertension. Revue Médicale de Liège 57(3):142–147

Leutholtz B C, Ripoll I 1999 Exercise and disease management. CRC Press, Boca Raton, FL

Liebson P R, Grandits G, Prineas R et al 1993 Echocardiographic correlates of left ventricular structure among 844 mildly hypertensive men and women in the treatment of mild hypertension study (TOMHS). Circulation 87:476–486

Lilly L S 1997 The pathophysiology of heart disease, 2nd edn. Lippincott Williams & Wilkins, Philadelphia

Lutoslawska G 2000 The influence of physical exercise on glucose transport into the muscle. Medicina Sportiva 5(1):9–15

Mahmud A, Feely J 2001 Acute effect of caffeine on arterial stiffness and aortic pressure waveform. Hypertension 38(2):227–231

Meredith I T, Jennings G L, Esler M D et al 1990 Time-course of the antihypertensive and autonomic effects of regular endurance exercise in human subjects. Journal of Hypertension 8:859–866

Meredith I T, Friberg P, Jenning G L et al 1991 Exercise training lowers resting renal but not cardiac sympathetic activity in humans. Hypertension 18:575–582

Meyer R, Meyer U, Weiss M et al 1988 Sympathoadrenergic regulation of metabolism and cardiocirculation during and following running exercise of different intensity and duration. International Journal of Sports Medicine 9(suppl 2):S132–S140

Narloch J, Brandstater M 1995 Influence of breathing technique on arterial blood pressure during heavy weight lifting. Archives of Physical Medicine and Rehabilitation 76(5):457–462

National Cancer Institute 1995 The smoking cessation action area. Clearing the air. NIH: Publication No. 95–1647

National Center for Health Statistics 1994 Plan and operation of the third national health and nutrition examination survey, 1988–1994. Vital Health Statistics 1(32):US Department of Health and Human Services publications (PHS) 94–1308

National Center for Health Statistics 1995 Health. United States Public Health Service, Hyattsville, MD

National Nutritional Survey 1998 National nutritional survey of the people of the Kingdom of Saudi Arabia. Annals of Saudi Medicine 18(5):401–407

Nobel B J, Borg G A, Jacobs I et al 1983 Category ratio perceived exertion scale: relationship to blood and muscle lactates and heart rate. Medicine and Science in Sports and Exercise 15:523–528

Okuno T, Sugiyama T, Tominaga M et al 2002 Effects of caffeine on microcirculation of the human ocular fundus. Japanese Journal of Ophthalmology 46(2):170–176

Paffenbarger R S, Wing A L, Hyde R T et al 1983 Physical activity and incidence of hypertension in college alumni. American Journal of Epidemiology 117(3):245–247

Pouliot M C, Despres J P, Lemineux S et al 1994 Waist circumference and abdominal sagittal diameter: best simple anthropometric indexes of abdominal visceral adipose tissue accumulation and related cardiovascular risk in men and women. American Journal of Cardiology 73:460–468

Preuss H G 1997 Effects of glucose/insulin perturbations on aging and chronic disorders of aging: the evidence. Journal of the American College of Nutrition 16:397–403

Primary Care Clinical Effectiveness Guidelines 2000 Classifications for blood pressure and follow up recommendations. NHS, UK

Quinn T J 2000 Twenty-four hour, ambulatory blood pressure responses following acute exercise: impact of exercise intensity. Journal of Human Hypertension 14(9):547–553

Rankin L I, Henry D P, Weinberger M H et al 1981 Sodium intake alters the effects of norepinephrine on the renin system and the kidney. American Journal of Kidney Disease 1(3):177–184

Roman O, Cuevas G, Badilla M et al 2002 Morbidity and mortality of treated essential arterial hypertension in a 26 years follow up. Revista Medica de Chile 130(4):379–386

Sadowski R H, Falkner B 1996 Hypertension in pediatric patients. American Journal of Kidney Disease 27:305–315

Saruta T, Tominaga T, Yamakawa H et al 1995 Blood pressure sensitivity to salt, calcium metabolism and insulin sensitivity in essential hypertension. Clinical and Experimental Pharmacology and Physiology 22(12):S406–S411

Secretaria de Salud 1996 Encuesta Nacional de Estadistica Cronicas. DF: SSA, Mexico

Singh J P, Larson M G, Manolio T A et al 1999 Blood pressure response during treadmill testing as a risk factor for new-onset hypertension. The Framingham study. Circulation 99(14):1831–1836

Stewart K J, Effron M B, Valenti S A et al 1990 Effects of diltiazem or propranolol during exercise training of hypertensive men. Medicine and Science in Sports and Exercise 22:171–177

Vander A J, Sherman H, Luciano D S 1990 Human physiology, 5th edn. McGraw-Hill, New York

Vanhees L, Fagard R, Lijnen P et al 1984 Influence of physical training on blood pressure, plasma renin, angiotensin and catecholamines in patients with ischaemic heart disease. European Journal of Applied Physiology and Occupational Physiology 53(3):219–224

Vescovi J, Fernhall B 2000 Cardiac rehabilitation and resistance training: are they compatible? Journal of Strength and Conditioning Research 14(3):350–358

WHO (World Health Organization) 1986–1995 World health Statistics Annual. WHO, Geneva

Wilson M F, Sung B H, Pincomb G A et al 1990 Exaggerated pressure response to exercise in men at risk of systemic hypertension. American Journal of Cardiology 66:731–736

Wofford W R, Davis M M, Harkins K G et al 2002 Therapeutic considerations in the treatment of obesity hypertension. Journal of Clinical Hypertension 4(3):189–196

Zarnke K B, McAlister F A, Campbell N R et al 2002 The 2001 Canadian recommendations for the management of hypertension: Part one – assessment for diagnosis, cardiovascular risk, causes and lifestyle modification. Canadian Journal of Cardiology 18(6):604–624

Chapter 6

Overweight and obese adults

CHAPTER CONTENTS

Introduction 95
Prevalence 96
Diagnosing 96
Adipose tissue 97
Influences upon body weight 97
  The hypothalamus, pituitary and thyroid gland 97
  Metabolic rate 98
  Thermogenesis 98
  Leptin 98
Aetiology of overweight and obesity 98
  Energy balance 98
  Physical inactivity 98
  Physical fitness 99
  Diet and patterns of eating 99
    High-fat diets 99
    High-carbohydrate diets 100
    Eating patterns 100
  Genetics, genetic disorders and metabolic rate 100
  Illnesses 100
    Hypothyroidism 100
  Medications 101
Physiological effects of overweight and obesity 101
  Aerobic capacity and anaerobic threshold 101
  Lipid metabolism 101
  Thermogenesis 101
  Sodium-potassium (Na⁺-K⁺) pump 102
  Sex hormones 102
  Heart and vasculature 102
  Insulin insensitivity 102
  Respiration 103
  Musculoskeletal problems 103
  Gallstones 103
Treatment 103
  Pharmacological 103
  Surgical procedures 103
  Diet control 104

Physical activity/exercise 104
  Abdominal fat 104
  Appetite 104
  Metabolic rate 105
  Fat-free mass 105
  Insulin resistance 105
  Lipoprotein lipase activity 105
  Leptin 105
  Exercise effect on hypothalamus 105
  Weight management 106
  Exercise and diet 106
  Insulin resistance 106
Pre-exercise prescription 106
Physical activity/exercise prescription 106
  Intensity 106
  Frequency 107
  Duration 107
  Types of physical activity/exercise 107
Considerations and contraindications 108
  Medication 108
  Absolute contraindications for exercise 108
Summary 108
Suggested readings, references and bibliography 109

INTRODUCTION

In the developed world, the incidences of obesity are now estimated to be similar in number to those suffering from hunger in developing countries (Campbell & Dhand 2000). In many countries, overweight and obesity have reached epidemic levels and obesity is now well recognized as a disease in its own right. Obesity induces diseases such as type II diabetes (p. 65) and heart and vascular diseases (p. 10), and increases the risk of several types of cancer, gallbladder disease, musculoskeletal disorders and respiratory problems. Findings from the third NHANES, (2002) estimate that as many as 47 million Americans may exhibit a cluster of medical conditions, termed 'metabolic syndrome', which is characterized by insulin resistance in the presence of obesity, and high levels of abdominal fat, blood glucose, cholesterol and triglyceride and high blood pressure. For the majority of these individuals this is largely preventable, through changes in lifestyle; and it has been stated that the diverse and extreme impact of obesity should be regarded as one of the greatest neglected public health problems of our time (WHO 1997).

PREVALENCE

Recent studies have shown that overweight and obesity affect over half the adult population in many countries. Obesity is common in industrial nations and is rapidly increasing in many developing countries. In the UK rates of obesity have been related to the increase in number of cars and televisions per household (Prentice & Jebb 1995). The prevalence of obesity in adults is around 10–25% in most countries of Western Europe, and 20–25% in some countries in the Americas. This figure increases up to 40% for women in Eastern Europe and Mediterranean countries and black women in the USA, with probably the highest rates in the world among Melanesians, Micronesians and Polynesians (WHO 1997).

The financial burden of overweight and obesity is of extreme concern to many countries, especially those with already overstretched resources, and if obesity rates continue to rise, most countries will be unable to meet the demands for health care. In 2000, for example, the financial cost of obesity for the treatment of US adults was estimated at around $117 billion (CDP 2003). In the UK the indirect cost of obesity for the National Health Service was around £4.4 billion per annum (Josling 2000). Therefore, since obesity is largely preventable, government strategies to tackle overweight and obesity are vital.

DIAGNOSING

High abdominal fat is highly related to cardiovascular disease (Pihl & Jurimae 2001), diabetes and hyperlipidaemia (Ramachandran et al 2000, Idzior-Walus et al 2001) and even as long ago as the 1940s is was believed that it was excess fat (adipose tissue) rather than body weight per se that was related to greater risk of cardiovascular disease and type II diabetes (Vague 1947). Thus, it has been suggested that high abdominal circumference be used as an indicator for identification of not only obesity but also related diseases (WHO 1997).

There are many methodologies for determining degrees of adiposity, and those that are most easily employable

Table 6.1 BMI in normal males and females of different ages from a Saudi population (data from El-Hazmi & Warsy 1997)

Age groups (years)	Male		Female	
	Number	Mean	Number	Mean
14–15	219	18.8	198	16.3
16–20	177	22.3	202	19.7
21–25	93	25.0	138	24.4
26–30	81	24.8	131	27.2
31–35	52	27.6	104	28.4
36–40	73	26.4	80	29.4
41–45	42	27.1	41	30.8
46–50	41	28.6	29	32.3
51–55	32	28.9	27	33.1
56–60	27	28.2	15	27.7
61–65	14	27.3	11	29.8
66–70	9	27.1	6	27.7
>70	3	29.6	10	21.8

Table 6.2 Overweight and obesity classifications in BMI (kg/m²) (not gender specific) (adapted from WHO 1997)

Overweight and obesity classifications	BMI
Pre-obese (overweight)	25–29.9
Obese	30
Class I obese	30–34.9
Class II obese	35–39.9
Class III obese	≥40

are bioelectrical impedance, the measurement of skin folds, waist circumference, waist to hip ratio (WHR) and body mass index (BMI) (weight (kg) divided by the square of height (metres) (kg/m²)). Arguably, BMI, waist circumference and WHR are the easiest and quickest methods for classifying adiposity and risk to health.

Waist circumferences of greater than 102 cm (~40 inches) for men, for example, and 88 cm (~35 inches) for women are seen as risk factors (if the adult is not too short in stature) (CDC 2003). So is a WHR ratio of 1.0 or higher, whereas ratios less than 0.9 for men and 0.8 women indicate lower risk to health.

Body mass index is a commonly used method for quick assessment and although BMI may vary between genders, different age groups and within different populations (Table 6.1), for the majority of the population BMI is generally a good indicator of overweight and obesity (Table 6.2), and a high BMI is associated with many health risks (Table 6.3). However, BMI assumes that the muscle-to-fat ratio is normal. Thus, for certain athletic groups who possess high proportions of fat-free mass (muscle weighing more per unit volume than adipose tissue) BMI may not be a suitable method of determining adiposity. The body of the average male, for instance, comprises around 15–16% fat and that of the normal

Table 6.3 BMI and health risk (data from Huskey 1998)

Health risk		BMI	% increase in risk
Death/all causes (BMI <19)	vs	27–29:	60
		29–32:	10
		32–35:	120
Death/cancer (BMI <19)	vs	27–32:	80
		32–35:	110
Death/heart disease (vs. BMI <19)	vs	27–29:	210
		29–32:	360
		32–35:	480
Type II diabetes (BMI <22–23)	vs	27–29:	1480
		29–31:	2660
		31–33:	3930
		33–35:	5300
High blood pressure (BMI <23)	vs	26–28:	180
		29–31:	260
		32–35:	350
Degenerative arthritis (BMI <25)	vs	30–35:	400
Gallstones (BMI <24)	vs	27–29:	150
		30–35:	270
Neural birth defects (BMI 19–27)	vs	29–35:	90

Table 6.4 Classifications for percentage body fat

Classification	Men	Women
Low	6–10	14–18
Optimal	11–17	19–22
Moderate	18–20	23–30
Obese	>20	>30

female around 19–22% (Table 6.4), whereas athletes may reduce their body fat to less than 9% but still have normal body weight. Therefore, for certain athletic individuals other methods, such as WHR or skin fold measures may be more appropriate (Groer & Shekleton 1989).

ADIPOSE TISSUE

Adipose tissue is a collection of adipocytes and has been described as an organ acting in response to various hormones, such as those of the sympathetic nervous system. Adipose tissue acts as storage for excess consumed calories when the energy needs of the body are less than the calorie intake. The converted food molecules are carried as fatty acids by lipoproteins from the liver (p. 35) and taken up by the adipocytes. Adipocytes are situated predominantly in the subcutaneous tissues and mesentery, and are found in collections throughout the body, which contribute to around

10 to 20 kg of body weight. The absolute amount of adipose tissue can increase by hypertrophy of the adipocytes, which can swell by up to ten times their normal size, beyond which the cells divide and increase in total number, termed hyperplasia (increase in number). For fat cells to divide it appears that they need to reach this critical volume and probably require some adipogenic signal. Once formed, adipocytes are thought to remain for life. It is believed that there are critical stages of human development when hyperplasia of adipocytes occurs. These stages are during infancy and early childhood, adolescence and pregnancy, and only in response to excess calorie intake. Hence, excess calorie intake in childhood may predispose the individual to obesity. It may also be that some individuals are more prone to adipocyte hyperplasia in response to excess calorie intake than others, thus causing greater predisposition toward obesity. In adults, however, obesity generally occurs in response to excess calorie intake and hypertrophy of the adipocytes (Groer & Shekleton 1989).

Adipocytes are not uniform in structure or function, which is dependent upon their anatomical location. Gender influences the deposition of adipose tissue, which is related to sex hormones; men, for example, tend to collect fat in the upper body and abdomen, whilst women generally store fat peripherally in the thighs, arms and buttocks (Groer & Shekleton 1989). Central fat deposition is metabolically more active, contributing to the risk of many diseases associated with obesity, such as hyperlipidaemia (Lean 2000), insulin resistance and diabetes (Idzior-Walus et al 2001). Whereas the gluteofemoral fat in females is less lipolytically active (Bjorntorp 1989), other than during pregnancy, and appears not to contribute toward these diseases.

INFLUENCES UPON BODY WEIGHT

Body weight is influenced by many biological functions and although these contribute toward overweight and obesity, they are not considered to be the direct or primary cause. This section will outline some of these influencing factors.

THE HYPOTHALAMUS, PITUITARY AND THYROID GLAND

The influence of the hypothalamus upon the pituitary and thyroid gland is important in the effect that it has upon body weight and other biological processes. The hypothalamus and pituitary are both positioned at the base of the brain, where the hypothalamus secretes hormones that affect anterior pituitary hormones, which in turn affects the thyroid gland. The pituitary is an endocrine gland, supplying numerous hormones (including growth hormone) that govern many vital processes. The hypothalamus is a portion of the brain that controls the appetite, and therefore has a significant influence upon body weight. The hypothalamus also controls and integrates the peripheral autonomic nervous system, body temperature, sleep and appetite, which all have an influence upon body weight (for greater explanation refer to Vander et al 1990).

The thyroid gland is positioned at the front of the neck and the pituitary thyrotrophic hormone activates the thyroid. Thyroid hormones have numerous functions, many of which affect body weight. For instance, thyroid hormones increase the rate of metabolism, which affects body temperature; regulate protein, fat and carbohydrate catabolism in all cells; and maintain growth hormone secretion and skeletal maturation. They also affect cardiac rate, force and output, promote central nervous system development, stimulate the synthesis of many enzymes, and are necessary for muscle tone and vigour. Hence, it can be seen that anything that affects the function of the pituitary, hypothalamus and thyroid potentially affects the function of the body including body weight (Vander et al 1990).

METABOLIC RATE

Basal metabolic rate (BMR) can have a significant effect upon weight loss and gain, and can be influenced by factors such as environmental temperature, nutrition, muscular work, emotions and disease. Generally, males have a higher BMR than females, due in part to their usually greater body surface area. Basal metabolic rate increases during muscular exercise, when food is ingested, during fever, in response to sympathetic nervous system stimulation and as a result of a hyperactive thyroid, where the latter may increase BMR by around 40–80%. Conversely, BMR may be reduced by as much as 25–40% of normal as a consequence of hypothyroidism. Thus, BMR is a significant factor in determining body weight (Groer & Shekleton 1989).

THERMOGENESIS

The metabolism of food molecules in the body supplies heat required for thermoregulation, and excess is given off into the environment. Seventy per cent of energy in food becomes heat energy in the formation of ATP, and more is lost when ATP hydrolysis and cellular work occurs (Groer & Shekleton 1989).

LEPTIN

The hormone leptin is a product of the leptin gene and is considered to be a major player in the regulation of body fat (Chen et al 1996). It is produced by adipocytes (Xiong et al 2001) and appears to act directly on the brain to increase metabolism and eating behaviour, regulating pituitary hormones, thus affecting the release of growth hormone. Although increased leptin levels appear to result in reduction in body weight (Sone & Osamura 2001), high levels of circulating levels of leptin in overweight and obese individuals represent insensitivity to leptin, which may be a cause of overweight and obesity (Misra et al 2001). Additionally, plasma leptin is found to be markedly increased in obese individuals suffering from hypothyroidism and hyperinsulinaemia (Kautzky-Willer et al 1999), and may be linked to metabolic syndrome. Treatment of hypothyroidism also results in a reduction in raised plasma leptin levels, supporting the link between leptin and pituitary function (Pinkney et al 1998). Furthermore, diet appears to be an important regulator of leptin levels, as shown in animals fed different types of diets, though dietary fat does not appear to be the influence (Haynes et al 2003).

AETIOLOGY OF OVERWEIGHT AND OBESITY

The principal causes of the acceleration in obesity are sedentary lifestyles and high-fat and energy-dense diets, which reflect the profound changes in behavioural patterns of communities over the last 20 to 30 years. Despite obesity having strong genetic determinants, the genetic composition of the population does not change rapidly. Therefore, the sudden rise in obesity must reflect major changes in non-genetic factors (Hill & Trowbridge 1998). The fundamental causes of the obesity epidemic therefore are changing behaviours and lifestyle, particularly diet (WHO 1997).

ENERGY BALANCE

Overweight and obesity primarily result from energy imbalance, which involves eating too many calories and not being sufficiently physically active. Body weight is basically the result of metabolism, genetics, behaviour, environment, culture and socio-economic status. Behaviour and environment play a large role in causing people to be overweight or obese and these are the most important areas for prevention and treatment (US Surgeon General 2001). Whilst it is clear that these are important factors, how they affect energy balance still requires more investigation (Goran 2000).

PHYSICAL INACTIVITY

Physical inactivity and adiposity have been shown to be important determinants of mortality risk (Katzmarzyk et al 2003), and a sedentary lifestyle has also been shown to be an independent risk factor for overweight and obesity (Astrup 2001) and associated diseases. The increase in fat mass with age is also strongly related to a decrease in leisure time physical activity, suggesting that maintaining or increasing physical activity levels may blunt the age-related increases found in total and central fatness (Poehlman et al 1995). Whilst a sedentary lifestyle contributes toward a positive energy balance, resulting in increased adiposity, regular physical activity may contribute toward a neutral or negative energy balance as well as other important components of health.

PHYSICAL FITNESS

Epidemiological evidence suggests that risk of disease and all-cause mortality is lower in the physically fit (i.e. those with a high aerobic capacity), and research has shown that physically fit men with a higher waist girth possess a lower risk of disease and all-cause mortality than unfit men with smaller girths (Lee et al 1999). Moreover, a review of studies carried out by Blair & Brodney (1999) showed that physical activity appeared not only to attenuate the health risks of being overweight and obese, but active obese individuals actually had lower morbidity and mortality rates than normal weight sedentary individuals, thus suggesting that it is better to be physically fit and overweight than slim and unfit. Nevertheless, being physically fit does not completely reverse the increased risks associated with excess adiposity (Stevens et al 2002) and the greatest health benefits of leanness appear to be conferred on fit individuals (Lee et al 1999). The possible mechanism for this may be related to the fact that physically fit individuals have been shown to possess a higher resting metabolic rate (RMR) and high rates of fat oxidation (Sjodin et al 1996) from daily physical activity (Kriketos et al 2000), which would contribute toward lower body fat levels. Additionally, since there is a high genetic component that contributes to aerobic capacity, it might be that this is also linked to a higher RMR and lower body fat levels.

DIET AND PATTERNS OF EATING

Dietary recommendations change over time, but play a significant role in health and the development of overweight and obesity. Whilst a well-balanced diet is important for health, including sufficient hydration, vitamins and minerals, and appropriate proportions of proteins, carbohydrates and fats (Table 6.5), both high-fat and high-carbohydrate diets appear to be detrimental to health. It is clear, however, that lower total energy intake is necessary for weight loss, and although most diets can achieve this short-term, in order to sustain a healthy body weight, a balanced diet should be incorporated within a healthy lifestyle, inclusive of regular physical activity (Hensrud 2004).

Table 6.5 Recommended human dietary proportions of carbohydrates, fats and proteins

Foodstuff	Percentage of normal diet
Carbohydrates	45–50
Fats	30–40
Proteins	12–24

High-fat diets

High-fat diets are largely responsible for weight gain (WHO 1997, Jequier & Bray 2002). High-fat diets are energy dense and therefore greater in calorie content but also have a weak satiating effect and promote a passive over-consumption of energy relative to need. In addition, metabolically, fat intake does not measurably stimulate fat oxidation; rather dietary fat above energy requirements is stored as adipose tissue (Jequier & Bray 2002, Peters 2003). Thus, fat requires less metabolic energy expenditure than carbohydrate, promoting a positive energy balance (Peters 2003). Nonetheless, overweight individuals do appear to metabolize fat differently from non-obese individuals. For instance, a study carried out on obese and normal-weight women observed that the obese individual had an exaggerated lipid and hormonal postprandial response compared to normal-weight individuals, which was regardless of the type of fat ingested (Jensen et al 1999).

It has been speculated that not all saturated fats are equally cholesterolaemic, particularly with regard to the ingestion of palm oil. However, evaluation of the effect of palm oil on blood lipids and lipoproteins suggests that diets incorporating palm oil, as the major dietary fat, do not raise plasma total and low-density lipoprotein cholesterol (p. 39) to the extent expected from its fatty acid composition (Chandrasekharan 1999, Jensen et al 1999). Conversely, ingestion of trans fatty acids has been shown to result in lower serum high-density lipoprotein cholesterol and raised low-density lipoprotein cholesterol (p. 39–40) (Chandrasekharan 1999). Nonetheless in the animal model, fasting blood insulin levels appear to vary with regard to the type of ingested fat. For example, palm oil fed mice were found to have better glycaemic control, with more favourable glucose responses from ingestion of fish oil. Additionally, obesity and higher intake of linoleic acid have been found to be independent risk factors for glucose intolerance (Ikemoto et al 1996), indicating that the type of fat ingested may have a potential influence upon health.

The potential influence of diet upon health is important, especially as there is a fashion for high-fat diets for weight reduction. A study carried out on obese and lean rats fed an energy-restricted high-fat (60% energy) low-carbohydrate (15%) diet was assessed. In obese rats, it was found that the diet failed to improve impaired glucose tolerance, hyperinsulinaemia and hypertriglyceridaemia in the presence of lower visceral fat mass and liver lipid content. In the lean rats, the restricted intake of the high-fat diet actually impaired glucose tolerance and increased visceral fat mass and liver content (Axen et al 2003). This study indicates that the fashion for high-fat diets for weight reduction may not be good for health in overweight or lean individuals.

High-carbohydrate diets

Diets high in carbohydrate may also contribute toward the pathogenesis of obesity and metabolic syndrome. The quantity and quality of carbohydrates have a high insulinogenic effect, with the potential to raise insulin levels. A high insulinogenic response to diet represents a chronic stimulus to the beta cells of the pancreas, which may induce an adaptive hypertrophy and progressive dysregulation of these cells, resulting in postprandial hyperinsulinaemia, especially in genetically predisposed individuals. Evidence suggests that postprandial hyperinsulinaemia promotes weight gain and the development of insulin resistance and metabolic syndrome (Kopp 2003). Therefore, for those predisposed to insulin resistance and diabetes, a diet high in carbohydrate should be avoided.

Eating patterns

Obese individuals are often characterized as being hyperphagic (excessive, erratic and uncontrolled eating), though this may only be seen in a small proportion of these individuals. Environmental and psychological factors contribute greatly toward eating patterns, and emotional eating has been found to be a strong predictor of binge eating (Wiser & Telch 1999). Therefore, emotions may explain weight gain in a small subset of overweight individuals (Golay et al 1997). However, no consistent differences have been found between obese and non-obese individuals in terms of depression and anxiety. Depression has mainly been associated with severe obesity (Dixon et al 2003, Onyike et al 2003). Therefore, any reduction in obesity may lessen anxiety and depression (Dixon et al 2003, Jorm et al 2003) and any associated emotional eating.

Early research reported food intake in the obese to be the same as in non-obese people. However, latterly some overweight individuals have been found to underestimate their calorie intake. For instance research based on 11 663 individuals found that 31% under-reported their energy intake; those who under-reported tended to be less well-educated and heavier individuals (Klesges et al 1995). Numerous studies have observed greater underreporting of calorie intake in the obese compared to the non-obese (Bandini et al 1990, Schoeller et al 1990). Whilst obese individuals tend to under-report the most, the factors that influence this appear to be complex (Hill & Davies 2001).

GENETICS, GENETIC DISORDERS AND METABOLIC RATE

A small proportion of the population may become obese as a result of genetic predisposition to gaining weight when exposed to unhealthy diets and lifestyle (Barash et al 2000), which may make it more difficult for them to sustain a healthy weight. Conversely, there are also individuals who appear not to gain weight even when consuming excess calories, and it has been suggested that males in particular tend to lose excess calories through enhanced body heat loss (Seo 1996). Furthermore, studies have indicated that genetics play a role in body weight since research carried out on identical twins reared apart suggests that around 60% of the variability in BMI is due to genetic factors, though 12% of this variability may be related to metabolic rate. Notwithstanding this, the genetic component may be largely mediated by the behavioural factors such as energy intake and expenditure through physical activity and exercise (Ravussin & Bogardus 2000). Furthermore, research suggests that those with a family history of obesity have lower metabolic rates than lean individuals (Shah et al 1988).

There are numerous disorders that can cause overweight and obesity, such as a genetic disorder, Prader–Willi syndrome, which is predominantly found in children and young adults (Kiess et al 2001). This is a metabolic syndrome characterized by congenital hypotonia (lack of tone or tension in the body structure), hyperphagia, obesity and mental retardation. This syndrome is also associated with a below normal secretion of gonadotropic hormones by the pituitary glands. Fat mass of these individuals has, however, been found to be inversely related to levels of physical activity (van Mil et al 2001), indicating that physical activity (PA)/exercise intervention may assist in reduction of weight gain.

ILLNESSES

Endocrine disorders such as Cushing's syndrome and hypothyroidism may lead to overweight and obesity. Cushing's syndrome is a rare metabolic disorder characterized by an abnormal increase in adrenocortical steroids, which results in accumulations of fat on the abdomen, chest and upper back and a predisposition toward diabetes and hypertension (Nieman 2002).

Hypothyroidism

Hypothyroidism often results in overweight and obesity (Dale et al 2001) and is often found in obese individuals (Mehta et al 2001). Hypothyroidism is characterized by decreased activity of the thyroid gland, which may be caused by part removal or atrophy of the thyroid gland, overdose of anti-thyroid medication, a decreased effect of thyroid-releasing hormone by the pituitary gland and/or peripheral resistance to thyroid hormone, all of which can lead to weight gain.

MEDICATIONS

A number of drugs are capable of changing body weight as an adverse effect of their therapeutic action, and weight gain is more of a problem than weight loss. For some individuals weight gain, during drug treatment, for any disease may be a reflection of improvement of the disease itself. It is drug-induced obesity that is of primary concern. Drug-induced obesity may be the result of alterations in neurotransmitter systems acting on several hypothalamic nuclei, which are pivotal in the regulation of body fat stores. Most drugs that are capable of changing body weight interfere with these neurotransmitter systems and the extent of their effect will depend upon the type and dose of the drug concerned. Some antidepressants induce weight gain, which may amount to up to 20 kg over several months of treatment (Pijl & Meinders 1996, Zimmermann et al 2003). Therefore, it is important to establish the person's medication prior to any PA/exercise prescription. Lithium, for example, a drug often used for psychotic individuals, may cause large increases in body weight, whereas selective serotonin reuptake inhibitors may actually cause weight loss. Anticonvulsants and insulin therapy (for diabetic patients) tend to induce weight gain in a considerable percentage of patients, as may some antineoplastic agents used for treatment of breast cancer and several drugs used as prophylaxis in migraine (Pijl & Meinders 1996, Zimmermann et al 2003).

PHYSIOLOGICAL EFFECTS OF OVERWEIGHT AND OBESITY

The onset of overweight and obesity tends to alter certain physiological processes and this section highlights some of the known processes that it appears to affect. An understanding of these alterations is especially important for the exercise practitioner, since these may not only affect the overweight or obese individual's PA/exercise ability, but may in certain instances be considered to contraindicate particular types of PA/exercise prescription.

AEROBIC CAPACITY AND ANAEROBIC THRESHOLD

Since the calculation of aerobic capacity, relative to body weight, involves body weight as a component of its measure ($ml\,kg^{-1}\,min^{-1}$), the aerobic capacity of overweight and obese individuals is generally limited. However, the nature of this limitation, in obese individuals in particular, is also related to being less mechanically efficient and suffering greater musculoskeletal pain compared to non-

obese individuals, which also appears to affect their peak effort and achievable load (Hulens et al 2001). Furthermore, fat distribution has an effect on anaerobic threshold, so that those with upper body obesity tend to have lower anaerobic thresholds than those with lower body obesity (Li et al 2001). Obese individuals tend also to take longer to recover after exercise than lean individuals (Hulens et al 2001).

LIPID METABOLISM

Hyperlipidaemia is often found in overweight and obese individuals, usually in the form of high blood triglyceride, cholesterol and fatty acid levels (Ch. 3). In the obese individual, the normal regulation of free fatty acid (FFA) mobilization is disturbed. It appears that lipolysis in the adipocytes is increased, causing excessive mobilization of fatty acids. The regulation of lipolysis and esterification of fatty acids, to form triglycerides, is abnormal, and enzymatic disturbances have also been reported in obese individuals. Normal weight individuals generally experience blood elevations in FFA in response to fasting. However, in obese individuals this response is minimal or absent, despite the basal FFA level being increased above normal. The net synthesis of triglycerides from fatty acids in the liver is also increased and poorly regulated, and insulin regulation of triglyceride formation is disturbed. Hence it may be that the lipid defects are the result of insulin resistance and hyperinsulinaemia (p. 64). The obese person also appears to make more lipids from ingested carbohydrate than the non-obese, indicating that the triglyceride that is formed is not removed normally from the plasma. Furthermore, some believe that obese individuals have a greatly elevated satiety set point and the elevated fatty acids result from the fact that the obese person is always hungry, and therefore would eat more often. Others, though, suggest that satiety is not involved at all, and that obese individuals eat in response to cues, which possibly are far more than for non-obese individuals (Groer & Shekleton 1989).

THERMOGENESIS

In the animal model, obese mice have been found to be metabolically 'efficient', in that the calories they consume are more readily stored as fat and less readily used for thermogenesis when compared to their lean counterparts (Groer & Shekleton 1989). Experiments on mice also suggest that cold sensitivity related to deficient heat production is a characteristic of the obese mouse (Romsos 1981) and findings from studies carried out on adult humans suggest that a low metabolic response to cold can partly explain an increased risk for the development of obesity (van Marken Litchenbelt & Daanen 2003). In non-obese individuals during energy consumption there is an associated transient increase in energy expenditure, most of which is related to the process of food digestion and heat loss. However, in obese individuals, their 'metabolic efficiency' means less energy is lost as heat and the majority of energy is used for processing food (Groer & Shekleton 1989).

SODIUM–POTASSIUM (Na⁺-K⁺) PUMP

It is postulated that obese people may have a defect related to alterations in sodium-potassium ATPase concentrations. Sodium-potassium ATPase mediates the Na⁺-K⁺ pump of cells required for maintaining electrochemical gradients across cell membranes and controls the osmotic pressure of many cells (energy is required for this activity) (Fig. 6.1), and it appears that the thyroid hormone L-T_3 acts mainly through stimulation of the production of this enzyme (Groer & Shekleton 1989, Chin et al 1998). Hormonal control of the Na⁺-K⁺ pump therefore modulates membrane potential in mammalian cells, which in turn drives ion-coupled transport processes and maintains cell volume and osmotic balance (Sweeney & Klip 2001). Genetically obese mice have been shown to be deficient in sodium-potassium ATPase in their skeletal muscle and liver (Lin et al 1980) and over-feeding has been shown to result in unfavourable metabolic alterations in the skeletal muscle glycolytic-to-oxidative enzyme ratio (Ukkola et al 2003). Sodium-potassium pump regulation is particularly important in the musculoskeletal, cardiovascular and renal systems, where decreased Na⁺-K⁺ pump activity can result in a rise in intracellular Na⁺ concentrations, which in turn increases Na⁺/Ca²⁺ exchange, thereby raising intracellular Ca²⁺ levels. In cardiac and skeletal muscle, this may interfere with normal contractile activity, and would therefore have an influence on PA/exercise ability. Similarly, in vascular smooth muscle the result would be resistance to vasodilation, contributing toward hypertension (Sweeney & Klip 2001). Hence, any alterations or abnormalities in the

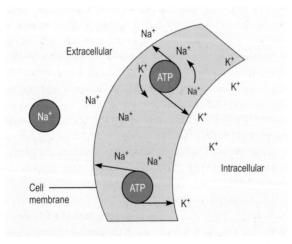

Figure 6.1 Sodium-potassium pump. (From Anderson et al 2002, with permission of Mosby.)

Na⁺-K⁺ pump may result (i) in an underactive thyroid and thyroid hormones, which are often found in the overweight and obese, and (ii) in hypertension and abnormalities in cardiac and skeletal muscle function.

SEX HORMONES

Alterations in the metabolism of endogenous hormones, including sex steroids, may lead to weight gain and may be related to increased risk of breast cancer in women (Bianchini et al 2002, Key et al 2003), which appears to be related to an increase in oestrogens (Key et al 2003). Additionally, in men visceral adipose tissue has been shown to correlate with male sex hormones (Phillips et al 2003).

HEART AND VASCULATURE

Overweight and obese individuals are prone to many cardiovascular and related problems, such as heart and vascular disease (Ch. 2), hypertension (Ch. 5), and insulin resistance and diabetes (Ch. 4). Hence overweight and obese individuals will have many cardiovascular disease risk factors, which should be determined as they will affect the PA/exercise prescription for these individuals.

Notwithstanding this, in severe obesity the sheer stress of the excess burden on the heart to supply blood to the additional tissue causes an increase in both stroke volume and circulating blood volume. Congestive heart failure, hypertension, stasis ulcerations and dyspnoea are all commonly found in the morbidly obese (Groer & Shekleton 1989).

INSULIN INSENSITIVITY

Hyperinsulinaemia and insulin resistance is common in obese individuals (Shafrir & Ziv 1998, Lewis et al 2002) who often possess hypertrophied pancreatic beta cells (Groer & Shekleton 1989) and show diminished insulin clearance (Lewis et al 2002), thus contributing toward hyperglycaemia and a predisposition toward diabetes. Nonetheless, the exact origin of hyperinsulinaemia and insulin resistance in obese individuals has still to be fully determined. It may result from abnormal insulin cell membrane receptors (Shafrir & Ziv 1998), and/or response of the tissues to constant exposure to high levels of insulin, with the tissues becoming more tolerant to insulin, and/or the pancreas compensating for primary insulin resistance by increasing insulin output, leading to hyperinsulinaemia. It is thought that insulin antagonists, such as glucagon and/or growth hormone, may also exert an effect (Groer & Shekleton 1989), though glucagon has been reported to be normal in obese Zucker rats (Fiebig et al 2002). It is also thought that hyperinsulinaemia may be the primary defect that causes obesity, although others consider it to be a response.

The normal role of insulin in lipid metabolism is to promote lipogenesis and fat storage. Thus if insulin resistance is present, there may be increased production of triglycerides, which in insulin-resistant individuals cannot then be taken up normally by the liver, adipose tissue and muscle. The normal stimulatory effect of insulin on lipoprotein lipase activity is also depressed in obesity (Ljung et al 2002). Therefore insulin resistance may actually cause the hyperlipidaemia in obese individuals. Additionally, carbohydrates are insulinogenic; thus high-carbohydrate diets tend to aggravate this situation. However, physical exercise and weight reduction appears to improve the situation (Groer & Shekleton 1989). Therefore, the case for weight loss through diet and physical activity is compelling (p. 104).

RESPIRATION

Obesity can profoundly alter pulmonary function and diminish exercise capacity as a result of the adverse effects upon respiratory mechanics, resistance within the respiratory system, respiratory muscle function, lung volume, work and energy cost of breathing, control of breathing and gas exchange. Weight loss can reverse many of these alterations. Obesity places the individual at risk of aspiration pneumonia, pulmonary embolism and respiratory failure. Obesity is also the most common precipitating factor in obstructive sleep apnoea and a factor in obesity hypoventilation syndrome, both of which are associated with morbidity and increased mortality (Koenig 2001).

Obesity–hypoventilation syndrome can be found in extremely obese individuals (BMI $>30\,kg/m^2$), generally men over 50 years, and is a major consideration when prescribing PA/exercise, since exercise-induced breathlessness is a constant finding. This condition is characterized by high $Paco_2$ as a result of alveolar hypoventilation and is primarily caused by the high cost of work of respiration, dysfunction of the respiratory centres and repeated episodes of nocturnal obstructive apnoea (the absence of spontaneous respiration) (Weitzenblum et al 2002). Research carried out on obese monkeys found that they breathe faster with lower tidal volume, and their functional residual capacity was related to their percentage body fat (Young et al 2003). Interestingly, a study carried out on 164 morbidly obese women found that those with upper body obesity had a greater oxygen requirement and showed more rapid and shallow breathing with higher ventilatory demand, and a lower anaerobic threshold during progressive cycle ergometry than those with lower body adiposity, affecting their cardiopulmonary endurance to exercise (Li et al 2001). This indicates that fat distribution may be an important factor in the exercise capacity of obese individuals, and may affect their anaerobic threshold. The effect of obesity on total lung capacity, end-expiratory lung volume and exercise capacity, during graded cycle ergometry, was also investigated in 9 obese women and 8 lean matched controls. The researchers found that total lung capacity was significantly reduced in the obese women, as was end-expiratory lung volume at ventilatory threshold. However, this did not appear to limit exercise capacity, suggesting that non-mechanical factors also have an influence upon the regulation of end-expiratory lung volume during exercise (Babb et al 2002).

MUSCULOSKELETAL PROBLEMS

Degenerative arthritis may develop as a mechanical compliance to obesity, and although obesity per se has not been determined as an independent risk factor for osteoarthritis (p. 161) (Felson et al 1988, Mehrotra et al 2003, Wendelboe et al 2003), BMI has been related to hip and knee replacement surgery (Wendelboe et al 2003). The Wisconsin Behavioural Risk Factor Surveillance System 2000–2001 found that 28% of those with arthritis had a BMI $>30\,kg/m^2$ (Mehrotra et al 2003).

GALLSTONES

Gallstone development is often associated with obesity (Hainer et al 1997) and those with high blood lipid levels (Laakso et al 1990), although the exact cause and effect relationship has yet to be fully determined.

TREATMENT

The control and treatment of overweight and obesity is of increasing concern and highlighted in this section are various types of interventions that are commonly employed.

PHARMACOLOGICAL

Although the use of drugs to control overweight and obesity are generally effective in the short term, as a method of long-term control the results have been disappointing (Sjostrom et al 1998, Williamson 1999). Moreover, most prescription drugs are for short-term use only, of a few weeks or months, and the effect of longer terms beyond a year are generally not known (NIH 2003). Additionally, these types of drugs frequently result in unpleasant side effects that can also be detrimental to health and may affect the individual's ability to carry out PA/exercise (Ch. 14, p. 229).

SURGICAL PROCEDURES

Surgical procedures, such as the gastric band, gastric bypass and stapling of the stomach, to reduce its capacity for food, or wiring the jaws to prevent solid food intake, are usually only employed to help the morbidly obese to lose weight. These are extreme methods and generally only employed when other interventions fail.

DIET CONTROL

A plethora of studies have shown that diet management is important in body weight control and reductions in high-fat, energy-dense foods have been shown to be very effective. However, an energy-restricted diet is known to result in loss not only of body fat but also of fat-free mass (FFM) (i.e. skeletal muscle), and reductions of between 24% and 28% have been found in FFM after diet alone (Ballor & Poehlman 1995), as more protein is used for energy and less for muscular development and repair. Furthermore, since adipose tissue is not metabolically active and skeletal muscle is, the loss of FFM tends to result in a reduction in metabolic rate and hence fewer calories being used. Therefore, progressive weight loss through an energy-restricted diet alone may gradually result in a lower metabolic rate, thus making it more difficult over time to lose weight. A study looking into the effects of 8 weeks of dietary restriction in 28 healthy obese women (mean age 38 years) found that body weight was reduced by a mean of 10.8 kg, consisting of 8.6 kg of fat mass and 2.2 kg FFM. The study also found significant reductions in basal respiratory exchange ratio, sleeping metabolic rate and exercise-induced thermogenesis, indicating a reduction in energy metabolism. There were, however, no changes in muscle fibre type distribution or activities of enzymes reflecting beta-oxidation and mitochondrial density (Kempen et al 1998).

PHYSICAL ACTIVITY/EXERCISE

Physical activity/exercise is a large contributor toward a 'healthy' energy balance (p. 98). Nonetheless, daily physical activity only accounts for around 20–25% of daily energy expenditure, whereas RMR accounts for the other 75–80%. Therefore, simply increasing energy expenditure through physical activity is, on its own, unlikely to be sufficient to reduce body fat to healthy levels, particularly in obese people. King & Tribble (1991) reviewed 55 studies carried out on adults that employed exercise intervention alone. They found that on average there was only a 1.6% reduction in body fat. It was only those studies that employed long-term vigorous exercise that found large losses in body weight. Considering that this type of activity would be inappropriate for the vast majority of overweight and obese individuals, the study concluded that the volume of physical activity required to reduce weight to healthy levels in obese individuals would be extremely difficult to achieve. Nonetheless,

although exercise alone may not be deemed sufficient for weight loss in the obese, it can have some effect. For example, a study carried out on 120 overweight men and women (aged 40 to 65 years), who were randomly selected into three groups that underwent 8 months of jog/walk of various intensities and durations, or a control group, found that weight loss was related to the amount of PA/exercise, with weight loss ranging between 0.6 and 4.8 kg in the exercise groups, whereas the controls gained weight. Thus modest amounts of weight loss can be achieved in overweight individuals through walking around 30 minutes per day (Slentz et al 2004).

Abdominal fat

It is known that abdominal obesity is highly related to morbidity and a review of studies between 1966 and 1998, to determine whether abdominal fat was preferentially reduced as a consequence of weight loss, found very little research specifically in this area. However, in those studies that did look at reductions in abdominal fat induced by regular PA/exercise, only modest reductions of around 3 cm in response to weight loss of about 3 kg were found (Ross & Janssen 1999). Notwithstanding this, a more recent study (Samaras et al 1999) looking at the relationship between PA/exercise and total-body and abdominal fat in 970 female twins found that central abdominal fat levels were lower with higher levels of PA/exercise. Total-body and central abdominal fat levels were between 5.6 kg and 0.44 kg lower, respectively, in those who participated in vigorous weight-bearing activity. Regression analysis, including age, diet, smoking, hormone replacement therapy and socio-economic status, found that physical activity was the strongest independent predictor of total-body and central fat, thus indicating that PA/exercise is indeed important in determining levels of body fat.

Appetite

There has been some criticism with regard to exercise intervention increasing appetite, and therefore compensating any excess energy expenditure (van Baak 1999). However, research has shown that a single bout of 20 minutes' brisk walking can reduce appetite and produce higher satiety and fullness perceptions, which may be associated with serum leptin levels (p. 98 and 105). But no post-PA/exercise differences in subsequent food consumption were found when compared to controls (Tsofliou et al 2003). Regular physical activity has also been shown to regulate appetite levels (Mayer & Bullen 1974, Shephard 1989, Long et al 2002), thus supporting the case for habitual PA/exercise as part of body weight control.

Metabolic rate

When placed in the context of total daily energy demands, the effects of PA/exercise interventions are relatively small. There is therefore the suggestion that PA/exercise produces energetic benefits in other components of the daily energy budget, thus generating a net effect on energy balance much greater than the direct exercise cost of the PA/exercise alone (Speakman & Selman 2003). Active individuals, for instance, often have higher RMR than sedentary individuals (Poehlman 1989), which is probably as a result of the metabolic cost of resynthesizing glycogen stores and repairing tissue damage (Poehlman et al 1997) and as a result of increased FFM (Speakman & Selman 2003).

Resting metabolic rate is generally the largest component of the daily energy budget. Hence any increases in RMR in response to exercise are potentially of great importance to the overweight and obese (Speakman & Selman 2003). Melby et al (1993) reported resistance exercise to produce greater post-exercise oxygen consumption than endurance exercise and it appears that short-term elevations in RMR have two phases, one that lasts less than 2 hours and a smaller, prolonged phase lasting up to 48 hours. However, the extent of the post-PA/exercise increase in RMR ultimately depends on the intensity and duration of the prior activity (Boreder et al 1991, van Baak 1999); for example, a single bout of PA/exercise has been found, in a group of exercise beginners, to increase metabolic rate beyond resting levels by around 5–7 times (Andersen 1996).

The associated loss of FFM with weight loss has a significant effect on RMR and a possible mechanism for this may be related, in part, to the relationship between FFM and thyroid hormones. Changes in thyroid hormones have been found to reduce RMR in relation to the loss of FFM (Cavallo et al 1990, Kiortsis et al 1999), highlighting the integrated and complex nature of body composition and the endocrine system.

Fat-free mass

A review of studies looking at the effect of aerobic and resistance exercise on fat mass and FFM in individuals aged over 55 years found that whilst aerobic exercise intervention produced a decrease in fat mass of between 0.4 and 3.2 kg it had little effect on FFM. The change in fat mass was significantly related to the duration of the exercise intervention programmes. Moreover, resistance exercise intervention also showed reductions in fat mass of between 0.9 and 2.7 kg, with additional increases in FFM of 1.1–2.1 kg (Toth et al 1999). This suggests that in order to retain FFM, and therefore attenuate any potential reductions in RMR often seen with reductions in body weight, it would be beneficial for overweight and obese individuals to include resistance training within their PA/exercise regimen.

Insulin resistance

Skeletal muscle insulin resistance entails the dysregulation of both glucose and fatty acid metabolism (Ch. 4, p. 61). The effect of physical activity on glucose tolerance and insulin resistance in relation to obesity has been reviewed, and it has been shown that physical activity has a favourable effect in reducing insulin resistance in obesity and among type II diabetics. The probable mechanisms for this are outlined (Ch. 4, p. 69). The effect of PA/exercise on glucose tolerance, however, has been less consistently observed, which appears to be related to variations in PA/exercise intensity between the different studies, changes in adiposity, the interval between PA/exercise, testing of glucose tolerance and baseline severity of glucose intolerance (Kelley & Goodpaster 1999).

Lipoprotein lipase activity

Physical activity/exercise is known to increase lipoprotein lipase activity, which enhances lipid metabolism (p. 36).

Leptin

Exercise is associated with fluctuations in energy sources, systemic hormone levels and energy expenditure, which may contribute to the regulation of plasma leptin levels and its action. Initial studies have found variable findings in the leptin–exercise relationship, and whilst cross-sectional studies have provided mixed findings regarding the relationship between aerobic capacity or habitual physical activity and plasma leptin, studies investigating acute bouts of PA/exercise and PA/exercise training have, with few exceptions, suggested that exercise does not alter systemic leptin independent of changes in fat mass (Hickey & Calsbeek 2001). Therefore, it would seem that whilst an acute bout of PA/exercise does not appear to affect leptin levels, the effect of habitual PA/exercise has yet to be fully determined.

Exercise effect on hypothalamus

It has been shown that the hypothalamus has a significant effect upon body weight (p. 97). However, there is limited research into the effect that PA/exercise may have upon the function of the hypothalamus, especially in human subjects. Nonetheless, it has been shown that intermittent exercise at 90% of aerobic capacity in a group of males (mean age 25 years) increased circulating hormones of the hypothalamus–pituitary–adrenal axis (Golan 1993), which would result in an increase in metabolic rate.

Weight management

The intervention of PA/exercise and diet combined has been shown to be one of the most effective ways of managing weight control, and Kayman et al (1990) found that 90% of women who lost weight, and kept the weight off, carried out regular exercise. Furthermore, a one-year follow-up of 40 women who lost weight after a 16-week programme found that the most active third had lost additional weight, the middle third, whose physical activity was irregular, maintained their weight loss, whereas the least active third actually gained weight (Andersen et al 1999), indicating the importance of regular PA/exercise in the maintenance of weight loss. The psychological impact of PA/exercise is also a key element to weight management and those who exercise regularly are less likely to be depressed, have higher self-esteem, and have an improved body image (Brownell 1995).

Exercise and diet

For overweight and obese individuals, exercise in combination with a healthy diet can result in optimal changes in body composition by contributing toward a negative energy balance whilst preserving FFM. Ballor & Poehlman (1995) reported that while diet alone resulted in FFM reductions of around 24–28%, exercise and diet resulted in FFM loss of around 11–13%, thus, illustrating how PA/exercise attenuates the loss of lean body tissue when losing body weight.

Insulin resistance

Although PA/exercise alone has been reported to be effective in the enhancement of insulin sensitivity (p. 69), many interventions looking at insulin resistance in obese individuals employ interventions of PA/exercise with diet control. For example, the results from a study carried out on 9 obese men and 16 obese women (age 39 ± 4 years), who underwent 16 weeks of moderate-intensity physical activity with a calorie-reduced diet, found that rates of resting fat oxidation were enhanced, with greater proportions of resting energy being derived from fat, which was also found to be the strongest predictor of improved insulin sensitivity (Goodpaster et al 2003). Physical activity/exercise and diet combined is thus effective in enhancing insulin sensitivity.

PRE-EXERCISE PRESCRIPTION

As for all individuals undertaking an intervention of PA/exercise, those who are overweight and obese should undergo a thorough screening process in order to detect associated risk factors and other co-morbidities. During the screening process it is important to determine the level of overweight or obesity, as this will probably affect the extent of any associated metabolic abnormalities, thereby affecting the type of PA/exercise prescribed. The screening process should involve the completion of medical and pre-PA/exercise activity screening questionnaires, and where applicable appropriate assessments should be carried out (Appendix A). The exercise practitioner should, however, be particularly empathetic to overweight or obese individuals when carrying out any assessments, as embarrassment or humiliation may jeopardize the whole programme. If this is considered to be likely, then simply monitoring the individual's progress, in terms of walking longer and further, for example, may initially provide sufficient markers of progression. However, the omission of certain assessments should not be to the detriment of determining any co-morbidity that might contraindicate PA/exercise, as consideration of all factors will be required in order to prescribe appropriately.

PHYSICAL ACTIVITY/EXERCISE PRESCRIPTION

The characteristics that contribute toward weight gain and obesity may be the result not only of excess energy intake in relation to energy expenditure, but also of other factors, such as hormones, drugs, illness and environmental and psychological issues. Hence overweight and obesity is indeed a complex issue. Therefore, the role of the exercise practitioner is to consider not only the physiology of weight reduction but also the psychological, environmental and practical aspects which may significantly affect the client/patient's responses to the PA/exercise prescription.

Although it has been suggested that initially the exercise practitioner should focus on improving metabolic profile (Poirier & Despres 2001), since the vast majority of physiological problems associated with overweight and obesity tend to diminish with weight reduction to healthier levels, weight loss should be the primary goal. Realistic goals should be set at around 0.25 kg to 0.5 kg (~ 0.5 to 1.0 pound) a week, and it should be made clear to the client/patient, particularly those who are obese, that it usually takes years to reach a certain level of body weight. Therefore, with weight loss of such a modest weekly amount it will take time to reach a healthy level. Hence, weight loss of this weekly amount should be considered part of a lifestyle change (Andersen 1999).

INTENSITY

The intensity of the prescribed PA/exercise will ultimately be dependent upon the level of overweight and obesity, and any existing co-morbidities. Obese individuals often find that they become breathless with normal daily activities (p. 103), such as climbing stairs, and the mere physical effort and energy required for physical movement means that they tire easily. These individuals may also become overwhelmed by the idea of PA/exercise beyond this level of exertion. Hence, initially, intense vigorous exercise (60–90% aerobic capacity) should be avoided and the programme should commence with light exercise working at low to moderate levels (30–50% aerobic capacity).

FREQUENCY

In order to maximize the effect of PA/exercise on increased metabolic rate (p. 105) and energy expenditure it is suggested that overweight individuals carry out PA/exercise on a daily basis, and a minimum of 5 days per week. However, to reduce the risk of 'burn out' and enhance long-term lifestyle maintenance, it is probably better to incorporate a rest from structured PA/exercise within the week (Andersen 1999). Additionally, due to the fact that obese individuals in particular tend to tire easily, an interval approach to each PA/exercise session may be acceptable (short bouts of PA/exercise interspersed with short rests). Moreover, research carried out on the effect of post-exercise oxygen consumption on five obese and five normal weight women found interval exercise produced greater post-exercise oxygen consumption than steady-state exercise (Melton 1994). This indicates that interval training may increase post-exercise RMR, thereby increasing energy expenditure, an important consideration within a weight loss programme.

The accumulation of short bouts of PA/exercise throughout the day (Pate et al 1995) may also be a suitable intervention for the overweight and obese individual. However, the effectiveness of short accumulative bouts compared to longer continuous bouts (of similar volume and intensity) with regard to weight loss has still not been fully determined, and current research into the health benefits of accumulative compared to the traditional longer single daily PA/exercise bouts is limited and conflicting. Nonetheless, whilst some studies have found accumulative bouts to show greater adherence (Jakicic et al 1995), currently this author has not (unpublished data). Furthermore, several studies have found both accumulative and 'traditional' single daily bouts of PA/exercise to produce similar changes in aerobic capacity (Ebisu 1985, Jakicic et al 1995, Coleman et al 1999). However, these changes are not necessarily concurrent with other parameters. For example, Ebisu (1985) found that accumulated shorter bouts of running, an activity inappropriate for the vast majority of overweight and obese individuals, was more effective than longer single bouts at producing improvements in blood lipid profile, whereas research using the more suitable exercise mode of brisk walking found short accumulative bouts to be less potent than a single longer bout (Woolf-May et al 1997, 1998). Nevertheless, with regard to weight management it has been shown that any PA/exercise, even irregular PA/exercise, is much better than no PA/exercise at all (Andersen et al 1999).

DURATION

Factors that affect the prescribed PA/exercise duration will depend upon the individual's co-morbidities. This may influence mechanical and/or physiological restrictions to the duration of PA/exercise. The intensity of the PA/exercise currently being undertaken will also affect the duration of the PA/exercise bout, i.e. the more intense the PA/exercise bout the shorter the duration. Nonetheless, since increasing energy expenditure, for the majority of overweight and obese individuals, is the prime factor that results in weight loss, one should aim for each PA/exercise session to be as long in duration as is possible to maximize energy expenditure.

TYPES OF PHYSICAL ACTIVITY/EXERCISE

Finding a type of PA/exercise that a particular overweight and obese individual enjoys and is capable of carrying out is of great importance, especially if one is looking to maintain a high level of adherence to the PA/exercise. Overweight and obese individuals often intrinsically dislike exercise, and barriers to PA/exercise have been identified as lack of time, embarrassment at taking part in an activity, inability to exercise vigorously and lack of enjoyment of exercise (Andersen 1999). Initially increasing daily physical activities, such as walking rather than using the car, and for the class III obese (Table 6.2) especially, changing the television channel by not using the remote control, are small but important lifestyle changes, and may for certain individuals be the start of their PA/exercise intervention.

Aerobic activities are effective at increasing energy expenditure and thereby assist in the reduction of body weight. For example, a study carried out on 40 obese women (mean BMI ~40 kg/m^2, mean age 43 years) showed that after 16-week interventions of diet control and structured aerobic PA/exercise versus 'diet and lifestyle physical activity', 'diet and aerobic PA/exercise' resulted in greater mean reductions in body weight (8.3 kg) compared to the 'diet and lifestyle' group (7.9 kg). But only a mean of 0.5 kg of the weight loss in the 'diet and aerobic PA/exercise' group was attributed to loss of body fat, compared to 1.4 kg from the 'diet and lifestyle' group (Andersen et al 1999).

Furthermore, a study of obese women comparing the effects of aerobic training ($n = 10$, 60–70% HRmax 60 minutes a day, 6 days a week) and combined aerobic with resistance training ($n = 10$, resistance training 3 days plus 3 different days of aerobic training, as for other group) versus controls ($n = 10$) found that both intervention groups increased their aerobic capacity and improved their blood lipid profile. However, FFM was only increased in the combined group, and reductions in abdominal sub-cutaneous and visceral fat were only observed from aerobic training alone (Park et al 2003). Similarly a study comparing 10 weeks of aerobic and resistance inter-ventions, in 26 middle-aged men with abdominal obesity, found comparable reductions in WHR, but total body fat was only reduced in the resistance training group. However, high-density lipoprotein cholesterol was only increased in those who undertook the aerobic training (Banz et al 2003). In addition, a study carried out on 19 moderately obese women (mean age 38 years, mean body fat 37.5%) found similar increases in FFM from both a programme of 'resistance training' and 'walking plus resistance training' of around 1.9 kg, although aerobic capacity was only significantly increased in the 'walking plus resistance training' group (Byrne & Wilmore 2001). Thus a programme that integrates both aerobic and resistance PA/exercise will assist in body fat reduction, but can also maintain FFM, which is advantageous in preserving or enhancing metabolic rate and thereby energy expenditure.

CONSIDERATIONS AND CONTRAINDICATIONS

The exercise practitioner needs to consider numerous factors when designing a PA/exercise programme for overweight and obese individuals. This is especially so as behaviour and environmental factors play a large role in causing people to become overweight, and these are the greatest areas for prevention and treatment actions (US Surgeon General 2001).

When preparing the PA/exercise programme, the caloric expenditure is important and needs to be considered in conjunction with the person's caloric intake. It may therefore be a good idea, where possible, to liaise with a dietician and/or other health professionals in order to determine the person's eating behaviour and energy intake. Other aspects to consider are possible underlying factors that may be the cause of the overweight and obesity, such as illness (e.g. hypothyroidism) and certain medications. Also to be considered are co-morbidities, such as hyperlipidaemia, insulin insensitivity and diabetes, hypertension, arthritis and cardiovascular diseases, which are often found in overweight and obese individuals. Additionally, breathlessness and immobility are common factors which may affect an overweight or obese person's PA/exercise ability; all of which need to be taken into account when prescribing.

MEDICATION

Some drugs prescribed for weight loss can cause elevations in catecholamine levels and may increase heart rate and blood pressure (NIH 2003). If the client/patient already has elevated blood pressure, care should be taken that blood pressure does not exceed recommended levels (Ch. 5). Furthermore, if heart rate is affected by some

of these drugs, the heart rate and blood pressure should be monitored to reduce any risk to the person's health (Ch. 14).

ABSOLUTE CONTRAINDICATIONS FOR EXERCISE

Depending on any other co-morbidities, absolute contra-indications for exercise will be as for those cited for other individuals (Appendix A, Table A.1).

Suggested reading

SUMMARY

- Obesity is now recognized as a disease in its own right and can increase risk of:
  type II diabetes
  cardiovascular disease
  several types of cancer
  gallbladder disease
  musculoskeletal disorders
  respiratory problems.
- Despite obesity having strong genetic determinants, the principal causes of the rise in obesity are seden-tary lifestyles and high-fat and energy-dense diets.
- Overweight/obesity is a complex issue and factors that contribute are hormones, drugs, illness, environ-mental and psychological issues.
- Active obese individuals show lower morbidity and mortality rates than normal weight sedentary indivi-duals. Therefore, being physically fit and overweight may be less risky to health than being slim and unfit.
- Realistic weight loss goals should be set at around 0.25 kg to 0.5 kg and should be considered part of a lifestyle change.
- Physical activity/exercise intervention should commence with light PA/exercise.
- Increases in any lifestyle physical activity should be greatly encouraged.
- To maximize energy expenditure, interval and longer bouts of PA/exercise are effective. Accumu-lative shorter bouts may be a suitable alternative.
- A programme that integrates both aerobic and resis-tance PA/exercise is most effective at maintaining FFM and metabolic rate.
- Habitual appropriate PA/exercise intervention can result in:
  modification of associated disorders, such as coronary heart disease, diabetes and insulin resis-tance, blood lipids and blood pressure.
  ↓ rates of morbidity and mortality
  ↑ aerobic fitness
  ↓ body fat
  maintenance of FFM
  ↑ RMR and energy expenditure
  enhanced insulin sensitivity
  assistance in weight management.
- Co-morbidities and factors such as breathlessness and mobility should be considered within the PA/exercise programme.

Suggested readings, references and bibliography

Suggested readings

Groer M W, Shekleton M E 1989 Basic pathophysiology: a holistic approach, 3rd edn. Mosby, St Louis

Vander A J, Sherman J H, Luciano D S 1990 Human physiology. McGraw-Hill, New York

References and bibliography

Andersen R E 1996 Physiology of obesity. In: Cotton R T (ed) Lifestyle and weight management consultant manual. American Council for Exercise, San Diego, p 95–118

Andersen R E 1999 Exercise, an active lifestyle, and obesity. The Physician and Sports Medicine 27(10):41–42

Andersen R E, Wadden T A, Bartlett S J et al 1999 Effects of lifestyle activity versus structured aerobic exercise in obese women: a randomised trial. Journal of the American Medical Association 281(4):335–340

Anderson D M, Keith J, Novak P D et al (eds) 2002 Mosby's medical, nursing and allied health dictionary, 6th edn. Mosby, St Louis

Astrup A 2001 Healthy lifestyles in Europe: prevention of obesity and type II diabetes by diet and physical activity. Public Health Nutrition 4(2B):499–515

Axen K V, Dikeakos A, Sclafani A 2003 High dietary fat promotes syndrome X in nonobese rats. Journal of Nutrition 133(7):2244–2249

Babb T G, DeLorey D S, Wyrick B L et al 2002 Mild obesity does not limit change in end-expiratory lung volume during cycling in young women. Journal of Applied Physiology 92(6):2483–2490

Ballor D L, Poehlman E T 1995 A meta-analysis of the effects of exercise and diet restriction on resting metabolic rate. European Journal of Applied Physiology 71(6):535–542

Bandini L G, Schoeller D A, Cyr H N et al 1990 Validity of reported energy intake in obese and nonobese adolescents. American Journal of Clinical Nutrition 52(3):421–425

Banz W J, Maher M A, Thompson W G et al 2003 Effects of resistance versus aerobic training on coronary artery disease risk factors. Experimental Biology and Medicine 228(4):434–440

Barash G S, Farooqi S, O'Rahilly S 2000 Genetics of body-weight regulation. Nature 404:644–651

Bianchini F, Kaaks R, Vainio H 2002 Weight control and physical activity in cancer prevention. Obesity Reviews 3(1):5–8

Bjorntorp P A 1989 Sex differences in the regulation of energy balance with exercise. American Journal of Clinical Nutrition 17:55–65

Blair S N, Brodney S 1999 Effects of physical activity and obesity on morbidity and mortality: current evidence and research issues. Medicine and Science in Sports and Exercise 31(11 suppl): S646–S662

Boreder C E, Brenner M, Hofman Z et al 1991 The metabolic consequences of low and moderate intensity exercise with or without feeding in lean and borderline obese males. International Journal of Obesity 15(2):95–104

Brownell K D 1995 Exercise in the treatment of obesity. In: Brownell K D, Fairburn C G (eds) Eating disorders and obesity: a comprehensive handbook. Guilford Press, New York, p 473–478

Byrne H K, Wilmore J H 2001 The effects of a 20-week exercise training program on resting metabolic rate in previously sedentary, moderately obese women. International Journal of Sport Nutrition and Exercise Metabolism 11(1):15–31

Campbell P, Dhand R 2000 Obesity. Nature 404:631

Cavallo E, Armellini F, Zamboni M et al 1990 Resting metabolic rate, body composition and thyroid hormones. Short term effects of very low calorie diet. Hormone and Metabolic Research 22(12):632–635

CDC (Centers for Disease Control) 2003 Defining overweight and obesity. Online. Available: http://www.cdc.gov/bccdogo/dnpa/obesity/defining.htm February 2004

CDP (Chronic Disease Prevention) 2003 Preventing obesity and chronic disease through good nutrition and physical activity. Online. Available: http://www.cdc.gov/nccdphp February 2004

Chandrasekharan N 1999 Changing concepts in lipid nutrition in health and disease. Medical Journal of Malaysia 54(3):408–427

Chen G, Koyama K, Yuan X et al 1996 Disappearance of body fat in normal rats induced by adenovirus-mediated leptin gene therapy. Proceedings of the National Academy of Science USA 93:14795–14799

Chin S, Apriletti J, Gick G 1998 Characterization of a negative thyroid hormone response element in the rat sodium, potassium-adenosine triphosphatase α3 gene promoter. Endocrinology 139(8):3423–3431

Coleman K J, Raynor H R, Mueller D M et al 1999 Providing sedentary adults with choices for meeting their walking goals. Preventive Medicine 28:510–519

Dale J, Daykin J, Holder R et al 2001 Weight gain following treatment of hyperthyroidism. Clinical Endocrinology 55(2):233–239

Dixon J B, Dixon M E, O'Brien PE 2003 Depression in association with severe obesity: changes with weight loss. Archives of Internal Medicine 163(17):2058–2065

Ebisu T I 1985 Splitting the distance of endurance running: effect on cardiovascular endurance and blood lipids. Japanese Journal of Physical Education 30/31:37–43

El-Hazmi M A F, Warsy A S 1997 Prevalence of obesity in the Saudi population. Annals of Saudi Medicine 17(3):302–306

Felson D T, Anderson J J, Naimark A et al 1988 Obesity and knee osteoarthritis. The Framingham study. Annals of Internal Medicine 109(1):18–24

Fiebig R G, Hollander J M, Ney D et al 2002 Training down-regulates fatty acid synthase and body fat in obese Zucker rats. Medicine and Science in Sports and Exercise 34(7):1106–1114

Golan R 1993 Effects of thymopentin on the responses of hypothalamic-pituitary-adrenal axis to a high intensity dynamic exercise protocol. Microform Publications for Sport and Human Performance, Eugene, OR

Golay A, Hagon I, Painot D et al 1997 Personalities and alimentary behaviours in obese patients. Patient Education and Counselling 31(2):103–112

Goodpaster B H, Katsiaras A, Kelly D E 2003 Enhanced fat oxidation through physical activity is associated with improved insulin sensitivity in obesity. Diabetes 52(9):2101–2197

Goran M I 2000 Energy metabolism and obesity. Medical Clinics in North America 84(2):347–362

Groer M W, Shekleton M E 1989 Basic pathophysiology: a holistic approach, 3rd edn. Mosby, St Louis

Hainer V, Kunesova M, Parizkova J et al 1997 Health risks and economic costs associated with obesity requiring a comprehensive weight reduction program. Casopis Lekaru Ceskych 136(12):367–372

Haynes G R, Heshka S, Chadee K et al 2003 Effects of dietary fat type and energy restriction on adipose tissue fatty acid composition and leptin production in rats. Journal of Lipid Research 44(5):893–901

Hensrud DD 2004 Diet and obesity. Current Opinion in Gastroenterology 20(2):119–124

Hickey M S, Calsbeek D J 2001 Plasma leptin and exercise: recent findings. Sports Medicine 31(8):583–589

Hill J O, Trowbridge F L 1998 Childhood obesity: future directions and research priorities. Paediatrics 101(3 Pt 2):570–574

Hill R J, Davies P S 2001 The validity of self-reported energy intake as determined using the doubly labelled water technique. British Journal of Nutrition 85(4):415–430

Hulens M, Vansant G, Lysens R et al 2001 Exercise capacity in lean versus obese women. Scandinavian Journal of Medicine and Science in Sports 11(5):305–309

Huskey R J 1998 How's your BMI (body mass index)? Online. Available http://www.people.virginia.edu/~rjh9u/bmi.html February 2003

Idzior-Walus B, Mattock M B, Solnica B et al 2001 Factors associated with plasma lipids and lipoproteins in type I diabetes mellitus: the EURODIAB IDDM Complications Study. Diabetic Medicine 18(10):786–796

Ikemoto S, Takahashi M, Tsunoda N et al 1996 High-fat diet-induced hyperglycemia and obesity in mice: differential effects of dietary oils. Metabolism: Clinical and Experimental 45(12):1539–1546

Jakicic J M, Wing R R, Butler B A et al 1995 Prescribing exercise in multiple short bouts versus one continuous bout: effects on adherence, cardiorespiratory fitness and weight loss in overweight women. International Journal of Obesity 19:893–901

Jensen J, Bysted A, Dawids S et al 1999 The effect of palm oil, lard, and puff-pastry margarine on postprandial lipid and hormone responses in normal-weight and obese young women. British Journal of Nutrition 82(6):469–479

Jequier E, Bray G A 2002 Low-fat diets are preferred. American Journal of Medicine 113(suppl)9B:41S–46S

Jorm A F, Korten A E, Christensen H et al 2003 Association of obesity with anxiety, depression and emotional well-being: a community survey. Australian and New Zealand Journal of Public Health 27(4):434–440

Josling L 2000 Obesity: a curable epidemic. Online. Available: http://www.wsws.org/articles August 2001

Katzmarzyk P T, Jassen I, Ardern C I 2003 Physical inactivity, excess adiposity and premature mortality. Obesity Reviews 4(4):257–290

Kautzky-Willer A, Ludwig C, Nowotny P et al 1999 Elevation of plasma leptin concentrations in obese hyperinsulinaemic hypothyroidism before and after treatment. European Journal of Clinical Investigation 29(5):395–403

Kayman S, Bruvdd W, Stern J S 1990 Maintenance and relapse after weight loss in women: behavioural aspects. American Journal of Clinical Nutrition 52(5):800–807

Kelley D E, Goodpaster B H 1999 Effects of physical activity on insulin action and glucose tolerance in obesity. Medicine and Science in Sports and Exercise 31(11 suppl):S619–S623

Kempen K P, Saris W H, Kuipers H et al 1998 Skeletal muscle metabolic characteristics before and after energy restriction in human obesity: fibre type, enzymatic beta-oxidation capacity and fatty acid-binding protein content. European Journal of Clinical Investigation 28(12):1030–1037

Key T J, Appleby P N, Reeves G K et al 2003 Body mass index, serum sex hormones, and breast cancer risk in postmenopausal women. Journal of the National Cancer Institute 95(16):1218–1226

Kiess W, Galler A, Reich A et al 2001 Clinical aspects of obesity in childhood and adolescence. Obesity Reviews 2(1):29–36

King A C, Tribble D L 1991 The role of exercise in weight regulation in nonathletes. Sports Medicine 11(5):331–349

Kiortsis D N, Durack I, Turpin G 1999 Effects of low-calorie diet on resting metabolic rate and serum tri-iodothyronine levels in obese children. European Journal of Pediatrics 158(6):446–450

Klesges R C, Eck L H, Ray J W 1995 Who underreports dietary intake in a dietary recall? Evidence from the Second National Health and Nutrition Examination Survey. Journal of Consulting and Clinical Psychology 63(3):438–444

Koenig S M 2001 Pulmonary complications of obesity. American Journal of the Medical Sciences 321(4):249–279

Kopp W 2003 High-insulinogenic nutrition – an etiologic factor for obesity and the metabolic syndrome? Metabolism: Clinical and Experimental 52(7):840–844

Kriketos A D, Sharp T A, Seagle H M et al 2000 Effects of aerobic fitness on fat oxidation and body fatness. Medicine and Science in Sports and Exercise 32(4):805–811

Laakso M, Suhonen M, Julkunen R et al 1990 Plasma insulin, serum lipids and lipoproteins in gall stone disease in non-insulin dependent diabetic subjects: a case control study. Comment in Gut 32(2):339–340

Lean M E 2000 Review, Pathophysiology of obesity. Proceedings of the Nutrition Society 59(3):331–336

Lee C D, Blair S N, Jackson A S 1999 Cardiorespiratory fitness, body composition, and all-cause and cardiovascular disease mortality in men. American Journal of Clinical Nutrition 69(3):373–380

Lewis G F, Carpentier A, Adeli K et al 2002 Disordered fat storage and mobilization in the pathogenesis of insulin resistance and type 2 diabetes. Endocrine Reviews 23(2):201–229

Li J, Li S, Feuers R J et al 2001 Influence of body fat distribution on oxygen uptake and pulmonary performance in morbidly obese females during exercise. Respiration 6(1):9–13

Lin M H, Tuig J G, Romsos D R et al 1980 Heat production and Na^+-K^+ ATPase enzyme units in lean and obese (ob/ob) mice. American Journal of Physiology 238:E193–E199

Ljung T, Ottosson M, Ahlberg A C et al 2002 Central and peripheral glucocorticoid receptor function in abdominal obesity. Journal of Endocrine Investigation 25(3):229–235

Long S J, Hart K, Morgan L M 2002 The ability of habitual exercise to influence appetite and food intake in response to high- and low-energy preloads in man. British Journal of Nutrition 87(5):517–523

Mayer J, Bullen B A 1974 Nutrition, weight control and exercise. In: Johnson W R, Buskirk E R (eds) Science and medicine of exercise and sport. Harper & Row, New York

Mehrotra C, Chundy N, Thomas V 2003 Obesity and physical inactivity among Wisconsin adults with arthritis. Wisconsin Medical Journal 102(7):24–28

Mehta S, Mathur D, Chaturvedi M et al 2001 Thyroid hormone profile in obese subjects: a clinical study. Journal of the Indian Medical Association 99(5):260–261

Melby C, Schroll C, Edwards G et al 1993 Effect of acute resistance exercise on post exercise energy expenditure and resting metabolic rate. Journal of Applied Physiology 75(4):1847–1853

Melton C A 1994 The effect of exercise intensity on excess post-exercise oxygen consumption (EPOC) in normal and fat obese women. Microform Publications for Sport and Human Performance, Eugene, OR

Misra A, Arora N, Mondal S et al 2001 Relation between plasma leptin and anthropometric and metabolic covariates in lean and obese diabetic and hyperlipidaemic Asian Northern Indian subjects. Diabetes, Nutrition and Metabolism – Clinical and Experimental 14(1):18–26

NHANES (National Health and Nutrition Examination Survey) 2002 National Health and Nutrition Examination Survey. Department of Health and Human Services, US

Nieman L K 2002 Diagnostic tests for Cushing's syndrome. Annals of the New York Academy of Science 970:112–118

NIH (National Institutes for Health) 2003 Prescription medications for the treatment of obesity. Online. Available: http://www.niddk.nih.gov/health/nutrit/pubs/presmeds.htm March 2004

Onyike C U, Crum R M, Lee H B et al 2003 Is obesity associated with major depression? Results from the Third National Health and Nutrition Examination Survey. American Journal of Epidemiology 158(12):1139–1147

Park S K, Park J H, Kwon Y C et al 2003 The effect of combined aerobic and resistance exercise training on abdominal fat in obese middle-aged women. Journal of Physiological Anthropology and Applied Human Science 22(3):129–135

Pate R R, Pratt M, Blair S N et al 1995 Physical activity and public health: A recommendation from the Centers of Disease Control and Prevention and the American College of Sports Medicine. Journal of the American Medical Association 273:402–407

Peters J C 2003 Dietary fat and body weight control. Lipids 38(2):123–127

Phillips G B, Jing T, Heymsfield S B 2003 Relationships in men of sex hormones, insulin, adiposity, and risk factors for myocardial infarction. Metabolism: Clinical and Experimental 52(6):784–790

Pihl E, Jurimae T 2001 Cardiovascular disease risk factors in males with normal body weight and high waist-to-hip ratio. Journal of Cardiovascular Risk 8(5):299–305

Pijl H, Meinders A E 1996 Bodyweight change as an adverse effect of drug treatment. Mechanisms and management. Drug Safety 14(5):329–342

Pinkney J H, Goodrick S J, Katz J et al 1998 Leptin and the pituitary-thyroid axis: a comparative study in lean, obese, hypothyroid and hyperthyroid subjects. Clinical Endocrinology 49(5):583–588

Poehlman E T 1989 Exercise and its influence on resting energy metabolism in man. Medicine and Science in Sports and Exercise 21(5):515–525

Poehlman E T, Toth M J, Bunyard L B et al 1995 Physiological predictors of increasing total and central adiposity in aging men and women. Archives of Internal Medicine 155(22):2443–2448

Poehlman E T, Toth M J, Ades P A et al 1997 Gender differences in resting metabolic rate and noradrenaline kinetics in older individuals. European Journal of Clinical Investigation 27(1):23–28

Poirier P, Despres J P 2001 Exercise in weight management of obesity. Cardiology Clinics 19(3):459–470

Prentice A M, Jebb S A 1995 Obesity in Britain: glutton or sloth? British Medical Journal 311(7002):437–439

Ramachandran A, Snehalatha C, Satyayani K et al 2000 Cosegregation of obesity with familial aggregation of type 2 diabetes mellitus. Diabetes, Obesity and Metabolism 2(3)129–154

Ravussin E, Bogardus C 2000 Energy balance and weight regulation: genetics versus environment. British Journal of Nutrition 83(suppl)1:S17–S20

Romsos D 1981 Efficiency of energy retention in genetically obese animals and in dietary-induced thermogenesis. Federation Proceedings 40(10):2524–2529

Ross R, Janssen I 1999 Is abdominal fat preferentially reduced in response to exercise-induced weight loss? Medicine and Science in Sports and Exercise 31(11) (suppl 1):S568–S572

Samaras K, Kelly P, Chiano M N et al 1999 Genetic and environmental influences in total-body and central abdominal fat: the effect of physical activity in female twins. Annals of Internal Medicine 130(11):873–882

Schoeller D A, Bandini L G, Dietz W H 1990 Inaccuracies in self-reporting intake identified by comparison with the doubly labelled water method. Canadian Journal of Physiology and Pharmacology 68(7):941–949

Seo C 1996 Effects of ethanol on thermoregulation response during cold air exposure in male and female subjects. Microform Publications for Sport and Human Performance, Eugene, OR

Shafrir E, Ziv E 1998 Cellular mechanism of nutritionally induced insulin resistance: the desert rodent *Psammomys obesus* and other animals in which insulin resistance leads to detrimental outcome. Journal of Basic and Clinical Physiology and Pharmacology 9(2–4):347–385

Shah M, Miller D S, Geisslier C A 1988 Lower metabolic rates in post-obese versus lean women: thermogenesis, basal metabolic rate and genetics. European Journal of Clinical Nutrition 42(9):741–752

Shephard R J 1989 Nutritional benefits of exercise. Journal of Sports Medicine and Physical Fitness 29(1):83–90

Sjodin A M, Forslund A H, Westerterp K R et al 1996 The influence of physical activity and BMR. Medicine and Science in Sports and Exercise 28(1):85–91

Sjostrom L, Rissanen A, Andersen T et al 1998 Randomised placebo-controlled trial of orlistat for weight loss and prevention of weight regain in obese patients. European multicentre orlistat study group. Lancet 352:167–172

Slentz C, Duscha B D, Johnson J L et al 2004 Effects of the amount of exercise on body weight, body composition and measures of central obesity: STRRIDE – a randomised controlled study. Archives of Internal Medicine 164(1):31–39

Sone M, Osamura R Y 2001 Leptin and the pituitary. Pituitary 4(1–2):15–23

Speakman J R, Selman C 2003 Physical activity and resting metabolic rate. Proceedings of the Nutrition Society 62(3):621–634

Stevens J, Cai J, Evenson K R et al 2002 Fitness and fatness as predictors of mortality from all causes and from cardiovascular disease in men and women in the lipid research clinics study. American Journal of Epidemiology 156(9):832–841

Sweeney G, Klip A 2001 Mechanisms and consequences of Na$^+$-K$^+$-pump regulation by insulin and leptin. Cellular and Molecular Biology 47(2):363–372

Toth M J, Beckett T, Poehlman E T 1999 Physical activity and the progressive change in body composition with aging: current evidence and research issues. Medicine and Science in Sports and Exercise 31(11):S590

Tsofliou F I, Pitsiladis Y P, Malkova D I et al 2003 Moderate physical activity permits acute coupling between serum leptin and appetite-satiety measures in obese women. International Journal of Obesity 27(11):1332–1339

Ukkola O, Joanisse D R, Tremblay A et al 2003 Na$^+$K$^+$-ATPase alpha 2-gene and skeletal muscle characteristics in response to long-term overfeeding. Journal of Applied Physiology 94(5):1870–1874

US Surgeon General 2001 Call to action to prevent overweight and obesity, 2001. Online. Available: http://www.cdc.gov/nccdphp/dnpa/obesity/contributing_factors.htm February 2004

Vague J 1947 La différenciation sexuelle, facteur determinant des formes de l'obésité. Presse Med 30:339–340

van Baak M A 1999 Physical activity and energy balance. Public Health Nutrition 2(3A):335–339

Vander A J, Sherman J H, Luciano D S 1990 Human physiology. McGraw-Hill, New York

van Marken Litchenbelt W D, Daanen H A 2003 Cold-induced metabolism. Current Opinion in Clinical Nutrition and Metabolic Care 6(4):469–475

van Mil E G, Westerterp K R, Gerver W J et al 2001 Body composition in Prader–Willi syndrome compared with nonsyndromal obesity: relationship to physical activity and growth hormone. Journal of Pediatrics 139(5):708–14

Weitzenblum E, Kessier R, Chaouat A 2002 Alveolar hypoventilation in the obese: the obesity–hypoventilation syndrome. Revue de Pneumologie Clinique 58(2):83–90

Wendelboe A M, Hegmann K T, Biggs J J 2003 Relationships between body mass indices and surgical replacements of knee and hip joints. American Journal of Preventative Medicine 25(4):290–295

WHO (World Health Organization) 1997 Obesity epidemic puts millions at risk from related diseases. Online. Available: http://www.who.int/archives/inf-pr-1997/en/pr97-46.html February 2004

Williamson D F 1999 Pharmacotherapy for obesity. Journal of the American Medical Association 281:278–280

Wiser S, Telch C F 1999 Dialectical behavior therapy for binge-eating disorder. Journal of Clinical Psychology 55(6):755–768

Woolf-May K, Bird S, Owen A 1997 Effects of an 18 week walking programme on cardiac function in previously sedentary or relatively inactive adults. British Journal of Sports Medicine 31(1):48–53

Woolf-May K, Kearney E M, Jones D W et al 1998 The effect of two different 18 week walking programmes on aerobic fitness, selected blood lipids and factor XIIa. Journal of Sports Sciences 16:701–710

Xiong Y, Tanaka H, Richardson J A et al 2001 Endothelin-1 stimulates leptin production in adipocytes. Journal of Biological Chemistry 276(30):28471–28477

Young S S, Kseans S M, Austin T et al 2003 The effects of body fat on pulmonary function and gas exchange in cynomolgus monkeys. Pulmonary Pharmacology and Therapeutics 16(5):313–319

Zimmermann U, Kraus T, Himmerrich H et al 2003 Epidemiology, implications and mechanisms underlying drug-induced weight gain in psychiatric patients. Journal of Psychiatric Research 37(3):193–220

Chapter 7

Coagulation, fibrinolysis and risk of thrombosis

CHAPTER CONTENTS

Introduction 113
Thrombosis 113
Blood coagulation systems 114
    Blood coagulation (haemostasis) pathway 114
        Formation of a platelet plug 115
        Clotting 115
    The intrinsic and extrinsic pathways 115
        Intrinsic pathway 115
        Extrinsic pathway 116
Anticoagulation pathway 116
    Fibrinolytic system 117
Anti-clotting medication 117
Increased risk of thrombosis 117
    Increasing age 117
    Blood lipids, cardiovascular disease and obesity 118
    Diabetes 118
    Smoking 118
    Hormones and pregnancy 119
    Physical fitness 119
Single bout of physical activity/exercise and
    haemostasis 119
    Intensity 120
    Duration 120
Regular physical activity/exercise and haemostasis 121
Types of physical activity/exercise 121
Adverse cardiac events in response to physical
    activity/exercise 121
Those at increased risk of thrombosis from
    physical activity/exercise 121
    Physically unfit 121
    Age 122
    Cardiac patients 122
    Obesity 122
    Diabetes 122
Exercise prescription 122
    Considerations and contraindications 123
    Medication 123
Summary 123
Suggested readings, references and bibliography 123

INTRODUCTION

The objective of this chapter is to emphasize to the exercise practitioner how acute and habitual physical activity (PA)/exercise may alter the potential of the blood to coagulate or bleed. The aim is also to highlight those individuals who are at increased risk of thrombosis during and after PA/exercise as a result of increased blood coagulation potential (El-Sayed 1996, Gibbs et al 2001, Morris et al 2003).

THROMBOSIS

A thrombus is formed when the blood clotting mechanisms are activated and blood becomes a solid mass. The thrombus (blood clot) is formed inside the blood vessel, blocking the flow of blood within the vein or artery, and complete occlusion is termed thrombosis. Thrombosis can happen in any part of the body where there are blood vessels and is more likely to develop when (i) the blood is more viscous than normal, (ii) there is damage to the blood vessel wall, and/or (iii) the blood flow is reduced (Lifeblood 2003).

Thrombosis is generally classified as a blood clot either of the veins (venous thrombosis) or of the artery (arterial thrombosis). However, if an individual has thrombosis there is also risk of embolism, which is when part of a clot breaks off, known as an embolus, and travels within the vascular system becoming lodged at another site, blocking either an artery or vein. For example, when part of a clot from deep vein thrombosis (DVT) breaks off, it may travel up the leg, through the right side of the heart and lodge in the lung, which is known as a pulmonary embolism and is potentially fatal. Venous thrombosis is generally a blood clot to a deep vein, usually the leg and is known as DVT. It can also be a blood clot in the retinal vein of the eye termed retinal vein thrombosis. Arterial thrombosis, on the other hand, is generally a blood clot in the heart, and is the prime cause of a myocardial infarction (heart attack), or a blood clot in the brain, termed

Table 7.1   Main risk factors for venous and arterial thrombosis (data from Lifeblood 2003)

Venous thrombosis	Increasing age
	Immobility
	Myocardial infarction or stroke
	Recent operation, particularly the hips
	Previous DVT
	Previous family history of DVT
	Cancer and cancer treatment
	Pregnancy
	Combination oral contraceptive pill and hormone replacement therapy
	Long distance air travel
	Thrombophilia (range of conditions where an individual has viscous blood)
Arterial thrombosis	Smoking
	High blood pressure
	Hypercholesterolaemia
	Diabetes
	Increasing age
	Family history
	Poor diet
	Overweight or obesity
	Physical activity

a cerebrovascular accident, and the main cause of stroke (Lifeblood 2003) (Table 7.1).

BLOOD COAGULATION SYSTEMS

There are three main pathways involved in the coagulation system: the coagulation pathway, the anticoagulation pathway and fibrinolysis, as well as the *intrinsic* and *extrinsic* pathways. The intrinsic pathway is where everything necessary for clotting is within the blood, whereas the extrinsic pathway uses a protein (tissue factor (TF), also referred to as thromboplastin or factor (F) III) from the interstitial compartment outside of the bloodstream (the area surrounding the cells) (Vander et al 1990, King 1996) (Fig. 7.1) (p. 115).

BLOOD COAGULATION (HAEMOSTASIS) PATHWAY

The body's ability to control the flow of blood after vascular injury is extremely important for survival, and the process of blood clotting and, following repair of the injured tissue, the subsequent dissolution of the clot, is termed *haemostasis* (King 1996) (p. 115). A blood clot is formed by the same reactions that stop blood flow from a wound, and blood coagulation is triggered when the blood comes in contact with an acute (wound) or chronically (atherosclerotic) damaged vessel wall (Vander et al 1990). In general, contact with a wound or damaged vessel causes activation of enzymes. These enzymes normally exist in the bloodstream in an inactive form,

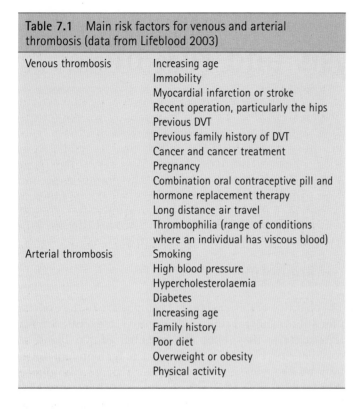

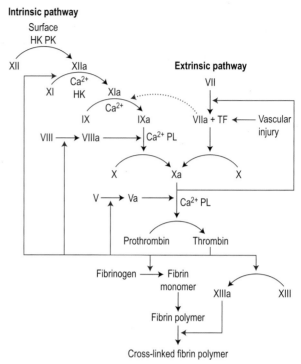

Figure 7.1   Intrinsic and extrinsic coagulation pathways. The intrinsic cascade is initiated when contact is made between blood and exposed endothelial cell surfaces. The extrinsic pathway is initiated upon vascular injury, which leads to exposure of tissue factor (TF) (also identified as factor III, sometimes referred to as thromboplastin), a subendothelial cell-surface glycoprotein that binds phospholipid. The dotted arrow represents a point of crossover between the extrinsic and intrinsic pathways. The two pathways converge at the activation of factor X to Xa. Factor Xa has a role in the further activation of factor VII to VIIa. Active factor Xa hydrolyzes and activates prothrombin to thrombin. Ultimately the role of thrombin is to convert fibrinogen to fibrin and to activate factor XIII to XIIIa. Factor XIIIa crosslinks fibrin polymers solidifying the clot. Ca2+, calcium; HK, high molecular weight kininogen; PK, prekallikrein; PL, phospholipid. (Reproduced with permission from King 1996.)

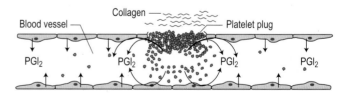

Figure 7.2   Events leading to vasoconstriction and platelet plug formation. Normal endothelium adjacent to a platelet plug produces prostacyclin I2 (PGI2) from platelet and endothelial cells, which inhibits platelet aggregation. This prevents spread of platelet aggregation from the damaged site. (From Vander A J, Sherman J H, Luciano D S 1990 *Human Physiology*, with permission of McGraw-Hill. ©The McGraw-Hill Companies, Inc.)

and once activated trigger a chain reaction, which amplifies the initial trigger but also localizes it to the area of vascular damage. This is accomplished by different proteins and phospholipids binding to cells, such as blood platelets, endothelial and smooth muscle cells. These bound substances keep the blood coagulation reaction restricted to the area of injury and prevent generalized coagulation, which otherwise would lead to widespread plugging of the circulatory system (Vander et al 1990) (Fig. 7.2).

Haemostasis is composed of four phases that occur in a set order:
1. The initial phase is vasoconstriction, which limits blood flow to the injured area.
2. Next, platelets become activated by *thrombin* and aggregate at the site of injury, forming a temporary loose *platelet plug*.
3. To ensure stability of the initially loose platelet plug, a fibrin mesh (clot) forms and entraps the plug.
4. Finally, following tissue repair, the clot must be dissolved in order for normal blood flow to resume. The dissolution of the clot, known as *fibrinolysis*, occurs through the action of *plasmin* (King 1996).

The intrinsic and extrinsic pathways both lead to the formation of a fibrin clot, and although the intrinsic and extrinsic pathways are initiated by distinctly different mechanisms, the two converge on a common pathway that leads to clot formation. The formation of a clot in response to an abnormal vessel wall in the absence of tissue injury is the result of the intrinsic pathway. However, the formation of a fibrin clot in response to tissue injury is the result of the extrinsic pathway (King 1996).

Formation of a platelet plug

Platelets adhere to surfaces but not to normal endothelial cells, which line the blood vessels. The protein fibrinogen is mainly responsible for stimulating platelet clumping, and platelets clump by binding to collagen that becomes exposed following rupture of the endothelial lining of vessels. Platelets adhere to the collagen, which triggers calcium (Ca^{2+}) release and secretary vesicles (granules). These granules contain a variety of chemical agents, such as serotonin, phospholipids, lipoproteins and other proteins important for the coagulation cascade, resulting in changes in the surface and shape of the platelets, to accommodate the formation of the plug. Furthermore, upon activation of the platelet granules there is a release of adenosine-5'-diphosphate (ADP) and thromboxane A_2 (TXA_2). Adenosine-5'-diphosphate further stimulates platelets, increasing the overall activation cascade, and also modifies the platelet membrane in such a way as to allow fibrinogen to adhere to two platelet surfaces, resulting in fibrinogen-induced platelet aggregation. TXA_2 also stimulates platelet aggregation, thus further strengthening the platelet plug. Platelets stimulate not only their own aggregation but also vasoconstriction, which leads

to compression and strengthening of the platelet plug. Whilst the platelet plug is being formed, the vascular smooth muscle in the vessel around the plug is being stimulated to contract, thereby decreasing blood flow to the area (Fig. 7.2).

The adherence of platelets to the damaged vessel is facilitated by the protein known as von Willebrand factor (vWF), which is secreted by the endothelial cells, and produced and stored by the granules of platelets, forming a physical link between the vessel wall and the first platelet layer. The vWF binds to the collagen and then platelets bind to the vWF protein. In addition to its role as a bridge between the platelets and exposed collagen on endothelial surfaces, vWF binds to and stabilizes coagulation factor (F) VIII (Vander et al 1990, King 1996).

Clotting

Clotting can occur in the absence of all cells except platelets. Clotting occurs around the original platelet plug when the plasma protein fibrinogen is converted to fibrin. Fibrinogen is a rod-shaped protein produced in the liver and in the healthy individual is always present in blood plasma. Circulating in the blood the protein pro-thrombin, in response to a stimulus, is enzymatically converted to thrombin. At the site of damage, the enzyme thrombin catalyzes a reaction that causes some poly-peptides to break from fibrinogen to bind and form fibrin. The enzyme FXIII is then converted from its inactive form to the active form FXIIIa by thrombin. Thrombin is the enzyme that converts fibrinogen to fibrin (which stabilizes the fibrin network) and activates FXIII. Cells within the blood, such as erythrocytes, become trapped in the fibrin network forming the clot or thrombus (Vander et al 1990, King 1996) (Fig. 7.1). Table 7.2 describes the various factors involved in clotting.

THE INTRINSIC AND EXTRINSIC PATHWAYS

The common point in both the intrinsic and extrinsic pathways is the activation of FX to its active form FXa (a represents the active form). Factor Xa activates prothrombin (FII) to thrombin (FIIa). Thrombin in turn converts fibrinogen to fibrin (Fig. 7.1). Thrombin also activates thrombin-activatable fibrinolysis inhibitor, thus modulating fibrinolysis (degradation of fibrin clots). Thrombin also leads to impaired plasminogen (p. 117) activation, thus reducing the rate of fibrin clot dissolution (King 1996).

Intrinsic pathway

The intrinsic pathway requires the clotting factors VIII, IX, X, XI and XII, the proteins prekallikrein and high-molecular-weight kininogen in addition to calcium ions and phospholipids secreted from the platelets (Fig. 7.1).

Table 7.2 Functional classification of clotting factors (adapted from King 1996)

Factors	Pathway	Activities
FXII (Hageman factor)	Intrinsic	Binds to exposed collagen at site of vessel wall injury
FXI	Intrinsic	Activated by FXIIa
FIX	Intrinsic	Activated by FXIa and in presence of Ca^{2+}
FVII	Extrinsic	Activated by thrombin in presence of Ca^{2+}
FX	Both	Activated on surface of activated platelets by FVIIa and in presence of tissue factor and Ca^{2+}
FII (prothrombin)	Both	Activated on surface of activated platelets by prothrombinase complex*
FVIII	Intrinsic	Activated by thrombin; FVIIIa is a cofactor in the activation of FX by FIVa
FV	Both	Activated by thrombin; FVa is a cofactor in the activation of prothrombin by FXa
FIII (tissue factor)	Extrinsic	A subendothelial cell-surface glycoprotein that acts as a cofactor for FVII
FI (fibrinogen)	Both	Essential for coagulation
FIV (calcium)	Both	Leads to the activation of certain enzymes
FXIII	Both	Activated by thrombin in presence of Ca^{2+}; stabilizes fibrin clot by covalent cross-linking
Regulatory and other proteins		
vWF		Associated with subendothelial connective tissue; serves as a bridge between platelet glycoprotein and collagen
Protein C		Activated to Ca by thrombin bound to thrombomodulin; then degrades FVIIIa and FVa
Protein S		Acts as a cofactor of protein C
Thrombomodulin		Protein on the surface of endothelial cells; binds thrombin, which then activates protein C
Antithrombin III		Most important coagulation inhibitor; controls activities of thrombin, and FIXa, FXa, FXIa and FXIIa

* prothrombinase complex is composed of various substances such as platelet phospholipids, Ca^{2+}, FVa, FXa and prothrombin, plus others.

These components lead to the conversion of inactive FX to its active form FXa. The intrinsic pathway is initiated when prekallikrein, high-molecular-weight kininogen, FXI and FXII are exposed to a negatively charged surface, termed the contact phase. Exposure to collagen is the primary stimulus for the contact phase (King 1996), though negatively charged triglyceride-rich lipoproteins may also cause initiation of the contact phase (Mitropoulos et al 1989, Schousboe 1990), thus predisposing individuals with high triglyceride levels (hypertriglyceridaemia) to risk of thrombosis.

The initiation of the contact phase leads to the conversion of prekallikrein to kallikrein, which activates the FXII to FXIIa, which can, through positive feedback, further hydrolyze prekallikrein to kallikrein. Factor XIIa also activates FXI to FXIa, which results in the release of bradykinin (potent vasodilator) from high-molecular-weight kininogen. In the presence of Ca^{2+}, FXIa activates FIX to FIXa, which leads to activation of FX to FXa. The activation of FX to FXa takes place through the production of phospholipids by the platelets. The exposure of these phospholipids by the platelets allows the *tenase complex* (the grouping of Ca^{2+} and factors VIIIa, IXa and X) to form. In this process FVIIIa acts as a receptor for FIXa and FX and as a cofactor in the clotting cascade. The activation of FVIII to FVIIIa occurs in the presence of minute quantities of thrombin. As the concentration of thrombin increases, FVIIIa is eventually cleaved by thrombin and inactivated. Thus thrombin not only activates the cascade but also deactivates it. This dual action, of thrombin upon FVIII, acts to limit the extent of the tenase complex formation and the coagulation cascade (Vander et al 1990, King 1996) (Fig. 7.1).

Extrinsic pathway

The intrinsic and extrinsic pathways converge at the site of FX activation to FXa (Fig. 7.1). The extrinsic pathway is initiated by the release of TF (FIII), which is released at the site of and in response to injury. Tissue factor is a cofactor in FVIIa activation of FX to FXa. Factor Xa has the ability, through the action of thrombin, to activate FVII and is a link between the intrinsic and extrinsic pathways. Another link between the two pathways is through the activation of FIX through tissue factor and FVIIa, and the complex between tissue factor and FVIIa is thought to be a major aspect in the clotting cascade. This is indicated from the fact that individuals with genetic defects in the contact phase of the intrinsic pathway do not exhibit problems with clotting. Inhibition of the extrinsic pathway occurs at the tissue factor–FVIIa–Ca^{2+}–FXa complex, where the protein lipoprotein-associated coagulation inhibitor binds to FXa, and only in the presence of FXa, to FVIIa, inhibiting coagulation (King 1996).

ANTICOAGULATION PATHWAY

The anticoagulation pathway involves prostacyclin (prostaglandin I_2 – PGI_2), protein C and antithrombin III. Prostacyclin is a prostaglandin which inhibits platelet

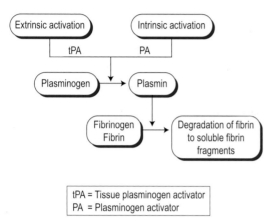

tPA = Tissue plasminogen activator
PA = Plasminogen activator

Figure 7.3   The basic fibrinolytic system.

aggregation and is produced by the endothelial cells. Additionally, protein C and antithrombin III both inhibit the positive feedback system and directly inhibit clotting, thus keeping the platelet plug within the area of vessel damage and preventing the coagulation process from spreading throughout the system (Fig. 7.2). The secondary inhibitory mechanism is thrombin. Thrombin activates a plasma protein, protein C, which then deactivates FVIII and V. Therefore, thrombin not only directly activates FVIII and V, but also deactivates them indirectly through the activation of protein C. The formation of the plasma protein antithrombin III inhibits the activities of FIXa, FXa, FXIa and FXIIa and deactivates thrombin. In order for antithrombin III to deactivate thrombin it requires the presence of heparin. Heparin is present on the surface of the endothelial cells and binds antithrombin III, the effect being that of anticoagulation (Vander et al 1990, King 1996).

FIBRINOLYTIC SYSTEM

The physiological mechanism responsible for removing a blood clot and the regulation of the enzymatic lique-faction of fibrin is the fibrinolytic enzyme system, and both the intrinsic and extrinsic pathways can initiate blood fibrinolysis. The ultimate liquefaction of fibrin works through a cascade of functions in a similar way to that of coagulation and this process allows the body to degrade a fibrin clot. The main phase of blood fibrinolysis is the enzymatic conversion of plasminogen to the proteolytic enzyme plasmin (El-Sayed 1996). Plasminogen circulates in the blood in its inactive form. Plasminogen binds to both fibrinogen and fibrin, thus becoming incorporated into the clot as it is formed. Primarily tissue plasminogen activator (tPA) converts plasminogen to plasmin. Inactive tPA is released from vascular endothelial cells following injury, it binds to fibrin and is consequently activated. Activated tPA cleaves plasminogen to plasmin which then digests the fibrin; the result is a soluble degradation product to which neither plasmin nor plasminogen can bind (Fig. 7.3). Following the release of plasminogen and plasmin, their

respective inhibitors rapidly inactivate them. There are several distinct inhibitors and the two that are thought to be of most physiological significance are plasminogen activator inhibitors type 1 (PAI-1) and type 2 (PAI-2) (King 1996).

ANTI–CLOTTING MEDICATION

There are several types of medications that are clinically employed to prevent or reverse blood coagulation. The most commonly used drugs are warfarin, heparin, aspirin, clopidogrel and streptokinase.

Heparin is a useful anticoagulant because it binds and activates antithrombin III, which inhibits the coagulation cascade (p. 115). Heparin is naturally abundant in the granules of the mast cells of the endothelium that line the vasculature, and in response to injury heparin is released and inhibits coagulation. Nevertheless, the drug heparin is generally administered to inhibit blood coagulation. The coumarin drugs, such as warfarin, inhibit coagulation by interfering with the action of vitamin K. Vitamin K is required for the function of thrombin and FVII, FIX and FX, as well as the proteins C and S. However, the action of coumarin drugs means that it takes several days for them to reach maximum effect, and because of this heparin is usually administered initially, followed by warfarin or warfarin-related drugs (Vander et al 1990, King 1996).

Plasminogen activators are also used for controlling coagulation. Since tPA is highly selective at degrading fibrin clots, it is extremely useful in restoring the patency of coronary arteries following thrombosis, and particularly in the short period immediately following myocardial infarction. The plasminogen activator is streptokinase, an enzyme from the *Streptococcus* bacterium, and is often used as a 'clot buster'. However, it is less selective than tPA, as it activates circulating plasminogen as well as that bound to fibrin. Aspirin, which works to inhibit platelet activation, is often used as a long-term anticoagulant. Aspirin works by reducing the production of TXA_2 (p. 115) and endothelial cell production of PGI_2 (Fig. 7.2), the outcome of which is to inhibit platelet aggregation; PGI_2 also induces vasodilation (King 1996).

INCREASED RISK OF THROMBOSIS

Normally there is a balance between blood coagulation and fibrinolysis. There are, however, several reasons why an individual may be more predisposed toward increased risk of thrombosis, and these result from multiple interactions between non-genetic and genetic factors (Tomoriova et al 1993, Marz et al 2000). The most common of the non-genetic factors are age, tissue damage, oral contraception, pregnancy, smoking, obesity, cardiovascular disease, hypertriglyceridaemia, hyper- and hypothyroidism, diabetes and/or lack of physical fitness. It is therefore important for the exercise practitioner to be aware of these factors and the risk that may arise for these individuals, especially during or after PA/exercise (p. 121).

INCREASING AGE

The haemostatic system can be affected by increasing age, and research carried out by Meade et al (1979) on 1601 men (aged 18 to 64 years) and 707 women (aged 18 to 59 years) showed that fibrinolytic activity became steadily reduced in men up to the age of 58 years, with a slight increase in fibrinolytic activity after this age. Women showed an increase in fibrinolytic activity up to the age of 40 years, with a slight decrease in activity from the age of 40 to 49 years. Research also indicates that regulated endothelial tPA appears to decline with age in sedentary individuals (Stratton et al 1991). These data therefore indicate a slight increased risk of thrombosis with age. The decrease in the fibrinolytic activity observed in the women over 40 years (Meade et al 1979) may possibly be connected with the change in hormones, due to the menopause in women over this age. Meade et al (1979) also observed that women on oral contraceptives showed the greatest amount of fibrinolytic activity, linking fibrinolytic activity with hormone levels (Cano & Van Baal 2001). Similarly Dotevall et al (1994) also observed an increased risk of thrombosis with age, where plasma levels of fibrinogen were positively related to age. Dotevall et al (1994) also found positive correlations with fibrinogen and body mass, waist to hip ratio, systolic blood pressure, serum cholesterol and triglyceride levels, and a negative correlation with plasma levels of high-density lipoproteins. Hence, since many of these variables are also interrelated, these findings highlight how numerous variables affect the balance between blood coagulation and fibrinolytic activity.

BLOOD LIPIDS, CARDIOVASCULAR DISEASE AND OBESITY

As long ago as 1852 it was first suggested by Carl von Rokitansky that the thrombotic processes were involved in atherogenesis. The opinion was held for many years that an atheroma was due primarily to hypercholesterolaemia, and the haemostatic system had no significant role in the pathogenesis of cardiovascular disease or other atherosclerotic disorders (Chandler et al 1974). However, in more recent times this view has changed. Pathological elevations in the plasma concentration of triglyceride-rich lipoproteins, which are often found in overweight and obese individuals (Phillips et al 1981, Connor et al 1982), appear to affect the natural anticoagulation properties of the endothelial cells, the adhesive and aggregatory responses of the platelets and the behaviour of the coagulation and fibrinolytic pathways, in a manner which promotes the growth of the atheromatous plaques and thrombus formation (Miller 1994) (Ch. 2).

Lipolysis of triglyceride-rich lipoproteins at the endothelial cell surface leads to transient activation of the coagulation mechanism with activation of FVII. Factor VII is the first enzyme in the extrinsic pathway (Fig. 7.1). Activation of FVII is generally achieved by tissue factor (thromboplastin), a substance formed during the earlier stages of blood coagulation. It acts as an enzyme, eventually converting inactive prothrombin to the enzyme thrombin, resulting from the conversion of FVII to FVIIa. Blood coagulation is then initiated by the subsequent activation of FIX and FX (Vander et al 1990).

There is increasing evidence that raised levels of FVII lead to increased thrombin production, where FVII has been found to be a strong risk factor for fatal coronary heart disease (Meade 1994, Miller 1994). There is also some evidence that triglyceride-rich lipoproteins influence the coagulation pathway in ways that do not involve the endothelium of the vessel walls (Constanton et al 1977, Miller et al 1985, Folsom et al 1991). For instance, a positive relationship has been found between FVII and coagulant activity and plasma concentration of triglyceride (Constanton et al 1977, Miller et al 1985, Folsom et al 1991), and a relation between FXIIa concentration and triglyceride-rich lipoproteins has also been reported (Mitropoulos et al 1989, Kelleher et al 1992, Woolf-May et al 2000). Factor XIIa is the active form of FXII (Hageman factor) and plays a key role in the early phase of intrinsic coagulation (Ratnoff 1966) and fibrinolysis (Niewiarowski & Prou-Watelle 1959). The autoactivation of FXII to FXIIa has been initiated by the negative charge on the membrane surface of triglyceride-rich lipoprotein particles (Mitropoulos et al 1989, Schousboe 1990).

DIABETES

In the rested state, for the well-controlled diabetic, hypercoagulation should not be a problem. However, hypercoagulation can be a characteristic of ketosis (Alakhverdian & Koev 1987, Golubiatnikova et al 1987) and complications such as hypertension, arteriosclerosis (often found in diabetics) and smoking tend to influence blood fluidity and contribute toward the development of microcirculatory blood flow disorders, which can cause platelet hyperactivity and hypercoagulation. Hypercoagulation is common in diabetics who display deterioration of blood flow, and these individuals tend to show raised fibrinogen levels (diabetics 442.4 ± 86.9 mg/dl, non-diabetics 349.2 ± 35.3 mg/dl) (Acang & Jalil 1993), which have been linked with increased plasma viscosity and erythrocyte aggregation (Volger 1986), as well as increased risk of cardiovascular disease (Imhof & Koenig 2001). Furthermore, obese type II diabetics have been shown to possess elevated levels of PAI-1 compared to non-obese type II diabetics (Aso et al 2002). In addition, hypertriglyceridaemia (p. 65) is often found in hyperinsulinaemic (p. 64) individuals and given that triglyceride-rich lipoproteins have been found to stimulate blood coagulation (Mitropoulos et al 1989, Kelleher et al 1992), this may further increase their risk of thrombosis.

SMOKING

Although it is the general consensus that cigarette smoking is bad for one's health and predisposes an individual to lung cancer (WHO 2003) and cardiovascular disease (Kawachi et al 1993) and impairs the healing of wounds (Whiteford 2003), the data are conflicting as to the effect of cigarette smoking on the haemostatic system. Nevertheless, there is evidence to indicate that smoking increases fibrinogen levels and the activation of platelets, leading to a prothrombotic state (Tsiara et al 2003).

HORMONES AND PREGNANCY

Steroid (Feuring et al 2002), thyroid (Erem et al 2002) and the stress hormones (Rosenfeld et al 1998) appear to affect the haemostatic system, as does pregnancy where there is a tendency toward hypercoagulation (Adachi et al 2002). For example, Koh et al (1999) observed a total of 71 pregnant women during their mid-trimester and found them all to be in a state of hypercoagulation. It would appear that the sex hormones, progesterone and oestrogen, affect platelet (Feuring et al 2002) and fibrinolytic activity (Cano & Van Baal 2001). For instance, a study investigating the effect of various types of hormone replacement therapy (which is primarily based on increasing the levels of oestrogen) in menopausal women found significant decreases in antithrombin and protein S (Table 7.2). Thus in thrombosis-prone individuals, hormone replacement therapy may cause a propensity toward blood coagulation (Sidelmann et al 2003). Although the oral contraceptive has been found to show enhanced fibrinolytic activity (Meade et al 1979), it has also been found to induce procoagulation activity, but the extent of this will be dependent upon the type of drug taken (Fruzzetti 1999, Martinelli et al 2003). Furthermore, fluctuations in the steroid hormones, progesterone and oestrogen, in response to the female ovarian cycle also appear to affect platelet function, due to their effect upon vWF concentrations (Feuring et al 2002).

Hyper- and hypothyroidism have both been reported to have an effect on haemostasis. Although there is still debate as to the effect of hyper- and hypothyroidism on haemostasis, several studies have found hyperthyroidism to cause abnormalities in blood coagulation and fibrinolysis, with increased levels of fibrinogen and vWF. A study investigating various haemostatic parameters in 41 hyperthyroid patients compared to 20 euthyroid controls found that compared to the controls the patients had significantly increased levels of fibrinogen, FIX, vWF,

antithrombin III and PAI-1, indicating decreased fibrinolytic activity (Erem et al 2002). Similarly, hypothyroidism has been reported to induce both hypo- and hypercoagulable states, where hypothyroidism has also been associated with atherosclerosis (p. 44) and increased risk of thrombosis. Research carried out to determine the various haemostatic parameters in 20 hypothyroid patients, compared to 20 euthyroid controls, found that plasma levels of fibrinogen, antithrombin III and PAI-1 were significantly greater in the hypothyroid patients, and FVIII and FX activity was decreased. The findings indicated a hypofibrinolytic status in the hypothyroid patients, which was mainly due to the enhanced levels of PAI-1 (Erem et al 2003), thus indicating the complex interaction of the thyroid hormones and the haemostatic system.

The effect of the stress hormones adrenaline (epinephrine), cortisol, glucagon, angiotensin II and vasopressin on the haemostatic system was assessed in a blind, placebo-controlled, crossover study carried out on 17 healthy subjects over a period of 24 hours. The results showed no significant increase in any measures of hypercoagulation in relation to these hormones. However, there were increases in tPA (Fig 7.3) and protein C (Table 7.2) activity (Rosenfeld et al 1998). These findings were indicative of an inhibition of coagulation and improved fibrinolytic state with these hormones. Since during PA/exercise there is an increase in circulating levels of stress hormones, this may explain the often-found increase in fibrinolytic activity during and immediately after PA/exercise (Ferguson et al 1987).

PHYSICAL FITNESS

Although much has still to be determined with regard to the beneficial effect of physical training upon the haemostatic system (Rauramaa et al 2001), it appears that those who are physically fit tend to be at reduced risk of thrombosis (Ferguson et al 1987). Whether this is due in part to other contributing factors, such as genetics and/or the status of the endothelium rather than the haemostatic system per se, has still to be fully determined. Nonetheless, a study carried out on 111 men aged between 51 and 53 years, who possessed normal blood lipid profiles, found physical fitness to negatively correlate with levels of fibrinogen and FX (Rankinen et al 1994). Similarly, unfavourable levels of physical fitness and adiposity were also found to correlate with levels of haemostatic markers in a study on 74 obese teenagers (Barbeau et al 2002). Furthermore, research looking at the differences between athletes and controls in responses of the haemostatic system after an acute bout of PA/exercise found that after exercise, the less physically fit individuals displayed greater propensity toward coagulation, even though both groups possessed a relatively high maximum oxygen uptake (athletes and controls

Table 7.3 Reported changes in coagulation and fibrinolytic parameters from an acute bout of PA/exercise (adapted from Prisco et al 1993)

Parameters	Changes
Fibrinogen	↑ or no change
vWF	↑
FIX	No change
FX	No change
FXI	No change
FXII	No change
FVII	↑
Antithrombin III	No change
Protein C	No change
TFPI	Variable
Fibrinolytic activity	↑
Plasminogen	No change
tPA	↑
PAI-1	↓

TFPI, tissue factor pathway inhibitor; tPA, tissue plasminogen activator; PAI-1, plasminogen activator inhibitor-1

68.4 and 52.6 ml kg^{-1} min^{-1}, respectively) (Kvernmo & Osterud 1997). Similar results were also found when physically active women were compared to their healthy, less active counterparts (DeSouza et al 1998). It also appears that after long-term physical training, for those at risk of cardiovascular disease and at greater risk of thrombosis there is a decrease in platelet aggregability and reduced platelet production of TXA$_2$ (Rauramaa et al 1984, 1986), thus indicating a link between physical fitness and risk of thrombosis (El-Sayed et al 2004).

SINGLE BOUT OF PHYSICAL ACTIVITY/EXERCISE AND HAEMOSTASIS

An acute bout of PA/exercise has been found to have a marked influence on the haemostatic system (Table 7.3) and, in healthy populations, there is a delicate balance between the activation of both coagulation and fibrinolysis (De Paz et al 1995, El-Sayed 1996). An acute bout of PA/exercise has been associated with a significant shortening of activated partial thromboplastin (tissue factor) time, and a marked increase in FVIII, which is related to PA/exercise intensity and the training status of the individual. Physical activity/exercise intensity and training status also influence fibrinolytic activity, where enhanced fibrinolysis is mainly the result of an increase in tPA and a decrease in PAI-1. Nonetheless, platelet count tends to increase with PA/exercise, which is probably due to the release of platelets from the spleen, bone marrow and lungs. However, the reports on the effects of PA/exercise on platelet aggregation and platelet activation markers have been conflicting; hence the exact effects of PA/exercise upon haemostasis still remain to be fully determined (El-Sayed et al 1996).

INTENSITY

During PA/exercise the haemostatic system appears to change from resting levels (Gunga et al 2002), which may be dependent upon PA/exercise intensity. However, short-term PA/exercise is known to induce shifts in plasma water into the interstitium with little change in the plasma protein concentration (Van Beaumont 1972), thus resulting in a greater cell volume after exercise, which will need to be corrected for in studies (De Paz et al 1992). Even so, studies have shown platelet aggregation (Joye et al 1978 (multistage treadmill exercise), van Loon et al 1992 (32 km run)) and fibrinolytic activity (Davis et al 1976 (cycle ergometry at less and more than 80% HR max), Szymanski & Pate 1994 (treadmill exercise at 50% and 80% aerobic capacity)) to decrease and increase, respectively, in relation to increases in PA/exercise intensity, which appear to be regardless of training status (De Paz et al 1992) or age (Gibelli et al 1972). However, not all studies have shown similar upward shifts in coagulation and fibrinolysis with increased PA/exercise intensity. Nevertheless, Andrew et al (1986) observed that graded exercise at 50 watt increments on a cycle ergometer caused a greater reduction in clotting time at lower intensities, suggesting lower-intensity PA/exercise to be less thrombotic than high-intensity PA/exercise. Similarly Prisco et al (1993) found the highest levels of thrombin after maximal treadmill exercise, which is supported by the findings of Herren et al (1992), who observed a significant correlation between coagulation activity and post-exercise lactate concentration, suggesting anaerobic metabolism favours activation of coagulation.

It has therefore been suggested that for individuals at greater risk of thrombosis, high-intensity PA/exercise may be detrimental (El-Sayed et al 2004) and may be a contributing factor to increased risk of sudden cardiac death in this group (van den Burg et al 1995). For instance, the tendency for increased coagulation following exercise is highlighted by a study on 29 sedentary, young (20–30 years) healthy males who underwent cycle ergometry tests at both 70% and 100% of their aerobic capacity. The findings revealed that whilst during the PA/exercise there were parallel increases in both coagulation (activated partial thromboplastin time) and fibrinolytic (tPA) activity, during recovery there was a sustained increase in coagulation and a decrease in fibrinolytic potential following both exercise intensities. Additionally, Prisco et al (1993) observed a small but significant increase in thrombin, in a group of healthy male subjects, 30 minutes after a standardized treadmill stress test, thus suggesting a post-exercise increase in risk of thrombosis (van den Burg et al 1995). Conversely, however, a study investigating the effects of high-intensity

PA/exercise (anaerobic Wingate test of 30-second duration) found that post-test markers for coagulation were increased, but to a greater extent, so were those of the fibrinolytic system (Gunga et al 2002). This highlights the need for additional research to determine the influence of PA/exercise upon coagulation and fibrinolysis systems and their clinical significance (Smith 2003).

DURATION

There are relatively few data regarding the effect of PA/exercise duration on the haemostatic system. However, from the little research that has been carried out, it would appear that the fibrinolytic system is activated fairly quickly after the commencement of maximal PA/exercise compared to coagulation. For example, a group of 15 healthy subjects underwent maximal cycle ergometry of 15, 45 and 90 seconds' duration, with 30-minute recovery between bouts. The results showed fibrinolytic activity to be stimulated after only 15 seconds of exercise whereas none of the exercise bouts caused a significant change in coagulation (Hilberg et al 2003). Aerobic PA/exercise of longer duration also appears to affect both coagulation and fibrinolytic activity as shown from studies carried out by Rock et al (1997) and van Loon et al (1992). Rock et al (1997), observed in a group of 14 healthy well-trained individuals, that 24 hours after a 42 km run indicators of coagulation were enhanced. Similarly van Loon et al (1992) found, in a group of well-trained diabetic and non-diabetic subjects, that after 32 km of running fibrinolytic activity continued to rise, and the findings were similar for both groups. Therefore, these data indicate that PA/exercise of long duration appears to stimulate both coagulation and fibrinolysis.

REGULAR PHYSICAL ACTIVITY/EXERCISE AND HAEMOSTASIS

Cross-sectional studies have shown differences in blood coagulation and fibrinolysis between trained and untrained individuals. For example, trained male distance runners have been shown to display greater resting and post PA/exercise fibrinolytic activity than matched less active individuals (De Paz et al 1992). In comparison to the effect of a single bout of PA/exercise on the haemostatic system, there is relatively little interventional research on the effect that habitual PA/exercise has on this system, and findings have been contradictory (Rauramaa et al 2001). From a review of studies on the effect of PA/exercise training on blood coagulation and fibrinolysis it would appear that for healthy young individuals, PA/training has little effect upon the haemostatic system. Nevertheless, it appears that physical training is of most benefit to older and cardiac populations whose haemostatic system is either less efficient and/or impaired (El-Sayed 1996). The possible mechanism for this may in part be related to

the effect of PA/exercise training on the endothelium to release tPA. For instance, Stratton et al (1991) found that after 6 months of endurance PA/exercise training, older ($n = 13$, 60–82 years) compared to young ($n = 10$, 24–30 years) men showed enhanced resting tPA and reduced fibrinogen and PAI-1 activity, with little change in the younger group. These findings are supported by those of Smith et al (2003), who carried out a study on 10 healthy older men (60 ± 2 years). They found that after 3 months of aerobic PA/exercise training, the capacity of the endothelium to release tPA was significantly increased by around 55% to levels similar to those of younger adult and older endurance-trained men, thus suggesting that regular aerobic exercise may not only prevent but also reverse the age-related loss of endothelial fibrinolytic function (Smith et al 2003). Furthermore, in middle-aged adults 18 weeks of brisk walking was found to result in a reduction in FXIIa levels (Woolf-May et al 2000).

TYPES OF PHYSICAL ACTIVITY/EXERCISE

The majority of research investigating the effect of PA/exercise on the haemostatic system has employed aerobic PA/exercise intervention, examples which have been cited above, and those few studies that have employed resistance training appear to show similar alterations in the haemostatic and fibrinolytic systems (El-Sayed 1993).

ADVERSE CARDIAC EVENTS IN RESPONSE TO PHYSICAL ACTIVITY/EXERCISE

In the healthy individual with intact endothelium and normal antithrombotic properties (Weiss et al 1998), vigorous PA/exercise is probably unlikely to present an increased risk of thrombosis or sudden cardiac event. Sudden cardiac death below the age of 35 years is rarely caused by thrombosis of a coronary artery, and in most cases are the results of anomalies in the coronary arteries and valves, and/or hypertrophic cardiomyopathy (Maron et al 1986). The majority of sudden deaths (70%) during PA/exercise are in those over 35 years, with the myocardial infarction (heart attack) attributed to the occlusion of a coronary artery by platelet-rich thrombi (Bartsch 1999).

INCREASED RISK OF THROMBOSIS FROM PHYSICAL ACTIVITY/EXERCISE

In general for the healthy young individual, a single bout of PA/exercise, carried out in favourable conditions, causes alterations in the haemostatic system that appear to maintain the balance between coagulation and fibrinolysis. However, for certain individuals, such as the physically unfit, cardiac patients, older individuals and diabetics, this balance may not be maintained, putting them at greater risk of hypercoagulation and thrombosis. It is therefore important that the exercise practitioner is able to identify those individuals who may be placed at risk from undertaking PA/exercise.

PHYSICALLY UNFIT

A bout of vigorous PA/exercise in the untrained individual can increase their risk of sudden death, and there is a 100-fold increase in risk of acute myocardial infarction (Siscovick et al 1984, Mittleman et al 1993). Although these data indicate enhanced risk, they do not show the direct cause and the exact physiological mechanisms still remain to be fully determined. However, platelet aggregation and activation is enhanced during a bout of vigorous PA/exercise (Wallen et al 1999) in conjunction with an increase in shear stress and increased concentration of catecholamines, adrenaline (epinephrine) and noradrenaline (norepinephrine), also known to activate platelets (Streiff & Bell 1994). Therefore, in comparison to the trained individual, with their higher PA/exercise tolerance, lower catecholamine concentration and less responsive platelets, the unfit individual will be at relatively greater risk of thrombosis. Physical training is also known to enhance the function of the endothelium, which may also play a role in protection from thrombotic development. Nevertheless, the risk is enhanced for the unfit individual and since vigorous PA/exercise poses a greater risk than moderate-intensity PA/exercise (Weiss et al 1998), the exercise practitioner should avoid vigorous PA/exercise in clients/patients who are currently unhabituated to PA/exercise.

AGE

Increasing age leads to many changes that affect optimum physiological function. In relation to risk of thrombosis, it appears that there is an age-related loss of endothelial fibrinolytic function, which would, in comparison to healthier younger individuals, predispose the older individual to increased risk of thrombosis from a single bout of PA/exercise. However, for the healthy physically trained older individual this risk may be reduced. For example, 3 months of aerobic PA/exercise training was found to enhance the capacity of the endothelium to release tPA to levels similar to those of younger adults and older endurance-trained men. Therefore, a healthy physically trained older individual may be at reduced risk of thrombosis from a single bout of PA/exercise. However, the older individual is also prone to other diseases, which may also affect their risk of thrombosis during physical exertion.

CARDIAC PATIENTS (Ch. 2)

In the healthy individual, a single bout of PA/exercise leads to a transient activation of both coagulation and fibrinolysis. However, in cardiac patients, whose fibrinolytic potential is reduced, there may be considerable risk of an acute cardiac event, especially in unfit individuals who are unaccustomed to strenuous physical exertion (Koenig & Ernst 2000, Imhof & Koenig 2001). For example, a study carried out by Kovalenko et al (1991) on 32 healthy and 35 myocardial infarction patients found that whilst a single bout of PA/exercise induced both enhanced coagulation and fibrinolytic activity in the healthy controls, for the cardiac patients there was a decrease in fibrinolysis and an enhancement of platelet aggregation. Furthermore, a study investigating the effect of treadmill walking to exhaustion in a group of 13 male chronic atrial fibrillation (AF) patients (65±11 years) compared to a group of healthy controls, found that following the PA/exercise, the AF patients had significantly raised plasma fibrinogen and reduced PAI-1 levels compared to the controls (Li-Saw-Hee et al 2001). Thus in the cardiac patients a single bout of PA/exercise induced a heightened coagulative state and increased risk of thrombosis.

The increased risk of thrombosis for cardiac patients occurs not only during the activity but appears to exist for some time after the PA/exercise has ceased. For instance, Gibbs et al (2001) investigated the effect of an acute bout of PA/exercise (treadmill exercised to exhaustion) in 17 male (65±9 years) stable chronic heart failure (CHF) patients, compared with 20 vascular disease patients free of CHF and 20 healthy controls. At baseline the CHF patients had significantly higher levels of vWF, and immediately and 20 minutes post-exercise plasma viscosity and fibrinogen were significantly increased. There was also a positive correlation between PA/exercise workload and maximal changes in plasma viscosity in the CHF patients. It was concluded that vigorous PA/exercise should be avoided in CHF patients in view of its prothrombotic potential (Gibbs et al 2001).

Although it is clear that PA/exercise training is beneficial to the cardiac patient (p. 18), it is important for the exercise practitioner to be aware of the increased risk of thrombosis, both during and after PA/exercise in the cardiac patient. The practitioner should therefore take care in determining the signs of an event and how to deal with one if it should occur (p. 22).

OBESITY (Ch. 6)

It would appear that during a bout of PA/exercise, obese individuals are at increased risk of thrombosis. This is highlighted by a study carried out by Morris et al (2003) who compared the effect of 30 minutes of walking (at 70% aerobic capacity) on haemostatic responses, in sedentary groups of 10 obese and 10 age-matched non-obese males. During and after the PA/exercise bout, the obese group showed lower fibrinolytic activity than the non-obese group, before returning to baseline values at 30 minutes post-PA/exercise, indicating heightened thrombotic risk over this time. However, the exact physiological link between obesity and reduced fibrinolytic activity is not clear and still remains to be determined.

DIABETES (CH. 4)

It is clear that diabetic individuals are prone to hypercoagulation (p. 65). However, there is little research to determine whether there is any increased risk of thrombosis during a bout of PA/exercise from diabetes per se and this is an area that requires investigation.

EXERCISE PRESCRIPTION

When prescribing to an individual at risk of thrombosis the issues will be similar to those for the cardiac patient (Ch. 2, p. 76), in conjunction with those discussed above.

CONSIDERATIONS AND CONTRAINDICATIONS

Any considerations and contraindications in relation to PA/exercise will be similar to those for cardiac patients (Ch. 2, p. 76).

MEDICATION

The effects that anticoagulation medication may have on PA/exercise are outlined in Chapter 14 (p. 227).

SUMMARY

- The process of blood clotting and the subsequent dissolution of the clot is termed *haemostasis*.
- Thrombosis may develop when (i) the blood is more viscous than normal, (ii) there is damage to the blood vessel wall and/or (iii) the blood flow is reduced.
- There are three main coagulation systems, the coagulation pathway, the anticoagulation pathway and fibrinolysis, as well as the intrinsic and extrinsic pathways.
- Clotting can occur in the absence of all cells except platelets.
- The normal balance between blood coagulation and fibrinolysis may be disrupted due to non-genetic and genetic factors. The most common of the non-genetic factors are increasing age, tissue damage, oral contraception, pregnancy, smoking, obesity, cardiovascular disease, hypertriglyceridaemia, hyper- and hypo-

thyroidism, diabetes and/or lack of physical fitness.
- An acute bout of PA/exercise has a marked influence upon the haemostatic system, the extent of which is related to the PA/exercise intensity, training status and health of the individual.
- There is greater risk of thrombosis at high-intensity PA/exercise, particularly for those prone to thrombosis.
- Physically unfit, cardiac patients, older individuals and diabetics are at greater risk of thrombosis from a single bout of PA/exercise.
- Physically trained individuals tend to display greater resting and post-PA/exercise fibrinolytic activity compared to less active individuals.
- Physical activity/exercise screening, prescription and PA/exercise considerations and contraindications are similar to those of cardiac patients.

Suggested readings, references and bibliography

Suggested reading
El-Sayed M S 1996 Effects of exercise on blood coagulation, fibrinolysis and platelet aggregation. Sports Medicine 22(5):282–298
King M W 1996 Blood coagulation. Online. Available: http://www.dentistry.leeds.ac.uk/biochem/thcme/blood-coagulation.html July 2004
Vander A J, Sherman J H, Luciano D S 1990 Human physiology, 5th edn. McGraw-Hill, New York

References and bibliography
Acang N, Jalil F D 1993 Hypercoagulation in diabetes mellitus. Southeast Asian Journal of Tropical Medicine and Public Health 24(suppl 1):263–266
Adachi T, Hashiguchi K, Matsuda Y et al 2002 A case of pregnancy with a history of paradoxical brain embolism. Seminars in Thrombosis and Hemostasis 28(6):525–528
Alakhverdian R, Koev D 1987 Fibrinogen-fibrin degradation products in diabetes mellitus. Vutreshni Bolesti 26(6):72–75
Andrew M, Carter C, O'Brodovich H et al 1986 Increases in factor VIII complex and fibrinolytic activity are dependent on exercise intensity. Journal of Applied Physiology 60(6):1917–1922
Aso Y, Matsumoto S, Fujiwara Y et al 2002 Impaired fibrinolytic compensation for hypercoagulability in obese patients with type 2 diabetes: association with increased plasminogen activator inhibitor-1. Metabolism: Clinical and Experimental 51(4):471–476
Barbeau P, Litaker M S, Woods K F et al 2002 Hemostatic and inflammatory markers in obese youths: effects of exercise and adiposity. Journal of Pediatrics 141(3):415–420
Bartsch P 1999 Platelet activation with exercise and risk of cardiac events. Lancet 354(9192):1747–1748
Cano A, Van Baal W M 2001 The mechanisms of thrombotic risk induced by hormone replacement therapy. Maturitas 40(1):17–38

Chandler A B, Chapman I, Erhardt L R et al 1974 Coronary thrombosis in myocardial infarction. Report of a workshop on the role of coronary thrombosis in the pathogenesis of acute myocardial infarction. American Journal of Cardiology 34:823–833

Connor S L, Connor W E, Sexton G et al 1982 The effects of age, body weight and family relationships on plasma lipoproteins and lipids in men, women and children of randomly selected families. Circulation 65:1290–1298

Constantin M, Mersky C, Kudzma D J et al 1977 Increased activity of vitamin K-dependent clotting factors in human hyperlipoproteinaemia – association with cholesterol and triglyceride levels. Thrombosis and Haemostasis 1:443–448

Davis G L, Abildgaard C F, Bernauer E M et al 1976 Fibrinolytic and hemostatic changes during and after maximal exercise in males. Journal of Applied Physiology 40:287

De Paz J A, Lasierra J, Villa J G et al 1992 Changes in the fibrinolytic system associated with physical conditioning. European Journal of Applied Physiology 65:388

De Paz J A, Villa J G, Vilades E et al 1995 Effects of oral contraceptives on fibrinolytic response to exercise. Medicine and Science in Sports and Exercise 27(7):961–966

DeSouza C A, Jones P P, Seals D R 1998 Physical activity status and adverse age-related differences in coagulation and fibrinolytic factors in women. Arteriosclerosis, Thrombosis and Vascular Biology 18(3):362–368

Dotevall A, Johansson S, Wilhelmsen L 1994 Association between fibrinogen and other risk factors for cardiovascular disease in men and women. Annals of Epidemiology 4:369–374

El-Sayed M S 1993 Fibrinolytic and hemostatic parameter response after resistance exercise. Medicine and Science in Sports and Exercise 25(5):597–602

El-Sayed M S 1996 Effects of exercise on blood coagulation, fibrinolysis and platelet aggregation. Sports Medicine 22(5):282–298

El-Sayed M S, El-Sayed A Z, Ahmadizad S 2004 Exercise and training effects on blood haemostasis in health and disease: an update. Sports Medicine 34(3):181–200

Erem C, Ersoz H O, Karti S S et al 2002 Blood coagulation and fibrinolysis in patients with hyperthyroidism. Journal of Endocrinological Investigation 25(4):345–350

Erem C, Kavgaci H, Ersoz H O et al 2003 Blood coagulation and fibrinolytic activity in hypothyroidism. International Journal of Clinical Practice 57(2):78–81

Ferguson E W, Bernier L L, Banta G R et al 1987 Effects of exercise and conditioning on clotting and fibrinolytic activity in men. Journal of Applied Physiology 62(4):1416–1421

Feuring M, Christ M, Roell A et al 2002 Alterations in platelet function during the ovarian cycle. Blood Coagulation and Fibrinolysis 13(5):443–447

Folsom A R, Wu K K, Davis C E et al 1991 Population correlates of plasma fibrinogen and factor VII, putative cardiovascular risk factors. Atherosclerosis 91:191–205

Fruzzetti F 1999 Hemostatic effects of smoking and oral contraceptive use. American Journal of Obstetrics and Gynecology 180(6 Pt 2): S369–374

Gibbs C R, Blann A D, Edmunds E et al 2001 Effects of acute exercise on hemorheological, endothelial and platelet markers in patients with chronic heart failure in sinus rhythm. Clinical Cardiology 24(11):724–729

Gibelli A, Morpurgo M, Giarola P et al 1972 Comparison study of coagulation fibrinolysis and cardiorespiratory function in elderly and young subjects after exercise. Journal of the American Geriatrics Society 20(2):59–62

Golubiatnikova G A, Valid B, Starosel'tseva L K et al 1987 Hemostasis and microcirculation in patients with diabetic ketosis. Terapevticheskii Arkhiv 59(7):109–111

Gunga H C, Kirsch K, Beneke R et al 2002 Markers of coagulation, fibrinolysis and angiogenesis after strenuous short-term exercise (Wingate-test) in male subjects of varying fitness levels. International Journal of Sports Medicine 23(7):495–499

Herren T, Peter B, Haeberli A 1992 Increased thrombin-antithrombin III complexes after 1 h of physical exercise. Journal of Applied Physiology 73:2499

Hilberg T, Prasa D, Sturzebecher J et al 2003 Blood coagulation and fibrinolysis after extreme short-term exercise. Thrombosis Research 109(5–6):271–277

Imhof A, Koenig W 2001 Exercise and thrombosis. Cardiology Clinical 19(3):389–400

Joye J, DeMaria A N, Giddens J et al 1978 Exercise induced decreases in platelet aggregation comparison of normals and coronary patients showing similar physical activity related effects. American Journal of Cardiology 41:432

Kawachi I, Colditz G A, Stampfer M J et al 1993 Smoking cessation in relation to total mortality rates in women. A prospective cohort study. Annals of International Medicine 119(10):992–1000

Kelleher C C, Mitropoulos K A, Imeson J et al 1992 Hageman factor and risk of myocardial infarction in middle-aged men. Atherosclerosis 97:67–73

King M W 1996 Blood coagulation. Online. Available: http://isu.indstate.edu/mwking/blood-coagulation.html July 2004

Koenig W, Ernst E 2000 Exercise and thrombosis. Coronary Artery Disease 11(2):123–127

Koh S C, Anaandakumar C, Bioswas A 1999 Coagulation and fibrinolysis in viable mid-trimester pregnancies of normal, intrauterine growth retardation, chromosomal anomalies and hydrops fetalis and their eventual obstetric outcome. Journal of Perinatal Medicine 27(6):458–464

Kovalenko V M, Shunkova E I, Goldberg G A et al 1991 The coagulating blood systems and thrombocyte aggregation in healthy subjects and patients with ischemic heart disease at rest and under physical loading. Terapevticheskii Arkhiv 63(4):69–71

Kvernmo H D, Osterud B 1997 The effect of physical conditioning suggests adaptation to procoagulant and fibrinolytic potential. Thrombosis Research 87(6):559–569

Lifeblood 2003 About thrombosis. Online. Available: http://www.thrombosis-charity.org.uk/aboutthromb.htm July 2004

Li-Saw-Hee F L, Blann A D, Edmunds E et al 2001 Effect of acute exercise on the raised plasma fibrinogen, soluble P-selectin and von Willebrand factor levels in chronic atrial fibrillation. Clinical Cardiology 24(5):409–414

Maron B J, Epstein S E, Roberts W C 1986 Causes of sudden death in competitive athletes. Journal of the American College of Cardiology 7:204–214

Martinelli I, Battagliolii T, Mannucci P M 2003 Pharmacogenetic aspects of the use of oral contraceptives and the risk of thrombosis. Pharmacogenetics 13(10):589–594

Marz W, Nauck M, Wieland H 2000 The molecular mechanisms of inherited thrombophilia. Zeitschrift für Kardiologie 89(7):575–586

Meade T W 1994 Haemostatic function and arterial disease. British Medical Bulletin 50(4):755–775

Meade T W, Chakrabarti R, Haines A P et al 1979 Characteristics affecting fibrinolytic activity and plasma fibrinogen concentrations. British Medical Journal 1(6157):153–156

Miller G J 1994 Lipoproteins and the haemostatic system in atherothrombotic disorders. Baillière's Clinical Haematology 7(3):713–732

Miller G J, Walter S J, Stirling Y et al 1985 Assay of factor VII activity by two techniques: evidence for increased conversion of VII to α VIIa in hyperlipidaemia, with possible implications for ischaemic heart disease. British Journal of Haematology 59: 249–258

Mitropoulos K A, Martin J C, Reeves B E A et al 1989 The activation of the contact phase of coagulation by physiological surfaces in plasma: the effect of large negatively charged lyposomal vesicles. Blood 73:1525

Mittleman M A, Maclue M, Tofler G H et al 1993 Triggering of acute myocardial infarction by heavy physical exercise. New England Journal of Medicine 329:1677–1683

Morris P J, Packianathan C I, Van Blerk C J et al 2003 Moderate exercise and fibrinolytic potential in obese sedentary men with metabolic syndrome. Obesity Research 11(1):1333–1338

Niewiarowski S, Prou-Watelle O 1959 Role du facteur contact dans la fibrinolyse. Thrombosis et Diathesis Haemorrhagica 3:593–598

Phillips N R, Havel R J, Kane J R 1981 Levels and interrelationships of serum and lipoprotein cholesterol and triglycerides. Association with adiposity and the consumption of ethanol, tobacco and beverages containing caffeine. Atherosclerosis 1:13–24

Prisco D, Paniccia R, Guarnaccia V et al 1993 Thrombin generation after physical exercise. Thrombosis Research 69:159

Rankinen T, Rauramaa R, Vaisanen S et al 1994 Relation of habitual diet and cardiorespiratory fitness to blood coagulation and fibrinolytic factors. Thrombosis and Haemostasis 71(2):180–183

Ratnoff O D 1966 The biology and pathology of the initial stages of blood coagulation. Progress in Haematology 5:204–245

Rauramaa R, Salonen J T, Kukkonen-Harjula K et al 1984 Effects of mild physical exercise on serum lipoproteins and metabolites of arachidonic acid: a controlled randomised trial in middle-aged men. British Medical Journal 288:603

Rauramaa R, Salonen J T, Seppanen K et al 1986 Inhibition of platelet aggregability trial in overweight men. Circulation 74:939

Rauramaa R, Li G, Vaisanen S B 2001 Dose-response and coagulation and hemostatic factors. Medicine and Science in Sports and Exercise 33(6 suppl):S516-S520

Rock G, Tittley P, Pipe A 1997 Coagulation factor changes following endurance exercise. Clinical Journal of Sports Medicine 7(2):94–99

Rosenfeld B A, Nguyen N D, Sung J et al 1998 Neuroendocrine stress hormones do not recreate the postoperative hypercoagulable state. Anesthesia and Analgesia 86(3):640–645

Schousboe J 1990 The inositol-phosphate-accelerated activation of prekallikrein by activated factor XII at physiological ionic strength requires zinc ions and high-Mr kininogen. European Journal of Biochemistry 193:495–499

Sidelmann J J, Jespersen J, Andersen L F et al 2003 Hormone replacement therapy and hypercoagulability. Results from the prospective collaborative Danish climacteric study. International Journal of Obstetrics and Gynaecology 110(6):541–547

Siscovick D S, Weiss N S, Fletcher R H et al 1984 The incidence of primary cardiac arrest during vigorous exercise. New England Journal of Medicine 311:874–877

Smith D T, Hoetzer G L, Greiner J J et al 2003 Effects of ageing and regular aerobic exercise on endothelial fibrinolytic capacity in humans. Journal of Physiology 546(Pt 1):289–298

Smith J E 2003 Effects of strenuous exercise on haemostasis. British Journal of Sports Medicine 37(5):433–435

Stratton J R, Chandler W L, Schwartz R S et al 1991 Effects of physical conditioning on fibrinolytic variable and fibrinogen in young and old healthy adults. Circulation 83(5):1692–1697

Streiff M, Bell W R 1994 Exercise and hemostasis in humans. Seminars in Hematology 31:155–165

Szymanski L M, Pate R R 1994 Effects of exercise intensity, duration and time of day on fibrinolytic activity in physically active men. Medicine and Science in Sports and Exercise 26(9):1102–1108

Tomoriova E, Takac I, Takac M 1993 Hypercoagulation states. Vnitrni Lekarstvi 39(11):1114–1119

Tsiara S, Elisaf M, Mikhailidis D P 2003 Influence of smoking on predictors of vascular disease. Angiology 54(5):507–530

Van Beaumont W 1972 Evaluation of hemoconcentration from hematocrit measurements. Journal of Applied Physiology 32:712–713

van den Burg P J, Hospers J E, van Vliet M et al 1995 Unbalanced haemostatic changes following strenuous physical exercise. A study in young sedentary males. European Heart Journal 16(12):1995–2001

Vander A J, Sherman J H, Luciano D S 1990 Human physiology. McGraw-Hill, New York

van Loon B J, Heere L P, Kluft C et al 1992 Fibrinolytic system during long-distance running in IDDM patients and healthy subjects. Diabetes Care 15(8):991–996

Volger E 1986 Hemorheologic findings in diabetes and their clinical relevance. Wiener Medizinische Wochenschrift. Journal Suisse de Medecine 136:5–10

Wallen N H, Goodall A H, Li N et al 1999 Activation of haemostasis by exercise, mental stress and adrenaline, effects on platelet sensitivity to thrombin and thrombin generation. Clinical Science 97:27–35

Weiss C, Seitel G, Bartsch P 1998 Coagulation and fibrinolysis after moderate and very heavy exercise in healthy male subjects. Medicine and Science in Sports and Exercise 30:246–251

Whiteford L 2003 Nicotine, CO and HCN: the detrimental effects of smoking on wound healing. British Journal of Community Nursing 8(12):S22–S26

WHO (World Health Organization) 2003 Cancer. Online. Available: http://www.who.int/whr/2002/en November 2003

Woolf-May K, Jones D W, Kearney E M et al 2000 Factor XIIa and triglyceride lipoproteins: responses to exercise intervention. British Journal of Sports Medicine 34(4):289–292

Chapter 8

Adults with asthma

Steve Bird and Kate Woolf-May

CHAPTER CONTENTS

Introduction 127
Definition 127
Symptoms 128
Diagnosis 128
Aetiology 128
  Classifications 128
    Allergic 129
    Childhood 129
    Intrinsic 129
    Exercise-induced asthma 129
    Nocturnal 130
    Occupational 130
    Steroid induced 130
Asthma attack 130
  Pathophysiology (non-EIA) 130
  Severity 132
Pharmacological treatment 132
Non-pharmacological treatment 132
  Breathing technique and aids 132
Reducing the risk of EIA 133
Physical activity/exercise 133
  Adaptations to physical training 133
Physical activity/exercise participation 133
Pre-physical activity/exercise participation 134
Exercise prescription 134
  Types of physical activity/exercise 134
    Water-based 134
    Intermittent physical activity/exercise 134
  Post-Physical activity/exercise 135
  Warming up and cooling down 135
Considerations 135
  What to do in an asthma attack 135
  Medications 135
  Physical activity/exercise environment 135
  Contraindications 135
Summary 136
Suggested readings, references and bibliography 136

INTRODUCTION

Many studies have suggested an increase in the prevalence of asthma (Mannino et al 1998, Rodrigo et al 2004), which has made it a global health concern (Yang 2000). However, changes in the diagnostic criteria (p. 128) and awareness make reliable estimations of these trends problematic. Hence the rise in prevalence may be due to a combination of increased detection rates, diagnosis and reporting, and/or changes in environmental factors, with the latter commonly being related to diet, local pollution and the indoor environment, particularly exposure to house dust mites. Taking these factors into consideration, it is therefore estimated that around 8–10% of the total US population suffers from asthma. Australia and New Zealand are reported to have the highest prevalence of childhood asthma in the world (>15%), whereas African and Asian countries have the lowest (about 5–10%). In general, countries in coastal, temperate and subtropical zones have the highest mite-sensitive asthma, and subarctic or semiarid areas have a lower prevalence (Yang 2000). The prevalence of asthma in adults has been increasing. In Australia, for example, the self-reported prevalence of doctor-diagnosed asthma increased from 5.6% in 1987 to 12.2% in 1997 (Ruffin et al 2001). Available data obtained from Canada and non-English speaking countries in Europe suggest that peak asthma prevalence has now been reached, at a level of 8–12% (von Hertzen & Haahtela 2005).

DEFINITION

Asthma is a disease of the lung that affects the bronchial tubes or airways (Ch. 9, p. 140). The term asthma comes from the Greek word 'to breath hard' and is defined as reversible obstructive airway disease, which is unlike other respiratory diseases, such as chronic obstructive pulmonary disease (COPD, p. 139), chronic bronchitis, emphysema or cystic fibrosis, where individuals are affected all of the time. The global strategy for asthma management and prevention (NHLBI/WHO 1993, 1995) describes asthma as intermittent and persistent with severe, moderate and mild degrees of the persistent disease.

SYMPTOMS

Asthma is characterized by episodes of transient airflow obstruction that make breathing difficult. These episodes are commonly referred to as asthma 'attacks' (p. 130) and are a result of the smooth muscle surrounding the bronchioles contracting (bronchoconstriction), and fluid (oedema) accumulating within these narrowed airways. The classic symptoms of an 'asthma attack' are therefore: a shortness of breath (dyspnoea), chest congestion and tightness, wheezing and coughing. Asthma severity ranges from mild occasional bouts of wheezing, to a life-threatening condition (CDCP 1996, D'Alonzo & Ciccolella 1999).

DIAGNOSIS

The identification of airflow obstruction is usually via simple pulmonary function tests of peak expiratory flow, in which reduced airflow is identified from reduced peak expiratory flow rates (PEFR), and a lower than normal forced expiratory volume exhaled in 1 second (FEV$_1$) (Ch. 9, Table 9.6). In some cases, for the purpose of diagnosis, bronchoconstriction may be deliberately provoked via an exercise challenge test (Nastasi et al 1995) or hyperventilation. In these tests, when compared to their pre-exercise or pre-test baseline values, asthmatics will exhibit significant post-exercise bronchoconstriction whereas non-asthmatics exhibit slight bronchodilation (Rees & Kanabar 2000).

AETIOLOGY

Asthma may develop in young babies and children (paediatric asthma), in which case the severity of the condition may abate with maturity, or it may not become apparent until adulthood. It can be associated with the living environment or occupation and may be exercise induced. It is a complex, multifactorial condition, for which there appears to be a genetic aspect that increases a person's predisposition to being asthmatic when exposed to environmental factors (Borrish 1999). This may be through inherited genes that code for increased interleukin and immunoglobulin E (IgE) responses to allergens and bronchial hyper-responsiveness (p. 130, 143). Additionally childhood exposure to allergens such as cigarette smoke (Charpin & Dutau 1999), air pollution (Nicolai 1999) and respiratory viruses (Martinez 1999) also increases the risk of children to becoming asthmatic.

CLASSIFICATIONS

Until recently asthma was classified into two clearly defined types, extrinsic (i.e. allergic) and intrinsic (non-allergic). Asthma is now classified into a variety of different categories, such as allergic, non-allergic, exercise-induced, nocturnal, occupational and steroid-resistant asthma (Table 8.1). Yet, despite the various classifications for asthma, generally these share aspects of common aetiology, pathology, clinical presentation, response to treatment and prognosis.

Table 8.1 Classifications and possible causes of asthma	
Classification	**Possible causes**
Allergic/extrinsic	Range of allergens: • Pet dander • Pollen • Dust mites • Pollutants • Wood dust • Smoke • Irritants • Chemicals • Viral infections • Bacteria
Childhood (allergic)	• Maternal cigarette smoking • Cigarette smoke can make people more prone to allergens, leading to allergic asthma
Non-allergic/intrinsic (typical onset over 40 years)	Respiratory irritants: • Perfumes • Cleaning agents • Fumes • Smoke • Cold air • Upper respiratory infections • Gastro-oesophageal reflux Intrinsic: • Stress • Emotion
Exercise induced asthma (EIA)	• Loss of heat and moisture in the lungs with strenuous physical exertion • Cold-dry environment
Nocturnal (sleep related)	• Allergens in the bedroom • Decrease in room temperature • Gastro-oesophageal reflux
Occupational	• Fumes • Irritants
Steroid resistant	• Overuse of asthmatic medication, 'status asthmaticus'

Allergic

Allergic asthma is triggered by substances that are capable of causing an allergic reaction (allergens), and 90% of all asthmatics have allergic asthma. A wide range of allergens, including pollen, pet dander and dust mites, can cause allergic asthma, as well as pollutants, wood dust, viral infections and bacteria (Clark et al 2000).

Childhood

The majority of childhood asthma is considered to be allergenic in origin and occurs more often in boys than girls. Research indicates that maternal smoking can contribute to asthma. Continued exposure of a child to cigarette smoke can irritate the respiratory tract and make infants and children more vulnerable to allergic asthma (Clark et al 2000). However, childhood asthma may abate during adulthood (Borrish 1999).

Intrinsic

In intrinsic asthma, allergens do not play a part, and it is not likely to develop in childhood, but typically occurs after the age of 40 years. The possible causes of intrinsic asthma are respiratory irritants, such as perfumes, cleaning materials, fumes and cold air. This type of asthma appears to be less responsive to treatment (Clark et al 2000).

Exercise-induced asthma

Exercise-induced asthma (EIA) affects about 4% of people who do not experience asthma symptoms at rest. Fortunately the risk of an asthma attack, both EIA and non-EIA, can be reduced by appropriate medication and behavioural choices (p. 132), thereby enabling asthmatics to safely include exercise in their lifestyle. Indeed, whilst severe asthmatics may be restricted in what they can participate in and may be advised to consider activities that are of a relatively low intensity, such as walking, bowls and golf, others can participate in more strenuous team sports and some can perform at an elite level in endurance sports, even to Olympic level (Voy 1986).

In addition to asthmatics exhibiting impaired lung function during an asthma attack (Table 8.2), about 80–90% of asthmatics are susceptible to EIA. Breathlessness is a normal response to sustained exercise of a strenuous intensity. However, it should not develop during or after exercise of a relatively mild or moderate intensity, but if it does, it may indicate that the person suffers from EIA. Exercise-induced asthma typically occurs 5 to 20 minutes after exercise and in most cases it will resolve spontaneously within 45 to 60 minutes (Lee et al 1983). Symptoms of breathlessness during exercise are generally attributed to poor conditioning and pre-existing obstruction rather than EIA, as respiratory assessments indicate bronchodilation rather than bronchoconstriction to dominate during exercise (McFadden & Gilbert 1994). A number of studies have

Table 8.2 Proposed factors that contribute toward classification of severity of asthma attack (adapted from Godfrey 2000)

Classification of asthma attack	Factors
Mild/moderate non-life-threatening	• Wheezing or coughing without severe distress • Able to talk normally • Little or no rapid (shallow) respiratory rate • PEFR >70% of predicted (See Table 9.6, p. 147) • No desaturation • Excellent response to beta$_2$-agonist therapy
Moderate/severe non-life-threatening	• Wheezing or coughing with moderate distress • Unable to talk normally, speak in phrases • Moderate rapid (shallow) respiratory rate • PEFR 50–70% of predicted • Modest response to beta$_2$-agonist therapy
Potentially life-threatening	• Severe respiratory distress/reactions • Unable to talk • Exhaustion/confusion • Cyanosis (bluish colour) of lips or tongue (in room air) • Poor respiratory effort • Marked rapid (shallow) respiratory rate and rapid heart rate • Saturation <90% • PEFR <33% predicted • No response to beta$_2$-agonist therapy

suggested that some individuals will exhibit a late EIA response that occurs 4 to 6 hours after exercise (Lee et al 1983, Boulet et al 1987). Others have suggested that the recorded respiratory constrictions are unrelated to the preceding exercise, but are a consequence of common daily variations in the participant's underlying asthma (Peroni & Boner 1996). Exercise-induced asthma can be effectively managed using beta agonists, cromolyn sodium and leukotriene antagonists, which not only enable the sufferer to undertake regular health-enhancing physical activity, but for those with the ability, to participate in elite sport.

Assessment of EIA

Clinical assessments for the diagnosis of EIA generally involve an exercise bout of 6 to 8 minutes at an intensity of 65–75% of predicted $\dot{V}O_2$max (75–85% of predicted maximum heart rate) (Morton & Finch 1993). Exercise-

Pathophysiology of EIA

According to the review by Storms (2003), the pathophysiology of EIA is yet to be fully understood, and at present there are two main theories: (1) the hyperosmolar theory and (2) the airway rewarming theory. D'Alonzo & Ciccolella (1999) report that 14% of high-performance athletes experience 'bronchial hyper-responsiveness, including bronchoconstriction' (exercise-induced bronchoconstriction – EIB). The symptoms of EIA and EIB are shortness of breath, cough and wheezing. Storms (2003) suggests that the pathophysiology of EIA may vary between sports and exercise scenarios. For example, the prevalence of EIA appears to be greater in cold weather athletes, at around 23% (Wilber et al 2000), compared with 16% in warm weather athletes (Weiler 1998). Additionally, cold weather athletes do not appear to respond to treatments such as beta$_2$ agonists (p. 229), which are effective for warm weather athletes. This, they suggest, indicates some form of chronic airway injury due to the inhalation of large volumes of cold air (Wilber et al 2000).

In accordance with the hyperosmolarity theory, EIA has been attributed to inhaling cold dry air, which as it is warmed within the lungs partially evaporates the fluid layer lining the airways, thereby causing an increase in osmolarity that results in the mast cells releasing histamine, neuropeptides, prostanoids and leukotrienes which cause bronchoconstriction (Hahn et al 1984, Anderson et al 1985, Howley & Franks 1997, Nicolet-Chatelain 1997) (Table 8.3). The second theory revolves around airway rewarming (McFadden et al 1986) in which it is proposed that the warm post-exercise air promotes a bronchodilation of the small airways, leading to fluid exudation from the blood vessels into the submucosa of the bronchioles. This then stimulates the release of mediators and results in bronchoconstriction. It is also evident that the greater the magnitude of difference in the temperature of the air inhaled during and after exercise the more severe the EIA response (McFadden et al 1986). In accordance with both of these explanations, running, during which large volumes of cold dry air are inhaled, is most likely to induce EIA, whereas swimming far less so, since the inhaled air is already saturated with water vapour and hence has little evaporative effect on the fluid within the lungs (Tan & Spector 1998). Even so, asthmatics with a mild condition, which is well managed, can still excel at endurance running (Freeman et al 1990).

Nocturnal

Nocturnal or sleep-related asthma (NA) affects people when they are sleeping, which may not necessarily be at night, though symptoms tend to be worse between midnight and 4 a.m. Nocturnal asthma is defined by a drop in FEV_1 (p. 147) of at least 15%, and may be triggered by allergens in bedding or bedroom, a decrease in room temperature and/or gastro-oesophageal reflux. It is estimated that around 75% of asthmatics are awakened by asthma symptoms at least once per week, and around 40% experience NA on a nightly basis (Clark et al 2000, Sutherland 2005).

Occupational

The prevalence of occupational asthma appears to be rising (Vigo & Grayson 2005), and is the direct result of the breathing of chemical fumes, wood dust or other irritants over long periods of time. In the West Midlands in the UK between 1990 and 1997, the annual incidence of occupational asthma was reported to be around 41.2 per million each year, and men were twice as likely as women to suffer from occupational asthma (Di Stefano et al 2004), mostly due to their increased exposure to these irritants.

Steroid induced

The overuse of steroid-based medications for the treatment of asthma can lead to 'status asthmaticus', which is a severe asthmatic attack that does not respond to medication and may require mechanical ventilation to reverse (Clark et al 2000).

ASTHMA ATTACK

Asthma attacks are reported to be most common at night or early in the morning, and when an attack does occur it can be resolved with bronchodilator drugs (p. 132) or will spontaneously abate over time. Asthmatics will experience attacks at rest and are also prone to the risk of an asthma attack when exercising (see 'Exercise-induced asthma', above). An asthmatic 'attack' is typically induced by a stimulus (trigger factor) such as allergens or irritants (D'Alonzo & Ciccolella 1999, Holcomb 2004). Asthmatics exhibit an increased responsiveness to these stimuli compared to non-asthmatics (Rodrigo et al 2004) a phenomenon termed as airway hyper-reactivity or airway hyper-responsiveness (AHR). Other factors that exacerbate asthma include viral infections, strong emotions and some medications such as aspirin. Due to their chronic susceptibility to airway inflammation, asthmatics will use anti-inflammatory medications to control their condition (p. 230).

PATHOPHYSIOLOGY (NON–EIA)

An asthma attack is caused by exposure to a trigger factor, such as dust, house mites, pollutants, pollen, che-

Table 8.3   Chemical and biological factors involved in asthma

Factor	Description
Bradykinin	A biologically active polypeptide, released from the mast cells during asthma attack, consists of nine amino acids, and forms from a blood plasma globulin; it acts on endothelial cells and mediates the inflammatory response. A potent but short-lived agent of arteriolar dilation and increased capillary permeability; also causes contraction of smooth muscle
Cytokines	Antibody protein messengers secreted by inflammatory leukocytes (white blood cells), macrophages or monocytes, involved in cell-to-cell communication, such as the interleukins and lymphokines. Released by the cells of the immune system and act as intercellular mediators in the generation of an immune response
Eosinophils	These are a type of white blood cell that constitutes 1–3% of white blood cells; they increase in number with allergy. Although the activities of eosinophils are not entirely understood, they are known to play a major role in allergic reactions. They also secrete chemical mediators that can cause bronchoconstriction in asthmatics
Histamine	A potent agent acting through receptors in smooth muscle and secretory systems. It is stored in the mast cells and released by antigens. Responsible for the early symptoms of asthma, such as bronchoconstriction
Immunoglobulin E (IgE)	One of the five major classes of immunoglobulins. Present primarily in the skin and mucous membranes, including those of the lungs. Produced by plasma cells and present in very low amounts in serum, mostly bound to mast cells. Takes part in various responses of the body to bacteria or foreign substances and responsible for allergic reactions
Interleukins	The generic name for a group of well characterized cytokines that are produced by leukocytes and other cell types. They are released from the mast cells, and have a broad spectrum of functional activities that regulate the activities and capabilities of a wide variety of cell types. They are particularly important as members of the cytokine networks that regulate inflammatory and immune responses
Leukotrienes	A family of biologically active compounds, released from the mast cells in reaction to an irritant. In asthmatics they participate in defence reactions and inflammation, and cause bronchoconstriction and mucus production. The mucus can block the smaller airways, resulting in coughing, wheezing and breathing problems
Macrophages	Large phagocytic cells of the reticuloendothelial system. Found in the lungs and ingest small inhaled particles resulting in the degradation of the antigen in immunocompetent cells
Mast cells	Cells of lung connective tissue, containing many granules rich in histamine, which is released, most significantly in susceptible individuals, in response to allergen or irritant
Neuropeptide	Any of various short-chain peptides found in brain tissue, such as endorphins. Released by neurons as intercellular messengers. Many are also hormones released by non-neuronal cells; can cause bronchoconstriction
Neutrophil	An abundant type of granular white blood cell that is highly destructive of microorganisms involved in fighting infection and disease
Prostanoid	Collective term for prostaglandins, prostacyclins and thromboxanes (see Glossary of terms). They are hormone like substances that act near the site of synthesis with altering functions throughout the body, and can cause bronchoconstriction
Serotonin	A neurotransmitter and hormone. An organic compound found in tissue, especially the brain, blood serum and gastric mucous membranes, and active as a neurotransmitter and in vasoconstriction, stimulation of the smooth muscles, and regulation of cyclic body processes
T lymphocytes	A subset of lymphocytes found in the blood, lymph and lymphoid tissues, constituting approximately 25% of white blood cells, which function in cellular immunity and can directly destroy target cells

micals, fumes, animal fur or feathers. Asthmatics are hypersensitive to one or a combination of these factors, which means that when they encounter them, the mast cells that line their bronchioles will release chemical mediators that initiate a chain of reactions leading to bronchoconstriction and inflammation (Figs 8.1 and 8.2). Whilst the exact aetiology of an asthma attack is not fully understood, it is evident that soon after exposure histamine, leukotrienes, bradykinin and serotonin are involved and cause increased vasopermeability of the bronchiole lining, contraction of bronchiole smooth muscle and increased mucus production. This causes oedema, airway constriction, wheezing and cough. Additionally, a number of hours after exposure, populations of white blood cells (eosinophils, neutrophils and macrophages) may be activated and T lymphocytes produce interleukins that further promote the inflammatory effect of eosinophils, thereby leading to an exacerbation of the inflammatory response (Table 8.3). Anti-inflammatory drugs suppress these responses and reduce the risk of exposure leading to a distressing attack.

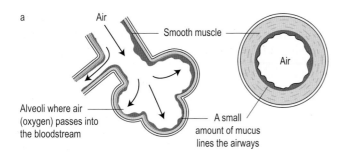

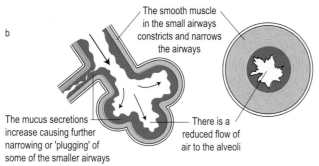

Figure 8.1 Diagram of cross-section of the small airway of the lung: (a) normal lung; (b) during an asthma attack (adapted from http://www.patient.co.uk.

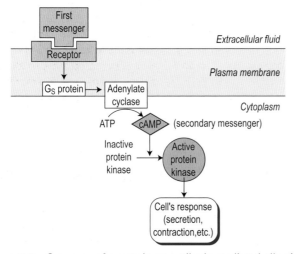

Figure 8.2 Sequence of events in an antibody-mediated allergic response through the second-messenger system. (After Vander A J, Sherman J H, Luciano D S 1990 Human physiology.© The McGraw Hill Companies, Inc.)

SEVERITY

The mechanisms that contribute toward the development of airway inflammation and changes in airway behaviours that contribute toward severe asthma are poorly understood. Severe asthma may develop over time, or shortly after the onset of the disease (Table 8.4). The pathology of severe asthma is fairly consistent; mucus plugs can form, blocking the airways, and with persistent inflammation the structure of the airways may be altered due

Table 8.4 Classifications for severity of exercise-induced asthma (EIA) (adapted from Morton & Finch 1993)

Classification	Percentage reduction in FEV_1 and PEFR
Mild	15–20
Moderate	30–44
Severe	>45

to membrane fibrosis (NHLBI 1997). Those with severe asthma often have air trapping and airway collapsibility (Wenzel 2003). The severity of airway inflammation is determined by the degree of histological change, including the number of eosinophils, lymphocytes and upregulation of certain cytokines (Table 8.3) in the layers of the airway wall membranes, the thickening of the wall, the epithelial damage and thickness of the base membrane (Woolcock et al 1998).

PHARMACOLOGICAL TREATMENT

Pharmacologically, the medications used to treat asthma may be broadly grouped as either bronchodilators or anti-inflammatories. The bronchodilators (beta agonists, methylxanthines and anticholinergics, p. 229) relax the smooth muscle of the airways whilst the anti-inflammatories (glucocorticoids, leukotriene blockers, cromolyn (cromoglicate) and nedocromil, p. 230) inhibit the release of the chemical mediators associated with the inflammatory response.

There are two aspects to the pharmacological treatment of asthma: chronic control of the condition and quick relievers that are taken 15 minutes prior to exercise as a means of prevention or in the event of an attack. The most common chronic controllers are the corticosteroids (p. 230). The most common quick relievers are the short acting $beta_2$ agonists (p. 229) such as albuterol (salbutamol). Fear of EIA is a common reason for asthmatics avoiding physical activity. But with the prophylactic use of inhaled beta agonists, or sodium cromoglicate and nedocromil (p. 229), EIA may be avoided (Tan & Spector 1998) and full participation in physical activity (PA)/exercise and sport may be possible for those with a mild or moderate condition. Storms (1999, 2003) suggests that if $beta_2$ agonists do not provide sufficient protection they may be taken in conjunction with cromolyn (cromoglicate).

NON-PHARMACOLOGICAL TREATMENT

There are several precautionary measures that may be taken to reduce the risk of asthma attack and EIA; these include breathing techniques and aids, and practical adjustments to where and when PA/exercise is performed.

BREATHING TECHNIQUE AND AIDS

One of the proposed causes of the bronchoconstriction and inflammation associated with an asthma attack is the inhalation of cold dry air (p. 130). So to prevent this, some authorities recommend that asthmatics should try to breathe through their nose during light exercise, as this will warm and humidify the inhaled air (D'Alonzo & Ciccolella 1999). However, during strenuous exercise, pulmonary ventilation will be very high, sometimes exceeding 150 litres per minute in fit athletes, and this rate far exceeds the ventilation rate that could be achieved through nasal breathing alone, which is approximately 40 litres per minute. Thus oral breathing is required during strenuous PA/exercise. To facilitate strenuous exercise in cold dry environments the asthmatic can try using a facemask that warms and humidifies the inhaled air. Some find these a useful aid although they obviously have limitations when participating in competitive sport.

REDUCING THE RISK OF EIA

To reduce the risk of EIA, it may be helpful to exercise at a time of day when the air is warmer, avoiding air pollution by exercising away from major roads and industrial areas that may have airborne chemicals. Likewise, exercising indoors on high pollen count days may be advocated if grasses or pollens are an allergen, and it is sensible to avoid exercising in areas where there may be cigarette smoke and dust. It is also suggested that participating in intermittent PA/exercise or team games is less likely to induce EIA than continuous hard physical activity such as running (Storms 2003). Additionally, recent research indicates that diets with a high salt content may also exacerbate airway inflammation (Mickleborough et al 2005) and therefore a diet with a lower salt content could be beneficial (Gotshall et al 2000).

PHYSICAL ACTIVITY/EXERCISE

Physical activity/exercise as a strategy to assist in the treatment of asthma is widely prescribed in rehabilitation programmes for asthmatics and has been shown to have health and quality of life benefits (Satta 2000). The health benefits gleaned by the asthmatic from PA/exercise participation are primarily the same as for non-asthmatics, i.e. a reduced risk of cardiovascular disease, improved musculoskeletal health, increased functional capacity, the facilitation of good mental health and social benefits (Cambach et al 1997). However, evidence for any potential benefits of PA/exercise upon the severity of the asthmatic condition are variable, as some research indicates that regular exercise does not improve resting lung function or the number of days of wheeze (Ram et al 2000), whilst other studies have reported a reduced demand for medication and a reduced number of Emergency Department presentations (Emtner et al 1996). Subjective reports also suggest that exercise can facilitate improvements in the quality of life of asthmatics, and perceptions of a reduced impact of asthma upon their life, although the review by Ram et al (2000) suggests that more evidence is required to verify these claims.

The physiological adaptations induced by exercise training for asthmatics are the same as those for non-asthmatics, including a reduction in the relative exercise intensity of a specific workload, such as a particular walking or jogging speed. One of the consequences of this is reduced pulmonary ventilation at each speed or workload, which will thereby reduce the likelihood of adverse evaporation and cooling of the airways (p. 130), and hence reduce the risk of an EIA attack being triggered (Ram et al 2000).

Adaptations to physical training

Regular physical activity improves the fitness of asthmatics, with similar physiological adaptations and improvements occurring in asthmatics and non-asthmatics (Strunk & Mascia 1991). Specific improvements following cardiovascular exercise training therefore include increased capacity to utilize oxygen ($\dot{V}O_2$max), maximum minute ventilation ($\dot{V}E$max), anaerobic threshold and oxygen pulse. These are manifested by a reduced perceived exertion, lower heart rate, lower pulmonary ventilation and lower concentrations of lactate at submaximal exercise intensities. It also produces improvements in exercise performance, such as walking distance within a set time limit and exercise capacity as demonstrated by increased time to exhaustion at specified cycle ergometer intensities. However, according to the review by Satta (2000), it is unclear whether the improvements include bronchiole responsiveness.

PHYSICAL ACTIVITY/EXERCISE PARTICIPATION

Fear of inducing an asthma attack represents a major barrier to PA/exercise for many asthmatics. Consequently by avoiding physical activity they will be at increased risk of cardiovascular disease as well as failing to gain the benefits of an enhanced physical capacity and psychosocial benefits. A combination of education and behavioural practices that ensure pharmacological control of their asthmatic condition and appropriate exercise choices will enable most asthmatics to gain the benefits of an active lifestyle without risk. Additionally, an improved level of fitness is likely to reduce the chances of EIA.

Exercise participation amongst asthmatics has, however, increased in recent decades along with improved medication and management, the myths of its dangers having been dispelled and its benefits more widely recognized. According to the review by Satta (2000) the apparent impairment of exercise performance and lack of fitness of many asthmatics is primarily due to their lack of participation in regular exercise, rather than being due to ventilatory limitations imposed by the disease (Emtner et al 1996). Lack of participation is often the result of fear of the consequences of exercise, particularly the risk of EIA, and this results in the avoidance of exercise (Clark 1993). However, with a comprehensive understanding of the condition and good management through appropriate medication, asthmatics with a mild condition can perform at the highest level, as evidenced by the large number of asthmatics who participate in elite sport (Larsson et al 1993) including Olympic champions (Wilber et al 2000). However, it is also recognized that those with a more severe condition will be limited in their level of participation, which in extreme cases will resemble hospital-based rehabilitation programmes that are similar to those prescribed for other respiratory diseases such as COPD (p. 149).

PRE-PHYSICAL ACTIVITY/EXERCISE PARTICIPATION

Most asthma sufferers will be aware of the type of allergens that trigger an attack, and it is important to make a note of these in order to avoid PA/exercise environments and situations that may predispose an attack. As for all individuals undertaking an intervention of PA/exercise, those with asthma should undergo a thorough screening process in order to detect associated risk factors and other co-morbidities. During the screening process it is important to determine the extent and severity of the asthma, as this will affect the type of PA/exercise prescribed. The screening process should involve the completion of medical and pre-PA/exercise activity screening questionnaires, and where applicable appropriate assessments should be carried out (Appendix A).

EXERCISE PRESCRIPTION

Given the large spectrum of severity for the asthmatic condition, exercise prescription will clearly relate to each individual's situation. For example, the goals of an exercise programme may be orientated towards participation in a particular sport and/or be directed towards increasing their capacity to perform activities of daily living and health-enhancing physical activity. Likewise, as for non-asthmatics, exercise adaptations will be in accordance with the type, intensity and duration of exercise undertaken. Therefore exercise programmes may be targeted towards improving cardiovascular and/or musculoskeletal fitness. As for non-asthmatics, prescription will be dictated by the individual's current exercise capacity, goals and ability to participate. Thus current fitness levels and aspirations need to be assessed for the purposes of both prescription and monitoring.

TYPES OF PHYSICAL ACTIVITY/EXERCISE

For adults whose asthma is classified as mild or moderate (Table 8.4), exercise prescription will be similar to that for non-asthmatics, with due attention being paid to the appropriate use of prophylactic medication. So for general cardiovascular health, the physical activity guidelines of the ACSM (1998) apply equally well to asthmatics as they do to asymptomatic adults. Thus, physical activity should involve the large muscle groups, be rhythmical in nature, performed at a moderate intensity for 30 to 40 minutes on most and preferably all days of the week. Walking, swimming, cycling, aerobics and similar activities are beneficial, as is general incidental physical activity such as household chores and gardening. For more severe asthmatics, exercise sessions may be designed as interval sessions with repeated intermittent bursts of activity separated by periods of low-intensity recovery.

The choice of exercise can also be guided by the same principles as those used for non-asthmatics, with the aim being to facilitate fitness, health and physical capacity, whilst promoting enjoyment and compliance with the levels of physical activity advocated for health. However, for those with severe asthma the goals are likely to be more oriented towards achieving a functional capacity that enables the performance of activities of daily living. Programmes for these individuals are likely to be of a lower intensity and resemble those prescribed for COPD patients (p. 151).

Progression and progressive overload are important in all training programmes in order to stimulate ongoing fitness improvements. For asthmatic individuals, these must be applied carefully and gradually in order to minimize the chances of an event that causes respiratory distress and thereby causes them to avoid further exercise sessions. For non-athletes, initial exercise sessions may include walking at a moderate intensity, and for those for whom further progression is deemed appropriate after a number of weeks, the walking may be interspersed with periods of jogging. The duration of these may commence at 10 to 30 seconds and be extended as fitness improves.

Water-based

Swimming is commonly prescribed for asthmatics, as it appears to be less likely to induce bronchoconstriction and EIA because the air is more saturated with water vapour than other environments (p. 130). Therefore swimming may be classified as an activity with low asthmogenicity, whereas running outdoors on a cold winter's day would be rated as having high asthmogenicity.

Intermittent physical activity/exercise

Participating in intermittent PA/exercise or team games is less likely to induce EIA than continuous hard physical activity such as running (Storms 2003), and for more severe asthmatics, exercise sessions may be designed as interval sessions with repeated intermittent bursts of activity separated by periods of low-intensity recovery.

POST–PHYSICAL ACTIVITY/EXERCISE

After PA/exercise, asthmatics should ensure that they do not become cold and should change into warm clothing, as they may be susceptible to sudden changes in temperature (Morton & Finch 1993). Respiratory infections will increase the asthmatic's susceptibility to EIA and therefore they should take precautions to minimize infection, such as avoiding people with colds and other upper respiratory tract infections.

It has been suggested that exercises for breathing control be included at the end of each exercise session, including diaphragmatic (abdominal) breathing and breathing against a resistance to increase the strength and endurance of respiratory muscles (Morton & Finch 1993).

WARMING UP AND COOLING DOWN

According to D'Alonzo & Ciccolella (1999) an extended warm-up can minimize the impact of EIA. They advocate initially warming up at a low intensity until a light sweat is induced and then performing close to maximum exertion for 5 minutes, and then resting. Others advocate using a routine of repeated short sprints to warm up (Schnall & Landau 1980). D'Alonzo & Ciccolella (1999) also suggest that accomplished athletes may perform this procedure recurrently for 30 to 40 minutes, with some needing to warm up for an hour, although for most people 10 minutes is usually adequate (Wright & Martin 1995). Likewise McKenzie et al (1994) also report that a high-intensity warm-up at 80–90% maximum will partially, if not entirely, reduce the severity of EIA. The underlying physiology of these practices may be related to the refractory period of 1 to 2 hours that is experienced by about 50% of asthmatics (Schoeffel et al 1980), during which adverse bronchoconstriction and other EIA responses are attenuated. Thus during the refractory period the risk of breathing difficulties during exercise is diminished and some athletes have been known to use this phenomenon (Reiff et al 1989). Tan & Spector (1998) report that the physiological basis for the refractory period has been linked to a depletion of catecholamines and perhaps also to the protective effect of prostaglandins released during the preceding exercise. They also emphasize that the refractory period is exercise specific since it does not apply to other stimuli such as allergens (McFadden & Gilbert 1994).

Following strenuous physical activity, moderate to low physical activity should be used as a gradual cool-down, in an environment that is not too cold. However, it should be remembered that one of the proposed stimuli for EIA is a large temperature differences between the inspired air during and after exercise, so this should not be too great. The rationale for using gentle exercise to cool down as a prophylactic for EIA is that by continuing to maintain a ventilation rate above resting values, the rate of airway rewarming will be slow and hence the stimuli for EIA reduced (McFadden 1995). Given the diversity of responses, each individual will need to try a variety of scenarios in order to establish the warm-up and cool-down procedures that best suit them.

CONSIDERATIONS

WHAT TO DO IN AN ASTHMATIC ATTACK

If a client/patient has an attack either during rest or PA/exercise, remain calm to avoid any additional anxiety that will make the situation worse; also encourage them to find a comfortable position and ask them to focus on their breathing and employ a technique known as 'pursed lip breathing'. Encourage the asthmatic to inhale as normal but to actively exhale the air through pursed lips. Most asthmatics will be familiar with this technique. The cause of this shortness of breath is the inability to exhale carbon dioxide (CO_2) through the constricted bronchial tubes. The active 'blowing out' stretches the bronchial tubes, allowing CO_2 to be exhaled (Lungdiseasefocus 2004).

MEDICATIONS

Most medications that are prescribed for asthmatics do not appear to limit their PA/exercise ability (p. 229), and provide no advantage during PA/exercise over non-asthmatic individuals. It is important for the vast majority of asthmatics that they take adequate medication prior to PA/exercise to avoid the onset of an attack.

PHYSICAL ACTIVITY/EXERCISE ENVIRONMENT

Since allergens and irritants trigger asthma, it is important for the client/patient and exercise practitioner to know what these are likely to be. This enables the avoidance of environments that will promote the onset of an asthma attack.

CONTRAINDICATIONS

Any PA/exercise contraindications are as stated in Appendix A, Table A.1. As a general rule, if prior to exercise an asthmatic records a forced vital capacity (FVC) or PEFR that is less than 80% of their best value, they may be advised not to exercise. Therefore, for moderate to severe asthmatics, it is important to check FVC prior to PA/exercise. According to Morton & Finch (1993), some asthmatics displaying these values will be able to exercise and their symptoms will improve, but the majority will not and are liable to worsen.

SUMMARY

- Asthma is a complex multifactorial condition resulting in airway hyper-responsiveness to inhaled irritants and allergens, causing bronchoconstriction and inflammation of the airways.
- An asthma attack is characterized by shortness of breath (dyspnoea), chest congestion and tightness, wheezing and coughing.
- There are several categories of asthma, such as allergic, non-allergic, childhood, exercise-induced asthma (EIA), nocturnal asthma (NA), occupational and steroid-resistant asthma (Table 8.1).
- Despite the different categories of asthma, generally they share aspects of aetiology, pathology, clinical presentation, response to treatment and prognosis.
- Exercise-induced asthma (EIA) may appear in those who do not suffer from asthma at rest.
- Cold weather appears to be a significant factor in EIA.
- The cause of severe asthma is not totally understood.
- Pharmacological treatment may prevent the onset of attack and treat the symptoms of asthma.
- Pre-PA/exercise the majority of asthmatics should take pharmacological prophylaxis to avoid the onset of an attack.
- Physical activity/exercise training assists asthmatics in enhancing their quality of life, and reduces pulmonary ventilation at similar pre-training workloads, but does not appear to improve lung function.
- Asthmatics adapt to PA/exercise training in a similar manner to healthy non-asthmatic individuals.
- Asthmatics may enjoy a wide range of PA/exercise, the extent and intensity being dependent upon their physical status and severity of asthma.
- Water-based and intermittent PA/exercise tend to be less asthmogenic.
- If prior to PA/exercise the asthmatic's FVC or PEER is <80% of their best value, PA/exercise should not be undertaken.

Suggested readings, references and bibliography

Suggested reading
Clark T H J, Godfrey S, Lee T H et al 2000 Asthma, 4th edn. Arnold, London

References and bibliography
ACSM (American College of Sports Medicine) 1998 Position stand. The recommended quantity and quality of exercise for developing and maintaining cardiorespiratory and muscular fitness, and flexibility in healthy adults. Medicine and Science in Sports and Exercise 30(6):975–991

Anderson S D, Schoeffel R E, Black J L et al 1985 Airway cooling as the stimulus to exercise-induced asthma – a re-evaluation. European Journal of Respiratory Diseases 67:20–30

Borrish L 1999 Genetics of allergy and asthma. Annals of Allergy and Asthma Immunology 82:413–424

Boulet L P, Legris C, Turcotte H et al 1987 Prevalence and characteristics of late asthmatic response to exercise. Journal of Allergy and Clinical Immunology 80:655–662

Cambach W, Chadwick-Straver R V M, Wagenaar R C et al 1997 The effects of a community-based pulmonary rehabilitation programme on exercise tolerance and quality of life: a randomized controlled trial. European Respiratory Journal 10:103–113

CDCP (Centers for Disease Control and Prevention) 1996 Asthma mortality and hospitalization among children and young adults – United States, 1990–3. Morbidity and Mortality Weekly Report 45:350–353

Charpin D, Dutau H 1999 Role of allergens in the natural history of childhood asthma. Pediatric Pulmonology 18(suppl):34–36

Clark C J 1993 The role of physical training in asthma. In: Casaburi R, Petty T L (eds) Principles and practice of pulmonary rehabilitation. Saunders, Philadelphia, p 424–438

Clark T H J, Godfrey S, Lee T H et al 2000 Asthma, 4th edn. Arnold, London

D'Alonzo G E, Ciccolella D E 1999 Asthma. In: Rippe J M (ed) Lifestyle medicine. Blackwell, Oxford, p 460–476

Di Stefano F, Siriruttanapruk S, McCoarch J et al 2004 Occupational asthma in a highly industrialized region of UK: report from a local surveillance scheme. Allergie et Immunologie 36(2):56–62

Emtner M, Herala M, Stålenheim G 1996 High-intensity physical training in adults with asthma: a 10-week rehabilitation program. Chest 109:323–330

Freeman W, Williams C, Nute M G L 1990 Endurance running performance in athletes with asthma. Journal of Sports Sciences 8:103–117

Godfrey S 2000 Childhood asthma. In: Clark T H J, Godfrey S, Lee T H et al Asthma, 4th edn. Arnold, London

Gotshall R W, Mickleborough T D, Cordain L 2000 Dietary salt restriction improves pulmonary function in exercise-induced asthma. Medicine and Science in Sports and Exercise 32:1815–1819

Hahn A, Anderson S D, Morton A R et al 1984 A reinterpretation of the effect of temperature and water content of the inspired air in exercise-induced asthma. American Review of Respiratory Disease 130(4):575–579

Holcomb S 2004 Asthma update. Dimensions of Critical Care Nursing 23(3):101–107

Howley E T, Franks B D 1997 Health fitness instructors handbook, 3rd edn. Human Kinetics, Champaign, IL, p 364–366

Larsson K, Ohlsen P, Larsson L et al 1993 High prevalence of asthma in cross country skiers. British Medical Journal 307:1326–1329

Lee T H, Nagakura T, Papageorgiou N et al 1983 Exercise-induced late asthmatic reactions with neutrophil chemotactic activity. New England Journal of Medicine 308(25):1502–1505

Lungdiseasefocus 2004 What is an asthma attack? Online. Available: http://www.lungdiseasefocus.com July 2005

McFadden E R 1995 Exercise-induced airway obstruction. Clinical Chest Medicine 16:671–682

McFadden E R, Gilbert I A 1994 Exercise-induced asthma. New England Journal of Medicine 330:1362–1367

McFadden E R, Lenner K A M, Strohl K P 1986 Post-exertional airway rewarming and thermally induced asthma. Journal of Clinical Investigations 78:18–25

McKenzie D C, Mcluckie S L, Stirling S R 1994 The protective effects of continuous and interval exercise in athletes with exercise-induced asthma. Medicine and Science in Sports and Exercise 26:951–956

Mannino D M, Homa D M, Pertowski C A et al 1998 Surveillance for asthma – United States, 1960–1995. Morbidity and Mortality Weekly Report. CDC Surveillance Summaries 47(1):1–27

Martinez F D 1999 Role of respiratory infection in onset of asthma and chronic obstructive pulmonary disease. Clinical and Experimental Allergy 29(suppl 2):53–58

Mickleborough T D, Lindley M R, Ray S 2005 Dietary salt, airway inflammation, and diffusion capacity in exercise-induced asthma. Medicine and Science in Sports and Exercise 37:904–914

Morton A R, Finch K D 1993 Asthma. In: Skinner J S (ed) Exercise testing and exercise prescription for special cases, 2nd edn. Williams & Wilkins, Baltimore, p 211–228

Nastasi K J, Heinly T L, Blaiss M S 1995 Exercise-induced asthma and the athlete. Journal of Asthma 32:249–257

NHLBI 1997 Guidelines for the diagnosis and management of asthma. Expert panel report II. Publication #97-4051. National Institutes of Health, Washington, DC

NHLBI/WHO (National Heart, Lung and Blood Institute/World Health Organization) 1993 Global strategy for asthma management and prevention. National Institutes of Health, Washington, DC

NHLBI/WHO 1995 Global initiative for asthma. Global strategy for asthma management and prevention. NHLBI/WHO

Nicklaus T M, Burgin W W, Taylor J R 1969 Spirometric tests to diagnose asthma. American Review of Respiratory Diseases 100:153–159

Nicolai T 1999 Air pollution and respiratory disease in children: what is the clinically relevant impact? Pediatric Pulmonology (suppl 18):9–13

Nicolet-Chatelain G 1997 Asthma induced by exercise. Revue Medicale de la Suisse Romande 117(6):465–470

Peroni D G, Boner A L 1996 Exercise-induced asthma: is there space for late-phase reactions? European Respiratory Journal 9:1335–1338

Ram F S, Robinson S M, Black P N 2000 Physical training for asthma. The Cochrane Database of Systematic Reviews 2000, Issue 1. Art. No.: CD001116. DOI: 10.1002/14651858.CD001116

Rees J, Kanabar D 2000 ABC of asthma, 4th edn. British Medical Journal Books, London

Reiff D B, Nozhat B C, Neil B P et al 1989 The effect of prolonged submaximal warm-up exercise on exercise-induced asthma. American Reviews of Respiratory Disease 139:479–484

Rodrigo G J, Rodrigo C, Hall J B 2004 Acute asthma in adults. Chest 125:1081–1101

Ruffin R, Wilson D, Smith B et al 2001 Prevalence, morbidity and management of adult asthma in South Australia. Immunology and Cell Biology 79(2):191–194

Satta A 2000 Exercise training in asthma. Journal of Sports Medicine and Physical Fitness 40:277–283

Schnall R P, Landau L I 1980 Protective effect of repeated short sprints in exercise-induced asthma. Thorax 35:828–832

Schoeffel R E, Anderson S D, Gillam I et al 1980 Multiple exercise and histamine challenge in asthmatic patients. Thorax 35(3):164–170

Storms W W 1999 Double-blind, placebo-controlled study of single doses of chlorofluorocarbon (CFC) and CFC-free cromolyn sodium for exercise-induced bronchoconstriction. Current Therapeutic Research 60:629–637

Storms W W 2003 Review of exercise-induced asthma. Medicine and Science in Sports and Exercise 35:1464–1470

Strunk R, Mascia A 1991 Rehabilitation of patient with asthma in the outpatient setting. Journal of Allergy and Clinical Immunology 87:601–611

Sutherland E R 2005 Nocturnal asthma: underlying mechanisms and treatment. Current Allergy and Asthma Reports 5(2):161–167

Tan R A, Spector S L 1998 Exercise-induced asthma. Sports Medicine 25:1–6

Vander A J, Sherman J H, Luciano D S 1990 Human physiology. McGraw-Hill, New York

Vigo P G, Grayson M H 2005 Occupational exposures as triggers of asthma. Immunology and Allergy Clinics of North America 25(1):191–205

von Hertzen L, Haahtela T 2005 Signs of reversing trend in prevalence of asthma. Allergy 60(3):283–292

Voy R O 1986 The US Olympic committee experience with exercise induced bronchospasm, 1984. Medicine and Science in Sports and Exercise 18:328–330

Weiler J M 1998 Asthma in the United States Olympic athletes who participated in the 1996 Summer Games. Journal of Allergy & Clinical Immunology 102:722–726

Wenzel S 2003 Mechanisms of severe asthma. Clinical and Experimental Allergy 33(12):1622–1628

Wilber R L, Rundell K W, Szmedra L et al 2000 Incidence of exercise-induced bronchospasm in Olympic winter sports athletes. Medicine and Science in Sports and Exercise 32:732–737

Woolcock A J, Dusser D, Fajac I 1998 Severity of chronic asthma. Thorax 53(6):442–444

Wright L A, Martin R J 1995 Nocturnal asthma and exercise induced bronchospasm. Postgraduate Medicine 97:83–90

Yang K D 2000 Childhood asthma: aspects of global environment, genetics and management. Chang Gung Medical Journal 23(11):641–661

Chapter 9

Chronic obstructive pulmonary disease

CHAPTER CONTENTS

Introduction 139
Prevalence and definition 140
Respiratory system physiology and anatomy 140
  Gas exchange 141
  Ventilation 141
Breathing mechanisms 141
Aetiology 142
  Emphysema 142
  Chronic bronchitis 143
  Asthma 143
  Host factors 143
    Genetic factors 143
    Airway hyper-responsiveness 143
    Lung growth 143
  Environmental exposure 143
  Respiratory infections 144
  Inflammation 144
  Oxidative stress 144
Pathophysiology 144
  Airflow limitation 145
  Pulmonary vascular changes 145
  Pulmonary hypertension 145
    Cor pulmonale 146
  Gas exchange 146
  Mechanical changes 146
Assessments 147
  Lung function 147
  Functional ability 147
Treatment 148
  Pharmacological 148
    Bronchodilators 148
    Corticosteroids 148
    Other drugs 148

  Non-pharmacological 149
    Pulmonary rehabilitation 149
    Smoking cessation 149
    Lung reduction surgery 149
    Lung function and lung reduction surgery 149
Physical activity/exercise 149
  Training and the lungs 150
  Training and lung function 150
  Airway inflammation 150
Pre-physical activity/exercise prescription 151
Physical activity/exercise prescription 151
  Types of physical activity/exercise 151
    Continuous versus interval physical activity/exercise 151
    Eccentric exercise 152
    Aerobic activities 152
    Resistance circuit training and weight training 152
    Upper body 152
    Water-based activities 152
  Physical activity/exercise intensity 152
Physical activity/exercise considerations 152
  Progression 153
  Lung sputum clearance and coughing 153
  Signs of disease progression 153
  Medication 153
  Absolute contraindications for exercise 153
  Physical activity/exercise limitations 153
    Hypercapnia 153
    Oxygen supplementation 153
    Oxygen saturation 154
    Muscle myopathy 154
    Lung hyperinflation 154
Summary 155
Suggested readings, references and bibliography 155

INTRODUCTION

In the past, chronic obstructive pulmonary disease (COPD) was thought to be untreatable, and though still incurable, the quality of life of these individuals may be enhanced by the development of various interventions (Crockett 2000), such as appropriate physical activity (PA)/exercise. Chronic obstructive pulmonary disease (COPD) is as common as asthma in adults over the age of 40, yet in comparison, receives relatively little attention. Nonetheless, the current available research will be reviewed and discussed with particular emphasis on PA/exercise.

Table 9.1 Terms that have been used to describe chronic obstructive pulmonary disease (adapted from Crockett 2000 and GOLD 2001)

Terms	Description
Emphysema	Destruction of the gas-exchanging surface of the lung alveoli, a pathological term that is often incorrectly used to describe only one of the several structural abnormalities present in COPD patients
Chronic bronchitis	The presence of a cough and sputum production for at least 3 months in each of two consecutive years. An epidemiological and clinical term
COAD	Chronic obstructive airways disease
COLD	Chronic obstructive lung disease
CAL	Chronic airflow limitation
CAO	Chronic airflow (or airways) obstruction
Chronic, irreversible asthma	

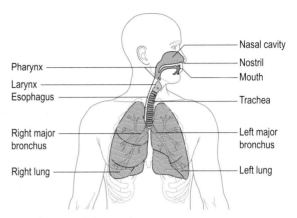

Figure 9.1 Layout of the respiratory system

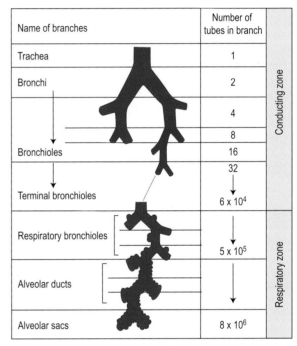

Figure 9.2 Branching of the airways (adapted from Vander et al 1990).

PREVALENCE AND DEFINITION

Chronic obstructive pulmonary disease is one of the most common respiratory diseases in the developed world and currently the fourth leading cause of death, accounting for around 5% of deaths worldwide (WHO 2000). However, due to inconsistencies in the definition and use of terminology for COPD (Table 9.1), it has been difficult to clearly determine the prevalence of this disease (WHO 2000). The problem with developing a definition for COPD is that the symptoms may be similar to that of other respiratory disorders. The characteristic symptoms of COPD are cough, sputum production and dyspnoea (breathlessness) and wheezing that worsens upon physical exertion, which may singularly and/or collectively be found in conditions such as asthma, emphysema, chronic bronchitis and pulmonary tuberculosis (Crockett 2000, GOLD 2001). This makes it difficult to determine the full prevalence of this disease. The current definition of COPD focuses more fully on the airflow limitation, which has the major impact on morbidity and mortality for COPD patients; it has recently been defined as:

> … a disease state characterised by airflow limitation that is not fully reversible. The airflow limitation is usually both progressive and associated with an abnormal inflammatory response of the lungs to noxious particles or gases. (GOLD 2001, p. 6)

RESPIRATORY SYSTEM PHYSIOLOGY AND ANATOMY

The purpose of the respiratory tract is to allow the body to absorb oxygen (O_2) and excrete carbon dioxide (CO_2). This is achieved as air is drawn into the body through the nose, where the air is filtered, warmed and moistened. From the nose the air passes through the pharynx and larynx into the lower respiratory tract (Crockett 2000). The larynx opens into the trachea, which branches into two bronchi; each bronchus then enters one of the two lungs. The lungs subdivide into more bronchi and smaller bronchioles (Vander et al 1990) (Figs 9.1 and 9.2).

A large bronchus may serve up to 65 000 bronchioles, which at the lower subdivisions may be less than 1 mm in diameter. The diameter of the bronchi and bronchioles is controlled by the smooth muscle in their walls, and their tone is subject to neural and hormonal factors. The final bronchioles have alveoli protruding from their walls, which are termed respiratory bronchioles. Further subdivisions and the respiratory bronchioles end in multiple alveoli. As the bronchi branch out, the cartilaginous plates that surround the bronchi tend to diminish, and at the smallest bronchioles there is no cartilage at all. The mucous glands that are also within the trachea and large bronchi diminish with the subdivision of the bronchioles. The submucous glands produce most of the airway secretions where the goblet cells, which are specialized epithelial cells that secrete mucus, are more prevalent. The mucus contains important antibacterial agents, such as immunoglobulin A (Ig A) (an antibody) and lysozyme (an enzyme with antiseptic actions that destroys some foreign organisms). The epithelial surfaces of the airways, at the end of the respiratory bronchioles, are also lined with cilia. These cilia beat continuously, moving the protective mucus layer upward toward the pharynx, getting rid of particulate matter such as dust contained in the inspired air that has stuck to the mucus. This is important in keeping the lungs clear of particulate matter and certain bacteria from entering the body on dust particles. However, many noxious agents, such as cigarette smoke, can repress these cilia, and a reduction in their activity can result in lung infection and/or airway obstruction by stationary mucus (Vander et al 1990, Crockett 2000). For a more in-depth description of the lungs, refer to Vander et al (1990, Ch. 14).

GAS EXCHANGE

The walls of the alveoli are the interface between alveolar gas and pulmonary capillary blood. The alveolar-capillary membrane is only 0.2 to 0.7 μm thick and composed of a single alveolar lining cell, a thin basement membrane and capillary endothelial cells, making diffusion of gases between the alveolar space and the capillary relatively easy. The final millimetre or two of gas movement to and from the alveolar-capillary membrane is entirely due to molecular diffusion. One of the important adverse effects of ventilatory obstruction on gas exchange is to impede the mass movement of the respiratory gases and increase the distance over which gas molecules have to travel by diffusion. Some alveolar walls have pores that permit the flow of air between alveoli. Though less efficient, this link between alveoli is important in cases of airway occlusion, as some of the air may still enter the adjacent alveolus by way of the connecting pores (Cole & Mackay 1990, Vander et al 1990,).

Factors that affect lung gas exchange are pulmonary ventilation, pulmonary blood flow and gaseous diffusion between the alveoli and pulmonary capillary blood. The partial pressure (P) of O_2 and CO_2 in arterial blood is an indicator of the effectiveness of gas exchange, and is a useful measure for determining abnormalities in response to respiratory diseases (Cole & Mackay 1990). The normal arterial blood P_{O_2} is between 95 and 100 mmHg, and P_{CO_2} between 35 and 45 mmHg.

VENTILATION

During the respiratory cycle the right ventricle of the heart pumps blood through the capillaries that surround each alveolus. In the average healthy adult, during rest, around 4 litres of air will enter and leave the alveoli each minute, while around 5 litres of blood will flow through the pulmonary capillaries. Airflow during heavy exercise may increase by 30 to 40 times that of rest, and blood flow by around 5 to 6 times. However, this quantity of air does not reach the alveoli, as part of each breath fills airways that have no role in gas exchange, known as dead space. Efficient respiration is achieved by maximal ventilation of the alveoli and adequate blood supply. There is also a slight difference between expired and inspired air. The alveolar air differs from inspired air in that CO_2 is continually added and O_2 removed by the blood perfusing the alveoli. In cases of hyperventilation (increased respiratory rate) there is a rise in alveolar O_2 tension and a fall in CO_2 tension, and during hypoventilation (decreased respiratory rate) a fall in O_2 tension and rise in CO_2 tension (Cole & Mackay 1990, Vander et al 1990, Crockett 2000).

BREATHING MECHANISMS

Inspiration is the result of the respiratory muscles contracting and the expansion of the diaphragm in a downward direction, and the upward and outward movement of the ribcage. This increases the volume of the chest, resulting in a fall in intrathoracic pressure across the walls of the airways. This causes air to be drawn into the smaller airways. Inspiration can be restricted by the calibre of the airways or by airway obstruction, particularly in the upper respiratory tract. The elastic recoil of the tissues and relaxation of the respiratory muscles causes contraction of the airways and an increase in pleural pressure (the tissue surrounding the lungs), which is above that of the pressure in the airways. The air is then forced out of the lungs, until the pressure in the airways equals the pleural pressure, which is when expiration ceases and inspiration commences. Expiratory airflow is not linear, as most of the air is expired during the first second of expiration. Hence, forced expiratory volume in one second (FEV_1) is a useful measure of airflow obstruction. FEV_1 is virtually completely dependent upon the elastic recoil of the lungs and chest walls, and degree of airflow obstruction, rather than on the effort of the individual. The latter part of expiration is less dependent upon elastic recoil, and during expiration, the pressure across the airway from the elastic recoil is greater than the pressure within the airway. In the bronchi, the bronchial wall cartilage inhibits the bronchial walls from collapsing and trapping air. The characteristic destruction of the lungs as a result of emphysema leads to the collapse of the walls of the airways, causing the trapping of air during expiration (Crockett 2000).

AETIOLOGY

The risk factors that potentially lead to COPD include both host factors and environmental exposure (Table 9.2) (GOLD 2001). Prolonged smoking and exposure to air pollutants, respiratory infections and allergies potentially lead to inflammation of the lungs (p. 144). This in combination with host factors, such as genetic predisposition, may result in diseases such as emphysema, chronic bronchitis, chronic asthma, which are outlined below, as well as bronchiectasis (irreversible dilation and destruction of the bronchial walls), silicosis (development of nodular fibrosis in the lungs as a result of long-term inhalation of dust from an inorganic compound) and pulmonary tuberculosis (chronic infection of the lungs); all of which are potential causes of COPD (Tamparo & Lewis 1995) (Fig. 9.3).

EMPHYSEMA

The main pathological sites of emphysema are the alveolar walls. Irritants to the lungs, such as cigarette smoke and other noxious environmental particles, cause lung inflammation, resulting in the release of proteolytic enzymes, such as elastase, from white blood cells called neutrophils. The enzyme elastase has the capacity to break down elastin, which is the elastic tissue of the alveolar walls. This results in the smaller individual alveoli coming together into larger sacs, leading not only to a reduction in the surface area of the lung but also to an increase in fibrosis and loss of the lung's elastic properties. Since a large proportion of expiration relies on elastic recoil, the loss of the elastic properties of the lung will have some effect upon expiration. In emphysema, the airways tend to close during expiration due to collapse of their walls, causing air to be trapped and an increase in residual volume (see Table 9.6). Breathing is therefore less efficient and the lungs become distended. There is therefore an increase in hypoventilation of the alveoli, resulting in a ventilation–perfusion mismatch and hypoxaemia (low arterial O_2 levels) (Cole & Mackay 1990, Crockett 2000).

There are two types of emphysema, which may coexist within an individual. Centrilobular emphysema is the destruction of the alveolar walls in the centre of the lung lobule, causing trapping of air; panacinar emphysema, which may be an advanced form of centrilobular, occurs when the majority of the alveolar walls within the lung lobule are destroyed, causing distended, irregular and unsupported airways and alveoli (Cole & Mackay 1990, Crockett 2000) (Fig. 9.4). This type of emphysema is generally seen in those with deficient alpha-1-antitrypsin (p. 143). Both types of emphysema lead to COPD.

Table 9.2 Major COPD risk factors (adapted from GOLD 2001)

Host factors	Environmental exposure
Genetic factors	Tobacco smoke
Airway hyper-responsiveness	Occupational chemicals and dust
Lung growth during gestation	Air pollution
	Infection
	Socio-economic status

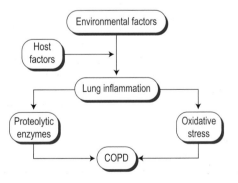

Figure 9.3 Factors that influence lung inflammation and the possible development of COPD (adapted from GOLD 2001).

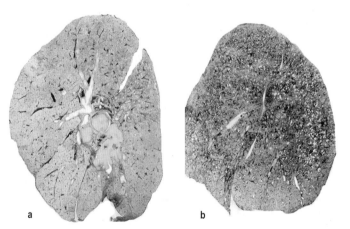

Figure 9.4 (a) A Gough–Wentworth paper-mounted whole lung section shows healthy lung parenchyma in which interlobular septa are focally seen as thin black lines, likely due to the patient dwelling in a city (a tumour is however noted, obstructing the airways in the lower lobes). (b): This compares with the parenchyma of a patient with emphysema whose lung section shows patchy loss of alveolar tissue represented by holes towards the centre of pulmonary acini. Changes are more marked in the upper lobe, typically of emphysema of centrilobular (mainly cigarette-related) type. (Images provided by Professor Andrew G. Nicholson, Royal Brompton Hospital, London, UK.)

CHRONIC BRONCHITIS

Chronic bronchitis is characterized by chronic inflammation of the bronchial endothelium, leading to a thickening of the mucosal lining of the bronchi. This is primarily due to an increase in goblet cells leading to hypertrophy of the mucous glands of the trachea and bronchi. The increase in goblet cells is most notable in the bronchioles, causing increased secretions and sputum production. Mucus viscosity is also increased, which destroys the cilia and impairs the efficiency of mucus clearance. In addition to this, airway hyper-responsiveness, to infection or inhaled irritant particles, causes bronchoconstriction (narrowing of the airways) and obstruction. Furthermore, since there is defective bronchial drainage, there is also an increased risk of chronic or recurrent inflammation, and irreversible structural damage (emphysema), which may lead to COPD (Cole & Mackay 1990, Crockett 2000).

ASTHMA

Similar to COPD, asthma is characterized by airflow limitation. However, while airflow limitation is reversible in asthma, currently it is not in COPD. Asthma may also coexist with COPD, though even without coexisting COPD, asthma is seen as a risk factor for COPD, especially chronic and poorly treated asthma. Asthma and COPD also display similar symptoms, such as airway hyper-responsiveness and susceptibility to lung infection. However, whilst the lung inflammation of COPD is mainly due to neutrophils (p. 142), the inflammation found in asthma is predominantly eosinophilic (Ch. 8, p. 131, Table 8.3) (Crockett 2000, GOLD 2001).

HOST FACTORS

Host factors include genetic factors, airway hyper-responsiveness and lung growth during the gestational period.

Genetic factors

Studies indicate that there may be a genetic link within families that may predispose an individual toward COPD (Joos et al 2002, Nishimura 2003, Molfino 2004), although it has been suggested that this may be due to shared environment rather than genetic factors per se (Nishimura 2003). Nonetheless, though only relevant to a small percentage of the world's population, the hereditary deficiency of alpha-1-antitrypsin (α-1-AT) is well documented as a contributor toward the development of COPD (Cole & Mackay 1990, GOLD 2001).

Alpha-1-antitrypsin protects the lungs against elastase. Elastase is an enzyme released from neutrophils (white blood cells) that breaks down elastin, a protein that makes up part of the lung tissue. Plasma concentrations of α-1-AT tend to rise in response to acute inflammation. It is when elastase exceeds the inhibitor, α-1-AT, that lung damage is likely to occur. Cigarette smoking is also inclined to inactivate α-1-AT (Hubbard et al 1987) and thus increase the amount of elastase. Therefore, for individuals who are α-1-AT deficient, smoking poses an enhanced risk of lung damage and emphysema-linked COPD. The imbalance between elastase and elastase inhibitors can also lead to bronchial and interstitial lung disease (Crockett 2000).

Airway hyper-responsiveness

Airway hyper-responsiveness is an inflammatory response of the lungs from exposure to tobacco smoke or other environmental and/or occupational dusts and chemicals. Airway hyper-responsiveness is also a risk factor for a decline in FEV_1, which is found in both COPD sufferers and asthmatics (Peat et al 1987), though its role in the development of COPD still remains uncertain (Silverman & Speizer 1996). Although asthma is still regarded as a risk factor for COPD, the airway hyper-responsiveness of asthma is unlike that of COPD, involving different inflammatory cells, mediators, inflammatory effects, and response to therapy. The inflammatory processes, and subsequent airway hyper-responsiveness of asthma, are mainly due to eosinophilic (leukocytes that are larger than neutrophils and constitute 1–3% of white blood cells, and increase in number with allergy) inflammation affecting the airways but not the lung tissue. The airway inflammation of COPD is basically due to neutrophilic inflammation (p. 142) (Barnes 2000).

Lung growth

Undernourishment of the fetus can impair lung growth and development (Stein et al 1997). Low birth weight and exposures during childhood (Table 9.2) can also affect lung growth. A reduction in lung function (as determined by spirometry, p. 143) may identify those who are at increased risk of developing COPD (Tager et al 1988, GOLD 2001).

ENVIRONMENTAL EXPOSURE

The prevalence of COPD is greater in areas of high industrial pollution (Ministry of Health 1954). For example, in London in December 1952, the air concentration of smoke and sulphur dioxide was more than 100 times greater than current levels, and caused an additional 4000 deaths.

Inhaled particles each pose a different risk to the individual, the extent of which will depend on the concentration, size and composition of the particle. An individual will be exposed to many inhaled substances throughout their life. However, research has found that only tobacco smoke (US Surgeon General 1984) and occupational dusts and chemicals, such as vapours, irritants and fumes (Kauffmann et al 1979, Becklake 1989), are known to be able to cause COPD on their own. An example of this can be seen in the rates of COPD in miners exposed to coal dust (CDCP 1995). Furthermore, these occupational exposures and tobacco smoke also appear to act additively to increase an individual's risk of developing COPD (Kauffmann et al 1979, GOLD 2001). However, only a small percentage (approximately 10–15%) of long-term smokers develop clinically significant COPD, and around half will never develop symptoms. The reasons why the protective inflammatory response, in some individuals, becomes exaggerated is still not fully understood, but it is presumed to be an interaction between host and environmental factors (Jindal et al 2003).

RESPIRATORY INFECTIONS

Chronic or recurrent respiratory infection in childhood has been associated with an increased risk of COPD in adulthood (Matsuse et al 1992, Hogg 1999, Kosciuch & Chazan 2003) and reduced adult lung function (Tager et al 1988, Johnston 1999), which are independent of exposure to cigarette smoke (Strachan 1990).

INFLAMMATION

Inflammation is a localized protective response in vascularized tissues induced by infection and/or cell and tissue damage (Pettersen & Adler 2002). The chronic inflammation that leads to permanent narrowing and fibrosis of the small airways and alveolar wall destruction (emphysema, p. 142) in COPD is characterized by an increase in the number of alveolar macrophages (a phagocyte that defends against infection), neutrophils (white blood cells) and foreign-cell-destroying T lymphocytes (white blood cells) (Barnes 2004a). The inflammatory initiated breakdown of lung tissue in COPD is a magnification of the normal inflammatory response (Barnes et al 2003). Since not all individuals will develop pathological inflammation, leading to COPD from excess exposure to certain airborne particles, the cause is thought to be the result of an interaction between environmental and host factors, such as genetic predisposition (Fig. 9.3 and Table 9.2).

Individuals with COPD have increased numbers of neutrophils and macrophages in their lungs (Traves et al 2002). Airway neutrophils are a central feature of COPD, and have been shown to be closely associated with the severity of peripheral airway dysfunction (O'Donnell et al 2004a). In the airways, the neutrophils are key cellular mediators of inflammation, and contain specific and highly regulated mechanisms for controlling the expression of adhesion molecules that allow them to tether and migrate into inflammatory sites. During normal conditions, circulating neutrophils roll along the blood vessel walls, and when an appropriate stimulus is present, these rolling neutrophils firmly adhere to endothelial cells. The neutrophils are then ready to migrate from the bloodstream to the site of injury. Adhesion molecules are not only activated by exogenous pollutants and irritant particles, but are also regulated by endothelial and epithelial cell signals. Lipid mediators, reactive oxygen and nitrogen species and cytokines from airway epithelial cells (Barnes 2004a) further control neutrophil functions, such as infiltration and activation, resulting in the release of the granule enzyme elastase (which in COPD sufferers is known to break down lung tissue). Furthermore, the products of viruses and bacteria affect inflammation by increasing secondary epithelial mediators. Nonetheless, once these endogenous and/or exogenous agents are disposed of, the neutrophil population are programmed to die and are cleared by macrophage phagocytosis (Pettersen & Adler 2002).

OXIDATIVE STRESS

Oxidative stress is a significant feature in the development of COPD, and there is increasing evidence that oxidant/antioxidant imbalance, in favour of oxidants, occurs in COPD (Guerin et al 2005). Oxidative stress contributes to both proteolytic imbalance and inactivating α-1-AT, and causes a dysfunction of pulmonary endothelial cells (Hoshino et al 2005), as well as mucus hypersecretion, increased infiltration of neutrophils into the pulmonary microvasculature, amplification of the inflammatory processes (MacNee 2001, Barnes et al 2003), and impairment of connective tissue repair, resulting in the structural and functional changes that are characteristic of COPD (Sanguinetti 1992). Hydrogen peroxide and nitric oxide are direct measures of oxidants generated from inflammatory leukocytes and epithelial cells. Hydrogen peroxide acts on the smooth muscle of the airways to cause constriction, contributing toward reversible airway narrowing (GOLD 2001). Furthermore, the oxidants generated by cigarette smoking, for example, have been found in the epithelial lining fluid, breath and urine of cigarette smokers and COPD sufferers (Hoshino et al 2005).

PATHOPHYSIOLOGY

The physiological abnormalities of COPD as a result of the pathological changes in the lungs include mucus hypersecretion, ciliary dysfunction, airflow limitation, hyperinflation, gas exchange abnormalities and, latterly, pulmonary hypertension and cor pulmonale (GOLD 2001). These also influence the mechanics of breathing and ultimately will have some effect on the individual's ability to perform PA/exercise, though the extent will be dependent upon the physical status of the individual and the stage of COPD.

AIRFLOW LIMITATION

The main characteristic of COPD is chronic airflow limitation. This is primarily due to a combination of airway disease, obstructing the small airways, and loss of pulmonary elastic recoil, from destruction of the lung tissue (parenchyma) (emphysema, p. 142) (Table 9.3). This is often accompanied by a chronic cough and sputum production, as a result of chronic bronchitis (p. 143). The probable mechanisms involved in the destruction of the lung parenchyma, for those with smoke-related and α-1-AT deficiency, is an imbalance between endogenous lung proteolytic enzymes (proteinases) and anti-proteinases; though oxidative stress and ensuing inflammation also appear to play a part (Repine et al 1997, GOLD 2001). Most COPD sufferers display some features of both emphysema and chronic bronchitis, with the magnitude of each varying between individuals (Crockett 2000, GOLD 2001).

The characteristic airflow limitation of COPD is generally progressive and irreversible, and whilst symptoms may be similar to those of asthma, the causes and responses to similar treatments are different (Crockett 2000, GOLD 2001) (p. 143). In the healthy lung, airway limitation of the smaller airways makes up a tiny percentage of the total resistance. In COPD sufferers, however, the total lower airways resistance almost doubles, which is mostly due to an increase in peripheral airways resistance (Hogg et al 1968).

The central (trachea, bronchi and bronchioles diameter >2–4 mm) and peripheral airways (small bronchi and bronchioles) (Figs 9.1 and 9.2) of the lungs, as well as the lung parenchyma, are affected in COPD. The symptoms of chronic cough and sputum production are due primarily to the pathological changes in the central airways, which may be present either on their own or in combination with changes in the peripheral airways and destruction of the lung parenchyma. The prime characteristic of change in the peripheral airways is airways narrowing, and is the major site of obstruction in COPD. Inflammation of the peripheral airways correlates with an early decline in lung function, which may also result from excess mucus production due to an increase in goblet cells. Another early symptom of COPD is ciliary dysfunction, due to metaplasia of the ciliated epithelial cells, and results in impaired mucociliary clearance mechanisms (GOLD 2001). Chronic inflammation of the airways also leads to a cycle of tissue injury and repair, causing tissue remodelling. This potentially alters the structure and function of the tissue, resulting in scar tissue formation and increased collagen content which narrows the lumen of the airways (Rennard 1999). The additional loss of elastic recoil and the mucus hypersecretion further contribute toward the obstruction of the airways (Table 9.3), all of which lead to an unequal patchy increase in airway resistance with trapping of the air (GOLD 2001).

As the severity of airflow limitation increases, expiration during normal breathing, or 'tidal breathing' (the volume of air that is inspired and expired during a normal breath at rest), becomes limited. Initially this is only apparent during physical exertion; however during the latter stages of COPD (see Table 9.4) this is also apparent during rest. Concurrently, there is an increase in the functional residual capacity (the volume of air in the lungs at the end of a normal breath) as a result of the decrease in elastic properties, premature airway closure, and altered breathing patterns that are assumed to cope with impaired lung mechanics (p. 146).

PULMONARY VASCULAR CHANGES

Structural alterations in the pulmonary vasculature are also observed in those with COPD. Early changes, such as vessel wall thickening, may be seen even at a time when lung function and pulmonary vascular pressures, during rest, are near to normal (Wright et al 1983, GOLD 2001). Risk factors for COPD, such as smoking and inflammatory mediators (Peinado et al 1999), affect endothelial function, which subsequently influences vascular tone leading ultimately to structural changes. These structural changes are also associated with an increase in pulmonary vascular pressure that is first displayed during exercise and latterly during rest (GOLD 2001). Chronic hypoxia (low O_2 levels) is more apparent as COPD progresses, and is a contributing factor for the development of pulmonary vascular remodelling and pulmonary hypertension (Presberg & Dincer 2003).

PULMONARY HYPERTENSION

Pulmonary hypertension usually develops in the latter stages of COPD, at around stage III (Table 9.4), and is associated with a worsening prognosis. Severe chronic hypoxia is a known cause of pulmonary vascular remodelling and pulmonary hypertension (Presberg & Dincer 2003). Damage to the pulmonary vasculature leads to impaired endothelial function, resulting in a reduction in nitric oxide (a potent vasodilator), which increases vasoconstriction in response to hypoxia. Enhanced vasoconstriction, pulmonary vascular remodel-

Table 9.3 Factors affecting airflow limitation in COPD (adapted from GOLD 2001)

Irreversible	Reversible
Narrowing of the airways (due to fibrosis)	Build-up of mucus and plasma exudate in bronchi
Elastic recoil loss (due to alveolar destruction)	Contraction of peripheral and central airways smooth muscle cells
Loss of airway patency (due to destruction of alveolar support)	Dynamic hyperinflation during exercise

Table 9.4 Stages of severity of COPD (adapted from GOLD 2001 and BTS 1997)

Stage	Lung function	Characteristics
Healthy	FEV$_1$ >80% predicted	Symptom free
0: At risk	Normal spirometry	Chronic cough and sputum production
I: Mild	FEV$_1$ ≥80% predicted FEV$_1$/FVC <70%	With or without chronic cough and sputum production Rarely presents for treatment except during infective exacerbation
II: Moderate	FEV$_1$ 40–59% predicted FEV$_1$/FVC <70%	Symptoms of deteriorating lung function Breathless on exertion With or without chronic cough and sputum production and breathlessness
III: Severe	FEV$_1$ <40% and <20% during final stages FEV$_1$/FVC <70%	Breathless on minimal exertion General wheezing and coughing Cyanosis and peripheral oedema in very severe cases Predicted respiratory failure Signs of right-sided heart failure Severely impaired quality of life

ling and destruction of the pulmonary capillary bed increase the pressure required to perfuse the pulmonary vascular bed. For some COPD sufferers, however, pulmonary hypertension may only be very slight during rest, though it is generally more marked during physical exertion.

Cor pulmonale

Pulmonary hypertension is related to cor pulmonale (enlarged right ventricle, due to lung disease) and poor prognosis (MacNee 1994), and is generally only seen in the advanced stages of COPD. Cor pulmonale leads to right-sided heart failure, and is associated with venous stasis and risk of thrombosis, which potentially may result in a pulmonary embolism and compromised pulmonary circulation (GOLD 2001).

GAS EXCHANGE

In the advanced stages of COPD there is a reduction in the lung's capacity for gas exchange. This is due to the combination of peripheral airway obstruction, destruction of the lung parenchyma, affecting the lung gas exchange surface, and pulmonary vascular changes. Although the correlation between lung function tests and blood gases is poor, hypoxaemia and hypercapnia (high blood CO_2 levels) are rare at FEV$_1$ >1.0 litre. Hypoxaemia is usually only present during physical exertion, and this is generally the result of a mismatch between the ventilation/perfusion ratio ($\dot{V}A/\dot{Q}$) (where ventilation refers to the movement of air in and out of the lungs, and perfusion to the flow of blood). The significant correlation between bronchiolar inflammation of the peripheral airways, and the disruption of ventilation is associated with $\dot{V}A/\dot{Q}$ mismatch. Furthermore, the destruction to the lung surface area, due to emphysema, also reduces the diffusing capacity of the lungs, affecting gas exchange (McLean et al 1992). The decrease in ventilation, as a result of loss of elastic recoil, together with loss of the capillary bed and general poor ventilation, consequently leads to a high $\dot{V}A/\dot{Q}$ ratio, indicating arterial hypoxia. Additional contributors to the mismatch in $\dot{V}A/\dot{Q}$ are abnormalities in the pulmonary vasculature. With vessel damage there is a reduction in the reversal of vasoconstriction in response to hypoxia (Barbera et al 1994), indicating pathological changes to the pulmonary arterial wall and loss of vascular response to hypoxia. Hypercapnia, on the other hand, reflects inspiratory muscle dysfunction and alveolar hypoventilation (GOLD 2001).

MECHANICAL CHANGES

The decrease in FEV$_1$ and vital capacity, and increase in residual volume with COPD, results in the mismatch in $\dot{V}A/\dot{Q}$, consequently leading to an increase in the energy cost of tidal breathing. This increase in energy required by the respiratory muscles (which include both expiratory and inspiratory muscles), simply to perform normal breathing, causes these muscles to fatigue more easily. Furthermore, hyperinflation of the lungs reduces the ability of the inspiratory muscles to generate power. Moreover, hyperinflation also leads to a shortening and flattening of the diaphragm, reducing the diaphragm's ability to generate power, further hindering inspiration and increasing the effort of tidal breathing (Fig. 9.5).

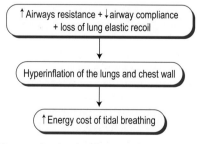

Figure 9.5 Factors that lead to increased energy cost of breathing in COPD (adapted from Crockett 2000).

COPD sufferers often adopt a 'sit forward' position that assists diaphragmatic function and thus normal breathing (Crockett 2000).

ASSESSMENTS

COPD is suspected on the basis of symptoms (Table 9.5) and signs of COPD. Physical signs of airflow limitation are rarely present until lung function is significantly impaired (GOLD 2001). Other measures that can be employed, both in the staging of COPD and in the follow-up of COPD sufferers, may be based upon the severity of symptoms, such as the level of disability, measure of arterial blood gases/pulse oximetry and/or the 6-minute walk test (Appendix A) (Jindal et al 2003).

LUNG FUNCTION

Spirometry is the gold standard and remains the most reproducible way of establishing the degree of airflow limitation, and for confirming the staging of COPD (GOLD 2001). Chronic airflow limitation of COPD results in a reduced maximum expiratory flow, as illustrated by the FEV_1, and slow forced emptying of the lungs (as shown by peak expiratory flow rate (PEFR); Table 9.6 and Fig. 9.6) (Crockett 2000, GOLD 2001). Airflow limitation that is not fully reversible is confirmed when, after the administration of a bronchodilator, FEV_1 is less than 80% of the predicted value in combination with a FEV_1/FVC <70% (GOLD 2001) (Fig. 9.7). Furthermore, reviews of the literature have consistently found reductions in FEV_1 and FVC in association with increased levels of systemic inflammatory markers (Gan et al 2004), thus providing support for the link between airflow limitation and inflammation.

Table 9.5 Symptoms of COPD

Main	Chronic cough, present on most days, for at least 3 months in the year, for two or more consecutive years
	Chronic sputum production
	Breathlessness (dyspnoea)
	Acute exacerbations – repeated episode of acute bronchitis
Hypercapnia (high blood CO_2 levels)	Bounding pulse
	Warm extremities
	Muscle tremor
Hypoxia (low blood O_2 levels)	Tremors
	Restlessness
	Confusion
	Cyanosis (blue discoloration of the skin)

Table 9.6 Assessment measures of lung function (adapted from Crockett 2000)

	Definition	
ERV	Expiratory reserve volume	Volume of air expired from the end of a normal breath to maximum expiration
FEV_1	Forced expiratory volume in 1 second	Volume of air expired in the first second of a forced expiration from a full inspiration (litres)
FRC	Functional residual capacity	Volume of air in the lungs at the end of a normal breath
IC	Inspiration capacity	Volume of air that can maximally be inhaled
IRV	Inspiratory reserve volume	Volume of air that could be inspired if the inspiration continued to the maximum from the end of a tidal inspiration
PEFR	Peak expiratory flow rate	The maximum flow rate that can be sustained for a period of 1 second
FVC	Forced vital capacity	The volume of expired during forced expiration, usually over a period of around 6 seconds
RV	Residual volume	Volume of air remaining in the lungs at the end of a maximum expiration
TLC	Total lung capacity	Volume of air in the lungs after a maximum inspiration
TV	Tidal volume	Volume of air that is inspired and expired during a normal breath at rest
VC	Vital capacity	Difference in volume of the lungs from full inspiration to full expiration

FUNCTIONAL ABILITY

Although FEV_1 is seen as the gold standard for determining degree of airflow limitation, it does not appropriately describe functional effects of pharmacological or non-pharmacological interventions. It has therefore been suggested that FEV_1 be performed in conjunction with assessments of PA/exercise capacity to determine functional ability (Magnussen 2004). Measures of aerobic capacity ($\dot{V}O_2max$) have been found to be less consistent in COPD patients, as markers of physiological adaptation to PA/exercise intervention, than in healthy individuals (Belman 1996). It has therefore been suggested that measures of blood lactate are more reliable indicators of changes in aerobic fitness, since blood lactate accumulates at higher levels of exertion and at a slower rate with increasing aerobic fitness (Mink 1997).

The type of assessment used to evaluate the functional capacity of COPD patients has also been an area of debate. Research has shown that exercise-induced hypoxaemia during both maximal and submaximal exercise appears

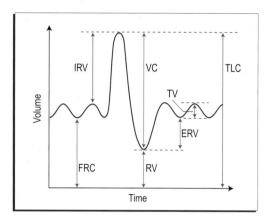

Figure 9.6 Lung volumes. ERV, expiratory reserve volume; FRC, functional residual capacity; IRV, inspiratory reserve volume; RV, residual volume; TLC, total lung capacity; TV, tidal volume; VC, vital capacity (see Table 9.2)

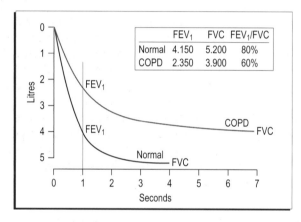

Figure 9.7 Normal spirometry and typical spirometry from a patient with mild to moderate COPD (GOLD 2001).

to be greatest during treadmill walking when compared to that of cycling. However, plasma lactate levels have been shown to be significantly higher during the cycling, with no difference in ratings of perceived exertion (Appendix B) between the two modes of exercise (Christensen et al 2004). Additionally, the type of test employed to determine functional capacity will ultimately depend on the physical status of the individual in terms of their disease stage. For instance, while the 6-minute walk test (Appendix A) may be an appropriate assessment of functional capacity for the majority of COPD patients, it would be unsuitable for those with stage III COPD and/or those who find ambulatory PA/exercise problematic.

TREATMENT

PHARMACOLOGICAL

The most commonly prescribed medications for COPD are bronchodilators, corticosteroids and antibiotics. For those in the more advanced stages of the disease, oxygen therapy may also be required (GOLD 2001).

Bronchodilators

Bronchodilators are central to the symptomatic management of COPD (Joos et al 2003, Pfeifer 2004), and inhaled drugs are preferred to oral preparations (Chabot 2004). Short-acting bronchodilators can be used when needed to relieve intermittent or worsening symptoms, and whilst long-acting bronchodilators may be of use to those in the later stages of COPD on continuous medication (Pfeifer 2004), they are not of great use during acute exacerbations of COPD (Lange et al 2004).

Although the use of bronchodilators just prior to PA/exercise may help to reduce dyspnoea and improve exercise capacity, this may not be seen in all COPD patients (Liesker et al 2002, Oga et al 2003, Oga 2004). Nonetheless, the client/patient and exercise practitioner should discuss and consider the use of bronchodilators just prior to any planned PA/exercise.

Corticosteroids

Currently there are no available treatments to reduce the progression or suppress the inflammation of COPD, and although understanding of the inflammatory and destructive processes involved in the development of COPD is better, there is still a need for new therapies for the treatment of COPD (Barnes 2004b). Nonetheless, corticosteroids are prescribed because of their anti-inflammatory effect, and work by breaking down phospholipids involved in the inflammatory process. Inhaled corticosteroids are used as a regular treatment for those with FEV_1 <50% predicted, and who suffer repeated exacerbations requiring treatment with antibiotics. Despite the debate over the effectiveness of corticosteroids for those with COPD (Barnes 2004b), oral or systemic treatment with corticosteroids has shown favourable responses during an acute exacerbation. However, chronic treatment with systemic corticosteroids should be avoided because of unfavourable side effects. The most frequently reported side effect is hyperglycaemia (AHRQ 2000); others are osteoporosis, muscle myopathy and peptic ulcer (BMA, RPS GB 2002).

Other drugs

Antibiotics are used to treat infectious exacerbations of COPD and bacterial infections, and the drug prescribed will depend on the type of infection (BMA, RPS GB 2002). Mucus-clearing treatments or mucolytic agents may also be prescribed to patients with viscous sputum production, and a Cochrane systematic review of 23 studies (Poole & Black 2003a) showed that mucolytic agents reduced acute exacerbations in those with COPD. Although the mechanisms by which they reduce exacerbations are not fully understood, their effectiveness may be by altering mucus production, reducing oxidative stress (p. 144) and/or bacterial infection and altering inflammatory processes. However, long term, they do not appear to affect the decline in lung function (Poole & Black 2003b), but have been shown to improve ventilatory function during acute exacerbation (AHRQ 2000). Those with COPD have also been reported to show abnormalities in the level of circulating anabolic hormones. It has therefore been suggested that this may be one of the causes of the often seen muscle myopathy (p. 154). Hence these hormones may be prescribed for some COPD patients (Casaburi 1998, 2001). Other drugs, such as sedatives and narcotics, are not recommended for those with COPD because they depress respiration, which may induce hypercapnia (BMA, RPS GB 2002).

NON-PHARMACOLOGICAL

In addition to pharmacological treatment of COPD, non-pharmacological treatments are of great benefit. The most effective is smoking cessation. Pulmonary rehabilitation is also a major aspect of treatment of COPD, including PA/exercise intervention.

Pulmonary rehabilitation

The Council of Rehabilitation Specialists state that the goal of rehabilitation is to restore patients to their fullest medical, mental, emotional, social and vocational potential possible. Pulmonary rehabilitation, similar to cardiac rehabilitation, is a multidisciplinary service which aims to control, alleviate and where possible reverse the symptoms and pathophysiological processes leading to, in this instance, respiratory impairment and to enhance and prolong the patient's life. Whilst early studies failed to find any changes in conventional measures of lung function after rehabilitation (Reardon et al 1994, Ries et al 1995), other outcome measures have shown positive changes in factors such as exercise capacity, quality of life, decreased dyspnoea and fewer hospital admissions. Any patient with symptoms of respiratory disease may enter into pulmonary rehabilitation, even those with severe disease. Pulmonary rehabilitation is now therefore considered the best treatment for patients with severe COPD. For instance, patients awaiting lung transplantation or lung volume reduction surgery have shown improvements and increased exercise endurance after pulmonary rehabilitation (Bartolome 1998). Physical activity/exercise intervention is a major aspect of pulmonary rehabilitation and programmes may include exercises not only to enhance general fitness but also for mobility and agility, breathing with low frequency, relaxation and inspiratory muscle training (Folgering & von Herwaarden 1994, Lotters et al 2002).

Smoking cessation

Smoking cessation is the only treatment that has unequivocally been shown to reduce the rate of decline in FEV_1 (Decramer et al 2005), and is thus the most important and effective step for slowing the advance of COPD (Jindal et at 2003).

Lung reduction surgery

Once adulthood is achieved, research has shown that, in the healthy adult, the lungs display no further growth. However, research on animals has shown that several years after lung resection changes in the lungs occur. The initial stimulus is thought to be due to stretching of the remaining lung tissue (Trone et al 1999). These changes involve both structural and functional growth of the remaining lung, predominantly at the alveolar level, though this does not appear to happen until around 50% of the lung has been removed. Furthermore, if compensatory hyperinflation of the remaining lung is prevented, then growth does not appear to occur to the same extent. Nonetheless, such growth does enable an increase in exercise capacity and improvement of pulmonary gas exchange (Wagner 2005). However, in the human, whilst there is some indication that there may be some lung growth after lung reduction (pneumonectomy) in children (Nakajima et al 1998), it has not been shown in adults (Trone et al 1999). Yet, despite the lack of evidence for lung growth in adults after surgery, research has shown an improvement in exercise tolerance and functional capacity, indicated by reported increases of between 20% and 25% in distance covered during the 6-minute walk test (Bousamra et al 1997, Matsuzawa et al 1998).

Lung function and lung reduction surgery

Improvements in lung function after lung surgery have been reported, which include increases in FEV_1 (range 29–59%) and FVC (range 24–37%), as well as a reduction in functional residual capacity (25%) and a decrease in perceived dyspnoea (O'Donnell et al 1996, Bousamra et al 1997, Matsuzawa et al 1998). The mechanisms for these post-surgical changes have been shown to be the result of reductions in hyperinflation (p. 146, 154), breathing frequency and mechanical constraints on lung volume expansion, in addition to enhanced elastic recoil (O'Donnell et al 1996, Sciurba et al 1996, Matsuzawa et al 1998). Furthermore, these improvements result in a decrease in arterial partial pressure of CO_2 (Sciurba et al 1996), thus reducing acidosis and consequent breathing frequency.

PHYSICAL ACTIVITY/EXERCISE

Regardless of the fact that the efficacy of exercise as an adjunct treatment has in the past been seen as equivocal (Berry & Walschlager 1998), the major benefits of PA/exercise training for those with COPD is through enhanced exercise tolerance, a decrease in ventilatory demands, and a reduction in symptoms (Casaburi et al 1997, Lisboa et al 2001). For instance, after 6 weeks of cycle ergometry (45 minutes, three times per week) 15 COPD patients, during a constant work rate, showed a reduction in ventilation and respiratory rate of about 10% and 19%, respectively, compared to controls (Casaburi et al 1997). Additionally, a study carried out by Lisboa et al (2001) found, in a group of 55 COPD patients, that after 10 weeks of exercise training there were significant improvements in maximal workload, aerobic capacity and endurance time (though no control group was employed). A review of 36 non-controlled studies also found that over 900 COPD patients displayed improvements in their exercise endurance after exercise training (Casaburi 1993). Furthermore, the greatest improvements have been seen in those with the lowest pre-training exercise capacity and FEV_1 (Casaburi et al 1991). Physical activity/exercise training also reduces ventilation at equivalent levels of oxygen consumption uptake, though the extent appears to be less in COPD patients than for healthy individuals (O'Donnell et al 1993). Nonetheless, the reduction in ventilation may ease the feeling of breathlessness, which is important as dyspnoea often compromises the COPD patient's ability to perform daily tasks. It has been suggested that while some of these changes, after training, reflect physiological adaptations such as a higher anaerobic threshold, a proportion are psychological. Thus the reduction in ventilation and dyspnoea may be due to a learning effect, and development of better performance strategies (Belman 1996, Mink 1997). It also appears that the PA/exercise training desensitized the individual to be able to tolerate breathlessness and reduce their fear of dyspnoea (Mink 1997, Gigliotti et al 2003). In addition, a review of the literature indicated that most types of PA/exercise intervention are effective at improving exercise tolerance in those with COPD, even from low-intensity activities (Killian et al 1992, Mink 1997). Furthermore, both endurance and resistance training have been shown to be beneficial in the reduction of muscle myopathy (p. 154) (Casaburi 2001, Storer 2001). However, despite PA/exercise intervention displaying measurable physiological adaptations as well as psychological benefits to these patients, it has not been shown to lengthen life expectancy (Mink 1997).

TRAINING AND THE LUNGS

In the healthy adult, whilst PA/exercise training enhances the oxygen transport functions of the heart, blood and muscles, training has little or no effect on the lungs. Therefore, the lack of trainability of the lungs may be seen as a limiting factor in exercise capacity, as after training they contribute little to the changes in maximal oxygen uptake ($\dot{V}O_2max$). However, the lack of lung trainability does not appear to affect gas exchange, and therefore in the healthy individual it can be said not to affect $\dot{V}O_2max$, as even unfit individuals show no reduction in arterial oxygenation during maximal exercise; it is rather an individual's reduced ability to utilize the available oxygen that affects $\dot{V}O_2max$ (Wagner 2005).

For those with COPD who suffer destruction of the lung, and show mismatch in the ratio of $\dot{V}A/\dot{Q}$, unlike healthy individuals, they will have impaired gas exchange resulting in severely compromised delivery of oxygen and $\dot{V}O_2max$. Furthermore, the increase in airway resistance and hyperinflation (p. 154) also raises the metabolic cost of breathing (Mink 1997). For instance, during low-intensity PA/exercise, the respiratory muscles of patients with pulmonary disease may use 40% of their total oxygen uptake compared to 10–15% in healthy individuals (Toshima et al 1990).

TRAINING AND LUNG FUNCTION

Physical activity/exercise training has been shown to decrease the sense of dyspnoea during exercise and enhance exercise tolerance and duration. However, it does not appear to have any significant effect upon traditional parameters of lung function, such as, FEV_1, VC, TLC and RV (de Lucas Ramos et al 1998, Grzanka et al 2004). Therefore, whilst one might expect to see changes in markers of physical fitness after PA/exercise intervention, it is unlikely that changes will be found in these measures of lung function.

AIRWAY INFLAMMATION

Neutrophils play a significant part in the airway inflammation found in patients with COPD (p. 142), and whilst appropriate PA/exercise training may be of overall benefit to these individuals, the effect of PA/exercise on airway inflammation has still to be fully determined. Nevertheless, studies have found that some endurance athletes have elevated levels of airway neutrophils, which have been shown to impair gas exchange (Wetter et al 2002). It is thought that the increase in airway neutrophils may result from hyperventilation-induced increase in airway osmolarity, stimulating bronchial epithelial cells to release cell migratory factors (Bonsignore et al 2003). Conversely, however, in atopic asthmatic mice, moderate-intensity aerobic exercise has been shown to attenuate airway inflammatory mediators (Pastva et al 2004). Nonetheless, the airway inflammation in asthmatics is different from that of COPD, thus potentially producing differing responses to PA/exercise. Additionally, studies on airway inflammation in horses have shown that oxidative stress during exercise correlated with lung function and airway inflammation (Kirschvink et al 2002). Similar results have been found from a human study on 10 COPD patients, who underwent dynamic quadriceps endurance exercise at 40% of their maximal strength. The findings showed that compared to the group of healthy controls ($n = 7$), the COPD patients showed greater plasma resting levels of inflammatory markers. Additionally, whilst 6 hours post-exercise both groups showed an increase in markers of oxidative stress, the extent of this increase was greater in the COPD patients (Koechlin et al 2004). Although the effect of exercise on airway cells requires further research, the possible implications for an increase in airway inflammation is a potentially important factor, especially as the lungs of COPD patients already suffer a degree of inflammation.

PRE-PHYSICAL ACTIVITY/EXERCISE PRESCRIPTION

As with any client/patient it is important to screen prior to PA/exercise. COPD sufferers vary greatly in the course of the development of the disease (GOLD 2001), and many have co-morbidities, such as cardiac complications (Ch. 2). Thus it is essential that before PA/exercise the COPD client/patient is evaluated to determine their functional or exercise capacity, level of hypoxia during rest and PA/exercise, as well as their cardiac risk, and the type and intensity of activities that will not induce arrhythmias (Mink 1997). It may also be necessary to establish if the client/patient requires supplemental oxygen during PA/exercise. If this is necessary, then it is advisable that the exercise practitioner works with the pulmonary rehabilitation team. Furthermore, since COPD is a progressive disease, clients/patients will need to be assessed regularly to determine any changes in their condition, so that if required, appropriate adjustments can be made to their PA/exercise prescription.

During any assessment of functional or exercise capacity it is important to use an appropriate protocol. The 6-minute walk test (Appendix A) is often employed, as is cycle ergometry and treadmill walking. Those with COPD can be very limited in their PA/exercise ability and it may be that all these assessment methods are unsuitable. Thus, simply determining a small level of progression from very low-intensity PA/exercise may be appropriate. The progression in PA/exercise of the COPD client/patient is often far slower than in other individuals, such as cardiac patients. However, even small improvements in physical status can make considerable differences to their ability to perform daily tasks, thus improving their quality of life (Mink 1997). Although measures of lung function are reported to show little change after PA/exercise intervention, it is useful to gain some indication of the patient's physical status. Thus simple spirometry measures are a useful guide to the patient's level of airways resistance and potential limitations. Furthermore, prior to PA/exercise prescription it is important to discuss the best type of PA/exercise for the particular individual, and any practical implications that may be imposed, so that coping strategies can be employed.

PHYSICAL ACTIVITY/EXERCISE PRESCRIPTION

For those with moderate and severe COPD, the prescription of exercise should be performed in collaboration with the pulmonary rehabilitation team. Individuals with milder COPD may present to the exercise practitioner independently, and in this instance, it is important that the exercise practitioner inform their general practitioner of this liaison.

TYPES OF PHYSICAL ACTIVITY/EXERCISE

The optimal type of training for those with COPD has still to be determined. There are still no clear PA/exercise guidelines specific for those with COPD, hence most programmes are still based on guidelines set out for healthy individuals (Casaburi 2001, Storer 2001). Nevertheless, numerous trials have been performed observing the effect of various types of PA/exercise on patients with COPD, and in general, PA/exercise of any type appears to have some beneficial effect. A review looking at various types of PA/exercise found both structured and unstructured PA/exercise improved patients' physical endurance; and upper body training was found to be of additional benefit. Improvements have also been gained from programmes that included three 1–2 hour sessions per week of low-intensity activity (Belman 1993). Both high- and low-intensity aerobic activities have been found to be effective at increasing PA/exercise endurance, but only high-intensity training has been found to produce gains in aerobic fitness (Rochester 2003).

Continuous versus interval physical activity/exercise

When prescribing PA/exercise to the individual with COPD, intermittent PA/exercise may produce better overall results than continuous activities. For example, a study carried out by Sabapathy et al (2004) found that when 10 patients with moderate COPD performed intermittent cycle ergometry (1 minute exercise and 1 minute rest) at the same power output (70% of peak power attained during an incremental test), subjects were able to complete a significantly greater total of work (56%), with significantly lower lung hyperinflation (p. 146). Similarly, Vogiatzis et al (2004) found that whilst COPD ($n = 27$) patients exhibited similar dynamic lung hyperinflation at the limit of exercise tolerance from both continuous (80% peak work capacity) and intermittent cycle ergometry (100% peak work capacity), exercise endurance time was significantly greater from interval (32.7 ± 3.0 minutes) than from continuous cycling (10.3 ± 1.6 minutes). Thus the implementation of interval PA/exercise may be preferable to continuous PA/exercise for COPD patients.

Eccentric exercise

The oxygen cost of eccentric exercise is lower than that of concentric at similar workloads. A study employing eccentric cycle training in COPD patients found similar changes in aerobic fitness to those found in subjects who underwent 'general' exercise training. Moreover, the eccentric exercise group were able to work at a higher intensity without becoming out of breath or requiring supplemental oxygen (Rooyackers et al 2003).

Aerobic activities

The vast majority of studies looking into the effect of PA/exercise in COPD patients employ a regimen of aerobic activities. For example, a study of 15 men and 10 women with COPD (mean age 68 years $\pm$ 6 years), who underwent 6 weeks of cycle ergometry (45 minutes, three times per week) at an intensity close to their maximal targets, showed improvements in aerobic fitness, and for an identical constant work rate, displayed reduced ventilation of about 10% and respiratory rate of about 19% (Casaburi et al 1997). Both high- and low-intensity aerobic activities have been shown to be effective at increasing PA/exercise endurance, though for changes in aerobic fitness to occur the regimen needs to be of a high intensity (Rochester 2003).

Resistance circuit training and weight training

Compared with endurance PA/exercise, resistance training has received relatively little attention. Nonetheless, a review of literature has shown resistance exercise to be beneficial for those with COPD. A study carried out by O'Hara et al (1984) on 14 COPD patients who underwent a home programme including weight lifting found that those who lifted the weights had reductions in minute ventilation and a 16% greater increase in cycle endurance, compared to their pre-training levels. Additionally, Simpson et al (1992) randomly assigned COPD patients to either a weight-lifting group ($n = 14$, upper and lower body muscle groups) or controls ($n = 14$). The researchers found that the trained subjects' muscle strength and endurance time, during cycling at 80% of maximum power output, increased by 73%, whilst the controls showed no change.

Upper body

Those with COPD display ventilatory constraints that limit their physical performance during unsupported arm exercise, which has been shown to be dependent upon respiratory muscle function (Lebzelter et al 2001). Although training employing both leg and arm exercises has been found to improve respiratory muscle function, only programmes that include specific unsupported arm training have shown reductions in the metabolic cost of unsupported arm exercise (Celli 1994). For instance,

Martinez et al (1993) randomly selected patients into a group of either unsupported (arm ergometry, $n = 17$) or supported arm exercise (raising weighted dowel, $n = 18$); both groups also performed 10 weeks of bicycle ergometry, treadmill walking and respiratory muscle training. The researchers found that it was the unsupported arm exercise group that showed the greatest reductions in $\dot{V}O_2$ (litres per minute) during arm exercise. They suggested that unsupported arm exercise training might be of greater clinical significance in COPD patients. Furthermore, upper body exercise has been shown to be very effective at improving task-specific performance (Reis et al 1988, Bartolome 1998), and since most daily life activities require the use of the arms this is extremely important. Thus incorporating upper body exercise into a PA/exercise programme will probably be of great benefit to the individual's daily life.

Water-based activities

Cold dry air can make breathing difficult; thus swimming in a heated pool is often recommended. However, since PA/exercise induces coughing and sputum clearance, for those with chronic bronchitis this type of activity may prove problematic and the exercise practitioner may need to discuss this with their client/patient.

PHYSICAL ACTIVITY/EXERCISE INTENSITY

The PA/exercise ability of each individual, even with similar levels of disease severity, may vary considerably. Therefore, clear guidelines for prescribing the intensity of PA/exercise are not readily available. Thus establishing each individual's PA/exercise capacity is important. Nonetheless, while structured high-intensity programmes have been found to be effective at producing a training effect (Casaburi et al 1997, Rochester 2003), less structured physical activity, which allows individuals to decide on their own level of intensity, has also shown improvements in exercise tolerance, reduction in minute ventilation and dyspnoea, even for those with quite severe disease (Killian et al 1992, Mink 1997).

PHYSICAL ACTIVITY/EXERCISE CONSIDERATIONS

There are many factors that require consideration when prescribing PA/exercise to those with COPD (Table 9.7). The majority will be related to the numerous PA/exercise limitations resulting from COPD. The extent of these will undoubtedly affect the individual's ability to perform PA/exercise and will require consideration when designing a PA/exercise programme.

Table 9.7 Physical activity/exercise considerations for those with COPD

Mode and intensity of PA/exercise
Progression of disease and subsequent programme adjustment
Social implications and of coughing
Social implications and strategies for coping with sputum clearance
Effects of medications, such as, bronchodilators
The need for oxygen supplementation during and after PA/exercise
Physical activity/exercise limitations:
Hypercapnia
Capillary oxygen saturation levels
Peripheral muscle myopathy
Lung hyperinflation

PROGRESSION

The increase in functional and exercise capacity in those with COPD is comparatively slow compared to other individuals. However, even small improvements can make considerable differences to the quality of life of these individuals (Mink 1997). COPD sufferers often go through cycles of relapse and recovery, which can make determining progression difficult.

LUNG SPUTUM CLEARANCE AND COUGHING

Although PA/exercise intervention does not appear to improve the degree of coughing and sputum production (Cox et al 1993), the onset of PA/exercise generally induces coughing, which may assist in the clearance of sputum (Oldenburg et al 1979, Thomas et al 1995, Nikolaizik et al 1998) and aid those with chronic bronchitis to clear their lungs. However, the exercise practitioner should be aware of and consider the social and practical implications of sputum clearance during PA/exercise, and strategies to cope with sputum clearance may need to be discussed.

SIGNS OF DISEASE PROGRESSION

Since COPD is a progressive disease, the exercise practitioner should be aware of signs of disease progression, such as cyanosis, drowsiness and confusion, peripheral oedema, increased dyspnoea, increased sputum production and weight loss, so that appropriate adaptations to any PA/exercise programme can be made and additional medical advice sought.

MEDICATION

The effect of the commonly prescribed medications for COPD (p. 148) upon PA/exercise ability will be discussed in Chapter 14 (p. 229).

ABSOLUTE CONTRAINDICATIONS FOR EXERCISE

In addition to the PA/exercise limitations for those with COPD, the absolute contraindications for exercise will be similar to those set out in Appendix A (Table A.1).

PHYSICAL ACTIVITY/EXERCISE LIMITATIONS

There are several factors that contribute toward exercise limitation in those with COPD, the major factor being airflow limitation, which is only partly reversible with the usual bronchodilator therapy. The inability of gas to move freely in and out of the lungs causes dyspnoea and exercise intolerance. The possible mechanisms for this exercise limitation under these conditions are the occurrence of expiratory flow limitation, and dynamic lung hyperinflation developing with the increase in minute ventilation during exercise (Palange et al 2005). Additional limitations during PA/exercise are from the cardiovascular system and/or peripheral muscle function. Additionally, those with FEV_1 values <40–60% of predicted value tend to show an increase in hypercapnia during PA/exercise. Oxygen uptake is also reduced in those with diffusion problems, severe $\dot{V}A/\dot{Q}$ mismatch or a reduced contact time between blood and alveolar gas. This leads to dyspnoea, which generally results in avoidance of all exertion, and thus a vicious circle of inactivity, low fitness and unpleasant physical sensations during exercise develops (Folgering & von Herwaarden 1994).

Hypercapnia

Although appropriate PA/exercise may be of benefit, even to those with severe COPD, great care should be taken during PA/exercise as this can lead to hypercapnia. A study of 7 severe COPD patients found that low-level steady-state exercise led to a fall in arterial O_2 pressure (P_{O_2}) of about 17% and mixed venous P_{O_2} by about 16%. There was also a rise in arterial CO_2 pressure (P_{CO_2}) of around 9%. A fall in oxygen saturation during PA/exercise is generally seen in healthy individuals (p. 154), but may require oxygen supplementation in some COPD individuals. The cause of worsening hypoxaemia with exercise has been suggested to be the inadequate ventilatory response to exercise, which leads to a rise in arterial P_{CO_2}, and the impact of $\dot{V}A/\dot{Q}$ mismatch (p. 146) (Dantzker & D'Alonzo 1986).

Oxygen supplementation

To assist in the ventilatory demands of PA/exercise, an intervention of breathing supplemental oxygen during exercise has been shown to reduce exercise ventilation. The supplementation of oxygen has been shown to maintain expiratory flow limitation within the tidal breathing range, resulting in a decrease in dyspnoea, allowing an increase in exercise intensity and duration (Palange et al 2005). However, not all studies have found similar results from oxygen supplementation. For instance, whilst the post-PA/exercise administration of oxygen does appear to reduce dynamic lung hyperinflation during recovery from exercise, it does not always relieve feelings of dyspnoea during PA/exercise recovery (Stevenson & Calverley 2004). Furthermore, the density of the gas administered also appears to have an influence on exercise capacity (Palange et al 2005), with the severity of the disease having an influence, as gas distribution tends tovary with disease severity (Cutillo et al 1981).

Oxygen saturation

In healthy individuals oxygen saturation during rest, at sea level, is rarely 100%, generally being between 95% and 98%. When oxygen saturation levels drop to values of 84% and 86%, however, an individual will start to become breathless (see McArdle et al 2000, pp. 230–258).

During PA/exercise, oxygen saturation generally drops from that at rest, and usually returns to normal after cessation of physical activity. However, for those with COPD who may have resting levels well below those found in healthy individuals, any drop in oxygen saturation may cause an increase in the discomfort associated with dyspnoea and require oxygen supplementation (p. 153).

Muscle myopathy

Peripheral and respiratory muscle myopathy is commonly seen in those with COPD, who often exhibit effort-dependent strength scores of 70–80% of those found in age-matched healthy subjects (Storer 2001). The causes of this myopathy are not fully understood. However, factors such as increased oxidative stress during PA/exercise (Couillard et al 2001, 2003), as well as generalized muscle weakening, due to low levels of anabolic steroids (Casaburi 1998), general physical deconditioning, malnutrition, electrolyte disturbances, cardiac failure, systematic inflammation and treatment with corticosteroids have been found to contribute (Table 9.8).

Muscle oxidative stress has been found to be associated with reduced quadriceps endurance. Couillard et al (2003), for example, examined the effect of repeated knee extension exercise of the dominant leg in 12 COPD patients,

Table 9.8 Factors affecting respiratory and peripheral muscle myopathy

Increased oxidative stress during PA/exercise
Low levels of anabolic steroids
General low physical fitness, due to inactivity
Malnutrition
Electrolyte disturbances
Cardiac failure (latter stages of disease)
Systemic inflammation
Long-term use of corticosteroids

compared to 10 healthy sedentary controls. The researchers found that quadriceps endurance was significantly reduced in the COPD subjects compared to the controls. Biopsies of the vastus lateralis muscle were also obtained 48 hours post-exercise, and showed a decrease in antioxidant activity in the COPD patients, suggesting that oxidative stress plays a part in myopathy during exercise. Additionally, Couillard et al (2001) found that during rest COPD patients exhibited significantly reduced levels of vitamin E (a known antioxidant) compared to healthy controls.

Microscopic muscle myopathy has been studied both in patients with COPD and in the animal model, and a generalized fibre atrophy was found, which does not appear to be confined to one particular fibre type (Decramer 2001). Histological data from quadriceps biopsies of COPD patients have also shown diffuse muscle fibre atrophy and necrosis, and an increase in the variation in the diameter of muscle fibres (Perez 2000). Moreover, abnormalities in both high-energy phosphate metabolism and a decrease in oxidative enzyme capacity have been found in the skeletal muscle of stable COPD patients. Irregularities in mitochondrial structure and function have also been observed during corticosteroid treatment. But a cross-sectional study performed by Pouw et al (2000) on 15 steroid-naive COPD patients, 14 COPD patients who had been taking corticosteroids for at least one year, and 10 healthy controls found that while adenosine triphosphate was significantly lower in the COPD patients on steroids, they did not differ in oxidative and glycolytic enzymes. Another study found steroid-induced myopathy to be associated with an increase in lactic dehydrogenase (Decramer et al 1996).

Lung hyperinflation

Chronic hyperinflation of the lungs shortens the inspiratory muscles, resulting in mechanical limitations. However, to counterbalance this mechanical disadvantage, the inspiratory muscles may adapt over time, and have been found to increase their proportion of type I fibres and mitochondrial density and show a decrease in sarcomere length (Perez 2000, Decramer 2001).

The role of dynamic lung hyperinflation in exercise limitation still remains to be fully determined. Nonetheless, a study on 105 COPD patients found that during exercise, dynamic hyperinflation restricted the peak, tidal volume response. Hyperinflation is thus considered to be a limiting factor in the responses to increased metabolic demand to exercise, and is a contributor toward exercise intolerance (O'Donnell et al 2001). Furthermore, those with severe COPD have also been shown to develop CO_2 retention during PA/exercise. This retention of CO_2 is thought to be due to hyperinflation, in addition to a reduction in gas exchange capabilities of COPD patients (O'Donnell et al 2002). However, bronchodilator-induced lung deflation can help to reduce the mechanical restriction imposed by hyperinflation and has been shown to increase ventilatory capacity and decrease respiratory discomfort, thus increasing PA/exercise endurance (O'Donnell et al 2004b, 2004c). Thus its administration should be considered during PA/exercise. Additionally, endobronchial valve placement has also been shown to reduce dynamic hyperinflation and prolong exercise time in patients with emphysema (Hopkinson et al 2005).

SUMMARY

- COPD is the most common respiratory disease in the developed world and accounts for around 5% of all deaths.
- COPD is characterized by airflow limitation of the lungs, and displays elements of both chronic bronchitis and emphysema, and may also show similar symptoms to other respiratory diseases.
- COPD is caused by both host factors and environmental exposure (Table 9.2).
- COPD results in pathological changes in the lungs including mucus hypersecretion, ciliary dysfunction, airflow limitation, hyperinflation, gas exchange abnormalities and latterly, pulmonary hypertension and cor pulmonale.
- Measures of lung function (Table 9.6) are used to determine certain stages of COPD (Table 9.4). Other measures of functional ability are better indicators of pharmacological and non-pharmacological interventions, such as PA/exercise programmes.
- Physical activity/exercise intervention generally enhances exercise tolerance, decreases ventilatory demand and reduces the symptoms of COPD, even in those with severe COPD. However, generally it produces little change to measures of lung function and does not appear to prolong life expectancy.
- Small improvements in physical function can make large differences in quality of life.
- Most types of PA/exercise have been shown to be of benefit to those with COPD, especially programmes that include specific unsupported upper body exercise.
- Intermittent compared to continuous PA/exercise has been shown to be more effective at enhancing functional capacity and PA/exercise endurance.
- Those with COPD suffer many limitations to exercise.
- Since COPD is progressive, COPD clients/patients will require regular assessment in order to adjust their PA/exercise programme.
- Due to the nature of COPD any progression is generally very slow.

Suggested readings, references and bibliography

Suggested reading

Bartolome R C 1998 Pulmonary rehabilitation for COPD. Postgraduate Medicine 103(4): April. Online. Available: http://www.postgradmed.com April 2005

Cole R B, Mackay A D 1990 Essentials of respiratory disease, 3rd edn. Churchill Livingstone, New York

Crockett A 2000 Managing chronic obstructive pulmonary disease in primary care. Blackwell Science, Oxford

GOLD (Global Initiative for Chronic Obstructive Lung Disease) 2001 Global strategy for the diagnosis, management, and prevention of chronic obstructive pulmonary disease. National Institutes of Health, Bethesda, MD

References and bibliography

AHRQ (Agency for Healthcare Research and Quality) 2000 Management of acute exacerbations of chronic obstructive pulmonary disease. AHRQ publication No. 01-E003

Barbera J A, Riverola A, Roca J et al 1994 Pulmonary vascular abnormalities and ventilation-perfusion relationships in mild chronic obstructive pulmonary disease. American Journal of Respiratory Critical Care Medicine 149:423–429

Barnes P J 2000 Mechanisms in COPD: differences from asthma. Chest 117(2 suppl):10S–14S

Barnes P J 2004a Mediators of chronic obstructive pulmonary disease. Pharmacological Reviews 56:515–548

Barnes P J 2004b COPD: Is there light at the end of the tunnel? Current Opinion in Pharmacology 4(3):263–272

Barnes P J, Shapiro S D, Pauwels R A 2003 Chronic obstructive pulmonary disease: molecular and cellular mechanisms. European Respiratory Journal 22(4):672–688

Bartolome R C 1998 Pulmonary rehabilitation for COPD. Postgraduate Medicine 103(4):Online. Available: http://www.postgradmed.com April 2005

Becklake M R 1989 Occupational exposures: evidence for a causal association with chronic obstructive pulmonary disease. American Review of Respiratory Disease 140(3 Pt 2):S85–S91

Belman M J 1993 Exercise in patients with chronic obstructive pulmonary disease. Thorax 48(9):936–946

Belman M J 1996 Therapeutic exercise in chronic lung disease. In: Fishman A P (ed) Pulmonary rehabilitation. Marcel Dekker, New York

Berry M J, Walschlager S A 1998 Exercise training and chronic obstructive pulmonary disease: past and future research directions. Journal of Cardiopulmonary Rehabilitation 18(3):181–191

BMA, RPS GB (British Medical Association & Royal Pharmaceutical Society of Great Britain) 2002 British National Formulary (BNF). Pharmaceutical Press, London

Bonsignore M R, Morici G, Vognola A M et al 2003 Increased airway inflammatory cells in endurance athletes: what do they mean? Clinical and Experimental Allergy 33(1):14–21

Bousamra M 2nd, Haasler G B, Lipchik R J et al 1997 Functional and oximetric assessment of patients after lung reduction surgery. Journal of Thoracic and Cardiovascular Surgery 113(4):675–681

BTS (British Thoracic Society) 1997 COPD group of the standards of care committee of the BTS. BTS guidelines for the management of chronic obstructive pulmonary disease. Thorax 52(suppl 5):S1–S28

Casaburi R 1993 Exercise training in chronic obstructive lung disease. In: Casaburi R, Petty T L (eds) Principles and practice of pulmonary rehabilitation. Saunders, Philadelphia

Casaburi R 1998 Rationale for anabolic therapy to facilitate rehabilitation in chronic obstructive pulmonary disease. Baillière's Clinical Endocrinology and Metabolism 12(3):407–418

Casaburi R 2001 Skeletal muscle dysfunction in chronic obstructive pulmonary disease. Medicine and Science in Sports and Exercise 33(7 suppl):S662–S670

Casaburi R, Patessio A, Ioli F et al 1991 Reductions in exercise lactic acidosis and ventilation as a result of exercise training in patients with obstructive lung disease. American Review of Respiratory Disease 143(1):9–18

Casaburi R, Porszasz J, Burns M R et al 1997 Physiologic benefits of exercise training in rehabilitation of patients with severe chronic obstructive pulmonary disease. American Journal of Respiratory and Critical Care Medicine 155(5):1541–1551

CDCP (Centers for Disease Control and Prevention) 1995 Criteria for a recommended standard: occupational exposure to respirable coalmine dust. National Institute of Occupational Safety and Health, Morgantown, Publication No. 95–106

Celli B R 1994 The clinical use of upper extremity exercise training in chronic obstructive pulmonary disease. Chest 93(4):688–692

Chabot F 2004 Health status in patients with chronic obstructive pulmonary disease. Revue du Practicien 54(13):1451–1454

Christensen C C, Ryg M S, Edvardsen A et al 2004 Effect of exercise mode on oxygen uptake and blood gases in COPD patients. Respiratory Medicine 98(7):656–660

Cole R B, Mackay A D 1990 Essentials of respiratory disease, 3rd edn. Churchill Livingstone, New York

Couillard A, Cristol J P, Chanes P et al 2001 Local exercise and oxidative stress in chronic obstructive broncho-pneumopathies: preliminary results. Journal de la Société de Biologie 195(4):419–425

Couillard A, Maltais F, Saey D et al 2003 Exercise-induced quadriceps oxidative stress and peripheral muscle dysfunction in patients with chronic obstructive pulmonary disease. American Journal of Respiratory and Critical Care Medicine 167(12):1664–1669

Cox N J, Hendricks J C, Binkhorst R A et al 1993 A pulmonary rehabilitation program for patients with asthma and mild chronic obstructive pulmonary diseases (COPD). Lung 171(4):235–244

Crockett A 2000 Managing chronic obstructive pulmonary disease in primary care. Blackwell Science, Oxford

Cutillo A, Bigler A H, Perondi R et al 1981 Exercise and distribution of inspired gas in patients with obstructive pulmonary disease. Bulletin Européen de Physiopathologie Respiratoire 17(6):891–901

Dantzker D R, D'Alonzo G E 1986 The effect of exercise on pulmonary gas exchange in patients with severe chronic obstructive pulmonary disease. American Review of Respiratory Disease 134(6):1135–1139

Decramer M I 2001 Respiratory muscles in COPD: regulation of trophical status. Verhandelingen – Koninklijke Academie voor Geneeskunde van Belgie 63(6):577–602, 602–604

Decramer M I, de Bock V, Dom R 1996 Functional and histologic picture of steroid-induced myopathy in chronic obstructive pulmonary disease. American Journal of Respiratory and Critical Care Medicine 153(6 Pt 1):1958–1964

Decramer M I, Grosselink R I, Bartsch P et al 2005 Effect of treatments on the progression of COPD: report of a workshop held in Leuven, 11–12 March 2004. Thorax 60(4):343–349

de Lucas Ramos P, Rodriguez G M, Garcia de Pedro J et al 1998 Training of inspiratory muscles in chronic obstructive lung disease. Its impact on functional changes and exercise tolerance. Archivos de Bronconeumologia 34(2):64–70

Folgering H, von Herwaarden C 1994 Exercise limitations in patients with chronic obstructive pulmonary diseases. International Journal of Sports Medicine 15(3):107–111

Gan W Q, Man S F, Senthilselvan A et al 2004 Association between chronic obstructive pulmonary disease and systemic inflammation: a systematic review and a meta-analysis. Thorax 59(7):574–580

Gigliotti F, Coli C, Bianchi R et al 2003 Exercise training improves exertional dyspnea in patients with COPD: evidence of the role of mechanical factors. Chest 123:1794–1802

GOLD (Global Initiative for Chronic Obstructive Lung Disease) 2001 Global strategy for the diagnosis, management, and prevention of chronic obstructive pulmonary disease. National Heart, Lung, and Blood Institute (NHLBI), National Institutes of Health, Bethesda, MD

Grzanka A, Pitsch T, Krzywiecki A et al 2004 Lung function and exercise tolerance after treatment with salmeterol or ipratropium bromide in chronic obstructive pulmonary disease. Polski Merkuriusz Lekarski 17(99):208–211

Guerin J C, Leophonte P, Lebas F X et al 2005 Oxidative stress in bronchopulmonary disease: contribution of N-acetylcysteine (SC). Revue de Pneumologie Clinique 61(1):16–21

Hogg J C 1999 Childhood viral infection and the pathogenesis of asthma and chronic obstructive lung disease. American Journal of Respiratory and Critical Care Medicine 160(5 Pt 2):S26–28

Hogg J C, Macklem P T, Thurlbeck W M 1968 Site and nature of airway obstruction in chronic obstructive lung disease. English Journal of Medicine 278(25):1355–1360

Hopkinson N S, Tudor P, Toma DM et al 2005 Effect of bronchoscopic lung volume reduction on dynamic hyperinflation and exercise in emphysema. American Journal of Respiratory and Critical Care Medicine 171:453–460

Hoshino S, Yoshinda M, Yano Y et al 2005 Cigarette smoke extract induces endothelial cell injury via JNK pathway. Biochemical and Biophysical Research Communications 329(1):58–63

Hubbard R C, Ogushi F, Fells G A et al 1987 Oxidants spontaneously released by alveolar macrophages of cigarette smokers can inactivate the active site of alpha 1-antitrypsin, rendering it ineffective as an inhibitor of neutrophil elastase. Journal of Clinical Investigation 80(5):1289–1295

Jindal S K, Gupta D, Aggarwal A N 2003 Guidelines for management of chronic obstructive pulmonary disease (COPD) in India: a guide to physicians (2003). Indian Journal of Chest Disease and Allied Sciences 46(2):137–153

Johnston I D 1999 Effect of pneumonia in childhood on adult lung function. Journal of Pediatrics 135(2 Pt 2):33–37

Joos L, Pare P D, Sandford A J 2002 Genetic risk factors of chronic obstructive pulmonary disease. Swiss Medical Weekly 132(3–4):27–37

Joos G F, Brusselle G, Derom E et al 2003 Tiotropium bromide: a long-acting anticholinergic bronchodilator for the treatment of patients with chronic obstructive pulmonary disease. International Journal of Clinical Practice 57(10):906–909

Kauffmann F, Drouet D, Lellouch et al 1979 Twelve years spirometric changes among Paris area workers. International Journal of Epidemiology 8:201–212

Killian K J, Leblanc P, Martin D H et al 1992 Exercise capacity and ventilatory, circulatory and symptom limitation in patients with chronic airflow limitation. American Review of Respiratory Disease 146(4):935–940

Kirschvink N, Smith N, Fievez L et al 2002 Effect of chronic airway inflammation and exercise on pulmonary and systemic antioxidant status of healthy and heaves-affected horses. Equine Veterinary Journal 34(6):563–571

Koechlin C, Couillard A, Cristol J P et al 2004 Does systemic inflammation trigger local exercise-induced oxidative stress in COPD? European Respiratory Journal 23(4):538–544

Kosciuch J, Chazan R 2003 The role of viruses in the pathogenesis of obstructive lung diseases. Polski Merkuriuz Lekarski 15(87):292–295

Lange C G, Scheuerer B, Zabel P 2004 Acute exacerbation of COPD. Internist 45(5):527–538

Lebzelter J, Klainman E, Yarmolovsky A et al 2001 Relationship between pulmonary function and unsupported arm exercise in patients with COPD. Monaldi Archives for Chest Disease 56(4):309–314

Liesker J J, Wijkstra P J, Ten Hacken N H et al 2002 A systematic review of the effects of bronchodilators on exercise capacity in patients with COPD. Chest 121(2):597–608

Lisboa C, Villafranca C, Caiozzi G et al 2001 Quality of life in patients with chronic obstructive pulmonary disease and the impact of physical training. Revista Medica de Chile 129(4):359–366

Lotters F, van Tol B, Kwakkel G et al 2002 Effects of controlled inspiratory muscle training in patients with COPD: a meta-analysis. European Respiratory Journal 20(3):570–576

McArdle W D, Katch F I, Katch V L 2000 Essentials of exercise physiology, 2nd edn. Lippincott Williams & Wilkins, USA, p 230–258

McLean A, Warren P M, Gillooly M et al 1992 Microscopic and macroscopic measurements of emphysema: relation to carbon dioxide gas transfer. Thorax 47:144–149

MacNee W 1994 Pathophysiology of cor pulmonale in chronic obstructive pulmonary disease: part two. American Journal of Respiratory Critical Care Medicine 150:1158–1168

MacNee W 2001 Oxidants/antioxidants and chronic obstructive pulmonary disease: pathogenesis to therapy. Novartis Foundation Symposium 234:169–185, 185–188

Magnussen H 2004 COPD: an inflammatory disease of the airways? Pneumologie 58(5):320–324

Martinez F J, Vogel P D, Dupont D N et al 1993 Supported arm exercise vs unsupported arm exercise in the rehabilitation of patients with severe chronic airflow obstruction. Chest 103(5):1397–1402

Matsuse T, Hayashi S, Kuwano K et al 1992 Latent adenoviral infection in the pathogenesis of chronic airways obstruction. American Review of Respiratory Disease 146(1):177–184

Matsuzawa Y, Kubo K, Fujimoto K et al 1998 Mechanism of short-term improvement in exercise tolerance after lung volume reduction surgery for severe emphysema. Nihon Kokyuki Gakkai Zasshi 36(4):323–329

Ministry of Health 1954 Mortality and morbidity during the London fog of December 1952. HMSO, London

Mink B D 1997 Exercise and chronic obstructive pulmonary disease: modest fitness gains pay big dividends. The Physician and Sportsmedicine 25(11): November

Molfino N A 2004 Genetics of COPD. Chest 125(5):1929–1940

Nakajima C, Kijimoto C, Yokoyama Y et al 1998 Longitudinal follow-up of pulmonary function after lobectomy in childhood – factors affecting lung growth. Pediatric Surgery International 13(5):341–345

Nikolaizik W H, Knopfli B, Leister E et al 1998 The anaerobic threshold in cystic fibrosis: comparison of V-slope method, lactate turn points, and Conconi test. Pediatric Pulmonology 25(3):147–153

Nishimura M 2003 Role of genetic factors in development of COPD. Japanese Journal of Clinical Medicine 61(12):2095–2100

O'Donnell D E, Webb K A, McGuire M A 1993 Older patients with COPD: benefits of exercise training. Geriatrics 48(1):59–66

O'Donnell D E, Webb K A, Bertley J C et al 1996 Mechanisms of relief of exertional breathlessness following unilateral and lung volume reduction surgery in emphysema. Chest 110(1):18–27

O'Donnell D E, Revil S M, Webb K A 2001 Dynamic hyperinflation and exercise intolerance in chronic obstructive pulmonary disease. American Journal of Respiratory Critical Care Medicine 164(5):770–777

O'Donnell D E, D'Arsigny C, Fitzpatrick M et al 2002 Exercise hypercapnia in advanced chronic obstructive pulmonary disease. American Journal of Respiratory and Critical Care Medicine 166:663–668

O'Donnell R A, Peebles C, Ward J A et al 2004a Relationship between peripheral airway dysfunction, airway obstruction and neutrophilic inflammation in COPD. Thorax 59:837–842

O'Donnell D E, Voduc N, Fitzpatrick M et al 2004b Effect of salmeterol on the ventilatory response to exercise in chronic obstructive pulmonary disease. European Respiratory Journal 24:86–94

O'Donnell D E, Fluge T, Gerken F et al 2004c Effects of tiotropium on lung hyperinflation, dyspnea and exercise tolerance in COPD. European Respiratory Journal 23:832–840

Oga T 2004 Exercise responses during endurance testing at different intensities in patients with COPD. Respiratory Medicine 98(6):515–521

Oga T, Nishimura K, Tsukino M et al 2003 A comparison of the effects of salbutamol and ipratropium bromide on exercise endurance in patients with COPD. Chest 123(6):1810–1816

O'Hara W J, Lasachuk B P, Matheson P et al 1984 Weight training and back packing in chronic obstructive pulmonary disease. Respiratory Care 29:1202–1210

Oldenburg F A Jr, Dolovich M B, Montgomery J M et al 1979 Effects of postural drainage, exercise and coughing on mucus clearance in chronic bronchitis. American Review of Respiratory Disease 120(4):739–745

Palange P, Crimi E, Pellegrino R et al 2005 Supplemental oxygen and heliox: 'new' tools for exercise training in chronic obstructive pulmonary disease. Current Opinion in Pulmonary Medicine 11(2):145–148

Pastva A, Estell K, Schoeb T R et al 2004 Aerobic exercise attenuates airway inflammatory responses in a mouse model of atopic asthma. Journal of Immunology 172(7):4520–4526

Peat J K, Woolcock A J, Cullen K 1987 Rate of decline of lung function in subjects with asthma. European Journal of Respiratory Disease 70:171–179

Peinado V I, Barbera J A, Abate P et al 1999 Inflammatory reaction in pulmonary muscular arteries of patients with mild chronic obstructive pulmonary disease. American Journal of Respiratory and Critical Care Medicine 159:1605–1611

Perez T 2000 Clinical investigation of diaphragmatic function. Relationship with the biology of muscle. Revue des Maladies Respiratoires 19(2 Pt 2):591–596

Pettersen C A, Adler K B 2002 Airways inflammation and COPD: epithelial-neutrophil interactions. Chest 121:142S–150S

Pfeifer M 2004 New therapeutic approaches to COPD. Internist 45(12):1395–1401

Poole P J, Black P N 2003a Mucolytic agents for chronic bronchitis or chronic obstructive pulmonary disease. Cochrane Database of Systematic Reviews (2):CD001287

Poole P J, Black P N 2003b Preventing exacerbations of chronic bronchitis in COPD: therapeutic potential of mucolytic agents. American Journal of Respiratory Medicine 2(5):367–370

Pouw E M, Koerts-de Lang E, Gosker H R et al 2000 Muscle metabolism status in patients with severe COPD with and without long-term prednisolone. European Respiratory Journal 16(2):247–252

Presberg K W, Dincer H E 2003 Pathophysiology of pulmonary hypertension due to lung disease. Current Opinion in Pulmonary Medicine 9(2):131–138

Reardon J, Awad E, Normandin E et al 1994 The effect of comprehensive outpatient pulmonary rehabilitation on dyspnea. Chest 105(4):1046–1052

Reis A L, Ellis B, Hawkins R W 1988 Upper extremity exercise training in chronic obstructive pulmonary disease. Chest 93(4):688–692

Rennard S I 1999 Inflammation and repair processes in chronic obstructive pulmonary disease. American Journal of Critical Care Medicine 160:S12–S16

Repine J E, Bast A, Lankhorst I 1997 Oxidative stress in chronic obstructive pulmonary disease. Oxidative stress study group. American Journal of Respiratory Critical Care Medicine 156:341–357

Ries AL, Kalan RM, Limberg TM et al 1995 Effects of pulmonary rehabilitation on physiological and psychosocial outcomes in patients with chronic obstructive pulmonary disease. Annals of Internal Medicine 122(11):823–832

Rochester C L 2003 Exercise training in chronic obstructive pulmonary disease. Journal of Rehabilitation Research and Development 40 (5 suppl 2):59–80

Rooyackers J M, Berkeljon D A, Folgering H T M 2003 Eccentric exercise training in patients with chronic obstructive pulmonary disease. International Journal of Rehabilitation Research 26(1):47–49

Sabapathy S, Kinglsey R A, Schneider D A et al 2004 Continuous and intermittent exercise responses in individuals with chronic obstructive pulmonary disease. Thorax 59:1026–1031

Sanguinetti C M 1992 Oxidant/antioxidant imbalance: role in the pathogenesis of COPD. Respiration 59(suppl 1):20–23

Sciurba F C, Rogers R M, Keenan R J et al 1996 Improvement in pulmonary function and elastic recoil after lung-reduction surgery for diffuse emphysema. New England Journal of Medicine 334(17):1095–1099

Silverman E K, Speizer F E 1996 Risk factors for the development of chronic obstructive pulmonary disease. Medical Clinics of North America 80(3):501–522

Simpson K, Killian K, McCartney N et al 1992 Randomised controlled trial of weightlifting exercise in patients with chronic airflow limitation. Thorax 47(2):70–75

Stein C E, Kumaran K, Fall C H et al 1997 Relation of fetal growth to adult lung function in South India. Thorax 52:55–58

Stevenson N J, Calverley P M A 2004 Effect of oxygen on recovery from maximal exercise in patients with chronic obstructive pulmonary disease. Thorax 59:668–672

Storer T W 2001 Exercise in chronic obstructive pulmonary disease: resistance exercise prescription. Medicine and Science in Sports and Exercise 33(7 suppl):S680-S692

Strachan D P 1990 Do chesty children become chesty adults? Archives of Disease in Childhood 65(2):161–162

Tager I B, Segal M R, Speizer F E et al 1988 Effect of cigarette smoking and respiratory symptoms. American Review of Respiratory Disease 138(4):837–849

Tamparo C D, Lewis M A 1995 Diseases of the human body, 2nd edn. Allied Health, Philadelphia

Thomas J, Cook D J, Brooks D 1995 Chest physical therapy management with cystic fibrosis: a meta-analysis. American Journal of Respiratory and Critical Care Medicine 151(3 Pt 1):846–850

Toshima M T, Kaplan R M, Ries A L 1990 Experimental evaluation of rehabilitation in chronic obstructive pulmonary disease: short-term effects on exercise endurance and health status. Health Psychology 9(3):237–252

Traves S L, Culpitt S V, Russell R E K et al 2002 Increased levels of chemokines GROα and MCP-1 in sputum samples from patients with COPD. Thorax 57:590–595

Trone F, Gregoire J, Leblanc P et al 1999 Physiologic consequences of pneumonectomy. Consequence on the pulmonary function. Chest Surgery Clinics in North America 9(2):429–473

US Surgeon General 1984 The health consequences of smoking: chronic obstructive pulmonary disease. US Department of Health and Human Services, Washington DC, Publication No. 84–50205

Vander A J, Sherman J H, Luciano D S 1990 Human physiology. McGraw-Hill, New York

Vogiatzis I, Nanas S, Kastanakis E et al 2004 Dynamic hyperinflation and tolerance to interval exercise in patients with advanced COPD. European Respiratory Journal 24:385–390

Wagner P D 2005 Why doesn't exercise grow the lungs when other factors do? Medicine and Science in Sports and Exercise 33(1):3–8

Wetter T J, Xiang Z, Sonette D A et al 2002 Role of lung inflammatory mediators as a cause of exercise-induced arterial hypoxia in young athletes. Journal of Applied Physiology 93(1):116–126

WHO (World Health Organization) 2000 World health report. WHO, Geneva

Wright J L, Lawson L, Pare P D et al 1983 The structure and function of the pulmonary vasculature in mild chronic obstructive pulmonary disease. The effect of oxygen and exercise. American Review of Respiratory Disease 128(4):702–707

Chapter 10

Adults with arthritis

CHAPTER CONTENTS

Introduction   159
Prevalence   159
Joint structure   160
   Synovial fluid   160
   Cartilage   160
Osteoarthritis   161
   Pathophysiology and symptoms   161
   Aetiology   161
      Physical activity/exercise   162
   Treatment   162
      Physical activity/exercise   162
Rheumatoid arthritis   163
   Pathophysiology   163
      Synovial fluid   164
   Aetiology   164
      Immune system   164
      Autoimmunity   164
      Autoimmunity and RA   165
      Endocrine system   166
   Treatment   166

Pharmacological   166
Rest   166
Physical activity/exercise   166
Immune response to physical activity/exercise   167
Types of physical activity/exercise   167
Pre-physical activity/exercise prescription for both OA and RA   167
Physical activity/exercise prescription   167
   Frequency   168
   Intensity   168
   Duration   168
   Types of physical activity/exercise   168
      Resistance training   168
      Water-based activities   168
   Warming up and cooling down   168
   Considerations and contraindications   169
      Absolute contraindications   169
      Medication   169
Summary
Suggested readings, references and bibliography   169

INTRODUCTION

Arthritis has long been known as one of the leading causes of disability in Western society (Kvalvik 1996), affecting people of all ages, but is especially prevalent in older individuals.

There are over 200 types of arthritis, some of which are found in younger individuals (ARC 2002). This chapter will, however, focus on adults who suffer from the most common forms of arthritis, namely osteoarthritis (OA) and rheumatoid arthritis (RA). Although both types of arthritis may be debilitating, the causes are different. Therefore, the known aetiology and pathology of these conditions will be dealt with separately, and will be looked into with particular reference to physical activity (PA)/exercise, and how PA/exercise prescription may affect those suffering from these conditions.

PREVALENCE

The term *arthritis* describes an inflammation of the joints characterized by pain, swelling, heat, redness and limitation of movement (Anderson et al 2002). However, there is often general confusion with regard to what constitutes arthritis, joint pain or musculoskeletal pain. The term *musculoskeletal condition* is used by the medical profession to cover arthritis and other forms of joint and bone disease, yet it is a term unfamiliar to most of the general public (ARC 2002). Due to this confusion in terminology, it is difficult to get a clear indication of the number of individuals who suffer from specific musculoskeletal conditions. Nonetheless, it was estimated by the Epidemiological Unit of ARC (2002) and CDC (1996) that around 7 million people in the UK and 40 million in the USA had long-term health problems associated with arthritis and

Table 10.1 Some additional complications associated with rheumatoid arthritis (adapted from Ebrahimi 1999)

Affected areas	Symptoms
Skin	Nodules
	Inflammation
Eyes	Dryness of the cornea
	Sloughing and inflammation of the sclera (white opaque membrane that covers the back of the eye)
Cardiovascular	Inflammation of the pericardium
	Nodules on the epicardium, myocardium, valves
	Conduction defects
Respiratory	Nodules
	Pleural effusion
	Inflammation
Neuromuscular	Muscle atrophy
	Neuropathies
	Myopathy
Haematological	Anaemia
	Increased blood platelets
Other	Enlarged spleen
	Accumulation of amyloid (starch-like glycoprotein) in tissues and organs, which impairs their function

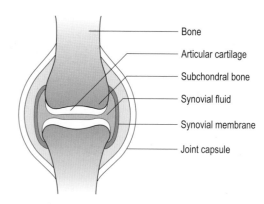

Figure 10.1   Healthy synovial joint.

related conditions. Similarly, arthritis affects about 3 million people in Australia, which is around 15% of the population (March & Bagga 2004). It has also been predicted that in the USA, by the year 2020, around 59.4 million individuals will suffer from arthritis and related conditions, mainly due to the ageing of the US population (NIAMS 1998).

JOINT STRUCTURE

Although RA in particular can affect various areas of the body (Table 10.1), arthritis in general is associated with inflammation of the joints. A brief overview of joint structure will therefore be given.

A joint is where two or more bones may articulate and there are three types of joints:

- *fibrous joints*, where bones are connected by collagenous tissues
- *cartilaginous joints*, where bones are connected by a mass of cartilage that acts as their growth centre

- *synovial joints*, where the junctions are enclosed by a fibrous capsule, which is lined with a synovial membrane and held together and stabilized by ligaments and tendons (Fig. 10.1), such as the knee and hip joints (Groer & Shekleton 1989).

SYNOVIAL FLUID

Synovial fluid is a diluted solution of blood plasma plus mucin, and its function is to lubricate the articulated surfaces and nourish the articular cartilage (Fig. 10.1). However, the status of the synovial fluid may be affected by its nutrient quality and ability to lubricate (Table 10.2). Therefore, any joint inflammation, bleeding, infection or trauma can potentially affect the quality of the synovial fluid (Groer & Shekleton 1989).

CARTILAGE

Cartilage is an essential component of the cartilaginous and synovial joints. Cartilage contains no blood vessels, lymphatics or nerves, and is therefore limited in its capacity to repair and regenerate. Thus, any damage or degeneration to the cartilage is generally permanent. Irregularities in or damage to the articular surface lead to progressive degenerative alterations in the surrounding cartilage, and ultimately to pain and limitation of movement. Even the normal stresses and strains of living cause wear and tear on the cartilage, causing it to be less resilient and increasing susceptibility to damage by enzymes released by certain types of infecting organisms (Groer & Shekleton 1989).

Table 10.2 Factors that affect the lubricant and nutrient quality of synovial fluid (information from Groer & Shekleton 1989)

Lubricant quality	Nutrient quality
Impaired secretory capacity of the synovial cells	Disruption or alterations in blood supply to the synovia
Dilution of synovial fluid	Change in fluid composition
Mixing of the synovial fluid with other substances	Barriers at the cartilage level, i.e. granulation of tissue
Breakdown of synovial fluid by chemicals, bacteria or enzymes	

OSTEOARTHRITIS

In the UK, between the years 1981 and 1991, there was a general rise, of around 13%, in people visiting their general practitioner for arthritis and related conditions (ARC 2002). It is thought that this general increase was related to the number of individuals with OA. Osteoarthritis is the most common form of arthritis, and in the years 1989–1991 affected around 12.1% of the US adult population (~20.7 million people) (NIAMS 1998). Osteoarthritis tends to affect people as they get older, and with the ageing population the prevalence of OA has increased. For example, the findings from the Epidemiological Unit of ARC (2002) showed that the ratio of young : middle-aged : elderly (young 16–44, middle-aged 45–64, elderly 65+ years) with OA was 1 : 6 : 9. Another reason for the increase in OA is related to the fact that one of the major risk factors, particularly for OA of the knee, is obesity (ARC 2002). Hence, the increases both in the aged population and in obesity play an important role in the increased prevalence of OA, and whilst exercise practitioners cannot alter the age of their clients, with appropriate PA/exercise prescription they may be able to assist them in reducing their body fat levels.

PATHOPHYSIOLOGY AND SYMPTOMS

Osteoarthritis, or degenerative joint disease, is characterized by degenerative alterations of the hyaline cartilage and hypertrophic changes in the articular bone ends. The affected bone becomes thickened and spreads outwards forming 'spurs' round the joint margins. Synovial fluid may enter the bone giving a cystic appearance. It is more common above the age of 60 years, and the most commonly affected sites are the hips, knees and spine. The joints that are affected become hypertrophied and there is a decreased flexibility, which leads to stiffness, pain and limitation in movement. Crepitus, or noise in the joints, on movement is common, and loose bodies (joint mice) may also be present. The joints most commonly affected by OA include the vertebrae, hips, knees, distal joints of the fingers, big toe and base of the thumb (Groer & Shekleton 1989) (Fig. 10.2).

AETIOLOGY

Although the exact aetiology of OA is unknown, primary or idiopathic OA is viewed as the inevitable effect of the ageing process, or a lifetime of wear and tear on the joints. The slowing of the metabolic and restorative capacity of the body tissues with ageing is also speculated to play a part. Some types of OA are hereditary, and this applies most particularly to OA of the finger joints. There are, however, four main categories of non-inherited risk factors: congenital abnormalities, trauma, overweight and obesity, and occupation (Silman & Hochberg 2001, ARC 2002) (Table 10.3). Inflammatory changes do not appear to be

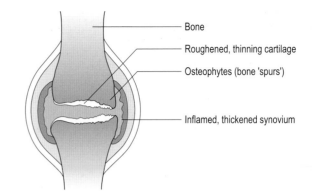

Figure 10.2 Synovial joint with osteoarthritis.

Table 10.3 Non-inherited risk factors of osteoarthritis (information from Groer & Shekleton 1989, ARC 2002)

Category	Major functions
Congenital abnormalities	OA may be late complication of congenital dislocation of the hip or hip dysplasia
Trauma	OA frequently develops in a joint that has been operated on, or previously experienced a serious injury, such as a fracture
Overweight and obesity	The strongest risk factor for developing OA of the knee. The compressive trauma to weight-bearing joints leads to cartilaginous erosion and osteolytic changes. Laxity or instability to the structural joint components also contributes to abnormal weight-bearing stresses, resulting in further cartilage damage
Occupation	OA is particularly common in the joints of those whose occupation involves the same continual repetitive movement and where there are unevenly distributed loads on the body. Particularly common in farmers and in the knees of those whose occupation involves a considerable amount of bending

significant in OA, but OA can be found in conjunction with RA, where inflammation plays a considerable part (Groer & Shekleton 1989, Gunn 1994).

Possible causes of OA have been attributed to imbalances in the catabolic and anabolic processes in the cartilage, which result in morphological changes and its destruction (Malemud & Goldberg 1999, Gibson et al 2001), as well as a degree of synovial inflammation (Fernandes et al 2002) (Fig. 10.2). Whether these are secondary to any damage, or the primary cause, thus initiating the OA process, is still not clear (Groer & Shekleton 1989). Nonetheless, this imbalance has been attributed to changes in the complex network of biochemical factors, including enhanced activity of proteolytic enzymes (enzymes that break down proteins) in OA cartilage, cytokines such as interleukin-1 (IL-1) and tumour necrosis factor (TNF)-alpha (produced by activated synoviocytes), mononuclear cells and/or the upregulation of the gene expression for metalloproteinases (MMP) by the articular cartilage itself (Fernandes et al 2002). Metalloproteinases are enzymes that catalyse metalloprotein, proteins that contain one or more metals, and have the capacity to degrade cartilage. Metalloproteinases are considered biomarkers for both physiological and pathological tissue remodelling because of their key role in articular cartilage homeostasis (Brama et al 2004). Furthermore, cytokines can blunt chondrocyte (cartilage cell) compensatory synthesis pathways, required to restore the integrity of the degraded extracellular matrix, and in the synovial fluid in OA there is a deficit in the production of natural antagonists of the IL-1 receptor. This, coupled with other factors, may contribute to the catabolic effect of IL-1 in this disease. However, certain cytokines, such as IL-10, have anti-inflammatory properties, which inhibit the synthesis of IL-1 and TNF-alpha, and are thought to be potential targets for therapy of OA (Fernandes et al 2002).

Physical activity/exercise

Considering that wear and tear and incorrect loading have been associated with OA, many have questioned whether regular participation in certain sports may actually increase the risk of developing OA. Several researchers have reviewed the literature, and taking into account animal experiments and occupational studies, there is a slight increase in risk of OA in weight-bearing joints, due to very frequent and heavy exercise over many years. However, for the less active exercisers and those participating in recreational physical activity, the risk of developing OA in normal joints does not appear to be increased (Lane 1995, Gross & Marti 1997). Several studies have compared the risk of developing OA between different sporting activities, and found certain sporting activities to produce a greater risk of OA than others. For instance, Kujala et al (1995) compared 117 former male athletes (aged 45 to 68 years) from a range of different sports with distinctly different loading conditions (28 long-distance runners, 31 soccer players, 29 weight lifters and 29 shooters). They found that soccer players had the highest percentage of tibiofemoral OA (26%), and weight lifters the highest percentage of femoropatellar OA (28%). The risk of OA of the knee was increased in those with previous knee injury, high body mass index at the age of 20 years, previous participation in heavy work, kneeling or squatting work and participation in soccer. Similar findings were also observed by Spector et al (1996) from a study carried out on 81 female former ex-elite athletes. They compared 67 middle- and long-distance runners and 14 tennis players, aged between 40 and 65 years, and found that tennis players tended to have greater risk of OA in the tibiofemoral joints and runners greater risk in the femoropatellar joints. However, when these women were compared to a group of 977 age-matched female controls, it was found that those women who were involved in weight-bearing sports activity had a 2–3-fold increase in risk of OA, as determined by radiography. Another study also compared a group of 22 former elite volleyball-players (age 34 ± 6 years) and 19 healthy untrained controls (35 ± 6 years), and found the athletes to have more radiological OA in the ankle joint compared to the controls (Gross & Marti 1999). Hootman et al (2003), however, looked at the physical activity levels of 5284 adults over a 12.8-year follow-up period, and found that the amount of walking and running was not associated with an increased risk of hip/knee OA.

TREATMENT

Treatment is aimed at dealing with the symptoms and retarding the inevitable effects of articular degeneration. Non-steroidal anti-inflammatory drugs (NSAIDs) (p. 166) are generally prescribed for pain relief, and depending on the extent of the incapacity, ambulatory aids such as walking supports, splints or braces may also be used. Other interventions involve physical therapies, such as manual therapy techniques, balance, coordination and functional retraining techniques. For those with OA of the knee-taping techniques, electrical stimulation and foot orthotics may also be used to assist in overcoming some of the barriers that make participation in PA/exercise difficult (Fitzgerald & Oatis 2004). When pain and deformity are severe, surgery may also be performed for the alteration or restoration of the articular surfaces (Groer & Shekleton 1989).

Physical activity/exercise

Regular PA/exercise is an important therapeutic intervention for all types of arthritis, as it can prevent deconditioning of the muscles, keep joints stable, improve joint function and flexibility, decrease pain, enhance aerobic fitness, improve balance and decrease risk of falls (Resnick 2001). For example, a study carried out by Kovar et al (1992) assessed the effect of an 8-week randomized controlled supervised fitness walking and patient education programme on functional status, pain and use of medication in patients with OA of the knee. At the end of the study, those assigned to the walking programme (47 patients) showed a statistically significant increase in their walking distance (18.4%) during a 6-minute walking test, and functional status, compared to the controls (45 patients). The walking group also experienced a decrease in arthritis pain and used medication less frequently. Similar results were also found by Hughes et al (2004), from a randomized controlled trial comparing the effects of a facility-based multiple component training programme, which consisted of range-of-motion, resistance training, walking and education, in 80 older adults with lower extremity OA, and a group of 70 controls. Hughes et al (2004) found that compared to the control group those in the PA/exercise group showed statistically significant increases in the 6-minute walking test (13.3%) and decreases in lower extremity stiffness and pain. Those in the PA/exercise group also showed greater post-programme home-based PA/exercise adherence (48%). Similar findings were also found in programmes looking at the effect of PA/exercise on OA of the hip (de Jong et al 2004), clearly indicating that PA/exercise may be beneficial for some individuals in the treatment of certain types of OA.

Overweight and obesity are contributors toward OA, and since weight reduction is commonly an outcome of PA/exercise programmes, this may, in part, be one of the mechanisms by which PA/exercise intervention can be effective in treating OA. Regardless of the fact that knowledge concerning the effect of PA/exercise on cartilage is still limited, it does appear that cartilage adapts to loading in a similar manner to other biological tissues, such as bone and muscle. Furthermore, whilst it seems that moderate loading is beneficial for both prevention and treatment of OA, mechanical loads that are either too high or low have been shown to decrease the proteoglycan content of the cartilage. It has been suggested that muscle weakness may be a contributor, indicating that physical inactivity as well as long-term vigorous activity may be a factor in the development of OA (Roos & Dahlberg 2004).

Although high-impact exercise may aggravate OA, most exercise interventions do not appear to produce adverse effects (Hughes et al 2004). In fact, dynamic PA/exercise, such as cycling and walking, have been shown to increase the rate of synovial blood flow in joints, which may be beneficial in inflamed joints that are chronically hypoxic (James et al 1994). Furthermore, research using horses has shown no increase in MMPs (p. 162) as a result of exercise (Brama et al 2004); and since MMPs have the capacity to degrade cartilage, this would suggest that appropriate PA/exercise is unlikely to be detrimental to those with OA.

RHEUMATOID ARTHRITIS

It is estimated that worldwide, 1 in every 100 people suffer from RA (Hartzheim & Gross 1998, Ebrahimi 1999), and in Western countries it affects 1–3% of the population. There are around 12 000 new cases of RA each year in the UK, affecting around 0.81% of the UK adult population (Symmons et al 2002). In Australia RA affects around 1.8 million people (Finocchiaro et al 1997), although RA is extremely rare amongst Australian Aboriginals (Douglas 1996, Roberts-Thompson et al 1998, Ebrahimi 1999).

Rheumatoid arthritis is found more often in women than in men, by a ratio of around 3 : 1 (Hartzheim & Gross 1998, Kumar & Clark 1998, Ebrahimi 1999), and research

indicates no increase in the incidence of RA with declining socio-economic status (Bankhead et al 1996, Ebrahimi 1999). However, RA appears to have some genetic foundations, and several generations of some families have been affected (Kumar & Clark 1998, Ebrahimi 1999).

PATHOPHYSIOLOGY

Rheumatoid arthritis is the most common of the connective tissue disorders, and presents itself with varying degrees of severity and disability (Akil & Amos 1996, Ebrahimi 1999). It is characterized by inflammation and destructive joint changes and inflammation to the tendon sheath (Fig. 10.3). The bones of affected individuals with RA also appear to have some erosion of the bone, joint deformity and a narrowed joint space, due primarily to inflammatory tissue forming over and destroying the articular hyaline cartilage (a type of connective tissue that thinly covers the articulating ends of bones), causing the joint to swell and limiting its degree of movement. Rheumatoid arthritis can affect several joints at once, the most common sites being the fingers, ankles, hips and knees (Gunn 1994) (Fig. 10.4). However, due to the inflammatory characteristic of RA many body tissues or organs may be affected (Dieppe et al 1985, Ebrahimi 1999), and people with RA often have a propensity toward respiratory and heart problems (Table 10.1).

Rheumatoid factors (RFs) also appear to play an important role in the pathophysiological process of RA. The RFs present in the majority of those with RA are antibodies of the IgG and IgM classes of gamma globulin. It is speculated that in RA, antibodies to one's own proteins may occur if their structure is altered, confusing the immune system. A configurational change might be caused by a viral infection, an abnormal metabolic reaction or a previous antigen–antibody reaction. Additionally, some bacterial antigens, such as *Streptococcus*, might be similar in structure to the human antigens, so that immunoglobulins specific to the bacterial antibodies could also attach and destroy certain human antigen-bearing cells. Furthermore, RFs themselves can provoke tissue damage, causing

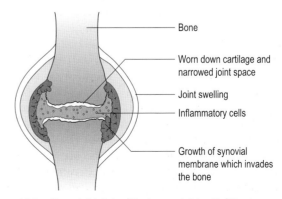

Figure 10.3 Synovial joint with rheumatoid arthritis.

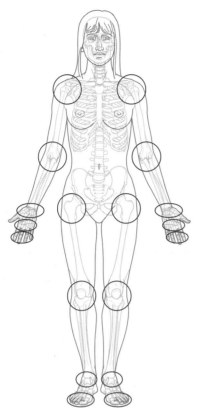

Figure 10.4 Common areas of joint pain (adapted from http://www.meritcare.com/hwdb/images/hwstd/medical/orthoped/n5 550622.jpg)

vasculitis (inflammation of the blood vessels), histamine release, and kinin activation (which can cause constriction of the visceral smooth muscle and vasodilation). Phagocytes may also be increased or decreased in response to the presence of RF, contributing toward the disease process. However, it is possible that the immune responses are only the result of the disease process of RA, rather than initiating it. Nonetheless, whatever the initial cause of RA, once the disease process is initiated it seems to be self-perpetuating (Groer & Shekleton 1989).

Synovial fluid

The synovial fluid of RA joints is also affected, and often infiltrated by lymphocytes (type of white blood cell) and plasma cells. It also demonstrates a sterile inflammation, with high neutrophil counts (white blood cells that remove and destroy bacteria, cellular debris and solid particles) and increased concentrations of proinflammatory cytokines. The plasma also shows a proinflammatory shift in T-cell populations (which stimulate other immune cells to proliferate and secrete) (Ahlqvist 1985). These cells, as well as the synovial membrane cells of the joint capsule, then release lysosomal enzymes (that cause self-digestion of the cell), which themselves act to perpetuate a chronic synovitis (inflammation of the synovial membrane of the joint), leading to eventual destruction of the articular car-

tilage, and the typical pain, stiffness and loss of function (Groer & Shekleton 1989). The immune complexes that are found within the synovial tissue are also presumably the result of high concentrations of RFs (Ahlqvist 1985), which are released into the synovium. It would therefore appear that in RA, inflammation, which normally serves a protective and self-limiting function, is a major contributor toward the RA disease process (Groer & Shekleton 1989).

AETIOLOGY

The exact cause of RA is still unknown, although it appears that immune responses play a significant part. Rheumatoid arthritis seems to arise from an autoimmune reaction by the immune system to normal body components, possibly triggered by bacterial or viral infection (Shephard & Shek 1997). It would appear that in RA some of these processes are misdirected against the body's own cells.

Immune system

The immune system is capable of recognizing and defending the body against foreign environmental or novel molecules, such as microorganisms (proteins) called immunogens. These microorganisms include viruses, bacteria, fungi and parasites, tumour growth, cell and tissue transplantation and allergens. The response of the system to any of these challenges involves a complex communication and coordination between cells, tissues and messenger molecules throughout the body (Mackinnon 1999).

The immune response in the healthy individual is generally initiated when an antigen (foreign substance that can evoke an immune response) breaks through the chemical and physical barriers protecting the body. The pathogen is usually engulfed by a phagocyte, which it then digests. The phagocyte processes the foreign protein, which then appears on the phagocyte's surface. The appearance of the foreign protein on the phagocyte's surface then stimulates the activation of T-helper lymphocytes, which subsequently stimulate other immune cells to proliferate and secrete substances that combat the microorganism. Antibodies are then produced against the foreign protein by mature B cells (Mackinnon 1999) (Table 10.4). Whilst in the healthy individual these responses are beneficial in immunity to disease and infection, for those with RA some of these reactions are part of the pathophysiology of the RA disease process, and the initiation of this immune response in RA has still to be determined.

Autoimmunity

The immune system includes two types of white blood cells, B and T cells (Table 10.4), which recognize the difference between 'self' molecules, belonging to the body, and 'non-self' molecules. Each B cell makes antibodies to one type of non-self molecule. However, it can only do so if

Table 10.4 Cells that mediate immune responses (adapted from Vander et al 1990)

Cells	Major functions
Leukocytes (white blood cells):	
Neutrophils	Phagocytosis (engulfment of particles by cell followed by the particle's digestion)
	Release chemicals involved in inflammation
Basophils	Functions similar in tissue to mast cells
	Enter tissues and transformed into mast cells
Eosinophils	Constitute 1–3% of white blood cells; they increase in number with allergy
	Destroy parasitic worms
Monocytes	In blood, similar function to macrophages in tissue
	Enter tissues and transformed into macrophages
Lymphocytes:	
B cells	Initiate antibody-mediated immune responses by binding specific antigens to their plasma-membrane receptors, which are antibodies
	During activation, are transformed into plasma cells, which secrete antibodies
T cells – cytotoxic T cells	Cell-mediated immunity, i.e. bind to antigens on plasma membrane of target cells and directly destroy the cells
Helper T cells	Secrete protein messengers (lymphokines) that activate B, cytotoxic T and NK cells and convert macrophages into effector macrophages (cells that have two distinct functions)
Suppressor T cells	Inhibit B and cytotoxic T cells
NK cells	Similar functions as cytotoxic T cells
Plasma cells	Secrete antibodies
Macrophages	Phagocytosis
	Process and present antigens to lymphocytes
	Secrete protein messengers involved in inflammation, activation of helper T cells, and systemic responses to infection or injury (the acute phase response)
Mast cells	Release histamine and other chemicals involved in inflammation

T cells recognize parts of the same non-self molecule. T cells are therefore seen as directing antibody production. Since T cells direct normal immunity, autoimmunity may start with T cells mistaking self for non-self molecules. However, autoimmunity in humans can be initiated by no obvious cause, and once initiated appears to be self-perpetuating. Furthermore, there is little evidence to suggest that anything from outside the body is fooling the T cells into confusing self and non-self molecules. Hereditary factors appear to make some individuals more at risk of this autoimmune response. Yet, even within these 'autoimmune families' there is still no way of determining those who will develop disease. This suggests that human autoimmunity may start with a chance event within the immune system, which then develops into a perpetual vicious cycle. It is believed that the chance event is the production of an autoantibody which has the very unusual ability to stimulate its own production (Edwards & Cambridge 1998).

The confusion with autoimmunity and disease is that even when autoantibodies are produced, they may in fact cause no harm. For instance, many individuals make sufficient autoantibodies to be measurable in a blood sample, and produce a positive RA autoantibody blood test, but never develop RA. Additionally, simply by becoming older we accumulate autoantibodies, which can stimulate their own production, but are harmless to tissue. Thus, in most cases, if an antibody attaches to a self-molecule, it is probably cleared away without any problems occurring. Nonetheless, certain autoantibodies are dangerous and can cause RA (Edwards & Cambridge 1998).

Autoimmunity and RA

In RA there is the perpetual cycle of antibodies against antibodies. There are five main types of antibodies; immunoglobulins (proteins that function as antibodies, and are formed in response to antigens) IgM, IgG, IgA, IgD and IgE. In RA the autoantibodies, known as rheumatoid factors (RFs), are antibodies against IgG. In RA some of the antibodies are IgG anti-IgG, i.e. they bind to themselves. These antibodies are difficult to measure and are thought to be important in the aetiology of RA. Pairs of stuck together IgG anti-IgG antibodies are dangerous because they are not cleared away. They are also small enough to pass out to the bloodstream and into the tissues. Once they have entered certain tissues they probably cause inflammation by stimulating macrophage cells (Table 10.4). They do this by binding to a receptor on the macrophage surface. Macrophages only carry this receptor in tissue affected by RA, such as the lining of the joints, the lungs and pericardial lining of the heart. Thus, inflammation from this cause only occurs in these tissues. The situation is worsened in the joints by the fact that, during inflammation, cells which make anti-IgG antibodies enter the joint lining and make autoantibodies inside the joint (Edwards & Cambridge 1998).

Endocrine system

Until relatively recently, it was considered that the endocrine system had little interaction with the system involved in immunity. However, it now appears that there are physiological interactions between the two systems. For instance, lymphocytes secrete several of the same hormones produced by endocrine glands (Vander et al 1990). Furthermore, several papers have cited abnormalities of cortisol and prolactin in RA patients (Pool & Axford 2001). Although the precise link between the immune and endocrine systems in RA has still to be determined, it appears that the endocrine system may play a role in the pathophysiology of RA.

TREATMENT

The vicious cycle that results in the production of large amounts of antibodies, and in damage to the body tissues, needs to be broken in order to slow or stop the progression of RA. Treatments are focused on breaking this cycle, by removing some of the cells that are involved (Edwards & Cambridge 1998). However, generally the major pharmacological treatment for RA is suppression of the inflammatory process with both non-steroidal anti-inflammatory agents and glucocorticoid steroids (Groer & Shekleton 1989).

Pharmacological

There are three main categories of drug therapies for those with RA, and generally sufferers are initially prescribed NSAIDs, which are used to reduce pain and joint stiffness but do not influence the underlying disease process (Capell et al 1983, Apley & Solomon 1993, Ebrahimi 1999). However, these types of medication may increase risk of ulcers or kidney damage in those with a history of stomach ulcers or kidney problems respectively (Arthritis Foundation 2004).

The second line of drug treatment is a group of drugs termed 'disease modifying anti-rheumatic drugs' (DMARDs), which directly affect immunopathological processes and can control disease progress (Apley & Solomon 1993). However, the use of these drugs has been contentious in the management of RA; whilst some researchers have found these drugs to produce unpredictable results with lethal side effects, suggesting they should therefore be reserved until all other interventions have failed, others have found DMARDs to be less toxic than some NSAIDs, and to reduce disability in the long term, suggesting that DMARDs should be used in the early stages of the disease (Ebrahimi 1999).

The third line of drug treatment involves the use of glucocorticoid steroids. These are very effective in relieving joint pain and stiffness. However, due to their adverse side effects, such as diabetes and osteoporosis, they are commonly reserved for when the condition is severe and incapacitating (Ebrahimi 1999). Glucocorticoid steroids increase the vasomotor activity of the vascular bed, so that capillary dilation is decreased and sensitivity to adrenaline-induced vasoconstriction is increased. These effects would oppose the normal increases in vascular supply and permeability during inflammation. Corticosteroids also alter the permeability characteristics of blood vessels directly. Inflammatory oedema and tissue swelling are therefore decreased by the administration of these drugs. Corticosteroids also inhibit certain types of white blood cells (polymorphonuclear chemotaxis, such as eosinophils, basophils or neutrophils, also known as granulocytes; Table 10.4) and decrease granulocyte adherence and fibroblast proliferation, collagen production and blood vessel growth at the inflamed site (Groer & Shekleton 1989).

Rest

Rest is frequently suggested as one of the most effective methods for reducing joint swelling and pain (Capell et al 1983, Apley & Solomon 1993). During flare-ups of RA symptoms, bed rest of around 2 to 3 weeks may settle acute inflammation (Apley & Solomon 1993). However, once these acute symptoms have settled, gentle mobilization may be introduced (Capell et al 1983).

Physical activity/exercise

In the healthy individual the synovial cavity has a negative pressure, and when the joint is exercised vascular patency is maintained. This allows for nutrition of the articular cartilage, which does not possess any blood vessels of its own. In RA the cavity pressure is higher than normal, and upon movement this pressure exceeds the capillary perfusion pressure, resulting in collapse of the blood vessels. This leads to what is termed 'hypoxic-reperfusion injury', which produces reactive oxygen species, and these may result in further damage within the synovial cavity. The reactive oxygen species may cause an increase in RFs (p. 163), alterations in immune function, and alterations in T cell/macrophage interactions (Mapp et al 1995). It might therefore be thought that any PA/exercise would be harmful or cause a progression in the disease. However, research into the effect of PA/exercise on RA has failed to show that appropriate PA/exercise accelerates the disease. Indeed, in most cases PA/exercise programmes have been shown to be of benefit to the RA sufferer. For instance, research has shown that dynamic PA/exercise can increase the rate of synovial blood flow in joints with effusions, possibly benefiting inflamed joints that are chronically hypoxic due to the elevated intra-articular pressure and chronic synovial ischaemia (James et al 1994).

Immune response to physical activity/exercise

Healthy individuals who regularly perform moderate PA/exercise tend to show little change in their pre-PA/exercise immune parameters. During and following PA/exercise there is a rise in proinflammatory cytokines IL-1, IL-6 and TNF-alpha (Haahr et al 1991), which is thought to be in response to micromuscular damage caused by the PA/exercise (Hoffman & Pedersen 1994), but these tend to return to pre-PA/exercise levels after the cessation of PA/exercise. Similarly, regular PA/exercise appears to have little effect on the resting immune state of RA sufferers. For example, a study carried out by Baslund et al (1993) on 18 RA patients found that after 8 weeks of cycle training, although aerobic capacity was significantly improved, resting levels of immune parameters did not significantly change. It therefore appears that whilst the immune system seems to respond during a bout of PA/exercise, these changes appear to return to pre-PA/exercise once the PA/exercise has ceased. Conversely, however, athletes who undergo long-term repetitive high-intensity training, such as marathon runners, tend to have lower than normal resting levels of immunoglobulins and circulating lymphocytes (Green et al 1981) and reduced lymphocyte responsiveness (Eskola et al 1978, Sharp & Koutedakis 1992, Pool & Axford 2001) (Table 10.4), suggesting that they may be more prone to infection.

Types of physical activity/exercise

Until relatively recently, dynamic PA/exercise was considered to be harmful to those suffering from RA. It was thought that dynamic PA/exercise would cause further damage to affected joints. However, this notion has now been dispelled (Pool & Axford 2001). For instance, Lyngberg et al (1988) employed a controlled cross-over designed study, using 18 RA patients. They looked at the effect of graduated progressive aerobic exercise and progressive strength training (twice a week for 8 weeks) on the increased activity of RA. The researchers found that although there was no change in the need for RA medication, training of the muscles acting over the swollen joint led to more than a 35% decrease in the number of swollen joints. Additionally, Nordemar et al (1981) found that after 4 to 8 weeks of home-based physical training, 23 RA patients showed a significant reduction in the progression of X-ray changes in the joints when compared to the control group. Furthermore, feelings of weakness were also more pronounced in the control group, who also experienced more discomfort from joints after physical exertion when compared to the active group (Nordemar 1981). Several researchers have reported

similar findings from interventions using dynamic PA/exercise (Van den Ende et al 1998), demonstrating the benefit of appropriate PA/exercise.

It is expected that dynamic exercise may be superior at improving aerobic capacity (Van den Ende et al 1996) than other types of PA/exercise. It also appears that dynamic PA/exercise may be more effective in increasing joint mobility and muscle strength (Stenstrom 1994). For instance, Van den Ende et al (1996) randomly assigned 100 RA patients either into a group who carried out full weight-bearing and cycle ergometry at 70–85% of maximum heart rate or into individual or home-based programmes of range-of-motion and isometric exercises, for a period of 12 weeks. The results showed that the dynamic training was more effective at increasing joint mobility, muscle strength and aerobic capacity than the other programmes.

Whilst studies demonstrate the beneficial effect of PA/exercise upon factors such as aerobic capacity, muscle strength and range-of-motion, PA/exercise may have little effect on markers of the disease. For example, Hansen et al (1993) found that a long-term (2-year) randomized trial involving 75 RA patients and using different training programmes had no effect on the disease activity or on the progression of the disease, though no detrimental effects were reported either.

It therefore appears that certain RA sufferers do appear to respond to training, without aggravating the disease, and although there is still a risk of overuse of RA-affected joints, it is now believed that, because of the other physiological and psychological benefits of PA/exercise, it is probably better to be overactive rather than the reverse (Nordemar et al 1981, Ettinger 1998).

PRE-PHYSICAL ACTIVITY/EXERCISE PRESCRIPTION FOR BOTH OA AND RA

All sufferers of OA and RA should be appropriately screened and assessed prior to any PA/exercise programme (Appendix A). Particular problem areas should be clearly identified to avoid incorrect PA/exercise prescription. Since the large majority of OA sufferers are likely to be elderly, they are also likely to have age-related co-morbidities, which need to be identified and accounted for within the PA/exercise programme.

PHYSICAL ACTIVITY/EXERCISE PRESCRIPTION

It is clear that with appropriate PA/exercise prescription, those suffering from OA and RA can safely participate in PA/exercise programmes (Ettinger 1998) and it has been recommended that a comprehensive PA/exercise programme should include stretching exercises followed by a range-of-motion programme for joints, muscle strength-

Table 10.5   Physical activity/exercise guidelines and considerations for those with arthritis (adapted from Roberts et al 1997)

Low-impact activities should be employed
PA/exercise should be of low to moderate intensity
PA/exercise sessions should be frequent
Reduce intensity and duration of sessions during periods of inflammation or pain
Modify intensity and duration according to the patient's PA/exercise responses, medication and disease and pain levels
If client/patient complains of pain during or following PA/exercise, suggest a couple of days' rest; if this persists client/patient should consult their general practitioner
Vary the type of dynamic PA/exercise
Enforce correct body alignment, as poor posture can predispose a client/patient to muscle pains, which may limit the type of PA/exercise they can perform
Since pain is quite normal in arthritis sufferers, they should be instructed to work just up to the point of pain, but not past it
If dynamic movements are too difficult, isometric exercises may be encouraged, as long as co-morbidities, such as hypertension, are not contraindicative
Encourage a daily routine incorporating a complete range of motion for all joints
Incorporate regular rest periods within a PA/exercise session
Consider other co-morbidities and accommodate accordingly

ening and aerobic exercise (Resnick 2001). Although knowledge regarding the optimal type, frequency, duration and intensity for those with OA and RA is still limited, there are certain PA/exercise guidelines that may assist in prescribing PA/exercise (Table 10.5).

Long-term compliance is important in achieving long-term benefits, and supervised classes appear to be as effective as treatments provided on a one-to-one basis. Thus, group-based exercise programmes not only provide a cost-effective alternative, but may also be more effective in general, especially since adherence to home-based programmes also appears to be lower (Kettunen & Kujala 2004).

FREQUENCY

It is important to maintain joint mobility. Therefore, all joints should be put through a full range of motion on a daily basis. Additionally, PA/exercise sessions should be frequent. However, if there is pain and inflammation a few days' rest may be required (Roberts et al 1997).

INTENSITY

The intensity of PA/exercise prescribed should be based on an individual's pain tolerance and physical capacity, with low- to moderate-intensity PA/exercise being preferred (Roberts et al 1997). High-impact loads or activities that have a high risk of injury (Kettunen & Kujala 2004) and quick and excessive movements should be avoided (Roberts et al 1997).

DURATION

The duration of a PA/exercise will depend upon the needs and physical status of the client/patient. However, initial sessions may start at around 10 to 15 minutes and gradually increase in duration (Roberts et al 1997).

TYPES OF PHYSICAL ACTIVITY/EXERCISE

In order to reduce joint stress, non-weight-bearing activities such as swimming and cycling are preferred (Roberts et al 1997). Particularly for those with RA, dynamic PA/exercise has been found to be more effective than other forms of PA/exercise (Stenstrom 1994, Van den Ende et al 1996). Dynamic PA/exercise such as cycling and walking has also been shown to increase the rate of synovial blood flow in joints, which may be beneficial to inflamed joints (James et al 1994).

Resistance training

For those with OA of the knee, progressive resistance exercises have been shown to be as effective as dynamic PA/exercise in producing improvements to the severity of disease, pain and walking time (Eyigor et al 2004).

Water-based activities

Water-based PA/exercise is recommended not only because it avoids quick movement, which is not recommended for those with arthritis (Roberts et al 1997), but also because it supports body weight and in warm water may help reduce pain. Additionally, it has been shown to be a good form of therapy for improving the strength of those with RA. For example, Danneskiold-Samsoe et al (1987) found that for eight RA sufferers, 8 weeks of a water-based PA/exercise programme, in a heated pool, resulted in a significant 38% improvement in isometric strength and 16% improvement in maximal isokinetic strength of the quadriceps. All patients showed improvement in aerobic capacity.

WARMING UP AND COOLING DOWN

Warming up before the PA/exercise session is an important part of most individuals' PA/exercise programme; and for those with arthritis there are other pre-PA/exercise interventions that may assist the arthritic individual during the PA/exercise session. For example, the Arthritis Foundation (2004) recommends that before structured exercise, heat or ice treatments should be applied to the area being exercised. The rationale behind this is that heat relaxes the joints and muscles and helps to relieve pain. Cold on the other hand can, for some individuals, reduce pain and swelling.

Those with arthritis also require an extended warm-up lasting at least 10 to 15 minutes. The warm-up should include gentle 'range-of-motion' and strength exercises before the aerobic/dynamic type activities. The cool-down should last around 10 minutes, and should incorporate gentle stretching (Arthritis Foundation 2004).

CONSIDERATIONS AND CONTRAINDICATIONS

Although it is clear that PA/exercise can be of great benefit to those with OA and RA, PA/exercise programmes should not include high-impact loads or activities that carry a high risk of injury (Kettunen & Kujala 2004), or quick and excessive movements (Roberts et al 1997). It is also important to balance rest with activity and passive PA/exercise (Apley & Soloman 1993), and during acute arthritic flare-ups PA/exercise should be avoided altogether (Roberts et al 1997) (Table 10.5).

In some individuals with OA of the knee, the quadriceps appears to have some impaired proprioception, particularly when the knee is in more extended positions. This results in a reduction in ability to accurately and steadily control submaximal force, and eccentric strength. Hence, this should be considered when designing PA/exercise and rehabilitation programmes (Hortobagyi et al 2004).

Absolute contraindications

The absolute contraindications for exercise will be similar to those set out for other individuals (Appendix A, Table A.1), in addition to those limitations imposed by the OA and RA.

Medication

Although there is very little research regarding the effect of medications for the treatment of arthritis upon PA/exercise ability, certain medications may have an influence (Ch. 14, p. 230).

SUMMARY

- There are over 200 types of arthritis, and it is one of the leading causes of disability in Western society, affecting people of all ages, especially older individuals.
- The most common forms of arthritis are osteoarthritis (OA) and rheumatoid arthritis (RA).

Osteoarthritis

- OA is the most common form and is termed degenerative joint disease. The exact aetiology is unknown, but it is viewed as the inevitable effect of the ageing process.
- OA is characterized by degenerative alterations of the hyaline cartilage and hypertrophic changes in the articular bone ends (Fig. 10.2).
- Treatment is aimed at dealing with the symptoms and retarding the inevitable effects of articular degeneration.

Rheumatoid arthritis

- RA is found more often in women than in men.
- The exact cause of RA is still unknown, though it appears to arise from an autoimmune reaction by the immune system to normal body components, possibly triggered by bacterial or viral infection.
- RA is characterized by inflammation and destructive joint changes and inflammation to the tendon sheath, with some erosion of the bone, joint deformity and a narrowed joint space. It is primarily due to inflam-

matory tissue forming over and destroying the articular hyaline cartilage, causing the joint to swell and limiting the degree of movement (Fig. 10.3).
- RA can affect several joints at once (Fig. 10.4) and due to the inflammatory characteristics of RA many body tissues and/or organs may be affected (see Table 10.1).
- There are three main categories of drug therapies: NSAIDs, DMARDs and glucocorticoid steroids.
- Rest is frequently suggested as one of the most effective methods for reducing joint swelling and pain during a flare-up.

Physical activity/exercise for OA and RA sufferers

- Regular PA/exercise is now an important therapeutic intervention for all types of arthritis, as it can:
  prevent deconditioning of the muscles
  keep joints stable
  ↑ joint function and flexibility
  ↓ pain
  ↑ aerobic fitness
  ↑ balance
  ↓ risk of falls.
- PA/exercise has little effect on disease markers of RA.
- Particular problem areas should be clearly identified prior to PA/exercise prescription. Since the large majority of OA sufferers are elderly, age-related co-morbidities need to be accounted for.

SUMMARY—*continued*

- Knowledge about the optimal type, frequency, duration and PA/exercise intensity for those with OA and RA is still limited. Nonetheless, certain PA/exercise guidelines may assist in the prescribing of PA/exercise (Table 10.5).
- A comprehensive PA/exercise programme should include stretching exercises followed by a range-of-motion programme for joints, muscle strengthening and aerobic exercise, carried out on a daily basis.
- Appropriate resistance training has been shown to be especially useful for those with OA of the knee, and dynamic PA/exercise is useful for RA sufferers. Water-based activities and activities that support body weight are also recommended.
- PA/exercise sessions should be preceded and followed by an adequate warm-up and cool-down.
- High-impact and vigorous PA/exercise is not recommended for either OA or RA.

Suggested readings, references and bibliography

Ahlqvist J 1985 On the structural and physiological basis of the influence of exercise, movement and immobilisation in inflammatory joint diseases. Annales Chirurgiae et Gynaecologiae 198:S10–S18

Akil M, Amos R S 1996 Rheumatoid arthritis: clinical features and diagnosis. In: Snaith M L (ed) ABC of rheumatology. BMJ Publishing, London

Anderson D M, Keith J, Novak P D et al (eds) 2002 Mosby's medical, nursing and allied health dictionary, 6th edn. Mosby, St Louis

Apley A G, Solomon L 1993 Apley's system of orthopaedics and fractures, 7th edn. Butterworth-Heinemann, Oxford

ARC (Arthritis Research Campaign) 2002 Arthritis the big picture. Online. Available: http://www.arc.org.uk/about _arth/default.htm September 2004

Arthritis Foundation 2004 Exercise and your arthritis. Online. Available: http://www.arthritis.org September 2004

Bankhead G, Silman A, Barret B et al 1996 Incidence of rheumatoid arthritis is not related to indicators of socio-economic deprivation. Journal of Rheumatology 23(12):2039–2042

Baslund B, Lyngberg K, Andersen V et al 1993 Effect of 8 weeks of bicycle training on the immune system of patients with rheumatoid arthritis. Journal of Applied Physiology 75(4):1691–1695

Brama P A, van den Boom R, DeGroott J et al 2004 Collagenase-1 (MMP-1) activity in equine synovial fluid: influence of age, joint pathology, exercise and repeated arthrocentesis. Equine Veterinary Journal 36(1):34–40

Capell H A, Daymond T J, Dick W C 1983 Rheumatic disease. Springer-Verlag, Berlin

CDC (Centers for Disease Control and Prevention) 1996 Prevalence and impact of arthritis by race and ethnicity – United States, 1989–1991. Morbidity and Mortality Weekly Report 45(18):373–378

Danneskiold-Samsoe B, Lyngberg K, Risum T et al 1987 The effect of water exercise therapy given to patients with rheumatoid arthritis. Scandinavian Journal of Rehabilitation Medicine 19(1):31–35

de Jong O R, Hopman-Rock M, Tak E C et al 2004 An implementation study of two evidence-based exercise and health education programmes for older adults with osteoarthritis of the knee and hip. Health Education Research 19(3):316–325

Dieppe P A, Doherty M, Macfarlane G M et al 1985 Rheumatological medicine. Churchill Livingstone, Edinburgh

Douglas W A 1996 Does rheumatoid arthritis exist in the indigenous Australian Aboriginal population? Medical Journal of Australia 164:191–192

Ebrahimi S 1999 Rheumatoid arthritis. Online. Available: http://www.podiatry.curtin.edu.au/encyclopedia/rheumatoid_arthritis/Oct 2004

Edwards J, Cambridge J 1998 Rheumatoid arthritis and autoimmunity: A new approach to their cause and how long term cure might be achieved. Online. Available: http://www.ucl.ac.uk. October 2004

Eskola J, Ruuskanen O, Soppi E et al 1978 Effect of sport stress on lymphocyte transformation and antibody formation. Clinical and Experimental Immunology 32:339–345

Ettinger W H Jr 1998 Physical activity, arthritis and disability in older people. Clinics in Geriatric Medicine 14(3):633–640

Eyigor S, Hepguler S, Capaci K 2004 A comparison of muscle training methods in patients with knee osteoarthritis. Clinical Rheumatology 23(2):109–115

Fernandes J C, Martel-Pelletier J, Pelletier P 2002 The role of cytokines in osteoarthritis physiology. Biorheology 39(1–2):237–246

Finocchiaro M, Abramson M J, Ryan P F 1997 Arthritis in Australian Aboriginal population? Medical Journal of Australia 166:352

Fitzgerald G K, Oatis C 2004 Role of physical therapy in management of knee osteoarthritis. Current Opinion in Rheumatology 16(2):143–147

Gibson G J, Verner J J, Nelson F R et al 2001 Degradation of the cartilage collagen matrix associated with changes in chondrocytes in osteoarthrosis. Journal of Orthopaedic Research 19(1):33–42

Green R L, Kaplan S S, Rabin B S et al 1981 Immune function in marathon runners. Annals of Allergy 47:73–75

Groer M W, Shekleton M E 1989 Basic pathophysiology: a holistic approach, 3rd edn. Mosby, St Louis

Gross P, Marti B 1997 Sports activity and risk of arthrosis. Schweizerische Medizinische Wochenschrift. Journal Suisse de Medecine 127(23):967–977

Gross P, Marti B 1999 Risk of degenerative ankle joint disease in volleyball players: study of former elite athletes. International Journal of Sports Medicine 20(1):58–63

Gunn C 1994 Bones and joints: a guide for students. Churchill Livingstone, New York

Haahr P M, Pedersen B K, Fomsgaard A et al 1991 Effect of physical exercise on in vitro production on interleukin 1, interleukin 6, tumour necrosis factor-alpha, interleukin 2 and interferon-gamma. International Journal of Sports Medicine 12:223–227

Hansen T M, Hansen G, Langgaard A M et al 1993 Longterm physical training in rheumatoid arthritis. A randomized trial with different training programs and blinded observers. Scandinavian Journal of Rheumatology 22(3):107–112

Hartzheim L A, Gross G L 1998 Rheumatoid arthritis: a case study. Nursing Clinics of North America 33(4):595–602

Hoffman G L, Pedersen B K 1994 Exercise and the immune system: a model of the stress response? Immunology Today 15:382–387

Hootman J M, Macea C A, Helmick C G et al 2003 Influence of physical activity-related joint stress on the risk of self-reported hip/knee osteoarthritis: a new method to quantify physical activity. Preventative Medicine 36(5):636–644

Hortobagyi T, Garry J, Holbert D, Devita P 2004 Aberrations in the control of quadriceps muscle force in patients with knee osteoarthritis. Arthritis and Rheumatism 51(4):562–569

Hughes S L, Seymour R B, Campbell R et al 2004 Impact of the fit and strong intervention on older adults with osteoarthritis. Gerontologist 44(2):217–228

James M J, Cleland L G, Gaffney R D et al 1994 Effect of exercise on 99m Tc-DTPA clearance from knees with effusions. Journal of Rheumatology 21(3):501–504

Kettunen J A, Kujala U M 2004 Exercise therapy for people with rheumatoid arthritis and osteoarthritis. Scandinavian Journal of Medicine and Science in Sports 14(3):138–142

Kovar P A, Allegrante J P, MacKenzie C R et al 1992 Supervised fitness walking in patients with osteoarthritis of the knee. A randomised, controlled trial. Annals of Internal Medicine 116(7):529–534

Kujala U M, Kettunen J, Paananen H et al 1995 Knee osteoarthritis in former runners, soccer players, weight lifters and shooters. Arthritis and Rheumatism 38(4):539–546

Kumar P, Clark M 1998 Clinical medicine, 4th edn. W B Saunders, Edinburgh

Kvalvik A 1996 Mortality in rheumatoid arthritis. Rheumatology Europe 25:9–14

Lane N E 1995 Exercise: a cause of osteoarthritis. Journal of Rheumatology 43:S3–S6

Lyngberg K, Danneskiold-Samsoe B, Halskov O 1988 The effect of physical training on patients with rheumatoid arthritis: changes in disease activity, muscle strength and aerobic capacity. A critically controlled minimised cross-over study. Clinical and Experimental Rheumatology 6(3):253–260

Mackinnon L T 1999 Advances in exercise immunology. Human Kinetics, Champaign, IL

Malemud C J, Goldberg V M 1999 Future directions for research and treatment of osteoarthritis. Frontier in Bioscience 4:D762–D771

Mapp P I, Grootveld M C, Blake D R 1995 Hypoxia, oxidative stress and rheumatoid arthritis. British Medical Bulletin 51(2):419–436

March L M, Bagga H 2004 Epidemiology of osteoarthritis in Australia. Medical Journal of Australia 180(5 suppl):S6–S10

NIAMS (National Institute of Arthritis and Musculoskeletal and Skin Diseases) 1998 Arthritis prevalence rising as baby boomers grow older, osteoarthritis second only to chronic heart disease in worksite disability. Online. Available: http://www.medscape.com/govmt/NIAMS/1998/05.98/NIAMS July 2001

Nordemar R 1981 Physical training in rheumatoid arthritis: a controlled long-term study II. Functional capacity and general attitudes. Scandinavian Journal of Rheumatology 10(1):25–30

Nordemar R, Ekblom B, Zachrisson L et al 1981 Physical training in rheumatoid arthritis: I. A controlled long-term study. Scandinavian Journal of Rheumatology 10(1):17–23

Pool A J, Axford J S 2001 The effects of exercise on the hormonal and immune systems in rheumatoid arthritis. Rheumatology 40:610–614

Resnick B 2001 Managing arthritis with exercise. Geriatric Nursing 22(3):143–150

Roberts S O, Robergs R A, Hanson P 1997 Clinical exercise testing and prescription. CRC Press, Boca Raton, FL

Roberts-Thompson P J, Hedger S, Bossingham D 1998 Rheumatoid arthritis and Australian Aboriginals. Medical Journal of Australia 165:92

Roos E M, Dahlberg L 2004 Physical activity as medication against arthrosis: training has a positive effect on the cartilage. Lakartidningen 10(25):2178–2181

Sharp N C, Koutedakis Y 1992 Sport and overtraining syndrome: immunological aspects. British Medical Bulletin 48:518–533

Shephard R J, Shek P N 1997 Autoimmune disorders, physical activity, and training, with particular reference to rheumatoid arthritis. Exercise Immunology Review 3:53–67

Silman A, Hochberg M C 2001 Epidemiology of the rheumatic diseases, 2nd edn. Oxford Medical Publications, Oxford

Spector T D, Harris P A, Hart D J et al 1996 Risk of osteoarthritis associated with long-term weight-bearing sports: a radiologic survey of the hips and knees in female ex-athletes and population controls. Arthritis and Rheumatism 39(6):988–995

Stenstrom C H 1994 Therapeutic exercise in rheumatoid arthritis. Arthritis Care and Research 7(4):190–197

Symmons D P M, Barrett F M, Bankhead C R et al 2002 The incidence of rheumatoid arthritis in the United Kingdom. British Journal of Rheumatology 33(8):735–739

Van den Ende C H, Hazes J M, le Cessie S et al 1996 Comparison of high and low intensity training in well controlled rheumatoid arthritis. Results of randomised clinical trial. Annals of the Rheumatic Diseases 55(11):798–505

Van den Ende C H, Vilet Vlieland T P, Munneke M et al 1998 Dynamic exercise therapy in rheumatoid arthritis: a systematic review. British Journal of Rheumatology 37(6):677–687

Vander A J, Sherman J H, Luciano D S 1990 Human physiology, 5th edn. McGraw-Hill, New York

Chapter 11

Adults with osteoporosis

CHAPTER CONTENTS

Introduction 173
Prevalence 173
Pathology 174
Bone structure 174
    Remodelling 175
Peak bone mineral density 176
    Physical activity/exercise during puberty 177
Classification 177
Assessment 177
Aetiology 178
    Gender 178
    Body weight 178
    Age 178
    Genetics 179
    Sex hormones 179
    Calcium levels 179
        Calcium and physical activity/exercise 180
    Vitamin D levels 180
    Medications 180
    Physical activity levels 180
    Smoking 181
    Alcohol 181
Prevention 181
Treatment 182
    Pharmacological 182
        Parathyroid hormone and vitamin D 182
        Bisphosphonates 182
        Calcitonin 182
        Oestrogen 182
        Selective oestrogen-receptor modulators 182
    Non-pharmacological 182
        Physical activity/exercise 182
        Falls prevention 183
Pre-physical activity/exercise prescription 183
Physical activity/exercise prescription 183
Single versus habitual physical activity/exercise 183

Physical activity/exercise intensity and impact 184
Duration and frequency of physical activity/exercise 184
Type of physical activity/exercise 184
    Aerobic activities 184
    Resistance training 185
    Chair-based exercise 185
Considerations and contraindications 185
    Absolute contraindications for physical activity/exercise 186
    Medications 186
Summary 186
Suggested readings, references and bibliography 186

INTRODUCTION

Osteoporosis can strike at any age, however, the risk rises with age, and since there is an increasingly aged population (p. 178) this chapter will primarily focus on adults suffering from this condition. However, some of the causes for osteoporosis may stem from childhood and adolescent lifestyle. Therefore, these factors will also be briefly addressed.

PREVALENCE

Osteoporosis is an increasing health care concern, and is a substantial cause of morbidity and mortality, as populations age throughout most of the developed world (Center & Eisman 1997). In the year 2000 osteoporosis was reported to be a health risk to around 28 million Americans, 80% of whom were women. Osteoporosis is annually responsible for more than 1.8 million fractures in the USA, approximately 300 000 of which will be fractures of the hip, and about 30–35% of these individuals will die within a year of their hip fracture (NIH ORBD-NRC 2000).

The social and economic costs of osteoporosis are mainly due to its clinical outcome of fracture, which increases exponentially with age (Center & Eisman 1997), in the USA contributing each day to around $38 million of national expenditure in hospitals and nursing homes (NIH ORBD-NRC 2000). Additionally, each day in 2001, around 177 Australians were hospitalized with osteoporotic fractures, amounting to indirect costs estimated at $5.57 million Australian dollars (between 2000 and 2001) (Osteoporosis Australia 2005). It is thus clear that osteoporosis is indeed both a significant economic and health problem to many societies.

PATHOLOGY

Osteoporosis is a systemic skeletal disease characterized by low bone mass and deterioration of the bone tissue micro-architecture, which leads to low bone density and an increase in bone fragility and susceptibility to fracture (NIH ORBD-NRC 2000) (Fig. 11.1a, b).

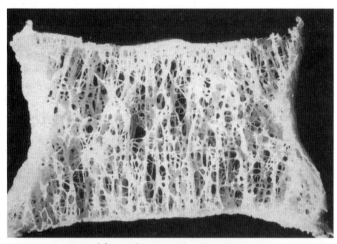

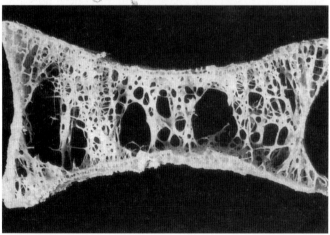

Figure 11.1 (a) Cross-section of normal bone. (b) Cross-section of osteoporotic bone. (From the International Osteoporosis Foundation website, http://www.osteofound.org/press_centre/bone_image.html, with permission.)

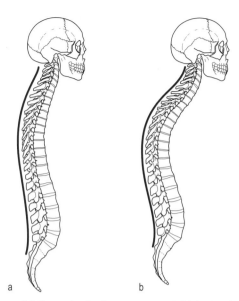

Figure 11.2 (a) Normal spinal curvature and (b) kyphosis of the spine due to osteoporosis.

Osteoporosis is often called a 'silent disease', since bone loss occurs without symptoms. An individual, for instance, may be unaware that they have the condition until they have a break, sometimes caused by as little as a sudden strain or bump. Signs of osteoporosis of the spine may be indicated by collapsed vertebrae, which can be felt or presented in the form of severe back pain, loss of height or spinal deformities, such as kyphosis (stooped posture) (Fig. 11.2) (NIH ORBD-NRC 2000).

BONE STRUCTURE

Bone is a rigid, non-elastic tissue and the bone matrix is mainly composed of calcium hydroxyapatite crystals. Hydroxyapatite is an inorganic compound composed of calcium, phosphate and hydroxide and in a crystallized lattice-like form gives the bone its structural rigidity (Groer & Shekleton 1989) (Fig. 11.1a). There are basically three types of cells that contribute toward bone homeostasis (osteoblasts which are bone-forming cells, osteoclasts that resorb or break down bone, and osteocytes which are mature bone cells), and two types of bone tissue, compact and spongy, so called to imply their different densities. The microstructure of bone consists of cells, osteocytes and a mineralized matrix that forms a complex array of the central structure of cortical bone and longitudinal miniature canals in the bone tissue (haversian canals) (Anderson et al 2002) (Fig. 11.3). Compact bone is often referred to as cortical bone and constitutes 80% of skeletal mass and is dense with comparatively narrow haversian canals (Fig. 11.4), which are penetrated by blood vessels, around which the osteocytes are regularly arranged. It forms the surface layer of all bones and the

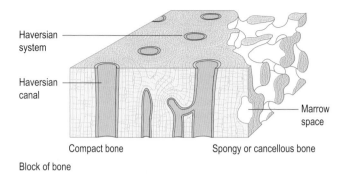

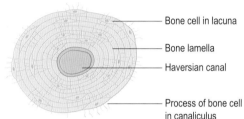

Figure 11.3 Basic structure of compact and spongy (cancellous) bone (adapted from Rowett 1990).

Figure 11.4 Transverse section of compact bone, showing a single haversian system.

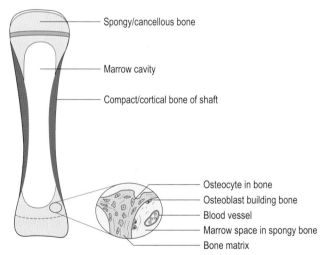

Figure 11.5 Basic structure of long bone, showing section of cancellous bone (adapted from Rowett 1990).

whole of the tubular shaft of long bones. Spongy bone may also be referred to as cancellous or trabecular bone, and is found inside cortical bone and has irregular spaces filled with red bone marrow (Rowett 1990) (Fig. 11.5). The cancellous bone makes up about 70% of the volume of the central skeleton. It consists of a honeycomb of vertical and horizontal bars called trabeculae, which are filled with varying amounts of marrow and fat. Even though remodelling is fairly similar for compact/cortical and cancellous/trabecular bone, the greater increased surface area in cancellous trabecular bone accounts for the fact that

changes in bone mass, in response to altered turnover, are generally earlier and more impressive in the cancellous/trabecular skeleton (Marcus 1987, Snow-Harter & Marcus 1991).

REMODELLING

Bone is an extremely active and dynamic tissue and is constantly undergoing remodelling according to the stresses put on it, so as to serve its major function, which is that of support (Groer & Shekleton 1989). It has been shown that the rate of bone reinforcement in an area of compressive stress concentration is much higher than the rate of bone resorption in an area of existing tension (Firoozbakhsh & Aleyaasin 1989), indicating the importance of compressive stress in the mechanisms involved in the adaptation of bone. However, research looking into the effect of both compressive and tensile force on bone mineral density (BMD) has found both to have an influence (Mayoux-Benhamou et al 1999). Muscle contraction, for example, has been found to be effective at enhancing BMD (Flodgren et al 1999), although not as effective as impact forces (Pettersson et al 1999). The frequency imposed by the impact forces may also have an influence on bone remodelling. For instance, systemic and local vibrations have been found to cause a reduction in BMD (Verbovoi 2001), conversely however, non-physiological mechanical stimulation in the form of low-intensity vibration (frequency 50 Hz, 30 minutes per day for 5 days per week), has also been shown to prevent early bone loss in postmenopausal rats. Indeed, Flieger et al (1998) observed that vibrated rats displayed statistically significantly higher BMD values compared to the rat controls, suggesting the frequency of the impact to be an important factor.

At various sites throughout the skeleton, microscopic areas of bone are being resorbed to be replaced by the formation and deposition of new bone. Both central hormonal (involving oestrogen production) and local mechanisms (such as mechanical forces of gravity and muscle contraction), which are closely related to physical activity patterns, are involved in this process (Kemper 2000) and play a critical role in calcium metabolism (Raisz & Kream 1983), though other factors may also influence the deposition and formation of bone (Table 11.1). Normally a steady state of deposition and resorption exists, thereby maintaining calcium metabolism and skeletal mass. However, this may be affected if there is disruption in this steady state. In the adult, when the normal ratio of resorption to formation is balanced and maintained, the skeletal mass will remain constant. If the ratio is altered in favour of resorption then loss of bone mass will occur (Groer & Shekleton 1989). Conversely, bone hypertrophy occurs when stress is applied in excess of normal levels. Osteoblasts then exceed osteoclastic resorption, which leads to a net gain in bone (Table 11.2).

Table 11.1   Factors that can influence bone resorption and deposition (adapted from Groer & Shekleton 1989)

	Increase	Decrease
Deposition	Physical activity/exercise, stress on bone Growth hormone Vitamin C Thyroid hormone Insulin Androgens Vitamin D metabolites Parathyroid hormone	Immobilization, disuse, bed rest Growth hormone deficiency Excess adrenocortical steroid Anticonvulsant medications
Resorption	Parathyroid hormone excess Vitamin D hormone Excess vitamin A Andrenocortical steroid excess Calcium deficiency Phosphorus deficiency Anabolic steroid deficiency Immobilization Acidosis Heparin Pregnancy and lactation Osteolytic neoplasms (including leukaemia) Prostaglandins (especially PGE_2)	Calcium Phosphorus Parathyroid hormone deficiency Calcitonin Magnesium deficiency Anabolic steroids Alkalosis Medications (mithramycin, bisphosphonates, colchicine)

Table 11.2   Types of bone cells

Bone cells	Function
Osteocytes	Mature bone cells Maintain normal bone structure by recycling calcium salts in the bony matrix Assist in repair
Osteoclasts	Large cells Their activity is influenced by parathyroid hormone, and is one mechanism by which calcium is removed from bone Acids secreted by osteoclasts dissolve the bony structure and release the stored minerals Help to regulate calcium and phosphate concentrations in body fluids
Osteoblasts	Responsible for production of new bone (osteogenesis)

Calcium is important in bone remodelling and a proportion of calcium in bone is exchangeable in the blood, and this exchangeable calcium pool is influenced by the activity of the hormone calcitonin, and the parathyroid hormone. Calcitonin is produced by the thyroid and is involved in the regulation of blood calcium levels and stimulates bone mineralization. It acts to reduce the blood levels of calcium and to inhibit bone resorption, whereas the parathyroid hormone acts to increase blood calcium levels and bone resorption (Anderson et al 2002).

This exchangeable pool of calcium, however, diminishes with age, and is, in part, why as we grow older bone becomes demineralized or less dense. Increasing demineralization with age causes the bone to become more brittle and prone to fracture when stressed (Groer & Shekleton 1989).

PEAK BONE MINERAL DENSITY

Peak BMD achieved early in adulthood determines the risk for pathological fractures and osteoporosis later in life (Sheth 2004). Around 90–95% of peak BMD is achieved during childhood and adolescent growth, predominantly due to the role of sex hormones (p. 179), and the other 5–10% during consolidation after this growth. Thus, increasing BMD in these early years may help to prevent or retard the onset of osteoporosis in later life (Bass et al 1998). Therefore, identifying the age when peak bone density is attained is essential in the development of strategies aimed at optimizing peak BMD. A study carried out on 274 healthy females aged between 11 and 32 years found that 95% of peak BMD was attained at 22.1 ± 2.5 years and by 26.2 ± 3.7 years 99% of peak BMD was attained (Teegarden et al 1995). However, peak BMD may be achieved at different stages for different types of bone, and it is thought that peak BMD is determined at around the average age of 34 to 40 years for cortical bone and earlier for cancellous/trabecular bone (Parfitt 1988). Other factors that influence peak BMD are gender (20–30% greater in males than females) and genetics (p. 179); and research using mice has shown male and female mice to display varying levels of BMD, which in the male appear to be dependent upon genetic factors such as stature and blood type and environmental influences (Orwoll et al 2001).

PHYSICAL ACTIVITY/EXERCISE DURING PUBERTY

Regular physical activity (PA)/exercise during puberty is associated with prevention of osteoporosis in later life and an increase in peak BMD, although excess PA/exercise during this period may contribute to amenorrhoea in females, and low peak BMD, and after puberty to secondary amenorrhoea and bone loss (Bass et al 1998). Amenorrhoea, as a result of excess PA/exercise, is primarily due to loss of body weight causing dysregulation of oestrogen (Felsenberg & Gowin 1998) (p. 178). Thus, excessive PA/exercise should be discouraged.

CLASSIFICATION

The World Health Organization (WHO 1994) has defined osteoporosis to be present when the bone density, as measured by dual energy X-ray absorptiometry (DXA), is more than 2.5 standard deviations below the mean value for young adults. Comparing values with a normal healthy population is seen as the most sensible way to achieve a comparable measure. However, the WHO definition was formulated for use with postmenopausal women and may not therefore be a suitable classification for men (Faulkner & Orwoll 2002). Furthermore, it has been shown that the classification for osteoporosis may also vary depending on the number and selection of sites being measured. For example, diagnosis of osteoporosis, using DXA, in a group of 206 men over the age of 50 years ranged from 1% to 39% depending on whether one or three sites, respectively, were measured (Stoch et al 2000). This indicates the need to clearly determine how an individual is assessed for the presence or risk of osteoporosis.

ASSESSMENT

Assessment of the risk and presence of osteoporosis can be done using a variety of laboratory and physical examinations. Measures of BMD and/or biochemical markers of bone turnover in the blood or urine can be used (Hu et al 1999, Rosen 2003). Tests for measures of 25-hydroxyvitamin D (p. 180), thyroid function, sex hormones (p. 179), parathyroid hormone (p. 176) and liver function may also be used as clinical indicators of osteoporotic risk. Biochemical bone markers, however, do not differentiate osteoporotic patients from healthy adults, as these markers suffer from large variability, thus negating their predictive value.

However, they can be useful in deciding on intervention, and/or in monitoring the efficacy of treatment (Kroger & Reeve 1998).

One of the most basic ways to diagnose osteoporosis is simply through the rate of fractures. However, generally the measure of BMD is the basis for the diagnosis of osteoporosis, and this can be assessed using several different techniques, including quantitative computer tomography, single and dual energy X-ray absorptiometry, radioabsorptiometry and ultrasound (Scheiber & Torregrosa 1998). Dual energy X-ray absorptiometry is at present the most precise and commonly used technique, and the most readily available method for assessing bone matter related risk of fracture (Felsenberg & Gowin 1999). Skeletal sites most commonly measured to determine BMD are the spine, hip, or total body (Fig. 11.6), though a combination of other sites are also assessed. Absorptiometry is a semi-quantitative method for determining BMD. The WHO (1994) classification is based upon DXA measured at central sites and the forearm. Dual energy X-ray absorptiometry uses two X-ray beams of differing energy levels to scan the area of interest. The attenuation of the beam is measured as it passes through the bone. The low-energy beams experience greater attenuation than high-energy beams, and bone attenuates X-rays to a greater extent than soft tissue. The discrepancy between these two measures allows for the correction of soft tissue, which is important as individuals vary with regard to soft tissue content. After the beam has passed, first through a known soft tissue equivalent filter and then through a known bone equivalent filter, it is possible to provide a quantitative measure of a specific site. When this value is compared to normal values, diagnosis can be made (American Medical Association 1995–2006).

Ultrasound of the bone may also provide a new measure of bone fragility, and broadband ultrasound has been shown to predict risk of hip fracture in elderly women. It is thought by some to be preferable, as ultrasound equipment is portable and unlike absorptiometry does not expose the individual to radiation. Other

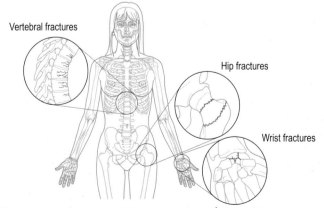

Figure 11.6 Common sites of osteoporosis (adapted from www.emirateshospital.ae/Images/news/19.gif).

techniques for diagnosis of osteoporosis are also being developed, but at present all involve a certain degree of error, both from the technique itself and in the interpretation of the data provided (Kroger & Reeve 1998).

AETIOLOGY

Numerous factors can contribute toward the onset and risk of osteoporosis and certain individuals are more likely to develop osteoporosis than others (Table 11.3). Outlined below are the major factors that influence risk of osteoporosis.

GENDER

Women, particularly postmenopausal women, are more prone to osteoporosis than men. This is mainly due to the fact that women have smaller and thinner frames than men, thus a smaller total bone mass and density, and the female postmenopause decline in oestrogen (p. 179). Many women by the age of 70 may have lost around 50% of skeletal mass to osteoporosis, whereas 70- to 80-year-old men may only just be beginning to show symptoms (Gordon & Genant 1985). Therefore it is apparent that the majority of research is carried out on postmenopausal women and adolescent girls. However, osteoporosis is also a problem for men, particularly those with low body weight and those who possess a genetic predisposition for osteoporosis, placing them at heightened risk (Stock et al 2004).

BODY WEIGHT

Numerous studies have identified the relationship between body weight and BMD for both men (Bell et al

---

Table 11.3 Risk factors for osteoporosis (adapted from NIH ORBD-NRC 2000)

Unchangeable risk factors
Female gender
Thin and/or small body frame
Advanced age
Family history of osteoporosis
Ethnic origin; Caucasian
Poor food absorption (gastrointestinal disorders – Crohn's disease, coeliac disease, cystic fibrosis)
Changeable risk factors
Sex hormones (postmenopause – including early or surgically induced menopause; abnormal absence of menstrual periods (amenorrhoea); low male testosterone levels)
Low body weight (anorexia nervosa or bulimia)
Low calcium and vitamin D levels (poor diet)
Use of medications, such as corticosteroids and anticonvulsants
Inactive lifestyle
Cigarette smoking
Excessive alcohol consumption

1995) and women, and a small frame and low body weight have been identified as risk factors for osteoporosis (NIH ORBD-NRC 2000).

For postmenopausal women, particularly, it appears that lean mass is the main determinant for bone mass, though fat mass and lean body mass both have a positive effect on BMD (Marone et al 1997). A review of the literature found fat mass to be most consistently important for postmenopausal women in protection against risk of osteoporosis (Reid 2002), and higher levels of lean mass and fat mass have been found to protect against the reduction of BMD during menopause. Hence postmenopausal women with low body weight are at greater risk of developing osteoporosis (Marone et al 1997).

Although there is a clear relationship between body weight and BMD, the effects of individual changes in body weight upon BMD are still not fully understood. In a study carried out by Pouilles et al (1995), 44 women of normal weight who had passed the menopause some 6 months to 5 years earlier, were followed for 40 months for the effects of changes in body weight on BMD (as determined by DXA). The researchers found a significant correlation between changes in body weight and changes in BMD at the vertebral and femoral sites. These changes remained significant even after adjustments for physical characteristics, such as age, years since menopause and initial BMD levels. Moreover, women who gained more than 1 kg during the 40-month follow-up period showed rates of bone loss that were two times less than those of the other women, highlighting the influence of body weight upon BMD (Pouilles et al 1995). Another study found that after 2 years of calcium supplementation postmenopausal women who were 106% of their ideal body weight had greater BMD of the spine and femoral neck than other women undergoing the same intervention (Harris et al 1992). This indicates that body weight may also influence mechanisms that relate to calcium metabolism. However, high body weight has not been found to show any protective action in the BMD of women who smoke (p. 181) (Broulik & Kapitola 1993); and considering the co-morbidities associated with excess body weight (Ch. 6) increasing body weight to excessive levels is not seen as a healthy intervention for the treatment of osteoporosis.

A number of mechanisms have been identified to explain the fat–bone relationship, and include the effect of soft tissue mass on skeletal loading, and the association of fat mass with the secretion of bone-active hormones from the pancreatic beta cells, such as insulin and the secretion of bone-active hormones, such as oestrogen (p. 179) and leptin, from the adipocytes. However, these factors alone do not fully explain these clinical associations (Reid 2002).

AGE

Increasing age is seen as a major determinant for risk of osteoporosis and there are numerous contributing factors. These include the decline in calcium absorption and other nutrients, a proportional increase in osteoclasts, possible fibrous and fatty infiltration of the haversian canals (contributing to the instability of the demineralized bone), postmenopausal reduction of oestrogen levels for women and a general reduction in physical activity levels (Groer & Shekleton 1989).

Age-related bone loss usually begins within a few years of achieving peak BMD and the average yearly loss of cortical bone is around 0.3% of peak BMD in males, and females up to menopause, which accelerates after menopause, mainly due to loss of oestrogen (Parfitt 1988, DoH 1991). Furthermore, osteoblasts are more sensitive to ageing than osteoclasts, and their reduction in numbers tips bone remodelling in favour of osteoclastic bone resorption, leading to increased bone fragility, as osteoblastic bone formation becomes unable to match the level of resorption (Eriksen & Kabgdagk 1997). Whilst age inevitably cannot be treated, other lifestyle changes, such as enhanced nutrition and increased physical activity, as well as medical interventions may help retard the age-related development of osteoporosis.

GENETICS

Genetic factors appear to have a significant influence upon BMD, and although hormonal, nutritional (Parfitt 1988, DoH 1991, Basu et al 2001) and physical activity status (Kemper 2000) cannot be ignored, studies on families and twins have found a strong genetic component (Klein et al 1998) accounting for around 80% of the variance in BMD (Giguere & Rousseau 2000). Research has also identified 10 chromosomal sites linked to peak bone mass development in the female mouse. Several of these identified sites map near genes encoding hormones, structural proteins and cell surface receptors that are intricately involved in skeletal homeostasis (Klein et al 1998, 2001), strongly suggesting the influence of genetic factors upon BMD.

More graphically, studies have shown Afro-Caribbean individuals to have greater peak BMD than white individuals, and in certain lower body sites, black men to possess higher BMD than white men (Bell et al 1995). White American women have also been found to have lower hip BMD and show higher rates of hip fracture than African-American women (Peacock et al 2004), though African-American women over the age of 50 years are also still prone to osteoporosis (NIH ORBD-NRC 2000).

SEX HORMONES

The mechanisms by which sex hormones regulate bone turnover have been investigated, and even though there is still much to be done to fully determine the many effects of sex steroid hormones on the skeleton, it appears that the major effect of sex steroid hormones is in preventing bone loss which results from inhibition of apoptosis in osteoblasts and the stimulation of apoptosis in osteoclasts (Lorenzo 2003). It appears that although testosterone, the major male sex hormone, has an anabolic effect on bone (Wimalawansa & Wimalawansa 1999), oestrogen, the major female sex hormone, has a greater effect in enhancing BMD than testosterone. A study looking at the relationship between sex hormones, bone geometric properties and BMD in 10- to 13-year-old girls, found oestrogen to have a positive effect on bone density geometric development, by suppressing bone turnover during the early pubertal period. This study also found that sex hormone-binding globulin, a protein that binds testosterone and oestradiol (naturally occurring oestrogen) in the plasma, has the opposite effect to oestrogen, and that testosterone appears to have no effect on these measured factors of bone geometry or density (Wang et al 2004). The effects of oestrogen are most graphically illustrated by the fact that postmenopausal women, whose oestrogen levels start to fall, show a decline in BMD, which after the administration of synthetic oestrogen has been shown to increase (Prelevic et al 2004). For some women, oestrogen replacement can prevent and possibly restore bone loss; however, studies have found mixed results with regard to its effectiveness (DoH 1991). Additionally, in the animal model, when sex-steroids are withdrawn there is rapid bone loss (Jilka et al 1992, Kousteni et al 2002).

CALCIUM LEVELS

In the average healthy adult, there is around 1.2 kg of calcium in the body, around 99% within the bones and teeth. The other 1% is in the tissues and fluids of the body, where it is essential for cellular structure and inter- and intracellular metabolic function and signal transmission. Dietary calcium is important in the development of peak BMD; thus too little calcium in early years can cause osteoporosis. Although some individuals can adapt to prolonged low intake, by increasing their efficiency of absorption (Malm 1958), it is generally recommended that in order for adults to maintain healthy bone they need to achieve absorption of around 160 mg (4 mmol) of calcium per day

Table 11.4 Dietary calcium mg/day (mmol/day) reference values for adults and adolescents (adapted from DoH 1991)

Age (years)	Estimated average requirement	Reference nutrient intake
Males:		
11 to 18	750 (18.8)	1000 (25.0)
Females:		
11 to 18	625 (15.6)	800 (20.0)
Pregnant	No increment	No increment
Lactating	No increment	+ 500 (14.3)
All adults:		
19–50+	525 (13.1)	700 (17.5)

1 mmol = 40 mg.

(DoH 1991) (Table 11.4). However, due to the endogenous secretion of calcium, mainly through renal excretion, but also through faeces, sweat, skin, hair and nails, the net absorption is less than the gross dietary absorption by around 100 mg (2.5 mmol) per day (DoH 1991). Additionally, as we become older our ability to absorb nutrients from our food is reduced (Dietze et al 1978) and therefore the intake of calcium may need to increase to combat the likelihood of calcium deficiency (DoH 1991).

In postmenopausal women, some attribute the increasing prevalence of osteoporosis, and associated fractures, to a deficiency in dietary calcium (Chan et al 1987). However, osteoporosis results from a loss of all components of bone not just calcium, and the postmenopausal increase in bone loss is mainly the result of oestrogen deficiency (p. 179).

Calcium and physical activity/exercise

A consideration is that calcium supplementation in addition to PA/exercise prescription may maximize the effect of the PA/exercise intervention, as studies have shown that calcium may influence the impact of PA/exercise on bone, with greater effects in calcium-replete subjects. Furthermore, comparative studies between Asian (high physical activity, low calcium intake) and US populations (low physical activity, high calcium intake) suggest that physical activity may permit an adaptation to low calcium intakes, though the interaction between physical activity and calcium still needs to be determined (Murphy & Carroll 2003).

VITAMIN D LEVELS

Vitamin D is a fat-soluble vitamin that is found in relatively few foods; it is also derived by the action of ultraviolet light upon the skin. Vitamin D is crucial in maintaining blood calcium within the normal range (total plasma calcium 90 to 105 mg/1 (2.25 to 2.60 mmol/l)), and normal plasma levels for adults (the plasma form being 25-hydroxyvitamin D) are between 15 ng/ml and 35 ng/ml in summer and 8 ng/ml and 18 ng/ml during winter. Since vitamin D is important in calcium homeostasis any deficiency would ultimately affect bone health. However, vitamin D deficiency is not uncommon. This is partly due to the fact that many foods have little or no vitamin D content, and as a result of insufficient exposure to sunlight. For individuals who live a normal lifestyle, supplementation is not required, but for those confined indoors an amount of 10 µg per day has been recommended (DoH 1991). It is also recommended that in order to achieve sufficient ultraviolet exposure and avoid skin damage, 5 to 10 minutes a day of sun exposure, without sunscreen, may provide an adequate amount of vitamin D (Holick 2004).

MEDICATIONS

Long-term use of medications prescribed for a wide range of diseases, such as arthritis, asthma, Crohn's disease, lupus and other diseases of the lungs, kidneys and liver, can lead to a loss of BMD, as can drugs used to treat seizures, certain cancers and endometriosis, resulting in enhanced risk of fracture (NIH ORBD-NRC 2000, Sheth 2004). For example, anti-seizure medications have been found to result in nearly 50% greater bone loss, which has been found regardless of other factors, such as calcium and vitamin D supplementation, smoking, height, weight or physical activity levels (Gross et al 2004). This indicates that intervention to combat risk of osteoporosis may not be as effective as it would be for individuals not taking medication. One of the most common forms of drug-induced osteoporosis is through glucocorticoids, and fractures have been found to occur in around 30–50% of chronic users, which appears to occur despite efforts to reduce the dose of these medications (Graves & Lukert 2004). These findings highlight the fact that bone loss can occur relatively quickly after taking some of these drugs. Therefore, whilst the processes by which these medications result in this side effect are varied and still remain to be fully determined, it is important that the exercise practitioner is aware of the potential for any drug-induced loss in BMD, especially since PA/exercise may not be able to retard these effects.

PHYSICAL ACTIVITY LEVELS

Bone like muscle is a living tissue, and adapts to certain stresses placed upon it. It is clear therefore that a regular lack of certain types of mechanical load, i.e. physical inactivity, can be a contributor toward risk of osteoporosis, especially during puberty and early adulthood when peak BMD is acquired (p. 177). The importance of PA/exercise has been dramatically illustrated by studies involving weightlessness (Pereira et al 2004, Shackelford et al 2004) and bed rest, where mechanical load has been reduced. Liu et al (2003), for example, observed the effect of 21 days of supine bed rest ($n = 5$), and supine bed rest plus 60 minutes per day of supine cycle ergometry ($n = 5$), in a group of healthy young men. The researchers found that on average femur BMD decreased by 5.8% and 0.9%, respectively. Similarly, Shackelford et al (2004) observed the effect of 17 weeks of supine bed rest ($n = 18$) and supine bed rest plus maximal resistance training ($n = 9$), in a group of healthy men and women. Whilst the exercising group showed positive gains in BMD, from various sites, the non-exercise group showed a reduction in BMD. These findings are interesting in that they not only demonstrate the loss of BMD through reduced mechanical load via bed rest, but also show how non-weight-bearing aerobic exercise can attenuate this effect, and how resistance exercise, in this instance, can enhance BMD. Additionally, although scuba diving is considered to be a physical sport, professional scuba divers, who undergo similar conditions of weightlessness as astronauts, have been shown to possess reduced BMD (Pereira et al 2004). These studies indicate the importance of specific types of mechanical load, and therefore specific types of PA/exercise, for enhancing, maintaining or attenuating the loss of BMD, and how lack of this mechanical load can increase risk of osteoporosis. Thus they highlight the importance of PA/exercise in terms of bone health during both the developmental and adult years.

SMOKING

Habitual cigarette smoking can increase the risk of osteoporosis in both men (Ortego-Centeno et al 1997, Vogel et al 1997, Szulc et al 2002) and women (Chapurlat et al 2001, Tanko & Christiansen 2004), and male smokers may increase their risk of fracture by around 10–30% per decade (Vogel et al 1997).

There are multiple mechanisms by which smoking can affect bone (Hadley & Reddy 1997), and smoking has been shown to reduce BMD to a greater extent in cancellous than in cortical bone (Vogel et al 1997). Although the mechanisms by which smoking results in lower BMD have yet to be fully established, smoking appears to have a significant effect upon calcium and vitamin D metabolism, and a depressant effect on serum vitamin D and the parathyroid hormone system, partly explaining some of the potential mechanisms by which smoking affects bone (Brot et al 1999). Furthermore, smokers have been shown to have higher levels of urinary markers of bone resorption, and lower serum levels of 25-hydroxyvitamin D (Brot et al 1999, Szulc et al 2002) (p. 180). While smokers may display lower BMD as measured from most areas of the skeleton, smokers are also more likely to suffer from spinal column degenerative disease, where the vertebrae of smokers have been shown to be less strong, mineral deficient, with reduced blood supply and with fewer and less functional osteoblasts (Hadley & Reddy 1997). Smoking also has an oestrogen-lowering effect, making postmenopausal women who smoke especially vulnerable. These women have been found to display significantly lower BMD than non-smoking postmenopausal women (Brot et al 1999). Moreover, even postmenopausal female smokers on oestrogen hormone therapy have been found to display only half the concentrations of matched non-smokers (Tanko & Christiansen 2004), thus demonstrating the deleterious effects of habitual cigarette smoking and how important it is to encourage smoking cessation.

ALCOHOL

Excess alcohol consumption has been associated with an increased risk of osteoporosis (NIH ORBD-NRC 2000), and the amount and duration of alcohol abuse probably has an effect with regard to the extent of bone damage. Although excessive alcohol consumption may be a risk factor for osteoporosis, a study on female twins found that moderate consumption was not harmful to health in women, as there was a positive association between alcohol consumption and BMD, and the markers of bone turnover were not associated with alcohol consumption (Williams et al 2005). In addition, a large epidemiological study, carried out in Denmark, showed that moderate intake (1–27 drinks per week for men and 1–13 for women) was not associated with fracture of the hip, but more than 27 drinks per week was a major risk factor for hip fracture in men (Hoidrup et al 1999).

Co-morbidities may also have an influence with regard to the effect of alcohol on bone. For instance, alcohol abusers tend to be less physically active, which may be a contributing factor to the heightened risk, especially since studies on male rats have found that reduced weight-bearing accentuated the detrimental effects of alcohol on cortical bone, by further inhibiting bone formation (Hefferan et al 2003). Liver disease is also an independent risk factor for bone loss (Odvina et al 1995) and since liver disease is associated with chronic alcohol abuse, the effect of alcohol on the liver may be one of the mechanisms by which alcohol consumption has an effect on bone health.

Chronic alcoholics have been shown to display deficiencies of active metabolites of vitamin D (p. 180), and exhibit other dietary, vitamin and electrolyte deficiencies (Medras & Jankowska 2000), which can affect bone health. Alcohol also has a toxic effect on bone marrow, affecting iron metabolism (Homann & Hasselbalch 1992) and other areas of health in addition to that of bone. Studies using the animal model have shown that 3 weeks of binge drinking in rats can significantly reduce cancellous BMD by stimulating bone resorption (Callaci et al 2004), possibly by inhibiting osteoblast activity (Rico et al 1987), thus reducing bone density and bone mass in both cortical (Sampson et al 1998) and cancellous bone (Hogan et al 2001). The diminishing effects also appear to be dependent upon the duration of alcohol use (Hogan et al 2001). Nonetheless, although some rat studies showed alcohol not to affect calcium regulation or sex hormones (Sampson et al 1998), other studies found alcohol to have a modulating effect on mineral-regulating hormones such as vitamin D metabolites, parathyroid hormone and calcitonin (Sampson 1997).

Thus it would appear that while moderate alcohol intake may not be detrimental to bone health, regular excessive consumption does appear to be harmful. Therefore, for those at risk or suffering from osteoporosis the amount of alcohol consumed should be carefully considered.

PREVENTION

By about the age of 20, most people have acquired around 98% of their bone mass, and building strong bones during childhood and adolescence can be the best defence against developing osteoporosis in later life (p. 176). Ways to prevent osteoporosis are to have a lifestyle that contains a balanced diet including sufficient calcium (p. 179) and vitamin D intake (p. 180), weight-bearing exercise (p. 180), no cigarette smoking (p. 180) and limited alcohol intake (p. 181) (NIH ORBD-NRC 2000).

TREATMENT

Once risk or presence of osteoporosis has been determined treatment may take the form of non-pharmacological strategies and/or pharmacological therapy (Follin & Hansen 2003).

PHARMACOLOGICAL

There are a variety of drugs that are prescribed for the treatment and prevention of osteoporosis, some of which are outlined below. These medications may include selective oestrogen-receptor modulators and calcitonin, which are options for both the prevention and treatment of osteoporosis; and medications prescribed for the treatment of osteoporosis may be oestrogens, bisphosphonates, vitamin D and parathyroid hormone (NIH ORBD-NRC 2000, Sambrook 2005). However, pharmacological treatments are continually progressing and developing, and the exercise practitioner should be aware of the changes in these treatments, particularly if they influence the ability of the individual to perform PA/exercise.

Parathyroid hormone and vitamin D

Parathyroid hormone (Follin & Hansen 2003, Sambrook 2005) and vitamin D both promote bone formation and given the appropriate dose have been shown to increase bone mass (NOF 2004).

Bisphosphonates

Bisphosphonates are anti-resorptive medications and have shown great benefit in reducing bone loss and increasing bone density, in both the spine and hip, and therefore reducing the risk of both spine and hip fractures. Bisphosphonates inhibit bone resorption and may have an anabolic effect on cancellous bone. They have also been found to be a useful treatment of bone loss from glucocorticoid medications, and are used to treat men with osteoporosis. Side effects are uncommon but may include abdominal or musculoskeletal pain (which may affect PA/ability), nausea, heartburn or irritation of the oesophagus. One of the biggest drawbacks of this type of medication is that in order to avoid irritation of the oesophagus, the individual is recommended to remain upright for at least 30 minutes after having taken it (NIH ORBD-NRC 2000, NOF 2004).

Calcitonin

Calcitonin is an anti-resorptive medication that inhibits the resorption of cancellous bone, though its effect on cortical bone still remains to be determined. Calcitonin is a naturally occurring non-sex hormone involved in calcium regulation and bone metabolism. In women who are at least 5 years beyond the menopause, calcitonin slows bone loss, and increases spinal bone density. Calcitonin may be injected or administered through a nasal spray. However, the injection may cause an allergic reaction and other side effects such as flushing of the face and hands, urinary frequency, nausea and skin rash. The only side effect of the nasal spray is a runny nose (NIH ORBD-NRC 2000, NOF 2004).

Oestrogen

Despite studies showing mixed results with regard to its effectiveness in slowing the progression of osteoporosis (DoH 1991), oestrogen therapy is known as an anti-resorptive medication and has been shown to reduce bone loss and increase BMD in both the spine and hip and reduce the risk of hip and spinal fractures in postmenopausal women (NOF 2004). However, when taken alone oestrogen can increase a woman's risk of developing cancer. Therefore, it has been recommended that oestrogen should not be used for the sole purpose of osteoporosis prevention. Nonetheless, short-term use is acceptable for women with vasomotor symptoms or when the benefits outweigh the risks (Follin & Hansen 2003).

Selective oestrogen–receptor modulators

Selective oestrogen-receptor modulators are used to reduce bone loss in women, and have been developed to provide the beneficial effect of oestrogens without their potential disadvantages, as they have been shown to reduce the risk of oestrogen-dependent breast cancer by 65% over 4 years (NOF 2004).

NON–PHARMACOLOGICAL

Non-pharmacological strategies include PA/exercise, appropriate dietary intake of calcium and vitamin D (p. 179, 180) and the discontinuation of tobacco (p. 181) and alcohol abuse (p. 181) (Follin & Hansen 2003).

Physical activity/exercise

Regular PA/exercise in youth is seen as a preventative measure against risk of osteoporosis in later life (p. 176). However, levels of PA/exercise tend to decline with increasing age and for most older individuals there is virtually no remaining benefit of PA/exercise performed in youth (Karlsson 2002). Nonetheless, the value of PA/exercise in adulthood is through its ability to maintain BMD or reduce age-related bone loss, and in some individuals BMD can be enhanced (Shackelford et al 2004). Furthermore, PA/exercise has very little in the way of adverse side effects, is low cost and confers additional benefits such as postural stability and fall prevention (Murphy & Carroll 2003). Therefore, PA/exercise is frequently promoted as part of the treatment for osteoporosis (Beck & Snow 2003).

Falls prevention

Falls are a major cause of mortality and morbidity in the elderly, affecting about one-third of those aged over 65 years, and around 10% of these falls will result in major injury or fracture (Masud & Morris 2001). Moreover, the rate of hospital admissions as a result of falls has risen in south east England for those aged over 85 years (Cryer et al 1996). Therefore, strategies to reduce the risk of falls are of prime concern to health authorities, and PA/exercise interventions have been shown to be effective.

PRE-PHYSICAL ACTIVITY/EXERCISE PRESCRIPTION

Individuals with osteoporosis should be appropriately screened and assessed prior to any PA/exercise programme (Appendix A). Although the primary objective in osteoporosis treatment is to retard further bone loss, because the large majority of those with osteoporosis are elderly, they are also likely to have age-related co-morbidities, which also need to be identified and accounted for within the PA/exercise programme.

PHYSICAL ACTIVITY/EXERCISE PRESCRIPTION

The aim of a PA/exercise programme for the osteoporotic individual is primarily, where possible, to enhance BMD, and reduce further bone loss and risk of fracture. Most osteoporotic individuals will suffer some level of pain, so the PA/exercise programme should also aim to reduce pain, as well as increase mobility, improve muscle strength and endurance, and improve balance and stability, in order to enhance independence and quality of life (Bass et al 2001, Beck & Snow 2003).

The optimal type and amount of PA/exercise required in order to reduce further bone loss and risk of fracture has yet to be fully determined, as are the effects of PA/exercise on bone size, shape, architecture and frequency of injurious falls. Nonetheless, lack of this evidence does not mean absence of effect (Karlsson 2002). For instance, a randomized controlled study looking into the effect of a community-based exercise programme (twice weekly exercise class for 20 weeks) in reducing risk of falls, in a group of 80 osteoporotic women aged between 65 and 75 years, found that compared to controls, those who participated in exercise experienced enhanced dynamic balance

and strength (both determinants of risk of falls) (Carter et al 2002). This is of particular importance as a fall for an osteoporotic individual may result in a serious fracture that could have long-term debilitating consequences. Furthermore, research comparing 9 months of home-based and supervised exercise, consisting of resistance and endurance training, found larger increases in total body BMD and significantly greater increases in lumbar spine BMD from the supervised exercise group compared to the home-based exercise group. The supervised group also showed greater decreases in body weight and fat mass and increases in muscle strength (Villareal et al 2003), thus indicating that both programmes can result in improvements in BMD in a particularly high-risk group, and that in terms of reducing further risk of osteoporosis, either may be advocated. In addition, an 18-month randomized controlled study, and 8-month follow-up, looking at the influence of twice weekly aerobic and step training, in a group of premenopausal women ($n = 30$ active and $n = 19$ controls), found improvements in BMD of the lumbar spine and various sites of the lower limbs (Heinonen et al 1999). High-impact PA/exercise is therefore effective in enhancing BMD. Different types of PA/exercise have different loading effects upon the skeleton, thus affecting its adaptation. Weight-bearing PA/exercise, for instance, appears to be most tive, and this was demonstrated in a group of adolescent female athletes, where activities such as running were associated with larger site-specific BMD than were swimming or cycling. Knee extension strength was only weakly correlated as an independent predictor of BMD in this group (Duncan et al 2002), thus suggesting that even though strength exercises can be effective at enhancing BMD, activities that place the bone under mechanical stress are most effective.

Physical activity/exercise is clearly beneficial to most postmenopausal women although it may not fully compensate for the negative effects of oestrogen and calcium deficiency (Baptista & Sardinha 1994), and even though the latter may be compensated by pharmacological interventions, continued bone loss may still occur despite PA/exercise intervention.

SINGLE VERSUS HABITUAL PHYSICAL ACTIVITY/EXERCISE

Most of the research looking into the effect of PA/exercise upon bone health has looked at habitual PA/exercise, and although there are relatively few studies on the acute effect of PA/exercise upon the markers of osteoporosis, some research has been carried out. A single bout of PA/exercise, for instance, can bring about acute hormonal alterations (Bunt 1986, 1990). In this context, oestradiol (naturally occurring oestrogen), which has been shown to suppress bone turnover and therefore help maintain BMD, may be one of the mechanisms by which PA/exercise affects bone health. One of the few studies looking into the effect of a single bout of PA/exercise found that in 25 early postmenopausal women, 2 hours after approximately 60 minutes of high-impact physical exercise, there was a 20% increase in oestradiol levels (Kemmler et al 2003). Additionally, a study looking into the effect of a single bout of 60 minutes of brisk walking found no significant changes in parathyroid hormone or calcitonin. However, there were changes in serum levels of bone collagen, markers that indicated an altered bone collagen turnover (Thorsen et al 1996).

The length of these changes appears to vary depending on which markers are being observed and the intensity, type and duration of the PA/exercise bout. Therefore, it is difficult to determine whether the chronic changes in markers of bone turnover are simply the accumulative effect of single bouts of exercise, or indeed the adaptive effect to longer-term PA/exercise. Nonetheless, a review of literature (Murphy & Carroll 2003) has shown that both acute and chronic exercise reduce bone resorption.

PHYSICAL ACTIVITY/EXERCISE INTENSITY AND IMPACT

It is clear that strenuous PA/exercise is associated with enhanced bone density; and a study looking at the effect of different modes of exercise in 171 male undergraduates found exercise intensity and history to positively correlate with values of BMD (Zhao 2001). However, of most interest to the exercise practitioner is the most effective PA/exercise intensity for those already at risk. Hatori et al (1993) carried out a study to determine the most effective PA/exercise intensity in a group of 33 postmenopausal women. The women were randomly selected into either a group of controls ($n = 12$) or two exercise groups (mainly walking for 30 minutes three times per week, for 7 months); one group worked at a speed just above their anaerobic threshold ($n = 12$), and the other ($n = 9$) just below. Whilst postintervention the controls and the lower-intensity group showed decreases ($1.7 \pm 2.7\%$ and $1.0 \pm 3.1\%$, not statistically significantly different) in BMD of the lumbar vertebrae (as determined by DXA), there were significant increases ($1.1 \pm 2.9\%$) for the higher-intensity group. These findings therefore indicate higher-intensity PA/exercise to be more effective. However, 24 weeks of high-impact moderate-intensity aerobic exercise has also been found to enhance BMD (Chien et al 2000), thus suggesting that the impact of the activity or the overall mechanical loading of the PA/exercise sessions may be more important than the overall intensity of the PA/exercise per se.

Whilst research generally shows intense weight-bearing PA/exercise to be most effective at enhancing peak BMD, it is important to understand that continual cyclic load during physical activity may lead to fatigue degradation of the bone and an increased risk of fracture. Those most prone to this are the young and elderly, and females prone to amenorrhoea (i.e. those who are extremely physically active or underweight). Cyclic loading of cancellous/trabecular bone (p. 174) can result in a reduction in the elastic properties of the bone and an accumulation of residual strain. These effects increase with augmenting stress levels, leading to a progressive reduction in point of bone fatigue. This reduction in point of bone fatigue has been related to an increase in residual strain accumulation rates at elevated stress levels (Gangualy et al 2004). Research has also shown exercise intensity and body mass index to be associated with an increased probability of stress fracture (Lauder et al 2000). Therefore, a balance with regard to the intensity of PA/exercise is required, highlighting the need for the exercise practitioner to account for each individual's risks and requirements.

DURATION AND FREQUENCY OF PHYSICAL ACTIVITY/EXERCISE

Although it has been shown that the duration of physical activity is positively correlated with the BMD of weight-loaded sites (Karlsson et al 2001), the optimal duration and frequency of PA/exercise to maintain and promote bone health in adults has still to be elucidated. A study carried out on 171 male undergraduates found that exercise performed more than three times per week improved BMD significantly. The researchers suggested that to increase peak BMD, PA/exercise should be higher in intensity and more than half an hour each session, and more than three times per week (Zhao & Zhang 2000, Zhao 2001). However, there may be a point where the duration and frequency of PA/exercise has no additional benefit. For example, a study on national male soccer players ($n = 67$, aged 17 to 35 years) found bone strength to be achieved by around 6 hours of exercise per week. Beyond this, additional exercise was found not to confer higher BMD. It was thus concluded that the skeleton adapts to the prevalent level of PA/exercise intensity required and no further (Karlsson et al 2001).

TYPE OF PHYSICAL ACTIVITY/EXERCISE

The types of PA/exercise found to promote bone health are varied in both their mode and their effectiveness. The responses to the various types of PA/exercise will ultimately depend on the status of the individual, something that the exercise practitioner should determine prior to PA/exercise prescription. Nonetheless, outlined below are some of the current findings regarding different types of PA/exercise and their effect upon bone health.

AEROBIC ACTIVITIES

Researchers have investigated the effects of a wide variety of aerobic activities upon bone health. From this it appears that the adaptation of the bone is very site specific, depending very much upon the activity (McDermott et al 2001), and it is clear that weight-bearing activities generally produce the most significant results (Torstveit 2002). For instance, when elite female cyclists, runners, swimmers and triathletes were compared to a group of controls, the runners were found to have larger site-specific BMD than the swimmers or cyclists (Duncan et al 2002). Furthermore, despite being highly trained and physically fit, master cyclists, with a long history of training exclusively in cycling, have been shown to possess lower total body BMD than their aged-matched peers (Nichols et al 2003). This indicates the need for mechanical loading upon bone. Similarly, another study found male runners to have greater BMD, particularly of the leg, compared to male cyclists, who also had reduced BMD of the spine. The researchers in this study also found that those athletes who regularly performed both running and cycling possessed greater total body and arm BMD (Stewart & Hannan 2000). However, findings from another study, on triathletes, showed that despite the generalized anatomical distribution loads of triathlon, the triathletes' total BMD was not significantly better than those of the runners (Duncan et al 2002). The importance of weight-bearing activities is further highlighted by research showing that in the absence of weight-bearing activity, nutritional or endocrine interventions appear unable to maintain bone mass (Murphy & Carroll 2003). Nonetheless, that is not to say that non-weight-bearing aerobic activities fail to enhance bone health. An extreme example can be seen from a study carried out on individuals who suffered spinal cord injury ($n = 10$, aged 35.3 ± 2.3 years) (Mohr et al 1997), who generally suffer substantial bone loss, particularly in the lower limbs. These individuals were given 30 minutes per day of electrical stimulated upright cycling, 3 days per week for 12 months. Post-intervention these individuals showed a 10% gain in BMD of the proximal tibia, thus indicating the influence of even non-weight-bearing aerobic PA/exercise on BMD. Research would suggest, however, that enhanced BMD is most likely the result of the overall mechanical loading placed upon the bone, rather than the mode of PA/exercise per se. For instance, Pettersson et al (1999) observed that high-impact activities tended to weaken the relationship between BMD and muscle strength, suggesting that impact forces may be of greater importance in regulating BMD.

RESISTANCE TRAINING

Generally, high-impact, weight-bearing activities are found to be most effective at enhancing BMD at the specific sites of impact. Nonetheless, it appears that resistance exercise is more effective at enhancing cortical bone than aerobic PA/exercise alone (McDermott et al 2001) and muscle contraction can result in site-specific increases in BMD. Flodgren et al (1999) observed the effect of muscular contraction and non-weight-bearing loading patterns on BMD in a group of kayakers ($n = 6$ male and $n = 4$ female, elite kayakers, median age 19 years) compared to controls. The researchers found that the kayakers had significantly greater BMD in most upper body sites, with no significant differences in the BMD of the total body, head or any of the lower body sites, except the pelvis, compared to the controls. Heavy resistance training has also been found to increase site-specific BMD in men, though, this has not been found to be as consistent in either pre- or postmenopausal women. Nonetheless, resistance training has been found to reduce the age-related losses of BMD in postmenopausal women (Hurley 1995), suggesting that muscular contractions as well as impact forces are important factors in bone remodelling.

Whilst resistance exercises are an important component of any PA/exercise programme for those with or at risk of osteoporosis, it is inadvisable for older individuals to use free weights. Loss of balance and a fall when using these weights may increase risk of fracture; therefore, other forms of resistance equipment would be preferable.

CHAIR-BASED EXERCISE

It is clear that weight-bearing and resistance forms of PA/exercise are important in maintaining BMD. However, some older individuals may find ambulatory and other types of PA/exercise difficult. The relatively recent development of chair-based exercise programmes now allows these elderly people the opportunity to engage in PA/exercise. Although this type of exercise has been found to enhance older individuals' functional activities (Allen & Simpson 1999), whether it is effective at reducing risk of osteoporosis and increasing BMD has still to be determined.

CONSIDERATIONS AND CONTRAINDICATIONS

The majority of osteoporotic individuals are over the age of 65 years and therefore are likely to suffer age-related co-morbidities. Hence these factors will also need to be considered in conjunction with those related to the osteoporosis. Whilst it is always advisable to start any PA/exercise at a lower intensity, high-impact PA/exercise is excellent for maintaining BMD in individuals with osteoporosis. However, the PA/exercise should not put any sudden or excessive strain on bones, especially as there is an increased risk of stress fracture with high-intensity exercise (Lauder et al 2000). Additionally, continual cyclic load during physical activity may lead to fatigue degradation of the bone and an increased risk of fracture (Gangualy et at 2004), so there needs to be a balance between the intensity, impact and mode of the PA/exercise in order to promote BMD without causing additional risk of fracture.

Some osteoporotic individuals may suffer from kyphosis (stooped posture, see Fig. 11.2). This will not only affect the biomechanics of any PA/exercise performed, but may also affect breathing, as the lungs, diaphragm and intercostal muscles are unable to function normally. The exercise practitioner will therefore have to select activities that allow for the resultant limitations (Bloomfield 1997).

Fear of falling is of great concern to some older and osteoporotic individuals, as this may result in fracture. Therefore, the PA/exercise programme should include activities that enhance balance and postural stability. The use of free weights should also be discouraged, as free weights generally require greater control and balance and thus place these individuals at greater risk of fall. Furthermore, due to the risk of falls it is a good idea for these individuals to perform their PA/exercise in an environment that will minimize the risk of fracture if a fall occurs (Bloomfield 1997).

ABSOLUTE CONTRAINDICATIONS FOR PHYSICAL ACTIVITY/EXERCISE

The absolute contraindications for exercise will be as for those cited for other individuals (Appendix A, Table A.1) in addition to those limitations imposed by osteoporosis.

MEDICATIONS

Certain medications can contribute toward bone loss (p. 231), and the exercise practitioner should be aware of the fact that continued bone loss, as a result of continued use of these medications, may be unavoidable and may continue despite the intervention of PA/exercise. Although cessation of certain medications may halt the pharmacologically mediated bone loss, research is limited in this area and it is not clear whether the rate of bone loss will slow down or continue. In addition, medications can affect the individual's ability to perform PA/exercise (Ch. 14, p. 231). For example, bisphosphonates can cause muscular pain, which may affect PA/exercise ability. Additionally, if the client/patient is injecting calcitonin, they may experience soreness at the site of injection and if this is in one of the active muscles it may affect PA/exercise ability. Physical activity/exercise may, however, enhance the effect of calcium supplementation (Murphy & Carroll 2003).

SUMMARY

- Osteoporosis is characterized by low bone mass and bone mineral density (BMD), which leads to increased risk of bone fragility and susceptibility to fracture.
- Risk of osteoporosis increases with age, and is a considerable public health problem in many societies.
- Osteoporosis affects both cortical and cancellous/trabecular bone.
- Peak BMD is achieved during adolescence and early adulthood and tends to diminish with increasing age.
- Enhanced BMD may protect against osteoporosis in late adult life.
- Risk factors associated with increased risk of osteoporosis are: age, gender, body weight, genetics, oestrogen levels, calcium and vitamin D levels, smoking, alcohol abuse, regular use of certain medications and PA/exercise levels.
- Physical activity/exercise may retard the loss of BMD and reduce the risk of osteoporosis; however, even PA/exercise intervention and other interventions may not be able to counteract the influence of other risk factors.
- Pharmacological interventions may reduce loss of BMD.
- Non-pharmacological interventions may be employed, which include PA/exercise.
- The optimal frequency, intensity, duration and type of PA/exercise to reduce risk and treat osteoporosis have yet to be determined. However, considering that bone adaptation is very site-specific, it does appear that the overall compressive and tensile stress placed on a particular bone is more important in its adaptation than the frequency, intensity, duration and type of PA/exercise per se.
- Continued cyclic loading or any sudden or excessive strain can result in fracture, especially for those at greater risk of osteoporosis. Therefore, a balanced PA/exercise programme, taking into account each individual's risks and needs, is required.

Suggested readings, references and bibliography

Suggested reading
Bloomfield S A 1997 Osteoporosis. In: ACSM's exercise management for persons with chronic diseases and disabilities. Human Kinetics, Champaign, IL

Snow-Harter C, Marcus R 1991 Exercise, bone mineral density, and osteoporosis. Exercise and Sport Sciences Reviews 19:351–388

References and bibliography
Allen A, Simpson J M 1999 A primary care based fall prevention programme. Physiotherapy Theory and Practice 15:121–133

American Medical Association 1995–2006 Recommendations for BMD testing. Online. Available: http://www.ama-cmeonline.com February 2005

Anderson D M, Keith J, Novak P D et al (eds) 2002 Mosby's Medical, nursing and allied health dictionary, 6th edn. Mosby, St Louis

Baptista F, Sardinha L 1994 The effects of exercise on bone density of postmenopausal women. Portuguese Journal of Human Performance Studies 10(2):63–79

Bass S, Pearce G, Bradney M et al 1998 Exercise before puberty may confer residual benefits in bone density in adulthood: studies in active prepubertal and retired female gymnasts. Journal of Bone and Mineral Research 13(3):500–507

Bass S, Forwood M, Larsen J et al 2001 Prescribing exercise for osteoporosis. International Sportmedicine Journal 1(5):February

Basu S, Michaelsson K, Olofsson H et al 2001 Association between oxidative stress and bone mineral density. Biochemical and Biophysical Research Communications 288(1):275–279

Beck B R, Snow C M 2003 Bone health across the lifespan – exercising our options. Exercise and Sport Science Reviews 31(3):117–122

Bell N H, Gordon L, Stevens J et al 1995 Demonstration that bone mineral density of the lumbar spine, trochanter, and femoral neck is higher in black than in white young men. Calcified Tissue International 56(1):11–13

Bloomfield S A 1997 Osteoporosis. In: ACSM's exercise management for persons with chronic diseases and disabilities. Human Kinetics, Champaign, IL

Brot C, Jorgensen N R, Sorensen O H 1999 The influence of smoking on vitamin D status and calcium metabolism. European Journal of Clinical Nutrition 53(12):920–926

Broulik P D, Kapitola J 1993 Interrelations between bodyweight, cigarette smoking and spine mineral density in osteoporotic Czech women. Endocrine Regulations 27(2):57–60

Bunt J C 1986 Hormonal alterations due to exercise. Sports Medicine 3(5):331–345

Bunt J C 1990 Metabolic actions of estradiol: significance for acute and chronic exercise responses. Medicine and Science in Sports and Exercise 22(3):286–290

Callaci J J, Juknelis D, Patwardhan A et al 2004 The effects of binge alcohol exposure on bone resorption and biomechanical and structural properties are offset by concurrent bisphosphonate treatment. Alcoholism: Clinical and Experimental Research 28(1):182–191

Carter N D, Khan K M, McKay H A et al 2002 Community-based exercise program reduces risk of falls in 65- to 75-year-old women with osteoporosis: randomised controlled trial. Canadian Medical Association Journal 167(9):997–1004

Center J, Eisman J 1997 The epidemiology and pathogenesis of osteoporosis. Baillière's Clinical Endocrinology and Metabolism 11(1):23–62

Chan G M, McMurray M, Westover K et al 1987 Effects of increased dietary calcium intake upon calcium and bone mineral status in lactating adolescent and adult women. American Journal of Clinical Nutrition 46:319–323

Chapurlat R D, Ewing S K, Bauer D C et al 2001 Influence of smoking on the antiosteoporotic efficacy of raloxifene. Journal of Clinical Endocrinology and Metabolism 86(9):4178–4182

Chien M Y, Wu Y T, Hsu A T et al 2000 Efficacy of a 24-week aerobic exercise program for osteopenic postmenopausal women. Calcified Tissue International 67(6):443–448

Cryer PC, Davidson L, Styles C P et al 1996 Descriptive epidemiology of injury in the south-east: identifying priorities for action. Public Health 110:331–338

Dietze F, Laue R, Schulz H J 1978 Digestion and absorption in elderly man. Zeitschrift für Alternsforschung 33(1):65–78

DoH (Department of Health) 1991 Dietary reference values for food energy and nutrients for the United Kingdom. HMSO, London

Duncan C S, Blimkie C J R, Cowell C T et al 2002 Bone mineral density in adolescent female athletes: relationship to exercise type and muscle strength. Medicine and Science in Sports and Exercise 34(2):286–294

Eriksen E F, Kabgdagk B L 1997 The pathogenesis of osteoporosis. Hormone Research 48 (suppl 5):78–82

Faulkner K G, Orwoll E 2002 Implications in the use of T-scores for the diagnosis of osteoporosis in men. Journal of Clinical Densitometry 5(1):87–93

Felsenberg D, Gowin W 1998 Bone densitometry: applications in sports-medicine. European Journal of Radiology 28(2):150–154

Felsenberg D, Gowin W 1999 Bone densitometry by dual energy methods. Radiologe 39(3):186–193

Firoozbakhsh K, Aleyaasin M 1989 The effect of stress concentration on bone remodelling: theoretical predictions. Journal of Biomechanical Engineering 111(4):355–360

Flieger J, Karachalios T, Khaldi L et al 1998 Mechanical stimulation in the form of vibration prevents postmenopausal bone loss in ovariectomised rats. Calcified Tissue International 63(6):510–514

Flodgren G, Hedelin R, Henriksson-Larsen K 1999 Bone mineral density in flatwater sprint kayakers. Calcified Tissue International 64(5):374–379

Follin S L, Hansen L B 2003 Current approaches to the prevention and treatment of postmenopausal osteoporosis. American Journal of Health-System Pharmacy 60(9):883–901

Gangualy P, Moore T L, Gibson L J 2004 A phenomenological model for predicting fatigue life in bovine trabecular bone. Journal of Biomechanical Engineering 126(3):330–339

Giguere Y, Rousseau F 2000 The genetics of osteoporosis: complexities and difficulties. Clinical Genetics 57(3):161–169

Gordon G, Genant H 1985 The aging skeleton. Clinics in Geriatric Medicine 1:95–118

Graves L, Lukert B P 2004 Glucocorticoid-induced osteoporosis: a clinician's perspective. Clinical Reviews in Bone and Mineral Metabolism, Drug-Induced Osteoporosis 2(2):79–90

Groer M W, Shekleton M E 1989 Basic pathophysiology: a holistic approach, 3rd edn. Mosby, St Louis

Gross R A, Gidal B E, Pack A M 2004 Antiseizure drugs and reduced bone density. Neurology. Online. Available: http://www.osteo.org February 2005

Hadley M N, Reddy S V 1997 Smoking and the human vertebral column: a review of the impact of cigarette use on vertebral bone metabolism and spinal fusion. Neurosurgery 41(1):116–124

Harris S, Dallal G E, Dawson-Hughes B 1992 Influence of body weight on rates of change in bone density of the spine, hip and radius of postmenopausal women. Calcified Tissue International 50(1):19–23

Hatori M, Hasegawa A, Adachi H et al 1993 The effects of walking at the anaerobic threshold level on vertebral bone loss in postmenopausal women. Calcified Tissue International 52(6):411–414

Hefferan T E, Kennedy A M, Evans G L et al 2003 Disuse exaggerates the detrimental effects of alcohol on cortical bone. Alcoholism: Clinical and Experimental Research 27(1):111–117

Heinonen A, Kannus P, Sievanen H et al 1999 Good maintenance of high-impact activity-induced bone gain by voluntary, unsupervised exercises. An 8-month follow-up of a randomised controlled trial. Journal of Bone and Mineral Research 14(1):125–118

Hogan H A, Argueta F M, Moe L et al 2001 Adult-onset alcohol consumption induces osteopenia in female rats. Alcoholism: Clinical and Experimental Research 25(5):746–754

Hoidrup S, Gronbaek M, Gottschau A et al 1999 Alcohol intake, beverage preference and risk of hip fracture in men and women. American Journal of Epidemiology 149(11):993–1001

Holick M F 2004 Sunlight and vitamin D for bone health and prevention of autoimmune disease, cancers and cardiovascular disease. American Journal of Clinical Nutrition 80(6 suppl):1678S–1688S

Homann C, Hasselbalch H C 1992 Haematological abnormalities in alcoholism. Ugeskrift for Laeger 154(32):2184–2187

Hu Y, Zhao X, Bai J 1999 Relationship between bone mineral density and blood and urine biochemical indices in women. Chinese Journal of Preventive Medicine 33(5):298–300

Hurley B 1995 Strength training in the elderly to enhance health status. Medicine, Exercise, Nutrition and Health 4(4):217–229

Jilka R L, Hangoc G, Girasole G 1992 Increased osteoclast development after estrogen loss: mediation by inter-leukin-6. Science 298:843–846

Karlsson M 2002 Is exercise of value in the prevention of fragility in men? Scandinavian Journal of Medicine and Science in Sports 12(4):197–210

Karlsson M K, Magnusson H, Karlsson C et al 2001 The duration of exercise as a regulator of bone mass. Bone 28(1):128–132

Kemmler W, Wildt L, Engelke K et al 2003 Acute hormonal responses of high impact physical exercise session in early postmenopausal women. European Journal of Applied Physiology 90(1–2):199–209

Kemper H C G 2000 Skeletal development during childhood and adolescence and the effects of physical activity. Paediatric Exercise Science 12(2):198–216

Klein R F, Mitchell S R, Phillips T J et al 1998 Quantitative trail loci affecting peak bone mineral density in mice. Journal of Bone and Mineral Research 13(11):1648–1656

Klein R F, Shea M, Gunness M E et al 2001 Phenotypic characterization of mice bred for high and low peak bone mass. Journal of Bone and Mineral Research 16(1):63–71

Kousteni S, Chen J R, Bellido T 2002 Reversal of bone loss in mice by nongenotropic signalling of sex steroids. Science 298:88–91

Kroger H, Reeve J 1998 Diagnosis of osteoporosis in clinical practice. Annals of Medicine 30(3):278–287

Lauder T D, Dixit S, Pezzin L E et al 2000 The relation between stress fractures and bone mineral density: evidence from active-duty women. Archives of Physical Medicine and Rehabilitation 81(1):73–79

Liu Y S, Huang W F, Li L P et al 2003 Preventive effects of exercise training on bone loss during 21 d –6 degrees head down bed-rest. Space Medicine and Medical Engineering 16(2):96–99

Lorenzo J 2003 A new hypothesis for how sex steroid hormones regulate bone mass. Journal of Clinical Investigation 111:1641–1643

Malm O J 1958 Calcium requirements and adaptation in adult men. Scandinavian Journal of Clinical and Laboratory Investigations 10(36S):1–290

Marcus R 1987 Normal and abnormal bone remodelling in man. Annual Review of Medicine 38:129–141

Marone M M, Gouveia C H, Lewin S et al 1997 Influence of body composition on the bone mass of postmenopausal women. Sao Paulo Medical Journal 115(6):1580–1588

Masud T, Morris R O 2001 Epidemiology of falls. Age and Ageing 30(suppl 4):3–7

Mayoux-Benhamou M A, Leyge J F, Roux C et al 1999 Cross-sectional study of weight-bearing activity on proximal femur bone mineral density. Calcified Tissue International 64(2):179–183

McDermott M T, Christensen R S, Lattimer J 2001 The effects of region-specific resistance and aerobic exercises on bone mineral density in premenopausal women. Military Medicine 166(4):318–321

Medras M, Jankowska E A 2000 The effect of alcohol on bone mineral density in men. Przeglad Lekarski 57(12):743–746

Mohr T, Podenphant J, Biering-Sorensen F et al 1997 Increased bone mineral density after prolonged electrically induced cycle training of paralysed limbs in spinal cord injured man. Calcified Tissue International 61(1):22–25

Murphy N M, Carroll P 2003 The effect of physical activity and its interaction with nutrition on bone health. Proceedings of the Nutritional Society 62(4):829–838

Nichols J F, Palmer J E, Levy S S 2003 Low bone mineral density in highly trained male master cyclists. Osteoporosis International 14(8):644–649

NIH ORBD-NRC (National Institutes of Health, Osteoporosis and Related Bone Diseases National Resource Center) 2000 Osteoporosis overview. Online. Available: http://www.osteo.org/osteo.html November 2001

NOF (National Osteoporosis Foundation) 2004 Medications to prevent and treat osteoporosis. Online. Available: http://www.nof.org February 2005

Odvina C V, Safi I, Wojtowicz C H et al 1995 Effect of heavy alcohol intake in the absence of liver disease on bone mass in black and white men. Journal of Clinical Endocrinology and Metabolism 80(8):2499–2503

Ortego-Centeno N, Munoz-Torres M, Jodar E et al 1997 Effect of tobacco consumption on bone mineral density in healthy young males. Calcified Tissue International 60(6):496–500

Orwoll E S, Belknap J K, Klein R F 2001 Gender specificity in the genetic determinants of peak bone mass. Journal of Bone and Mineral Research 16(11):1962–1971

Osteoporosis Australia 2005 What you should know about osteoporosis. Online. Available: http://www.osteroporosis.org.au January 2005

Parfitt A M 1988 Bone remodelling: relationship to the amount and structure of bone and the pathogenesis and prevention of fractures. In: Riggs B, Melton L (eds) Osteoporosis: etiology, diagnosis and management. Raven Press, New York

Peacock M, Keller D L, Hui S et al 2004 Peak bone mineral density at the hip is linked to chromosomes. Osteoporosis International 15(6):489–496

Pereira S J A, Costa D F, Fonseca J E et al 2004 Low bone mineral density in professional scuba divers. Clinical Rheumatology 23(1):19–20

Pettersson U, Nordstrom P, Lorentzon R 1999 A comparison of bone mineral density and muscle strength in young male adults with different exercise level. Calcified Tissue International 64(6):490–498

Pouilles J M, Tremollieres F, Ribot C 1995 Influence of body weight variations on the rate of bone loss at the beginning of menopause. Annals d'Endocrinologie 56(6):585–589

Prelevic G M, Markou A, Arnold A et al 2004 The effect of tibolone on bone mineral density in postmenopausal women with osteopenia or osteoporosis: 8 years follow-up. Maturitas 47(3):229–234

Raisz L G, Kream B E 1983 Regulation of bone formation. New England Journal of Medicine 309:29, 83

Reid J R 2002 Relationships among body mass, its components, and bone. Bone 31(5):547–555

Rico H, Cabranes J A, Cabello J et al 1987 Low serum osteocalcin in acute alcohol intoxication: a direct toxic effect of alcohol on osteoblasts. Bone and Mineral 2(3):221–225

Rosen H N 2003 Biochemical markers of bone turnover: clinical utility. Current Opinion in Endocrinology and Diabetes 10(6):387–393

Rowett H C Q 1990 Basic anatomy and physiology, 3rd edn. John Murray, London

Sambrook P N 2005 How to prevent steroid induced osteoporosis. Annals of the Rheumatic Diseases 64(2):176–178

Sampson H W 1997 Alcohol, osteoporosis and bone regulating hormones. Alcoholism: Clinical and Experimental Research 21(3):400

Sampson H W, Hebert V A, Booe H L et al 1998 Effect of alcohol consumption on adult and aged bone: composition, morphology and hormone levels of a rat animal model. Alcoholism: Clinical and Experimental Research 22(8):1746–1753

Scheiber L B, Torregrosa L 1998 Evaluation and treatment of postmenopausal osteoporosis. Seminars in Arthritis and Rheumatism 27(4):245–261

Shackelford L C, Le Blanc A D, Driscoll T B et al 2004 Resistance exercise as a countermeasure to disuse-induced bone loss. Journal of Applied Physiology 97(1):119–129

Sheth R D 2004 Bone health in paediatric epilepsy. Epilepsy and Behavior 5(suppl 2):S30–S35

Snow-Harter C, Marcus R 1991 Exercise, bone mineral density, and osteoporosis. Exercise and Sport Sciences Reviews 19:351–388

Stewart A D, Hannan J 2000 Total and regional bone density in male runners, cyclists and controls. Medicine and Science in Sports and Exercise 32(8):1373–1377

Stoch S A, Wysong E, Connolly C et al 2000 Classification of osteoporosis and osteopenia in men is dependent on site-specific analysis. Journal of Clinical Densitometry 3(4):311–318

Stock H, Schneider A, Strauss E 2004 Osteoporosis: a disease in men. Clinical Orthopaedics and Related Research 1(425):143–151

Szulc P, Garnero P, Claustrat B et al 2002 Increased bone resorption in moderate smokers with low body weight: The Minos study. Journal of Clinical Endocrinology and Metabolism 87(2):666–674

Tanko L B, Christiansen C 2004 An update on the antiestrogenic effect of smoking: a literature review with implications for researchers and practitioners. Menopause 11(1):104–109

Teegarden D, Prouix W R, Martin B R et al 1995 Peak bone mass in young women. Journal of Bone and Mineral Research 10(5):711–715

Thorsen K, Kristoffersson A, Lorentzon R 1996 The effect of brisk walking on markers of bone and calcium metabolism in postmenopausal women. Calcified Tissue International 58(4):221–225

Torstveit M K 2002 Does exercise improve the skeleton of young women? Tidsskrift for Den Norske Laegeforening 122(21):2112–2115

Verbovoi A F 2001 Effect of local and overall vibration on bone mineral density and phosphorus and calcium metabolism. Gigiena i Sanitariia 6:42–44

Villareal D T, Binder E F, Yarasheski K E et al 2003 Training added to ongoing hormone replacement therapy on bone mineral density in frail elderly women. Journal of the American Geriatrics Society 51(7):985–990

Vogel J M, Davis J W, Nomura A et al 1997 The effects of smoking on bone mass and the rates of bone loss among elderly Japanese-American Men. Journal of Bone and Mineral Research 12(9):1495–1501

Wang Q, Nicholson P H F, Suuriniemi M et al 2004 Relationship of sex hormones to bone geometric properties and mineral density in early pubertal girls. Journal of Clinical Endocrinology and Metabolism 89(4):1698–1703

WHO (World Health Organization) 1994 The WHO study group on osteoporosis. 1994 Assessment of fracture risk and its application to screening for post-menopausal osteoporosis. WHO, Geneva

Williams F M K, Cherkas L F, Spector T D et al 2005 The effect of moderate alcohol consumption on bone mineral density: a study of female twins. Annals of the Rheumatic Diseases 64(2):309–310

Wimalawansa S M, Wimalawansa S J 1999 Simulated weightlessness-induced attenuation of testosterone production may be responsible for bone loss. Endocrine 10(3):253–260

Zhao J 2001 Effects of exercise modes on peak bone mineral density in human subjects. Hong Kong Journal of Sports Medicine and Sports Science May: 64–72

Zhao J X, Zhang L 2000 Effect of exercise mode on peak bone mineral density in human bodies. Chinese Journal of Sports Medicine 19(2):163–166

Chapter 12

Adults with and surviving from cancer

CHAPTER CONTENTS

Introduction   191
Aetiology   192
    Chemical agents   192
    Tobacco smoking   192
    Diet   192
    Radiation   192
    Infectious agents   192
    Age   192
    Physical inactivity   193
Pathology   193
    Stages of cancer   194
Treatments   194
    Surgery   194
    Radiation   194
    Pharmacological   194
        Chemotherapy   194
        Hormone therapy   194
Physical activity/exercise   195
    Immune system   195
        Regular physical activity/exercise   195
        Single bout of physical activity/exercise   195

Hormones   196
Damage and repair   196
Insulin   197
Body composition   197
Treatment-related symptoms   197
Pre-physical activity/exercise prescription   197
    Newly diagnosed patients   197
    Survivors and patients undergoing treatment   198
Physical activity/exercise prescription   198
Current suggested guidelines   198
    Strength/resistance training   198
    Debilitated individuals   198
Considerations and contraindications   199
    Absolute contraindications   199
    Treatments   199
        Surgery   199
        Radiation   199
        Chemotherapy   199
        Hormone therapy   199
Summary   199
Suggested readings, references and bibliography   200

INTRODUCTION

Cancer is a collective term that refers to a group of diseases characterized by abnormal cell development, proliferation and the ability of the cells to migrate to distal tissue (ACS 2003). More than 10 million individuals are diagnosed with cancer each year, and it is estimated that by 2020 there will be, every year, around 15 million new cases. Cancer causes around 6 million deaths every year or 12% of deaths worldwide (WHO 2003). Yet, despite these high mortality rates increasing numbers of sufferers are surviving after treatment. It has been estimated that the 5-year relative survival rate in the USA, across all cancers and at all stages of the disease, is around 62%, and this figure increases to over 90% for early detection of the more common cancers, such as breast and colon cancer (ACS 2003). There is also growing evidence that physical activity at the various stages of cancer can be of great benefit to the quality of life of these individuals (Courneya 2003). Therefore, there is the need for an understanding of the requirements of these individuals at various stages of their treatment and recovery, of their particular type of cancer and the implication of their treatment and medications upon their physical capacity, so that appropriate physical activity (PA)/exercise may be prescribed. However, as there are many different cancers, it is beyond the scope of this chapter to address each individual type. Nonetheless, the aim will be to focus more generally on common cancers and the influence that PA/exercise may have both during and after treatment.

AETIOLOGY

Hereditary factors account for less than around 10% of cancers (ACS 2003) and enough is known about the causes to prevent about one-third of all cancers worldwide. The modifiable causes of cancer have been attributed to exposure to carcinogens such as tobacco smoking, ultraviolet and poor diet (WHO 2003), and lack of physical activity (Lee 2003).

CHEMICAL AGENTS

The association between cancer and exposure to chemicals was described as long ago as 1775 when Percivall Pott noted that chimney sweeps had a high incidence of cancer of the scrotum, which was attributed to exposure to soot. Since then many hundreds of chemical carcinogens have been implicated in the causation of cancer (Phillips et al 2001). These include asbestos, which can lead to lung cancer; aniline dyes, implicated in bladder cancer; and benzene, which has been found to cause leukaemia. Therefore, the prevention of occupational and environmental exposure to these and other chemicals is important in the prevention of cancer (WHO 2003).

The majority of chemical carcinogens modify the deoxyribonucleic acid (DNA) of exposed cells, inducing mutations. Some chemical agents are not themselves carcinogenic but are converted to carcinogenic derivatives by the body's metabolic enzymes. Chemical carcinogenesis is thought to occur through processes termed 'initiation' and 'promotion'. Initiation is the acquisition of a mutation by a cell following exposure to a carcinogen. Exposure to a carcinogen alone is not usually sufficient for tumour formation to occur. If the cell, however, is then exposed to a promoter then a tumour may form. Promoters are not themselves mutagenic but are potent mitogens and induce proliferation of cells, though application of a promoter without prior initiation will not lead to tumour formation (Phillips et al 2001).

TOBACCO SMOKING

Tobacco smoking is the single largest preventable cause of cancer, and in 2000 there were 1.1 million deaths from lung or bronchial cancer worldwide. While tobacco smoking is known to be the major cause, resulting in around 80–90% of all lung cancer deaths (including those from oral cavity, larynx, oesophagus and stomach cancer) (WHO 2003), occupational carcinogen exposure and possibly air pollution may also make a small contribution (Cohen 2003, Whitrow et al 2003).

DIET

There is a strong link between overweight/obesity and cancers of the oesophagus, colorectum, breast, endometrium and kidney. A diet high in fruit and vegetables may have a protective effect against many cancers. Conversely, excess consumption of red and preserved meat may be associated with an increased risk of colorectal cancer (WHO 2003).

RADIATION

Exposure to ionizing radiation is known to cause certain cancers. For instance, uranium miners have shown 10-fold increases in incidence of lung cancer and mortality rates from leukaemia. Ionizing radiations are carcinogenic because they can interact with DNA and induce mutations, as the rays disrupt the DNA's chemical bonds. Ultraviolet radiation reacts differently with DNA than ionizing radiation, but is also capable of causing skin cancer. Therefore, avoiding excessive exposure and the use of sunscreens and protective clothing are effective preventive measures (Phillips et al 2001, WHO 2003).

Damage caused by exposure to chemical carcinogens or radiation is not necessarily permanent as cells have the capacity to repair DNA. However, repair is required to take place prior to cell division to prevent the transmission of a potentially harmful mutation to the daughter cells (Phillips et al 2001).

INFECTIOUS AGENTS

Infectious agents are responsible for around 22% of cancer deaths in the developing world and 6% in industrial countries. For example, viral hepatitis B and C can result in cancer of the liver, human papilloma virus can lead to cervical cancer and the bacterium *Helicobacter pylori* increases risk of stomach cancer. In certain countries the parasitic infection schistosomiasis increases the risk of bladder cancer and in other countries the liver fluke increases the risk of cholangiocarcinoma of the bile ducts. Preventative measures include vaccination and prevention of infection and infestation (WHO 2003).

Virus-associated cancers occur in both immunocompetent and immunodeficient individuals, although the latter are at greater risk, such as those with AIDS, indicating that the immune system plays a role in preventing the development of cancer (p. 195). The development of virus-associated cancers in immunocompetent individuals suggests that the virus-infected tumour cell is also able to escape immune recognition (Phillips et al 2001).

AGE

Incidence of cancer increases with age, which may have more to do with lifestyle and increased years of exposure to carcinogens than age per se, although immune system function decreases with age and may be a contributing factor. Nonetheless, older individuals who regularly exercise have been found to show increased levels of T cells compared to age-matched controls (Mazzeo 1994).

PHYSICAL INACTIVITY

There is sufficient epidemiological evidence to associate lack of physical activity with many cancers, particularly common cancers such as colon and breast cancer (Mctiernan et al 1998, Thune & Furberg 2001). A symposium held by the ACSM, regarding physical activity and cancer, reviewed epidemiological studies from North America, Europe, England, Asia, Australia and New Zealand (Lee 2003), and they generally found that 'hard muscular work' was important for cancer prevention. At least 50 studies looking at the association between physical activity and risk of developing colon cancer found that despite the sparseness of data, around 30–60 minutes per day of moderate to vigorous intensity PA/exercise (Appendix B, Table B.3) appeared to be sufficient to decrease risk in both men and women; this may in part be due to the effect of physical activity on peristalsis, which reduces bowel transit time and probably diminishes exposure of the intestinal mucosa to faecal carcinogens (Marti 1992, Hardman 2001). Conversely, at least 30 studies showed no association between physical activity and risk of developing rectal cancer, finding rates to be similar among active and inactive men and women.

Most notably, Lee (2003) studied 53 papers that observed lower cancer rates among physically active women. Even though not all of the studies directly examined the duration of exercise bouts, women who expended ≥1500 kcal per week in moderate and vigorous PA/exercise (equivalent to about 3–4 hours per week) experienced 20% lower rates of breast cancer than women who expended <200 kcal per week. Additionally, 36 studies investigating the association between physical activity and risk of developing prostate cancer (the most commonly diagnosed cancer in men in Western countries) found as much as a 70% reduction in risk among the active compared to the least physically active men. Despite the confounding influence of factors such as cigarette smoking, 21 studies investigating risk of lung cancer reported lower rates among the physically active individuals. Other site-specific cancers were also investigated and although the data were limited, regular participation in PA/exercise may play a role in the prevention of endometrial, ovarian, testicular, pancreatic, kidney, bladder and haematopoietic cancers. Hence, although it was suggested that more studies are required to determine the shape of the dose–response curve and the optimal amount, intensity, duration and frequency to reduce one's risk of developing certain cancers, and also more studies from other subject populations, the epidemiological evidence strongly indicates that regular PA/exercise

is beneficial in preventing risk of cancer (Lee 2003). It is, however, important to note that individuals who are habitually physically active or work in physically demanding occupations are likely to adopt generally healthier lifestyles, thus reducing their risk of cancer-associated factors such as cigarette smoking or poor diets. Furthermore, common genetic factors may predispose an individual toward both a physically active lifestyle and low risk of cancer (Mackinnon 1999).

PATHOLOGY

The mechanism by which carcinogenic agents stimulate the development of cancer has been under extensive research for many years, and it appears that changes occur in the expression of cells' regulatory genes (DNA) that can lead to the development of cancer (Phillips et al 2001). Cancer is a cellular disorder and although there are several hundred different types of cancer, generally they share similar characteristics. Cancer cells experience uncontrolled and disorganized growth. Normal cells, for example, generally only divide around fifty times before they die. Cancer cells, however, continue dividing, tending to reproduce over and over again, never differentiating. In laboratory tissue cultures, cancer cells lack what is known as contact inhibition. Contact inhibition, exhibited by normal cells, is when a cell stops reproducing when it contacts another cell and/or the sides of a culture bowl. Normal cells, in a tissue culture, tend to grow in only one layer, as they stop growing once they contact either the side of the bowl or another cell. Cancer cells, however, do not display contact inhibition and grow in multiple layers. In vivo, a cancer cell will continue to divide and forms a growth, or tumour, that invades and destroys neighbouring healthy tissue. This new growth is termed neoplasia, and is made up of cells that are disorganized, a condition termed anaplasia. The cells are disorganized because they do not differentiate into the tissue or organ and never fulfil the function of the organ. To support their growth, cancer cells release a growth factor that causes vascularization of neighbouring blood vessels to branch into the cancer tissue. Furthermore, cancer cells may detach from the primary tumour and spread around the body. The cancer cells have receptors that enable them to adhere to the base membranes of blood and lymph vessels. They also produce proteolytic enzymes that degrade the membrane and allow them to invade the underlying tissues and cross over into the main vessel and enter the systemic and/or lymphatic circulation (Fig. 12.1).

Cancer cells also tend to be motile, which may be associated with their disorganized internal cytoskeleton and their lack of intact microfilament bundles. After travelling through the blood and/or lymphatic system, cancer cells may start a new tumour elsewhere in the body,

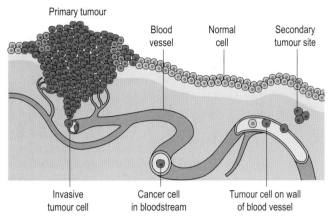

Figure 12.1 Process of tumour and metastasis (adapted from http://sciencemuseum.org.uk/exhibitions/lifecycle/77.asp).

through the process known as metastasis. Benign tumours are those that remain in one place and malignant tumours are those that metastasize. If the original tumour is found before metastasis has occurred the chances of survival after treatment are greatly increased (Cancer Information and Support International 2003).

STAGES OF CANCER

Cancer staging describes the size and extent and spread of a malignant tumour and is used to plan treatment and predict prognosis. This can be particularly useful in allowing the exercise practitioner to appropriately assist and prescribe to the patient/client. However, staging systems are different between countries; hence readers may need to refer to their local oncology centre for the method employed in their country.

TREATMENTS

The functional impact of cancer depends upon a variety of factors, including type, stage, pre-existing co-morbidities and overall health, age at time of diagnosis and treatment status. Irrespective of the location and functional impact of cancer, the goal of the treatment is to eradicate any cancerous cells and prevent subsequent proliferation and metastasis. This may be achieved through surgery, radiation therapy and systemic therapy (i.e. drugs), all of which have an effect on the patient's quality of life, are potentially toxic and have pronounced side effects (Salmon & Swank 2002, Courneya 2003). Combinations of these therapies are commonly employed in the treatment of cancer and will undoubtedly influence the patient's ability to carry out PA/exercise and the extent of this will need to be ascertained by the exercise practitioner.

SURGERY

Surgery can be used in diagnosis, treatment and cure, though diagnosis is increasingly done via non-surgical procedures. It is, however, common practice for certain cancers to have the primary tumour surgically removed (Souhami & Tobias 1998), and about 60% of cancer survivors will have had the primary tumour removed surgically (Courneya 2003). Surgery may in certain cases result in amputation, pain, diminished flexibility, and/or motor and sensory nerve damage (Salmon & Swank 2002), as well as diarrhoea, dyspnoea and lymphoedema (Courneya 2003).

RADIATION

More than 50% of cancer survivors undergo radiation therapy at some point during their treatment. This treatment is typically administered in small repeated doses over a period of 5 to 8 weeks, which is done in order to maximize the death of cancer cells and minimize normal cell damage (Courneya 2003). However, toxicity to normal tissue does occur and may result in diminished flexibility in exposed joints, scarring of heart and/or lungs (Salmon & Swank 2002), also potentially resulting in nausea, fatigue, dry mouth, diarrhoea and cardiomyopathy (Courneya 2003).

PHARMACOLOGICAL

Systemic treatment, such as the administration of certain drugs, is prescribed for the treatment of many different types of cancer. There are presently three main types of drug treatments; chemotherapy, endocrine or hormone therapy and biological or immunotherapy (Souhami & Tobias 1998, Salmon & Swank 2002, Courneya 2003).

Chemotherapy

Chemotherapy is usually administered intravenously or orally and given in repeated courses or cycles 2 to 4 weeks apart over a 3- to 6-month period (Courneya 2003). The side effects of this treatment may include peripheral nerve damage, cardiomyopathy, pulmonary fibrosis and anaemia; the latter is an especially common side effect of many anticancer drugs (Salmon & Swank 2002).

Hormone therapy

Hormone therapy, especially in the treatment of breast cancer, has been transformed in recent years, and knowledge of a tumour's hormone receptor status has become clinically important (Souhami & Tobias 1998). This type of treatment is usually administered orally. It also has significant side effects such as weight gain, fat accumulation to the trunk and face, loss of muscle mass, proximal muscle weakness, osteoporosis, fatigue, hot flushes and increased susceptibility to infection (Courneya 2003).

PHYSICAL ACTIVITY/EXERCISE

The relationship between PA/exercise and cancer is complex and not fully understood, and although the physical as well as psychological benefits of physical activity are beginning to be recognized for individuals suffering and surviving from cancer, it is not considered a treatment but more part of disease management. Nevertheless, PA/exercise may potentially influence several physiological mechanisms that affect the development and progression of cancer.

IMMUNE SYSTEM

Although the majority of cancers are non-immunogenic, evidence exists to suggest that the immune system is involved in defence against tumours of a viral origin (Janeway & Travers 1996). Physical activity/exercise is also known the have an effect on the immune system (Mackinnon 1999) and in order to understand the effect that PA/exercise might have a brief overview of this system is provided.

The immune system is capable of recognizing and defending the body against foreign environmental or novel molecules, such as proteins called immunogens. These include viruses, bacteria, fungi and parasites; tumour growth; cell and tissue transplantation and allergens. The response of the system to any of these challenges involves a complex communication and coordination between cells, tissues and messenger molecules throughout the body. The immune response is initiated when an antigen breaks through the chemical and physical barriers protecting the body. This pathogen is usually engulfed by a phagocyte, which then digests it. The phagocyte then processes the foreign protein, and the foreign protein appears on the phagocyte's surface. The appearance of the foreign protein on the phagocyte's surface then stimulates the activation of T-helper lymphocytes, which then stimulate other immune cells to proliferate and secrete substances that combat the pathogen. Antibodies are then produced against the foreign protein by mature B cells. In addition, during the early stages of the body's encounter with the foreign microbe, memory T and B cells are generally produced that respond quickly to subsequent infection by the same agent, in the majority of cases conferring immunity (Fig. 12.2). The combination of these processes is usually effective against most pathogens. However, in some instances the host's defences are ineffective or inappropriate and infection may persist (Mackinnon 1999).

Although infectious agents may in certain cases stimulate cancer (p. 192), cancer is not an infectious disease. Notwithstanding this, there is research to indicate that the immune system destroys cancerous cells (Phillips et al 2001) and stimulation of the immune system

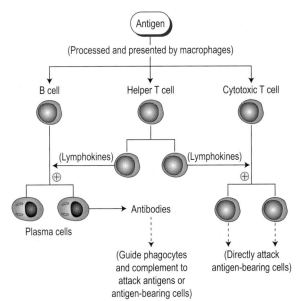

Figure 12.2   General scheme of the immune response to an antigen (adapted from Vander et al 1990).

through PA/exercise may help those being treated and recovering from cancer (Pedersen 1997, Mackinnon 1999).

Regular physical activity/exercise

Cancer treatments, such as surgery, radiotherapy and systemic therapy, can result in some degree of impairment to the immune system, which makes the individual undergoing such treatment more vulnerable to infection. Regular moderate PA/exercise, however, is known to enhance the immune system (Newsholme & Parry-Billings 1994), as it causes the release of cytokines, which, in this regard, coordinate antibody and T-cell immune interactions and amplify immune reactivity, which may assist the cancer sufferer to resist infection and/or further development of additional cancer. It has been suggested that cytokines play a role in the defence against tumour growth and metastasis through stimulating adhesion of tumour cells to extracellular proteins, which may enhance the interaction with cytotoxic T cells and natural killer cells. Natural killer cells are lymphocytes that are capable of binding and killing virus-infected cells and some tumour cells by releasing cytotoxins. Furthermore, PA/exercise has also been found to release interleukin-2 (which enhances T lymphocytes and natural killer cells), which may further assist in defence against cancer cells (Pedersen 1997, Mackinnon 1999).

Single bout of physical activity/exercise

In vitro experiments on animal cells have found that single bouts of PA/exercise enhance macrophage-mediated tumour cytotoxicity (Davis et al 1998), indicating that a single bout of PA/exercise stimulates immune system activity. Nonetheless, extreme PA/exercise can depress the immune system (Nieman 1994, Castell et al 1997) and for this and other reasons should be avoided in patients undergoing treatment and recovering from cancer.

HORMONES

The steroid hormones progesterone, oestrogen and testosterone are associated with both female and male reproductive cancers, and these hormones are known to have both a mitogenic and proliferative effect. One of the mechanisms by which regular physical activity may influence cancer is through its effect on these hormones (Westerlind 2003).

It has been suggested that exposure of oestrogen to the breast is a stimulus for breast cancer, and the number of menstrual cycles a women experiences has been related to breast cancer risk. Therefore, delay of menarche and establishment of menstrual cycle would decrease total steroid hormone exposure, thus hypothetically reducing risk (Apter 1996). It is also well known that menarche tends to commence later in girls who regularly participate in athletic activities (Berstein et al 1987) and delays have been observed in these girls' normal ovarian cycle (Apter 1996). This would therefore decrease their overall levels of oestrogen exposure and may be a potential mechanism for the observed reduction in rates of breast cancer in active women (Lee 2003). Reductions in oestrogen and progesterone have also been shown to reduce proliferative activity, and women who carry out vigorous exercise display reductions in serum levels of these hormones (Bullen et al 1985). However, vigorous PA/exercise would not generally be recommended for those women undertaking or recovering from cancer treatment. It is of interest to note that research has shown oestrogen supplementation in animals to reduce physical activity behaviour (Hoffman-Goetz et al 2001). Hence it could be speculated that girls who naturally have lower levels of oestrogen may be predisposed toward being more physically active (Westerlind 2003), and is an additional factor for consideration in the relationship between physical activity and cancer. Nonetheless, in laboratory adolescent rats, alterations have been shown in their mammary gland cell turnover in response to exercise training (Westerlind et al 2002). Whilst proliferation of these cells was observed in the first 4 weeks of training, this was followed by cell apoptosis in weeks 6 and 8. Since no hyperplasia was observed this suggested the increase in proliferation was compensated by the increase in cell apoptosis. Furthermore, a study carried out on women (Gram et al 1999) found moderate PA/exercise, of more than 2 hours per week, to be weakly inversely associated with risk of breast cancer, after adjustment for menopausal status and body mass. Thus PA/exercise intervention probably does have a beneficial effect upon breast cancer risk.

It has been speculated that more subtle, non-clinically detectable changes may occur as a result of regular PA/exercise that are not related to menstrual function or fertility, which may affect cancer risk (Westerlind 2003). Oestrogens are metabolized primarily through two mutually exclusive pathways, C-2 and C-16-α-hydroxylation (Zhu & Conney 1998). The C-2-hydroxylation pathway results in metabolites without oestrogen activity, whereas the C-16-α-hydroxylation pathway results in metabolites that are relatively potent oestrogens (Westerlind et al 1998). Research on female athletes has indicated that they possess increased levels of oestrogens via the 2-hydroxylation pathway (Snow et al 1989), which might be a mechanism by which regular PA/exercise reduces risk of certain cancers in active individuals. Furthermore, increases in 2-hydroxylation and/or decreases in 16-α-hydroxylation have also been associated with decreases in breast cancer and cervical cancer risk (Sepkovic et al 1995, Ho et al 1998). Additionally, increased 2-hydroxylation has been associated with decreased risk of prostate cancer in men (Muti et al 2002). Elevated levels of 16-α-hydroxylation have also been linked with obesity (Schneider et al 1983), which might, in part, explain the increased risk of cancer in obese individuals (Albanes 1990). Moreover, research has also found that exercise alters the 2-hydroxyoestrogens to yield 2-methoxyoestradiol, which is a powerful anti-angiogenic (De Cree et al 1998) and is currently being used in trials for chemotherapy (Westerlind 2003).

Male sex hormones are known to affect testicular and prostate tumours, and whilst some studies have found regular PA/exercise to show reductions in these hormones (Hackney et al 1998, Wheeler et al 2002) others have found no change (Lucia et al 1996). Nonetheless, regular PA/exercise may affect the ability of these hormones to bind to their specific receptor site, making them less available (Westerlind 2003). Conversely, however, studies have indicated that PA/exercise may actually increase risk of prostate cancer (Srivastava & Kreiger 2000), where incidence of prostate cancer has been found to be positively correlated with upper body muscle mass (Severson et al 1988). Since increased muscularity is associated with increased levels of male sex hormones, the larger muscle mass often found in physically active men might partly explain the link between PA/exercise and risk of prostate cancer. However, the effect of resistance exercise upon prostate cancer does not appear to have been specifically investigated and is an obvious area for future research, as is the effect of PA/exercise upon testicular cancer (Westerlind 2003).

DAMAGE AND REPAIR

Physical activity/exercise, especially of a vigorous and/or prolonged nature, may lead to cell and tissue damage, resulting in damage to lipids, proteins and DNA. During exercise the body is placed under enhanced oxidative stress as it increases the production of oxygen free radicals (Ji 1999). These oxygen free radicals are also capable of causing cell mutagenesis and induction of tumour cell proliferation. To counteract these free radicals the body possesses a free radical scavenger and antioxide system (Dreher & Junod 1996). Under resting, and low to moderate PA/exercise levels (Kido et al 1997), this system assists the body in defending itself against the production of these free radicals. However, during vigorous PA/exercise conditions, increased oxidative damage generally occurs (Poulsen et al 1996), despite antioxidant enzyme repair also being enhanced (Robertson et al 1991). Hence the beneficial or deleterious effect of prescribed PA/exercise may be dependent upon its intensity and duration, in addition to the person's physical and nutritional status. Furthermore, the efficiency of the antioxidant system tends to diminish with increased age, and habitual PA/exercise training has been found to attenuate this decline (Kretzschmar & Muller 1993). Hence the intervention of moderate PA/exercise may be able to slow the loss of antioxidants in this population (Westerlind 2003) and assist these individuals during treatment and recovery from cancer.

INSULIN

The role of insulin as a carcinogenic agent has been investigated (Westley & May 1995) and non-insulin-dependent diabetes mellitus (NIDDM) has been positively associated with incidence of cancer (Hu et al 1999). Indeed, serum levels have been found to be elevated in individuals with cancer without disease-related hyperinsulinaemia (Del Giudice et al 1998). Hence individuals suffering from insulin resistance and with NIDDM would potentially be at risk (Westerlind 2003). Given that insulin levels are also influenced by PA/exercise (p. 88), obesity and fat distribution (p. 83) (Bjorntorp 1991), and that PA/exercise appears to compensate for insulin resistance caused by a high-fat diet (Kraegen et al 1989), PA/exercise may be another mechanism for protection against cancer. During PA/exercise insulin-like growth factor (IGF-1) has been found to alter (Nguyen et al 1998) and this factor is thought to play a major role in carcinogenesis (Westley & May 1995). However, more research is required to establish the effect of different types of PA/exercise upon this factor.

BODY COMPOSITION

Body fat distribution, especially abdominal fat (Schapira et al 1990, Giovannucci et al 1995), and general obesity have been associated with numerous cancers (Albanes 1990); and since habitually physically active individuals tend to have lower abdominal fat levels (Pescatello & Murphy 1998) and not to be overweight or obese, this might explain the observed relationship between physical activity and cancer (Lee 2003). Physical activity/exercise has also been independently related to cancer risk when controlled for

body weight and body mass index (Albanes et al 1989, Slattery et al 1997). However, in rats whose energy metabolism was modulated by restricting dietary calories and/or by increasing energy expenditure through exercise, there was no conclusive cancer inhibition, despite the exercise groups displaying significant reductions in carcass fat (Gillette et al 1997). This is of interest as calorie restriction has been shown to be protective against tumour development (Kritchevsky 1999). Nonetheless, there are several possible physiological mechanisms by which PA/exercise might influence risk of cancer in overweight and obese individuals. For instance, obesity has been associated with altered oestrogen metabolism (Schneider et al 1983) (p. 196) and with insulin resistance and elevated levels of insulin-like growth factor (Ballard-Barbash et al 1997), all of which have been shown to have carcinogenic properties, and are influenced by PA/exercise. This highlights the complex relationship between PA/exercise, obesity and cancer.

TREATMENT-RELATED SYMPTOMS

Increasingly research is finding that PA/exercise prescription can assist the cancer patient in relief of treatment-related symptoms, although the exact frequency, type and dose has yet to be fully determined. In parts of the USA, administration of PA/exercise intervention is a concomitant part of cancer patients' treatment regimen and research carried out using individualized PA/exercise found a reversal in cancer treatment-related fatigue and increased muscular efficiency and mobility (Carter 2003), thus indicating the benefits of individualized PA/exercise programmes for this population.

PRE-PHYSICAL ACTIVITY/EXERCISE PRESCRIPTION

Identification of cancer risk factors is important in early detection and these may be incorporated into any pre-PA/exercise screening questionnaire (Appendix A, Fig. A.2). For those individuals who have cancer, the exercise practitioner should confirm with their doctor and/or cancer team that they are deemed well enough to undertake PA/exercise.

NEWLY DIAGNOSED PATIENTS

Pre-PA/exercise prescription assessment exercise testing is a valuable assessment tool for those individuals newly diagnosed with cancer, as it can establish a baseline functional capacity to help assess the subsequent impact of treatment, and may serve as a foundation for exercise prescription both during and following treatment (Salmon & Swank 2002).

SURVIVORS AND PATIENTS UNDERGOING TREATMENT

For survivors of cancer, who have not previously been assessed by the exercise practitioner, the treatment may cause deconditioning and the patient may be emaciated. Therefore, very low-level protocols will be required. Individuals who have received chest irradiation or chemotherapy, which is toxic to the heart and lungs, will require careful monitoring (Selby 1997).

PHYSICAL ACTIVITY/EXERCISE PRESCRIPTION

The effect of exercise on individuals diagnosed with cancer has only relatively recently undergone systematic research. There are at present comparatively few studies that have been carried out on human subjects and the amount and type of PA/exercise that produces optimal results still needs to be determined. Nonetheless, a review of PA/exercise studies carried out on women during breast cancer treatment showed that exercise had a significant beneficial effect on exercise capacity, body weight and composition, flexibility, fatigue, nausea, physical well-being, functional well-being, satisfaction with life and overall quality of life. The effect of PA/exercise after treatment for breast cancer was also reviewed and these studies showed improvements in aerobic capacity, number of monocytes, natural killer cell cytotoxic activity, depression, anxiety, mood, self-esteem, physical well-being, satisfaction with life and overall quality of life. The review also showed similar findings from a range of studies carried out on individuals with a variety of different cancers both during and after cancer treatment (Courneya 2003). The types of interventions differed in length (anywhere from 6 or more weeks) and mode (aerobic, strength and combined programmes) and were based upon traditional guidelines. For example, 22 cancer patients (57 ± 10 years) diagnosed with various types and stages of cancer and 19 controls (49 ± 11 years) underwent 6 months, 3 days per week of individualized PA/exercise prescription. Post-intervention, the experimental group were found to have significantly improved aerobic capacity, time on a treadmill and abdominal strength compared to the control group. Additionally, psychological measures of total fatigue were also significantly reduced compared to the controls (Carter et al 2003).

CURRENT SUGGESTED GUIDELINES

The PA/exercise prescription goal should be to improve strength, endurance and psychological status and maintain and improve physical status (Selby 1997), taking an integrative physiological and psychological approach to the prescription (Salmon & Swank 2002). Although there are currently no clear guidelines for individuals diagnosed with, undergoing treatment for or surviving from cancer, it has been suggested that PA/exercise practitioners should follow the current US Surgeon General's 1996 recommendations of 30 minutes of continuous exercise three to four times per week with attention to safely measures and general health maintenance (McNeill 1999). Moderate-intensity exercise for 20–30 minutes has been suggested with modifications as required, including very short PA/exercise bouts of around 3–5 minutes followed by rest periods (Salmon & Swank 2002). Walking and cycling, 3 to 5 times per week, have also been recommended as safe and generally well-tolerated forms of aerobic exercise; and for more deconditioned individuals, daily sessions of shorter duration and lower intensity (ACSM 2000, Courneya et al 2000). However, other researchers have suggested more detailed PA/exercise guidelines, especially for early stage cancer patients and survivors (Courneya et al 2000); and considering the extreme variability of the effects of cancer and treatment regimens on functional capacity, in addition to the possibility of other co-morbidities and factors such as increased age, it is recommended that the prescription should be more highly individualized (Selby 1997, Salmon & Swank 2002).

STRENGTH/RESISTANCE TRAINING

Some studies have employed strength training. For example, a study on 54 women aged 30 to 50 years who underwent 15 weeks of strength training found a reduction in insulin-like growth factor, a known cancer risk factor, compared to a control group (Schmitz et al 2002). However, there are currently few intervention studies with regard to cancer patients and strength/resistance training, and whether the exercise practitioner prescribes such an activity will depend on the patient's status.

DEBILITATED INDIVIDUALS

In extremely debilitated patients, the PA/exercise metabolic target may start from just above resting levels where the focus is simply on breathing and associated dyspnoea, a prime factor in management of lung cancer (Salmon & Swank 2002, ACS 2003). Physical activity may take the form of gentle yoga, stretching or gradual increase in weight-bearing. Even though these minimal interventions are unlikely to raise heart rate or fall within traditional training methods, such as 'training zone', they are important with regard to quality of life and palliative care; and may for some individuals lead to levels of PA/exercise that will eventually improve aerobic capacity and strength (Salmon & Swank 2002).

CONSIDERATIONS AND CONTRAINDICATIONS

The PA/exercise prescription for those with and surviving from cancer needs to be highly individualized owing to the extreme variability of the effects of cancer and treatment regimens on functional capacity, in addition to the possibility of other co-morbidities and factors such as increased age. Cancer and its treatment also has a profound psychological and emotional effect; therefore, the exercise practitioner should consider both psychological and physiological factors when prescribing PA/exercise (Salmon & Swank 2002).

ABSOLUTE CONTRAINDICATIONS

Absolute contraindications for PA/exercise would be similar to those cited for other individuals (Appendix A, Table A.1). However, it is always advisable to consult with the patient's doctor or cancer team when considering any form of PA/exercise.

TREATMENTS

Treatments may result in numerous side effects which will affect an individual's PA/exercise capacity and the exercise practitioner should take these as well as other co-morbidities into account.

Surgery

Surgery may in certain cases result in amputation, pain, diminished flexibility, and/or motor and sensory nerve damage (Salmon & Swank 2002), as well as diarrhoea, dyspnoea and lymphoedema (Courneya 2003).

Radiation

Radiation may result in diminished flexibility in exposed joints, scarring of heart and/or lungs (Salmon & Swank 2002), nausea, fatigue, dry mouth, diarrhoea and cardiomyopathy (Courneya 2003).

Chemotherapy

The side effects of chemotherapy treatment may include peripheral nerve damage, cardiomyopathy, pulmonary fibrosis and anaemia (Salmon & Swank 2002).

Hormone therapy

Hormone therapy may cause side effects such as weight gain, fat accumulation of the trunk and face, muscle loss, proximal muscle weakness, osteoporosis, fatigue, hot flushes and increased susceptibility to infection (Courneya 2003).

SUMMARY

- Cancer causes around 12% of deaths worldwide. Yet, increasing numbers of sufferers are surviving after treatment for cancer.
- Modifiable causes of cancer have been attributed to tobacco smoking, poor diet and exposure to carcinogens and lack of physical activity.
- Carcinogenic agents stimulate the development of cancer via changes in the DNA. Cancer is a cellular disorder and although there are many different types, generally they share similar characteristics. Cancer cells experience uncontrolled and disorganized growth.
- Epidemiological evidence associates lack of physical activity with many cancers, particularly colon and breast cancer.
- Individuals who carry out around 30–60 minutes per day of moderate to vigorous intensity PA/exercise have reduced rates of colon cancer; and active men have reduced risk of prostate cancer.
- Women who expended ≥1500 kcal per week in moderate and vigorous PA/exercise (equivalent to about 3–4 hours per week) experienced 20% lower rates of breast cancer compared to women who expended <200 kcal per week.
- PA/exercise may potentially influence several factors, such as the immune system, hormones, oxygen free radicals, insulin and body composition, that may affect the development and progression of cancer.
- PA/exercise may help relieve treatment-related symptoms.
- Sufferers and survivors of cancer show significant physiological, psychological and emotional benefits from individualized and appropriate PA/exercise intervention.
- The PA/exercise prescription for those with and surviving from cancer needs to be highly individualized owing to the extreme variability of the effects and treatment, in addition to the possibility of other co-morbidities and factors such as increased age.
- There are currently no clear guidelines for individuals diagnosed with or undergoing treatment for cancer or for survivors of cancer.
- Primary PA/exercise prescription goals should be to improve strength, endurance and psychological status and maintain and improve physical reserves, taking an integrative physiological and psychological approach to the prescription.

Suggested readings, references and bibliography

Suggested reading

Lee I-M 2003 Physical activity and cancer prevention – data from epidemiological studies. Medicine and Science in Sports and Exercise 35(11):1823–1833

Mctiernan A 2003 Physical activity, exercise, and cancer: prevention to treatment – symposium overview. Medicine and Science in Sports and Exercise 35(11):1821–1822

Mctiernan A 2003 Intervention studies in exercise and cancer prevention. Medicine and Science in Sports and Exercise 35(11):1841–1845

Pedersen B K 1997 Exercise immunology. Springer, Heidelberg

Phillips J, Murray P, Kirk P 2001 The biology of disease, 2nd edn. Blackwell Science, Oxford

Souhami R, Tobias J 1998 Cancer and its management, 3rd edn. Blackwell Science, Oxford

Westerlind K C 2003 Physical activity and cancer prevention – mechanisms. Medicine and Science in Sports and Exercise 35(11):1834–1840

References and bibliography

ACS (American Cancer Society) 2003 Cancer facts and figures 2003. American Cancer Society, Atlanta

ACSM (American College of Sports Medicine) 2000 ACSM's guidelines for exercise testing and prescription, 6th edn. Lippincott Williams & Wilkins, Philadelphia

Albanes D 1990 Energy balance, body size and cancer. Critical Reviews of Oncology and Hematology 10(3):283–303

Albanes D, Blair A, Taylor P R 1989 Physical activity and risk of cancer in the NHANES I population. American Journal of Public Health 79(6):744–750

Apter D 1996 Review. Hormonal events during female puberty in relation to breast cancer risk. European Journal of Cancer Prevention 5(6):476–482

Ballard-Barbash R, Birt D F, Kestin M et al 1997 Perspectives on integrating experimental and epidemiological research on diet, anthropometry and breast cancer. Journal of Nutrition 127 (5 suppl):S936–S939

Berstein L, Ross R K, Lobo R A et al 1987 The effects of moderate physical activity on menstrual cycle patterns in adolescence: implications for breast cancer prevention. British Journal of Cancer 55(6):681–685

Bjorntorp P 1991 Review. Metabolic implications of body fat distribution. Diabetes Care 14(12):1132–1143

Bullen B A, Skrinar G S, Beitins I Z et al 1985 Induction of menstrual disorders by strenuous exercise in untrained women. New England Journal of Medicine 312(21):1349–1353

Cancer Information and Support International 2003 Characteristics of cancer. Online. Available: http://www.cancer-info.com November 2003

Carter S D, Schneider C M, Dennehy C A et al 2003 Effects of prescriptive exercise intervention on cancer treatment-related systems. Online. Available: http://www.cancerfit.com/Research/research005.html December 2003

Castell L M, Poortmans J R, Leclercq R et al 1997 Some aspects of the acute phase response after a marathon race, and the effect of glutamine supplementation. European Journal of Applied Physiology and Occupational Physiology 75(1):47–53

Cohen A J 2003 Air pollution and lung cancer: what more do we need to know? Thorax 58(12):1010–1012

Courneya K S 2003 Exercise in cancer survivors: an overview of research. Medicine and Science in Sports and Exercise 35(11):1846–1852

Courneya K S, Mackey J R, Jones L W 2000 Coping with cancer: can exercise help? Physician and Sportsmedicine 28(5):49–73

Davis J M, Kohut M L, Jackson D A et al 1998 Exercise effects on lung tumour metastases and in vitro alveolar macrophages antitumour cytotoxicity. American Journal of Physiology 274(5 Pt 2): R1454–R1459

De Cree C, Ball P, Seidlitz B 1998 Responsiveness of plasma 2- and 4-hydroxycatecholestrogens to training and to graduate submaximal and maximal exercise in an untrained woman. International Journal of Sports Medicine 19(1):20–25

Del Giudice M E, Fantus I G, Ezzat S et al 1998 Insulin and related factors in premenopausal breast cancer risk. Breast Cancer Research and Treatment 47(2):111–120

Dreher D, Junod A F 1996 Review. Role of oxygen free radicals in cancer development. European Journal of Cancer 32A(1):30–38

Gillette C A, Zhu Z, Westerlind K C et al 1997 Energy availability and mammary carcinogenesis: effects of calorie restriction and exercise. Carcinogenesis 18(6):1183–1188

Giovannucci E, Ascherio A, Rimm E B et al 1995 Physical activity, obesity, and risk of colon cancer and adenoma in men. Annals of International Medicine 122(5):327–334

Gram I T, Funkhouser E, Tabar L 1999 Moderate physical activity in relation to mammographic patterns. Cancer Epidemiologic Biomarkers and Prevention 8(2):117–122

Hackney A, Fahrner C L, Gulledge T P 1998 Basal reproductive hormonal profiles are altered in endurance trained men. Journal of Sports Medicine and Physical Fitness 38(2):138–141

Hardman A E 2001 Physical activity and cancer risk. Proceedings of the Nutritional Society 60(1):107–113

Ho G H, Luo X W, Ji C Y et al 1998 Urinary 1/16 alpha-hydroxyestrone ratio: correlation with serum insulin-like growth factor binding protein-3 and a potential biomarker of breast cancer risk. Annals of the Academy of Medicine, Singapore 27(2):294–299

Hoffman-Goetz L, Fietsch C L, Mccutcheon D et al 2001 Effect of 17 beta-estradiol and voluntary exercise on lymphocyte apoptosis in mice. Physiology and Behavior 74(4–5):653–658

Hu F B, Manson J E, Liu S et al 1999 Prospective study of adult onset diabetes mellitus (type 2) and risk of colorectal cancer in women. Journal of the National Cancer Institute 91(6):542–547

Janeway C A, Travers P 1996 Immunobiology: the immune system in health and disease, 2nd edn. Current Biology, London

Ji L L 1999 Antioxidants and oxidative stress in exercise. Proceedings of the Society for Experimental Biology and Medicine 222(3):283–292

Kido Y, Tsukahara T, Rokutan K et al 1997 Japanese dietary protein allowance is sufficient for moderate physical exercise in young men. Journal of Nutritional Science and Vitaminology 43(1):59–71

Kraegen E W, Storlien L H, Jenkins A B et al 1989 Chronic exercise compensates for insulin resistance induced by a high-fat diet in rats. American Journal of Physiology 256(2 Pt 1):E242–E249

Kretzschmar M, Muller D 1993 Review. Aging, training and exercise: a review of effect on plasma glutathione and lipid peroxides. Sports Medicine 15(3):196–209

Kritchevsky D 1999 Review. Calorie restriction and experimental carcinogenesis. Toxicological Sciences 52(2 suppl):13–16

Lee I-M 2003 Physical activity and cancer prevention – data from epidemiological studies. Medicine and Science in Sports and Exercise 35(11):1823–1833

Lucia A, Chicharro J L, Perez L et al 1996 Reproductive function in male endurance athletes: sperm analysis and hormonal profile. Journal of Applied Physiology 81(6):2627–2636

Mackinnon L T 1999 Advances in exercise immunology. Human Kinetics, Champaign, IL

McNeill J A 1999 Health promotion for cancer survivors, In: Boyers K, Ford M B, Judkins A F et al Primary care oncology. W B Saunders, Philadelphia

Mctiernan A, Ulrich C, Slate S, Potter J 1998 Physical activity and cancer etiology: associations and mechanisms. Cancer Causes and Control 9(5):487–509

Marti B 1992 Exercise and cancer. An epidemiologic short review of the effects of physical activity on carcinoma risk. Schweizerische Medizinische Wochenschrift. Journal Suisse de Medecine 122(27–28):1048–1056

Mazzeo R S 1994 The influence of exercise and aging on immune function. Medicine and Science in Sports and Exercise 26(5):586–592

Muti P, Westerlind K C, Wu T et al 2002 Urinary estrogen metabolites and prostate cancer: a case-control study. Cancer Causes and Control 13(10):947–955

Newsholme E A, Parry-Billings M 1994 Effects of exercise on the immune system. In: Bouchard C, Shephard R J, Stephens T (eds) Physical activity, fitness and health: international proceedings consensus statement. Human Kinetics, Champaign, IL

Nguyen U N, Mougin M L, Simon-Rigaud J et al 1998 Influence of exercise duration on serum insulin-like growth factor and its binding proteins in athletes. European Journal of Applied Physiology 78(6):533–537

Nieman D C 1994 Exercise, upper respiratory tract infection, and the immune system. Medicine and Science in Sports and Exercise 26(2):128–139

Pedersen B K 1997 Exercise immunology. Springer, Heidelberg

Pescatello L S, Murphy D 1998 Lower intensity physical activity is advantageous for fat distribution and blood glucose among viscerally obese older adults. Medicine and Science in Sports and Exercise 30(9):1408–1413

Phillips J, Murray P, Kirk P 2001 The biology of disease, 2nd edn. Blackwell Science, Oxford

Poulsen H E, Loft S, Vistisen K 1996 Extreme exercise and oxidative DNA. Journal of Sports Sciences 14(4):343–346

Robertson J D, Maughan R J, Duthie G G et al 1991 Increased blood antioxidant systems of runners in response to training load. Clinical Science 80(6):611–618

Salmon P G, Swank A M 2002 Exercise-based disease management guidelines for individuals with cancer: potential applications in a high-risk mid-southern state. Journal of Exercise Physiology: Clinical Exercise Physiology. Online:5(4)

Schapira D V, Kumar, N B, Lyman G H et al 1990 Abdominal obesity and breast cancer risk. Annals of International Medicine 112(3):182–186

Schmitz, K H, Ahmed R L, Yee D 2002 Effects of nine-month strength training intervention on insulin, IGF-1, IGFBP1, and IGFBP-3 I, and IGFBP-3 in 30–50 year old women. Cancer Epidemiology, Biomarkers and Prevention 11(12):1597–1604

Schneider J, Bradlow H L, Strain G et al 1983 Effects of obesity on estradiol metabolism: decreased formation of nonuterotropic metabolites. Journal of Clinical Endocrinology Metabolism 56(5):973–978

Selby G 1997 Cancer. In: American College of Sports Medicine, Exercise management for persons with chronic diseases and disabilities. Human Kinetics, Champaign, IL

Sepkovic D W, Bradlow H L, Ho G et al 1995 Estrogen metabolite ratios and risk assessment of hormone-related cancers: assay validation and prediction or cervical cancer risk. Annals of the New York Academy of Science 768:312–316

Severson R K, Grove J S, Nomura et al 1988 Body mass and prostatic cancer: a prospective study. British Medical Journal 297(6650):713–715

Slattery M L, Potter J, Caan B et al 1997 Energy balance and colon cancer: beyond physical activity. Cancer Research 57(1):75–80

Snow R C, Barbieri R L, Frisch R E 1989 Estrogen 2-hydroxylase oxidation and menstrual function among elite oars-women. Journal of Clinical Endocrinology and Metabolism 69(2):369–376

Souhami R, Tobias J 1998 Cancer and its management, 3rd edn. Blackwell Science, London

Srivastava A, Kreiger N 2000 Relationship of physical activity to testicular cancer. American Journal of Epidemiology 151(1):78–87

Thune I, Furberg A S 2001 Review. Physical activity and cancer risk dose-response and cancer, all sites and site-specific. Medicine and Science in Sports and Exercise 33(6 suppl):S530–S550

Vander A J, Sherman J H, Luciano D S 1990 Human physiology, 5th edn. McGraw-Hill, New York

Westerlind K C 2003 Physical activity and cancer prevention – mechanisms. Medicine and Science in Sports and Exercise 35(11):1834–1840

Westerlind K C, Gibson K J, Malone P et al 1998 Differential effects of estrogen metabolites on bone and reproductive tissues of ovariectomized rats. Journal of Bone and Mineral Research 13(6):1023–1031

Westerlind K C, McCarty H L, Gibson K J 2002 Effect of exercise on the rat mammary gland; implications for carcinogenesis. Acta Physiologica Scandinavica 175(2):147–156

Westley B R, May F E 1995 Insulin-like growth factors: the unrecognised oncogenes. British Journal of Cancer 72(5):1065–1066

Wheeler G D, Wall S R, Belcastro A N et al 2002 Reduced serum testosterone and prolactin levels in male distance runner. Journal of the American Medical Association 252(4):514–516

Whitrow M J, Smith B J, Pilotto L S et al 2003 Environmental exposure to carcinogens causing lung cancer: epidemiological evidence from the medical literature. Respirology 8(4):513–521

WHO (World Health Organization) 2003 Cancer. Online. Available: http://www.who.int/whr/2002/en November 2003

Zhu B T, Conney A H 1998 Functional role of estrogen metabolism in target cells: review and perspectives. Carcinogenesis 19(1):1–27

Chapter 13

Exercise and the older adult

Steve Bird

CHAPTER CONTENTS

Introduction 203
Exercise and ageing 204
Exercise, functional capacity and quality of life in older people 204
Socio-economic implications of an ageing population 205
Older people, exercise and strength 206
  Changes in muscle mass, muscle quality, strength and power 206
  Functional strength and quality of life implications 206
  Exercise training for strength 207
  How much strength training is required? 208
    What frequency is required? 208
    What intensity is required? 208
    How many exercises and sets are required? 209

Training for balance and falls prevention 209
Exercising for bone health 210
Aerobic exercise, cardiovascular health and endurance 210
Ageing, exercise and flexibility 211
Physical activity, mental health, well-being and quality of life 212
Physical activity participation of older adults 212
Predictors, barriers and facilitators to physical activity in older adults 121
Interventions to promote physical activity in older people 213
Conclusion 214
Summary 215
Suggested readings, references and bibliography 215

INTRODUCTION

There is considerable evidence supporting the beneficial effects of exercise for older people (Bouchard et al 1994, ACSM 1998a, Taylor et al 2004). It can increase their physical capacity, promote good mental health, facilitate opportunities for social interaction, reduce the risk of disease and ameliorate the impact of existing pathologies. As with younger adults, whilst some benefits of physical activity may be gained from relatively short-term training regimens that target an acute problem, others will be derived from the prolonged participation in healthenhancing physical activity that is part of a healthy lifestyle.

To effectively promote exercise programmes and an active lifestyle to older people, those advocating exercise need to understand the issues around ageing and how they may impact on the individual. It is also vital to appreciate the diversity of older people, who will vary greatly in their physical capacities, past experiences, exercise histories, general health, beliefs in exercise and cultural backgrounds.

Since other chapters will address the impact of exercise upon reducing disease and ameliorating specific disease pathologies, this chapter will primarily focus on the benefits of exercise in maintaining functional capacity and reducing the risk of injury in older people. However, in doing so it is necessary to recognize that in the older age groups there is a greater prevalence of the aforementioned disease conditions and that exercise programmes will have to be designed accordingly. As a definition of older adults, this chapter will primarily consider the issues facing those aged 65 years and older, although some of the research studies referred to include younger age groups. Furthermore whilst the ageing continuum is recognized within the literature with the use of commonly applied terms such as 'young-old' (65–74 years), 'old' (75–84 years) and 'old-old' (>85 years), the health and exercise practitioner will appreciate that given the debilities suffered by some 65-year-olds compared with the physical abilities of some 85-year-olds, this is a gross simplification.

EXERCISE AND AGEING

Ageing is a complex phenomenon that affects individuals on many levels, from the molecular, physiological and morphological, to the behavioural and psychosocial. Consequently it is studied from a range of diverse perspectives from the medical and biological to the humanities and social sciences. For the exercise practitioner dealing with older people, each of these requires due consideration and it is of interest to consider the extent to which the changes that are typically observed with ageing are a result of immutable biological processes on the one hand or lifestyle such as diet and physical activity on the other, and how the expectations of society can influence lifestyle choices.

From a biological perspective ageing has been attributed to the accumulation of damage in the cells and to the DNA in particular, a limitation in the number of times a cell can replicate, and the exhaustion of body tissues. Each of these explanations has evidence to support it being a significant contributor towards biological ageing and there are many reviews of the topic (Harman 2001, Gavrilov & Gavrilova 2003, Hayflick 2001, Parsons 2003, Vina et al 2003).

To date, no known substance or lifestyle practice, including exercise, is capable of preventing primary ageing (Rose 1999, Holloszy 2000). Indeed in animal studies only severe sustained caloric restriction has been shown to have some effect and the implications of this for humans are unknown. That there may be genetic components to longevity is suggested from studies on nematode worms and fruit flies, which can be selected for longer lifespans. However, how these genes bring about their influence on the plethora of biochemical and physiological processes that may influence the ageing process has yet to be deduced. Furthermore, it is unclear how such findings relate to humans and to date there is little or no evidence for a human genotype that slows down primary ageing (Rose & Nusbaum 1994). But what is becoming increasingly evident is the potential role of a person's genotype in affecting their vulnerability to secondary ageing, through for example conveying protection against particular diseases. An example of this would be genotypes that ensure high levels of HDL-cholesterol and hence a reduced risk of cardiovascular disease. Furthermore, research to elucidate an understanding of the consequences of potential interactions between different genotypes and exercise on health and longevity is at a relatively early stage (Perusse et al 2003). But it may be expected that an eventual understanding of such interactions will contribute towards explaining some of the variability observed and assist with more effective exercise prescription on an individual basis.

So whilst it is widely accepted that exercise may not be effective against primary ageing, it should be remembered that few people live long enough to reach their absolute maximum lifespan and die of 'old age'. Instead, most of us will die from the effects of disease before such a time and en route will experience reduced functional capacity and morbidity. Therefore it is in this context that exercise and physical activity can have a profound influence upon longevity and quality of life. This has been clearly demonstrated in the context of diseases of the cardiovascular system, musculoskeletal degeneration and some cancers (Shephard 1996). It is also evident that whilst these benefits may be most efficacious if regular exercise is undertaken throughout life, benefits can be still be gained from the commencement of exercise at any age. Indeed Evans (1999), when reporting on a strength training study, stated that 'there is no segment of the population that can benefit more from exercise than the elderly'.

In terms of added years of life, studies generally find that those who are physically active have an increased life expectancy of 2–3 years (Pekkanen et al 1987, Paffenbarger & Lee 1996). The magnitude of this gain appears, not surprisingly, to relate to when an active lifestyle was commenced, with the findings of Paffenbarger et al (1986) suggesting a gain of more than 2 years if an active lifestyle was pursued from the fourth decade of life, but less than half a year if commenced in the eighth decade. In the case of the latter this may seem to be an almost negligible gain, but its value should not be underestimated when put into the context of gaining quality years, in which the individual is able to enjoy health and good functional capacity, with fewer years of morbidity prior to death. That is to say that when evaluating the benefits of exercise the emphasis should be on how it can improve quality of life through maintaining functional capacity rather than increased longevity per se. Indeed, as emphasized throughout this chapter, the maxim should be 'exercising to add life to your years rather than adding years to your life'.

EXERCISE, FUNCTIONAL CAPACITY AND QUALITY OF LIFE IN OLDER PEOPLE

It is evident that people usually reach their physical peak in their third decade, after which there is a decline in their physical capacity (senescence). As this progresses into their sixth, seventh and eighth decades, it can have a significant impact upon their functional ability and quality of life. However, whilst there are obvious declines in physical capacity between the ages of 20 and 70 years, it is also apparent that for many individuals a significant proportion of this decline is due to their sedentary lifestyle. This is demonstrated through studies that have shown appropriate exercise training to reverse some of the decline in physical capacity and is further supported by cross-sectional studies comparing sedentary older people with those who were long-term (12–17 years) chronic exercisers (~3 times per week) (Klitgaard et al 1990). Indeed, older people who remain physically active may have a physical capacity that is superior to that of less active individuals 20 or 30 years their junior.

Ageing brings about an increase in functional limitations, with nearly three-quarters of adults aged over 70 years experiencing some difficulties with basic activities (Lubitz et al 2003) and nearly half of older adults will have a problem with at least one of the following: stooping, crouching, kneeling, carrying 6 kg objects, grasping small objects, extending their arms above their shoulders and walking two to three blocks. If pronounced, these limitations will affect how the older person can cope with their 'activities of daily living' (ADL) such as: bathing, showering, dressing, eating, getting in or out of a chair or bed, using the toilet, housework, preparing meals, shopping, and managing money. It is estimated that between 10 and 20% of older people have difficulties with these activities, which will affect their independence and impact upon their quality of life. Such declines are also linked with an increased need for both inpatient and outpatient hospital services (Mor et al 1994), again affecting the individual's quality of life, as well as increasing demand upon health services. Therefore, if physical activity can have a positive influence upon functional capacity, its benefits will be manifest across the spectrum from the individual, their friends and family, to the health services that support them.

However, one of the difficulties associated with assessing the effects of exercise training upon functional performance is the sensitivity of the assessments. This is illustrated in the review by Seguin & Nelson (2003), where they comment on a study (Skelton et al 1995) that reported increases in muscle strength and power in older women aged >75 years yet did not find significant changes in functional tests. They suggest that the reasons for this may have been due to the sample group not suffering any limitations at baseline, and hence any actual improvements would not be detectable. Of course, this does not devalue the potential benefit of the intervention, as such activity may be prophylactic in preventing the occurrence of future disabilities. This is illustrated by Spirduso & Cronin (2001) who in their review concluded that the participation in long-term physical activity enhanced physical function and was associated with postponed disability and retention of independent living status, particularly in the oldest-old age group.

Likewise, there is also considerable evidence to support short-term interventions designed to ameliorate existing functional deficiencies. These include high-intensity strength exercises for preventing the deterioration of physical function to levels at which impairment is reported (Young & Skelton 1994). Furthermore, exercise regimens can also ameliorate the impact of existing conditions, as shown by Penninx et al (2001a), who found aerobic and strength training exercise regimens to be beneficial to older people with osteoarthritis as they reduced losses of function and enabled them to undertake their ADL more easily.

Thus, there is evidence from longitudinal interventions as well as cross-sectional data that exercise is beneficial to health and physical functioning. However, it is important to remember that a little caution is needed in the interpretation of the results from some studies. For example, a cross-sectional study that shows physically active older people to be healthier does not necessarily prove that it was the exercise which made them healthier. Indeed, the results could just as equally be interpreted as the healthy individuals being more inclined to exercise regularly. As indeed could be the case in the epidemiological investigation by Huang et al (1998), who in a 5-year study of more than 4500 men and women concluded that the more physically fit (assessed via treadmill test) and physically active had fewer functional limitations (assessed via a mailed survey on ability to perform daily household activities such as lifting, carrying, washing cars, digging in the garden and scrubbing floors). Such studies are important as indicators of the likely beneficial effects of physical activity, and are of real value when interpreted alongside randomized controlled trials that can demonstrate exercise to initiate changes in health status or health indicators. Even so, intervention studies necessarily involve volunteers and there is therefore an element of self-selection by the participants, and it may be that those who are more inclined to volunteer for such studies are more receptive and responsive to exercise than those who decline to become involved. However, despite these caveats, on balance when scientific reviewsendeavour to account for these limitations in the evidence, there is still a clear and overwhelming consensus supporting the contribution of exercise towards health, functional capacity and quality of life.

SOCIO-ECONOMIC IMPLICATIONS OF AN AGEING POPULATION

Many Western societies exhibit the demographics of an ageing population with a predicted doubling of the number of individuals aged over 85 years during the next few decades (Brock et al 1990, Harman 2001, Australian Bureau of Statistics 2004, United Nations 2004). One of the reasons for this is that with advances in medical science more people are living longer. Additionally, not only are there more older people in the population but when this is combined with a lower birth rate, it results in older people comprising an increasingly large proportion of the population. This shift in population demographics is causing policy planners considerable concern, as it is liable to place unprecedented demands on the health, medical and social services, which have never had to cope with so many older people. Furthermore, as there will be a reduced proportion of the population working to generate the economic wealth needed to fund these health and social support services, health planners view the envisaged socio-economic impacts with some apprehension.

It is also evident that the demands for health and social services are liable to be greater if a substantial proportion of the population are affected by age-linked debilities that impair their ability to perform ADL and/or make them more susceptible to injury and disease. Consequently initiatives that can promote health behaviours that reduce the likelihood of such debilities are important, not only for the individual's quality of life, but also from a population health and socio-economic perspective. Therefore given its aforementioned benefits, the promotion of physical activity for older adults has become a key population health issue.

OLDER PEOPLE, EXERCISE AND STRENGTH

CHANGES IN MUSCLE MASS, MUSCLE QUALITY, STRENGTH AND POWER

After the age of 30 years, adults generally experience a decline in muscle strength and power (usually measured as torque) (Lindle et al 1997, Metter et al 1999), with the magnitude and rate of decline being affected by lifestyle factors such as physical activity. In their review Young & Skelton (1994) reported that between the ages of 65 and 84 years people lose muscle strength at a rate of 1.5% per year and power at around 3.5% per year. These declines in muscle power are evident in both eccentric and concentric muscle peak torque (Lindle et al 1997), which therefore impacts upon lifting and lowering activities as well as walking and balance. One of the reasons for these declines in strength and power is a reduction in muscle mass (sarcopenia) (Roubenoff & Hughes 2000), which is reported to be in the region of 1% per year after the fourth decade of life (Lexell 1995) and may accelerate further with increasing age. Similarly a review by Pendergast et al (1993) reported that muscle strength remains relatively high until the age of 60 years, after which there can be dramatic reductions of around 10% per year. Thus, losses in muscle mass affect a significant proportion of older adults, with 13–24% of people aged 65–70 years and over 50% of those aged over 80 years affected by clinically significant sarcopenia (Taylor et al 2004). It is also evident that these losses in muscle mass may at least in part be concealed by increases in intramuscular and subcutaneous fat. This has been illustrated in MRI scans of the limbs of young and older men, in which the total limb volume may be similar, but the tissue composition markedly different (Overend et al 1992).

It is also suggested that independent of reductions in muscle mass, aged-related strength losses may be caused by changes in neural drive and muscle quality (Frontera et al 2000, Hunter et al 2004). Some of this has at least in part been attributed to the type II fibres experiencing greater atrophy than endurance-oriented type I fibres (Klitgaard et al 1990, Lexell 1995). This is illustrated in the findings of Larsson (1983) who reported a reduction in the vastus lateralis from 60% type II in young men aged 19–37 years to 30% type II in older men aged 70–73. Hence the ability of the older men to produce forceful contractions and powerful movements would be compromised. Other changes that may affect the strength of contractions include the ability to store and utilize elastic energy through the stretch-shortening cycle. Changes in these properties are linked to a stiffening of the tissues, although research by Lindle et al (1997) suggested that older women have an enhanced capacity to store and utilize elastic energy compared with similarly aged men as well as with younger women and men. However, the relative contribution of changes in muscle quality to loss of strength and power is subject to some debate, as Metter et al (1999) suggest that some of the findings may be attributable to the methodology used.

Losses of muscle strength and power of the magnitude of those reported above are liable to lead to a loss of function and independence, with a concomitant onset of frailty and an increased risk of falls as the person gets older. When combined with a weakened skeleton, falls may be particularly injurious to older people, resulting in disability, loss of independence, reduced quality of life and in some cases fatalities. Consequently, whilst strength training for older people was a novelty 30 years ago, recognition that it can reverse, prevent or ameliorate such losses has resulted in its endorsement by expert authorities (ACSM 1998a, Hunter et al 2004) and as a consequence it is becoming more widespread, as evidenced by the proliferation of many regional and national initiatives.

FUNCTIONAL STRENGTH AND QUALITY OF LIFE IMPLICATIONS

The functional consequences of declining strength and power were evident in the results of the Allied Dunbar National Fitness Survey (Sports Council and Health Education Authority 1992), in which it was concluded that 'the prevalence of a degree of leg weakness and loss of power among women likely to limit their mobility was greater than 50% in the 65–74 age group'. However, as with other aspects of declining physical capacity with age, some of the decline has been attributed to an inactive lifestyle, and participating in appropriate exercise training can help to reverse some of this decline and maintain strength (Young & Skelton 1994). Therefore, as stated in Seguin & Nelson's 2003 review of the benefits of strength training, many of the age-related decrements seen in older adults are not inevitable.

In the Framingham study, women were assessed on their ability to lift 4.5 kg. Those unable to do so increased from 40% of women aged 55–64 years, to 45% of women aged 65–74 years, and 65% of women aged 75–84 years. This reflected a similar increase in the number of women who reported that they were unable to perform some aspects of household work (Branch & Jette 1981, Jette & Branch 1981). In the Allied Dunbar National Fitness Survey (Sports Council and Health Education Authority 1992) the implications of deficiencies in strength were also illustrated by reference to functional activities and in the 65–74-year age group approximately 25% of men and over 50% of the women did not possess the leg power required to climb stairs without difficulty.

Since older women tend to have a smaller muscle mass and lower strength than men of a similar age (Hyatt et al 1990) they are more likely to have their quality of life and functional capacity adversely affected. Additionally, since women tend to live longer than men, they have more years in which to decline to debilitating levels of strength and may suffer the effects for longer. Hence, given this epidemiological evidence and the socio-cultural issues, some health-related strength-training initiatives are specifically targeted at women.

EXERCISE TRAINING FOR STRENGTH

As indicated above, poor muscle strength can be the limiting factor on the functional capacity of many older people (Hyatt et al 1990) and hence their potential to maintain independence and quality of life. Whilst general physical activity and aerobic exercise are important components of a holistic programme they do not induce the required changes in muscle function to rectify losses in muscle strength (Pendergast et al 1993) and therefore muscle strength training must be included specifically as a vital element in the prevention of disability in the elderly.

In their review, Seguin & Nelson (2003) present a summary of selected strength training studies that have demonstrated improvements in strength in older people. Additionally, a number of these studies also reported improvements in power, bone mineral density, endurance, gait speed, balance, sleep and depression. In another extensive review, Hunter et al (2004) report that many strength training intervention studies have demonstrated increases in muscle mass of 10–62% after 9–52 weeks of training. They also report on studies that indicate improvements in muscle quality through more effective motor unit activation.

It is now fairly widely accepted that older people are capable of strength training at fairly high intensities, subject to all the standard safety issues and the gradual progression from lower to higher intensities that would be applicable to exercisers of all ages. Likewise, it is also important to ensure that the workloads applied are individually tailored to the current strengths of the participants. Hence workloads are commonly expressed as a relative value and are calculated as a percentage of the maximum resistance/weight that the participant can move/lift. This is termed their 1 repetition maximum (1RM).

Many strength training studies pertaining to older people appear to follow a similar design, involving 6–10 exercises, using an intensity of ~65–80% 1RM, and sets of 8–12 repetitions repeated three times a week, although some variation exists between programmes in terms of whether each set of exercises is repeated once, twice or three times within each session. From the literature it appears that 8–12 weeks' participation is sufficient to produce measurable changes in strength and in reality these may be evident much sooner. The format of the training regimens vary from the classic laboratory-based clinical trial, to home-based settings, with both having their advocates and evidence to support them. The equipment used also varies from free weights, to exercise machines and elasticated bands.

Ferri et al (2003) conducted a 16-week study with older men (aged 65–81 years) in which the participants performed 1 set of 10 repetitions each of leg press and calf raise exercises, three times a week. The intensity was initially set at 50% of their 1RM and progressed to 80% during the first month of the study. Their results showed a 30% and 22% increase in knee extension and plantar flexion strength, respectively, with concomitant increases in torque (19% and 12%, respectively) and power (24% and 33%, respectively). In a similar 12-week study with men aged between 60 and 72 years who performed 3 sets of 8 repetitions at 80% 1RM for knee extension and leg curl, Frontera et al (1988) reported 10% gains in muscle mass and >100% increases in dynamic strength. Both studies concluded that muscle hypertrophy alone could not account for all the increases in torque, and it is likely that factors such as increased neural drive, improved coordination, decreased antagonist muscle co-activation and increases in individual fibre-specific tension may also have contributed.

Capodaglio et al (2002) investigated the efficacy of using elasticated bands (Theraband) in a home-based strength training programme for men aged 65–80 years. These men had already completed a 4-month supervised programme using isotonic machines three times a week. The home-based programme involved 20 repetitions of 6 exercises, three times a week. The relationship between the elongation of the bands and force had been previously calculated, which enabled the researchers to provide instructions to the participants in order for them to work at prescribed exercise intensities. These commenced at 40% of 1RM and progressed to 60% during the first month of home training. The results showed that the level of compliance was 78%, and compared to the control group who had completed the 4-month training programme but had opted not to continue training, the Theraband training group continued to increase their strength (mean increase ~5–15%), whereas the control group did not. They concluded that this low cost modality of using elastic bands at home was effective in maintaining strength and function in older men. Elastic bands were also used in another home-based study (Strong for Life) by Jette et al (1999) involving older men and women (75 ± 7 years) who performed 11 exercises to a 35-minute video tape. In this study the participants recorded strength gains of 6–12%, an improvement in tandem gait and an 18% reduction in disability.

Topp et al (1996) also used Theraband exercises (2 sets × 10 repetitions of 11 exercises) during a 14-week programme with older community-dwelling adults. They reported 44% increases in strength for the training group as well as an increase in gait velocity, but they did not find any statistically significant improvements in postural control. Some of these findings, particularly the increase in gait velocity, were in contrast to an earlier study (Topp et al 1993) in which the exercise group had a slower gait velocity after a 12-week exercise intervention compared with pre-intervention. In their 1993 paper, the authors suggest that the slower gait could have been due to better balance and control, since others have suggested that the increase in gait speed 'may reflect an attempt by the older adult to compensate for a shift forward in their centre of gravity'. The quicker gait is therefore a consequence of the older adult attempting to maintain their balance by 'catching up' with their centre of gravity. The 1993 study also failed to report significant improvements in balance in the control group. Consequently, these equivocal findings with alternative explanations illustrate the complexity of the topic and the need for caution when extrapolating clinical study findings to real world situations. Therefore the real-world validity of some assessments should be viewed carefully.

In their review Seguin & Nelson (2003) report that in addition to gains in muscle strength, strength training for older people (>50 years) has been demonstrated to increase bone mass, flexibility, dynamic balance, self-confidence and self-esteem. They also report that it reduces the symptoms of chronic diseases such as arthritis, depression, type II diabetes, osteoporosis, sleep disorders and heart disease, as well as reducing the risk of falls. Furthermore, Evans (1999) reported that a strength training regimen for elderly men and women in a care facility increased spontaneous activity as well as 1RM. This link between strength and functionality is also evident in other studies that have shown gains in muscle strength to be a predictor of improvements in mobility and other functional activities (Chandler et al 1998) and for leg power to be the strongest physiological predictor of functional status (Foldvari et al 2000).

HOW MUCH STRENGTH TRAINING IS REQUIRED?

As indicated above, many of the published intervention studies have utilized a prescription of 3 weekly sessions of 6–10 repetitions at around 80% 1RM for each of 6–10 exercises. However, whilst this seems to be the most popular prescription, there is some evidence to indicate that at least some of the benefits may be gained from a lesser dose, although this may of course be influenced by the baseline status of the participants.

What frequency is required?

A 6-month study by Taaffe et al (1999) examined the effects of 1, 2 or 3 strength training sessions a week at an exercise facility upon men and women aged 65–79 years. They found that those doing just one session a week exhibited improvements in strength, and that there were no statistically significant differences in the gains of the once a week group compared to the more frequent exercise groups. Thus benefits may be gained from strength training just once a week. This has implications for exercise prescription, compliance and safety, as even though there may be further benefits from more frequent sessions, and indeed more frequent sessions may be more efficacious for some groups, undertaking just one session a week may be more attainable for many older individuals, particularly if they need to travel to exercise facilities.

What intensity is required?

As indicated above, the exercise prescription for strength development commonly utilizes a regimen involving high-intensity training at 80% of 1RM. This appears to be effective, yet the work of Vincent et al (2002) would appear to suggest that improvements can be achieved via lower-intensity regimens. Their study involved a 6-month progressive, whole-body resistance training programme using resistance machines, in which older adults aged 60 to 83 years trained at either 50% of their 1RM for 13 repetitions (low exercise intensity) or 80% of 1RM for 8 repetitions (high exercise intensity). The participants completed one set of each of 12 exercises and both regimens were at a frequency of three times per week for 24 weeks. Thus the total amount lifted would have been similar in the two regimens. The results indicated an increase in total strength (sum of all 1RMs) of 17.2% in the low exercise intensity group and an almost identical 17.8% in the high exercise intensity group. Their results suggested that significant and similar improvements in strength, endurance, and stair climbing time could be obtained in older adults as a consequence of high- or low-intensity resistance exercise training. However, as an illustration of how studies can produce conflicting results, that by Beneka et al (2005) concluded that high-intensity (90% of 1RM) isokinetic exercise produced greater strength gains than low-intensity (50% 1RM) isokinetic exercise in older people when performed for 3 sessions per week for 16 weeks. So whilst some of the parameters required for effective strength training in older people are widely established and agreed upon, the finer points and details remain to be fully elucidated. For example, in the paper by Vincent et al (2002) the baseline values of the participants could be a factor and it is not known whether differences in the strength of the two groups would have developed given more time.

It should also be noted that a confounding factor that may affect the findings of many studies is the failure to readjust the training loads as the participants become stronger. Such an adjustment is needed since as the participants increase their strength, a load that corresponded to 80% of their baseline 1RM at the start of the programme will be less than 80% of their 1RM maximum as they become stronger 8–12 weeks into the programme. Hence they will no longer be training at such a high relative exercise intensity and to continue at the same relative exercise intensity the resistance or weight needs to be increased progressively and in accordance with the results of regular assessments of 1RM values.

How many exercises and sets are required?

The American College of Sports Medicine (ACSM 1998b) suggest that 1 set of 8–10 repetitions of each exercise will condition the major muscle groups. However, they go on to surmise that multiple set regimens may provide greater benefits, if time allows. Furthermore, whilst the consensus may be that around 8 exercises are required to utilize all the major muscle groups Henry et al (1999) sound a note of caution that care should be taken not to prescribe too many exercises, as in their study with older people this reduced their compliance in terms of correct alignment and quality of movement. Therefore, even when undertaking 8 exercises, exercise instructors should ensure that appropriate monitoring occurs and provide correction when required, although this issue is of course not unique to older people.

TRAINING FOR BALANCE AND FALLS PREVENTION

According to Khan et al (2001), 15% of people over the age of 65 years fall recurrently. This is a major health risk, particularly since a substantial proportion of older people have osteopenic and osteoporotic skeletons, which increases the risk of fracture. Indeed 90% of hip fractures are due to falls (Parkkari et al 1999) and in 12–20% of cases the outcome of such a fall will be fatal (Peck et al 1988). Even when not as severe, falls and fall-related injuries are responsible for 25% of admissions to nursing homes and a loss of the ability to maintain balance will reduce the safe execution of ADL and affect independence (Judge 2003).

In their review, Pendergast et al (1993) say that after age 60 years, there are dramatic decreases in muscle strength (approximately 10% per year), which leads to an approximately 4-fold increase in the likelihood of falls. They conclude that exercise programmes utilizing 'aerobic' exercise activities do not lead to an increase in muscle

function, whereas programmes designed specifically for muscle strengthening can increase function and according to other studies will reduce the risk of falls and injuries. This is supported by Gardner et al's (2000) review of 11 trials involving exercise intervention or interventions that included an exercise component, which concluded that exercise was effective in lowering the risk of falls and should be included in falls prevention programmes. However, it should be remembered that balance is a complex attribute, requiring sensory input from touch/pressure sensors on the plantar surface of the feet, joint position sense, visual acuity and vestibular input. All of these may deteriorate with age and consequently deterioration of motor control is a key factor associated with changes in balance with age (Thelen et al 1998). Indeed, whilst many studies have demonstrated improvements in balance alongside strength gains, it is not always the case (Bellew et al 2003) and they cannot be assumed to occur concurrently. It would therefore be remiss in a falls prevention programme to rely entirely upon strength training and strength gains alone to optimize the outcomes, but instead such programmes should include specific falls prevention training, balance exercises and appropriate education. This multidimensional approach was used in a large study (Day et al 2002) with over 1000 older people aged over 70 years and assessed the effects of the combined intervention of group-based exercise, home hazard management and vision improvement. Each aspect was deemed to be important and from the overall outcome it was concluded that the exercise-training component reduced the falls rate by about 18%.

In a series of studies conducted in New Zealand, a home-based exercise programme for people aged over 80 years was found to be effective in reducing falls. The programme included four home visits by a nurse or physiotherapist in the first 2 months of the programme, followed by booster visits every 6 months (Gardner et al 2001). The exercises incorporated the use of ankle cuff weights for strengthening, balance exercises and walking to improve endurance. The exercises were prescribed to be performed at a frequency of three or more times a week and the reduction in falls was calculated to be around 30% (Campbell et al 1997, 1999a, 1999b, Robertson et al 2001a, 2001b).

Judge (2003) concluded that both home- and class-based training programmes can reduce fall rates by up to 40%. He also advocates studies investigating the potential benefits of tai chi and social dance. Accordingly the 15-week tai chi programme used by Kutner et al (1997) was shown to improve confidence in balance and movement in older people (aged over 70 years). Likewise Wolf et al (2003) reported that although the risk ratio of falling was not statistically different between a tai chi group and a Wellness Education group, over the 48 weeks of intervention, 46% of the participants did not fall; and the percentage of participants who fell at least once was 60.3% for the Wellness Education group compared with only 47.6% for the tai chi group. They therefore considered these results to be encouraging and to warrant further investigation.

EXERCISING FOR BONE HEALTH

Bone is composed of a protein collagen matrix upon which minerals, primarily calcium and phosphorus, are deposited. It is a metabolically active tissue that remodels and adapts to the stresses it experiences. This is achieved via the combined action of osteoblastic cells that deposit the minerals and osteoclastic cells that resorb them. Adding or removing quantities of these minerals makes the bone more or less dense. Bone mineral density (BMD) is commonly used as an indicator of the health and strength of bone. It is assessed using dual energy X-ray absorptiometry (DXA or DEXA) and for a comprehensive assessment of a person's skeletal health, the BMD should be measured at a number of different sites, since the BMD at one site may not be representative of the entire skeleton (Faulkner et al 1999, Lu et al 2001). The density of the bone is then compared to the mean for young healthy people in the population and ascribed a T score, which indicates how far below or above the average the person's BMD is. To relate the person's BMD to the population of their own age and gender, Z scores can also be calculated. Osteoporosis is defined as a BMD more than 2.5 standard deviations below the young adult mean (T < −2.5) and values that are between 1.0 and 2.5 standard deviations below the young adult mean (T −1.0 to −2.5) are referred to as osteopenic (World Health Organization 1994).

With ageing there is a loss of bone density. The exact time-course of this loss varies between individuals and skeletal sites, but is likely to have commenced by the age of 40 years. Losses are at a rate of around 1% per year, with women experiencing an accelerated decline after the menopause due to oestrogen deficiency.

Since there is a loss of BMD with ageing, older adults are at increased risk of becoming osteopenic and osteoporotic, with the associated increased risk of osteoporotic fractures (Cummings et al 1993, Marshall et al 1996). Osteoporotic fractures occur in both men and women, but are more common in women as the peak average values for women, usually attained between 18 and 35 years of age, are below those of men and they are therefore more likely to decline to osteoporotic values with ageing. Additionally, because women tend to live longer, they have more years in which to deteriorate to osteoporotic levels. It is reported that 30–40% of women will suffer an osteoporotic fracture in their lifetime (Melton 2000), which is about three times the prevalence in men.

Due to the remodelling properties of bone, exercise is capable of promoting a high peak BMD, ameliorating the age-associated decline in BMD and perhaps reversing the decline in some older people (ACSM 1995). Whilst the optimal training regimens and prescription have yet to be elucidated, it would appear that the type of exercise required to stimulate these beneficial responses must be high intensity, require strong muscular forces and according to some authorities should preferably be high impact. It is also evident that the osteogenic benefits of the exercise are specific to the skeletal sites experiencing the stresses. Hence non-weight-bearing activities such as swimming and bicycling are unlikely to be beneficial, and even low-impact weight-bearing activities such as walking may have a limited effect (ACSM 1995). However, whereas higher-impact activities are likely to be beneficial for younger adults, additional care and consideration should be given concerning their potential risk–benefit for older adults who may possess already weakened skeletons. For non-weight-bearing bones strength training is recommended and there is a link between BMD and muscle mass. Indeed there is some evidence that high-intensity strength training may benefit both weight-bearing and non-weight-bearing bones.

Sartorio et al (2001) investigated the effects of high-intensity strength training upon indices of bone turnover in men aged 65–81 years. Their training regimen involved 6 sets of exercise (2 lower limb and 4 upper limb), with 10 repetitions of each exercise. For the lower limb exercises, the loads for each exercise commenced at 50% 1RM and increased to 80% during the first month of the study and from 40% to 65% of the 1RM for the upper body exercises. The exercise sessions were performed 3 times a week and for 16 weeks. Their results showed an improvement in the ratio of bone formation to bone resorption, suggesting a positive effect upon bone health. Likewise Nelson et al (1994) conducted a one-year strength-training programme (3 sets × 8 repetitions of 5 exercises at 80% 1RM, performed twice a week) with women aged 50–70 years. The aims of the study were to assess whether strength training could reduce the risk factors associated with osteoporotic fractures and the results showed that the exercise group, in addition to increasing their muscle mass and strength, also increased their bone density and improved their balance. In a similar study by Cussler et al (2003) (2 sets × 6–8 repetitions of 8 exercises at 70–80% of 1RM) beneficial changes in bone density were also observed and appeared to be dose dependent upon the amount of weight lifted during the year of the study.

AEROBIC EXERCISE, CARDIOVASCULAR HEALTH AND ENDURANCE

Regular moderate-intensity physical activity is recommended for people of all ages, including older adults (WHO 1997, ACSM 1998a). The rationale for promoting moderate-intensity aerobic exercise to older people is based upon the evidence of its efficacy in reducing the risk of disease and promoting cardiovascular fitness, which is a key component in determining a person's functional ability. It can also provide the opportunity for social interaction and facilitate good mental health. A key indicator of cardiovascular fitness is a person's capacity to utilize oxygen as indicated by their $\dot{V}O_2$max. As well as being a predictor of cardiovascular health and a reduced risk of cardiovascular disease, a good $\dot{V}O_2$max provides the capacity to perform moderate-intensity activities with relative ease. This includes walking, general household tasks and ADL. It also provides the basic fitness needed to enjoy active recreational pursuits.

A person's $\dot{V}O_2$max generally peaks in their third decade, after which it declines by approximately 0.6–1% per year. As with other health- and fitness-related factors, the rate of this decline is greater if the individual assumes a sedentary lifestyle. Therefore even though large volumes of endurance training cannot prevent an age-linked decline, aerobic exercise can ensure that the decline is not further accentuated by inactivity. Indeed, if an older person has been inactive, they can increase their $\dot{V}O_2$max to a level constrained by age-related factors, and research shows that the $\dot{V}O_2$max of older people can be increased by 20–30% (Lakatta 1993), which is similar to the level of trainability seen in younger adults.

Using a value of ~60% $\dot{V}O_2$max as an indicator of an exertion level that could be maintained, but above which would cause fatigue, the results of the Allied Dunbar National Fitness Survey (Sports Council and Health Education Authority 1992) indicated that over 20% of women aged 55–64, and over 40% of women aged 65–74 would find it difficult to maintain a steady walking speed (3 miles per hour) on level ground and for many it would not be possible. The results for the men were substantially better, with around 5% and 10%, respectively, being categorized as unlikely to be able to maintain steady walking on the flat. When the data were related to walking up a 5% gradient at 3 miles per hour, less than 10% of women aged 55–64 years and less than 5% aged 65–74 years were deemed to be able to achieve this, with the results for 55–64-year-old and 65–74-year-old men being 50% and 25%, respectively. Consequently the prevalence of low levels of aerobic fitness in the older age groups indicates that a large proportion would find walking in their locality difficult. At a more severe level of functional disability, this supposition is supported by the results of the 1998 Health Survey of England (DoH Health 2000), in which 2% of those aged 65–74 years reported not being able to walk at all, a figure that increased to 7.6% in the over 80–84 years age group and 12.7% in the over 85 years age group. Furthermore, since self-reported walking pace has been linked to the risk of premature mortality (Manson et al 2002), it is a concern that so few adults (~20%) aged over 65–69 years reported walking at the brisk or fast pace that is associated with reduced risk. In accordance with other fitness measures, this value declined

further with increasing age.

The aims of endurance training within a health-enhancing physical activity programme for older adults is to maximize their aerobic capacity and prevent it from declining to debilitating levels. Additionally, aerobic exercise conveys a reduction in the risk of cardiovascular disease in the elderly (Wenger 1996) and the American College of Sports Medicine (1998a) position statement on exercise and physical activity for older adults indicates a beneficial effect upon insulin sensitivity, blood pressure, lipoprotein lipid profiles (Reaven et al 1990) and body composition (ACSM 1998a). The recommended levels of aerobic exercise for older adults are similar to those for young adults (Pate et al 1995). That is, it should be undertaken on most and preferably every day of the week, at a moderate intensity (3–6 metabolic equivalents (METs)), with an emphasis upon activities involving the repetitive contractions of large muscle groups, such as brisk walking, swimming and cycling. The generally prescribed intensity used in health-enhancing aerobic exercise intervention studies with older adults is typically 50–70% $\dot{V}O_2$max (Taylor et al 2004). However, it is possible that benefits may be gained at lower intensities, as suggested by the observation that the greatest difference in all-cause mortality is between the lowest fitness quintile and the next (below-average age-related fitness) (Blair et al 1989). Hence doing some form of regular, albeit low-intensity activity, could convey considerable health benefits, compared to being completely sedentary (ACSM 1998b).

AGEING, EXERCISE AND FLEXIBILITY

One factor that determines a person's flexibility is the extensibility of the collagen fibres in their tendons and ligaments. Ageing reduces the extensibility of the collagen fibres due to an increase in the crystallinity of these fibres (ACSM 1998a). The Allied Dunbar National Fitness Survey (Sports Council and Health Education Authority 1992) indicated an increased loss of shoulder mobility (abduction) with increasing age and that in ~15% of men and ~20% of women aged 65–74 years, it was liable to impair their ability to perform functional tasks such as washing their hair, reaching up to high shelves or pegging out laundry.

The American College of Sports Medicine position statement on exercise and physical activity for older adults (1998a) suggests that, partly due to methodological issues and study designs, interventions have not provided clear unequivocal evidence for the dose–response effects of flexibility exercises. However, the review does indicate that flexibility exercises could be a useful component for the older adult who has reduced mobility (ACSM 1998b) and recommends that flexibility exercises should be incorporated into overall fitness programmes, and that the exercises should stretch all major muscle groups and be performed two to three times a week. They also advocate a combination of static and dynamic stretching techniques.

PHYSICAL ACTIVITY, MENTAL HEALTH, WELL-BEING AND QUALITY OF LIFE

According to the American College of Sports Medicine (1998a) review, the prevalence of depression and depressive symptoms amongst older people (15%) is a major public health issue. It is not only associated with a reduced quality of life (Copeland 1999) but is also linked to increased risk of disability and cardiac mortality (Penninx et al 2001b). According to the review by Taylor et al (2004), epidemiological studies indicate an inverse relationship between depression scores and level of physical activity, and Biddle & Faulkner (2002) conclude that overall, the evidence is in favour of physical activity having an antidepressant effect. Not unsurprisingly, therefore, exercise is commonly prescribed for mild depression.

Other changes in psychological function associated with ageing include declines in cognitive function and self-efficacy (ACSM 1998a). According to the American College of Sports Medicine (1998a), studies using cross-sectional data indicate superior cognitive function amongst exercisers (Boutcher 2000), although as previously stated this does not prove cause and effect, and it is somewhat unfortunate that to date the longitudinal intervention studies conducted into the efficacy of exercise in improving cognitive function are equivocal, thereby leaving the issue largely unresolved (Boutcher 2000, Biddle & Faulkner 2002).

Studies on the effects of physical activity on anxiety in older adults appear to suggest some benefit, but as yet remain somewhat equivocal (Taylor 2000). Likewise, whilst positive mood state and psychological well-being appear to be higher in regular exercisers (Skelton et al 1999, Biddle & Faulkner 2002) as does self-esteem (Fox 2000), establishing definitive proof of cause and effect requires further research.

PHYSICAL ACTIVITY PARTICIPATION OF OLDER ADULTS

Whilst the prevalence of inactivity at all ages is a cause for concern for many countries, it is evident that the lowest activity levels occur in the older age groups and are lower amongst women than men (Sports Council and Health Education Authority 1992, USDHHS 1996, Armstrong et al 2000). Taylor et al (2004) present data suggesting that more than half of adults aged 65–69 years do not participate in sufficient physical activity to convey health benefits,

and this figure increases to over 90% in those aged over 85 years. Even in terms of brisk walking, usually deemed to be the most accessible form of physical activity, only 22% of adults aged 65–69 years walked for a least 60 minutes a week and less than 12% completed this at a brisk pace. These figures fell still further with increasing age and were only 5.2% and 1.4%, respectively, in the over 85 years age group. Similar trends are apparent in data for the United States (USDHHS 1996), and in Australia whilst the activity patterns appeared to be slightly better, albeit any comparison being subject to the vagaries of different measurement tools, still only 37% of people aged 60–75 years reported walking five or more times a week, and only 7% of this age group reported participating in vigorous activity three or more times a week (Armstrong et al 2000). Therefore in accordance with the aforementioned concerns about the prospect of an increasingly large number of dependent older people within the populations of many countries, numerous public health initiatives are being instigated to encourage increased physical activity in this sector of society, with the aim of reducing the burden of disease and morbidity caused by inactivity.

PREDICTORS, BARRIERS AND FACILITATORS TO PHYSICAL ACTIVITY IN OLDER ADULTS

In order for active lifestyle initiatives to be successful, it is necessary to appreciate the barriers and facilitators to physical activity. In this older age group, many of these are the same as those given by younger adults, such as lack of time (Biddle & Mutrie 2001), but others are more specific to older people and consequently exercise programmes should be tailored to the lifestyle, age-specific obligations, and set of values of this target group (Schneider et al 2003).

According to Grossman & Stewart (2003), the motivators to exercise in the over 75 years age group include health, independence, family and appearances, whereas the barriers are poor health, lack of time, ageing and adverse environments. These are similar to the results of Kolt et al's (2004) study of regular older exercisers (aged 55–93 years) in which the most common motives for participation were to keep healthy, liking the activity, to improve fitness, and to maintain joint mobility, while the barriers to participation included poor health and physical condition, misconceptions about exercise and what they should be doing, and a lack of knowledge of the likely benefits. Other reasons are a perception that it is inappropriate and even ineffective for older people to exercise, fear of injury and illness (O'Brien Cousins 2000), perceived lack of ability and transportation problems (King et al 1998). King et al (1992) grouped the factors that influence whether an older person is liable to be physically active under three headings: (i) personal, (ii) environmental and (iii) programme- or regimen-based. The personal characteristics that are commonly reported to be associated with lower levels of physical activity are: female sex, lower educational attainment, lower income, smoking and being overweight, particular ethnicities, increasing age and lower self-efficacy (Sallis et al 1992, Booth et al 2000, King et al 2000). Other personal factors affecting exercise participation include: exercise beliefs, exercise benefits, past experiences of exercise, goals and personality (Resnick & Spellbring 2000). Research amongst older women has also identified a continuing commitment to caring roles as a reason for a lack of time to commit to personal exercise programmes (O'Brien Cousins & Keating 1995). However, whilst surveys consistently report lower activity amongst women compared with men at all ages, Emery et al (1992), in a study of older adults aged 67±5 years, did not find gender to be a predictor of exercise behaviour. Hence differences in research findings such as these reaffirm the complexity of the issues, the variability of the population and circumstances, and the need for interventions to be cognizant of local features if they are to have maximum impact. It is also interesting to note that both sedentary and active people report similar barriers to being physically active. Therefore of key practical interest is an understanding of why and how active people overcome these barriers whereas sedentary individuals do not.

The environmental factors known to influence participation in physical activity include: absence of enjoyable scenery (inverse), fears about safety (inverse), lack of footpaths (inverse), rarely seeing others exercising in one's neighbourhood (inverse), convenience of facilities, the 'walkability' of the neighbourhood and the weather (Sallis et al 1992, Booth et al 2000, Ball et al 2001, Giles-Corti & Donovan 2002a, King et al 2003, Salmon et al 2003, Humpel et al 2004). With respect to access and use of facilities it is important to consider the availability and convenience of both formal facilities that are primarily for exercise, such as gyms and swimming pools, and informal facilities where exercise may occur, such as local parks, the beach and pedestrian/bicycle friendly routes. Additionally, having shops and other facilities within a 'walkable' distance (~20 minutes) is also recognized as a factor promoting walking (King et al 2003).

The programme- or regimen-based factors that affect participation include difficulty in accessing the facilities, particularly if travel is an issue, a lack of familiarity with exercise environments such as gyms and physical activity in general, which is particularly prevalent amongst older women (O'Brien & Vertinsky 1991, Lee 1993), and a lack of appreciation that older people can benefit from regular exercise. Some of the latter facility issues are being addressed through home-based programmes, although on the negative side these may deprive the participants of the potential benefits of social interaction that may be gained from group sessions.

Indeed a number of studies have highlighted the importance of the social factors in motivating older people to exercise. Booth et al (2000) identified factors such as exercising with friends or family, and/or friend and family support as being of key importance. Likewise, owning a dog is linked to greater walking frequency (Ball et al 2001), which for older people living alone may also facilitate social contact. Indeed, whilst not specifically focusing upon older people, a number of studies investigating both the environmental and social environment have found the social environment to be the strongest predictor of physical activity participation (Ståhl et al 2001, Giles-Corti & Donovan 2002b). Particular ethno-cultural groups may also be less familiar with the concepts of exercise and participation by women and older adults. Studies in Australia, which has a large multicultural population, have emphasized the necessity for considering cultural factors in behavioural and social health theory building (Lupton 1994, Manderson & Reid 1994). This is also evident in the work of Giles-Corti & Donovan (2002a, 2002b) who in a study based in Western Australia recommended that whilst emphasis should be placed on creating a physical environment that enhanced physical activity, it needed to be complemented by effective strategies that influenced social factors. Thus group sessions for 'seniors' may not only overcome some of the barriers, but also provide an important social environment. This point was evident in a study of older people aged 74–85 years (Cohen-Mansfield et al 2004) in which participants who were not married were more interested in social aspects than those who were. Additionally, and not unsurprisingly, factors such as cost were more of a consideration for those with fewer resources and lower levels of education.

Thus it is evident that from a population health perspective, health and physical activity promotion cannot be fully effective unless it targets the facilitators and barriers that affect the individual and is aligned with policies relating to the built environment, local planning, transport and social factors.

INTERVENTIONS TO PROMOTE PHYSICAL ACTIVITY IN OLDER PEOPLE

In their review, van der Bij et al (2002) reported that home-based, group-based and educational interventions could all be effective in increasing the physical activity of older people. However, they went on to conclude that whilst adherence was often high in the short term it declined in the long term and a number of studies have demonstrated declines to former levels of inactivity once a formal programme of activity concludes (Robinson & Rogers 1994, Rhodes et al 1999). This feature is of course not unique to programmes involving older people. King et al (1998) suggested that greater maintenance could be attained with ongoing support, which was a characteristic of many of the successful strength training and falls prevention programmes, which used booster visits by nurses and telephone calls (Gardner et al 2001). However, according to the review by van der Bij et al (2002), it would appear that the long-term effectiveness of such behavioural reinforcement strategies is variable. Indeed, of the 38 studies that they reviewed, only one appeared to effectively maintain long-term (10-year) higher activity levels and it used a combination of birthday and get-well cards, newsletters, telephone reminders, meetings and rewards (Pereira et al 1998).

Satariano & McAuley (2003) emphasize how participation in physical activity is dependent upon the interaction between the individual and their environment. Hence, as previously indicated, personal, social and environmental factors will all contribute towards determining the likely outcome. Resnick & Spellbring (2000) suggest increasing pleasant sensations associated with exercise as a means to improving adherence, whilst Deforche & De Bourdeaudhuij (2000) advocate exercising in the company of family or friends as an intervention strategy, since it provides important supporting social influences.

As previously indicated, positive health and physical functioning outcomes have been attained through both home-based and facility-based or externally based interventions. There are pros and cons for both, and therefore some consideration needs to be given to the desired outcomes of an initiative and what are the likely barriers to its successful implementation, recruitment and compliance. From a public health perspective providing home-based programmes may capture those who are unable or disinclined to participate in traditional group-based interventions. However, regardless of the programme type, sustaining health-enhancing levels of participation remains a problem and to maintain participation multi-level interventions that consider a combination of environmental, safety, facility, community, transport, educational and socially oriented strategies are required. One particular strategy that has received some interest has been the role of the older person's physician, who is perceived to be relatively influential and may prescribe exercise (Cohen-Mansfield et al 2004). However, to optimize its effectiveness the prescription needs to be supported by education and access to either suitable environments or facilities that are appropriately supported by staff who understand the issues around older people and exercise. Hence the linking of physicians with suitably accredited exercise facilities, to which they may direct their patients, is becoming more common (Sims et al 2004).

Given the already acknowledged diversity and heterogeneity of older people, it is evident that different initiatives will be more or less suitable and efficacious depending on the circumstances and needs of the individual. For example, home-based interventions and initiatives obviously have the advantage of not requiring travel, but do not have in-built social interaction with others and the possible reinforcing effects. However, it is largely advocated that to be effective, home-based programmes should include a component of initial educational and technique instruction and regular follow-up visits and/or telephone calls to promote compliance (Gardner et al 2001). According to van der Bij et al (2002) both home-based and group-based interventions initially have a high participation rate, but they are not sustained in the long term (>1 year), with some indication that the decline may be greater in the home-based interventions. Resnick (2000) states that approximately 50% of adults who commence an exercise programme will stop within the first 6 months. To reduce this attrition they suggest a seven-step approach that includes: education, exercise pre-screening, goal setting, exposure to exercise, role models, verbal encouragement and verbal reinforcement. Whilst this model was instituted for an older person's care facility, it would seem that the elements could usefully inform other programmes in the wider community setting.

CONCLUSION

As evidenced throughout this chapter, older adults will benefit from regular physical activity, with optimal holistic benefits being derived from a programme that combines specific exercises for strength and BMD, brisk aerobic activity to promote cardiovascular health and reduce the risk of disease, flexibility exercises to maintain joint mobility and balance training to reduce the risk of falls. Whilst some form of physical activity should be undertaken on all days of the week, a total of three sessions per week that includes both strengthening and cardiovascular exercises can enhance functional fitness and will have more holistic benefits than just strengthening or cardiovascular exercise training alone (Wood et al 2001). Participating in the above can also promote good mental health and provide opportunities for positive social interaction. However, the low numbers of older people attaining the recommended levels of physical activity means that particular attention needs to be directed towards strategies for promoting, maintaining and sustaining long-term adherence to physical activity regimens. Personal, environmental, programme/regimen and social factors that may be barriers or facilitators to participation must all be considered in the planning process; otherwise an initiative will fail to fully achieve its intended outcomes.

In conclusion, evidence of the potential benefits of exercise for older people is considerable, yet is clearly not a new concept, as illustrated by this statement attributed to Hippocrates (470–360 BC).

In a word, all parts of the body which were made for active use, if moderately used and exercised at the labour to which they are habituated, become healthy, increase in bulk, and bear their age well, but when not used, and when left without exercise, they become diseased, their growth is arrested, and they soon become old.

Yet we are often faced with the attitudes expressed by Oscar Wilde:

To get back my youth I would do anything in the world, except take exercise, get up early, or be respectable. (The Picture of Dorian Gray, 1891)

And ultimately the musings of Eubie Blake, who lived to be 100 years old

If I'd known I was gonna live this long, I'd have taken better care of myself. (Quoted in The Observer, *13 February 1983)*

SUMMARY

- There is considerable evidence supporting the beneficial effects of exercise for older people. It can increase their physical capacity, promote good mental health, facilitate opportunities for social interaction, reduce the risk of disease and ameliorate the impact of existing pathologies.
- Relatively few older people attain the advocated levels of physical activity.
- To effectively promote exercise programmes and an active lifestyle to older people, those advocating exercise need to understand the physical, psychological, social and cultural issues around ageing.
- In many older people a significant part of their functional decline is due to inactivity and may be prevented or reversed through exercise.

- Strength training is important for older people.
- Effective strength training regimens commonly have the format of 6–10 exercises, at an intensity of ~65–80% 1RM, with sets of 8–12 repetitions repeated three times a week.
- Falls prevention is also important in older people and exercise regimens should include specific components targeting this.
- Regular moderate-intensity physical activity aimed at improving cardiovascular health and fitness, such as walking, cycling and swimming, are recommended for older adults and should be undertaken on most and preferably all days of the week.

Suggested readings, references and bibliography

ACSM (American College of Sports Medicine) 1995 Position stand. Osteoporosis and exercise. Medicine and Science in Sports and Exercise 27(4):i–vii

ACSM 1998a Position stand: exercise and physical activity for older adults. Medicine and Science in Sports and Exercise 30:992–1008

ACSM 1998b Position stand: the recommended quantity and quality of exercise for developing and maintaining cardiorespiratory and muscular fitness, and flexibility in healthy adults. Medicine and Science in Sports and Exercise 30:975–991

Armstrong T, Bauman A, Davies J 2000 Physical activity patterns of Australian adults. Results of the 1999 National Physical Activity Survey. Australian Institute of Health and Welfare, Canberra

Australian Bureau of Statistics 2004 Australian demographic statistics (Cat. no. 3101.0). Online. Available: http://www.abs.gov.au December 2004

Ball K, Bauman A, Leslie E et al 2001 Perceived environmental aesthetics and convenience and company are associated with walking for exercise among Australian adults. Preventive Medicine 33:434–440

Bellew J W, Yates J W, Gater D R 2003 The initial effects of low-volume strength training on balance in untrained older men and women. Journal of Strength and Conditioning Research 17(1):121–128

Beneka A, Malliou P, Fatouros I et al 2005 Resistance training effects on muscular strength of elderly are related to intensity and gender. Journal of Science and Medicine in Sport 8(3):274–283

Biddle S, Faulkner G 2002 Psychological and social benefits of physical activity. In: Chan K-M, Chodzko-Zajko W, Frontera W et al (eds) Active aging. Lippincott Williams & Wilkins, Hong Kong, p 89–164

Biddle S J H, Mutrie N 2001 Psychology of physical activity: determinants, well-being, and interventions. Routledge, London

Blair S N, Kohl H W 3rd, Paffenbarger RS Jr et al 1989 Physical fitness and all-cause mortality. A prospective study of healthy men and women. Journal of the American Medical Association 262(17):2395–2401

Booth M L, Owen N, Bauman A et al 2000 Social-cognitive and perceived environmental influences associated with physical activity in older adults. Preventive Medicine 31:15–22

Bouchard C, Shephard R J, Stephens T (eds) 1994 Physical activity and health: international proceedings and consensus statement. Human Kinetics, Champaign, IL

Boutcher S H 2000 Cognitive performance, fitness and ageing. In: Biddle S J H, Fox K R, Boutcher S H (eds) Physical activity and psychological well-being. Routledge, London, p 118–129

Branch L G, Jette A M 1981 The Framingham Disability Study: I. Social disability among the aging. American Journal of Public Health 71(11):1202–1210

Brock D B, Guralnik J M, Brody J A 1990 Demography and epidemiology of aging in the United States. In: Schneider E L, Rowe J W (eds) Handbook of the biology of aging, 3rd edn. Academic Press, San Diego, CA, p 3–23

Campbell A J, Robertson M C, Gardner M M et al 1997 Randomised controlled trial of a general practice programme of home based exercise to prevent falls in elderly women. British Medical Journal 315(7115):1065–1069

Campbell A J, Robertson M C, Gardner M M et al 1999a Falls prevention over 2 years: a randomized controlled trial in women 80 years and older. Age and Ageing 28(6):513–518

Campbell A J, Robertson M C, Gardner M M et al 1999b Psychotropic medication withdrawal and a home-based exercise program to prevent falls: a randomized, controlled trial. Journal of the American Geriatrics Society 47:850–853

Capodaglio P, Facioli M, Burroni E et al 2002 Effectiveness of a home-based strengthening program for elderly males in Italy. A preliminary study. Aging – Clinical and Experimental Research 14:28–34

Chandler J M, Duncan P W, Kochersberger G et al 1998 Is lower extremity strength gain associated with improvement in physical performance and disability in frail, community-dwelling elders? Archives of Physical Medicine and Rehabilitation 79:24–30

Cohen-Mansfield J, Marx M S, Biddison J R et al 2004 Socio-environmental exercise preferences among older adults. Preventive Medicine 38(6):804–811

Copeland J R M 1999 Depression of older age. British Journal of Psychiatry 174:304–306

Cummings S R, Black D M, Nevitt M C et al 1993 Bone density at various sites for prediction of hip fractures. Lancet 34:72–75

Cussler E C, Lohman T G, Going S B et al 2003 Weight lifted in strength training predicts bone change in postmenopausal women. Medicine and Science in Sports and Exercise 35(1):10–17

Day L, Fildes B, Gordon I et al 2002 Randomised factorial trial of falls prevention among older people living in their own homes. British Medical Journal 325(7356):128–133

Deforche B, De Bourdeaudhuij I 2000 Differences in psychosocial determinants of physical activity in older adults participating in organised versus non-organised activities. Journal of Sports Medicine and Physical Fitness 40(4):362–372

DoH (Department of Health) 2000 Health Survey for England 1998. The Stationery Office, London

Emery C F, Hauck E R, Blumenthal J A 1992 Exercise adherence or maintenance among older adults: 1-year follow-up study. Psychology and Aging 7(3):466–470

Evans W J 1999 Exercise training guidelines for the elderly. Medicine and Science in Sports and Exercise 31:12–17

Faulkner K G, von Stetten E, Miller P 1999 Discordance in patient classification using T-scores. Journal of Clinical Densiometry 2:343–350

Ferri A, Scaglioni G, Pousson M et al 2003 Strength and power changes of the human plantar flexors and knee extensors in response to resistance training in old age. Acta Physiologica Scandinavica 177(1):69–78

Foldvari M, Clark M, Laviolette L C et al 2000 Association of muscle power with functional status in community-dwelling elderly women. Journals of Gerontology Series A – Biological Sciences and Medical Sciences 55(4):M192–199

Fox K R 2000 The effects of exercise upon self-perceptions and self-esteem. In: Biddle S J H, Fox K R, Boutcher S H (eds) Physical activity and psychological well-being. Routledge, London, p 88–117

Frontera W R, Meredith C N, O'Reilly K P et al 1988 Strength conditioning in older men: skeletal muscle hypertrophy and improved function. Journal of Applied Physiology 64(3)1038–1044

Frontera W R, Suh D, Krivickas L S et al 2000 Skeletal muscle fiber quality in older men and women. American Journal of Physiology – Cell Physiology 279(3):C611–618

Gardner M M, Robertson M C, Campbell A J 2000 Exercise in preventing falls and fall related injuries in older people: a review of randomised controlled trials. British Journal of Sports Medicine 34(1):7–17.

Gardner M M, Buchner D M, Robertson M C et al 2001 Practical implementation of an exercise-based falls prevention programme. Age and Ageing 30(1):77–83

Gavrilov L A, Gavrilova N S 2003 The quest for a general theory of aging and longevity. Science of Aging Knowledge Environment 2003(28):RE5

Giles-Corti B, Donovan R J 2002a Socioeconomic status difference in recreational physical activity levels and real and perceived access to a supportive physical environment. Preventive Medicine 35:601–611

Giles-Corti B, Donovan R J 2002b The relative influence of individual, social and physical environment determinants of physical activity. Social Science and Medicine 54:1793–1812

Grossman M D, Stewart A L 2003 'You aren't going to get better by just sitting around': physical activity perceptions, motivations, and barriers in adults 75 years of age or older. American Journal of Geriatric Cardiology 12(1):33–37

Harman D 2001 Aging: overview. Annals of the New York Academy of Sciences 928:1–21

Hayflick L 2003 Living forever and dying in the attempt. Experimental Gerontology 38:1231–1241

Henry K D, Rosemond C, Eckert L B 1999 Effect of number of home exercises on compliance and performance in adults over 65 years of age. Physical Therapy 79(3):270–277

Hippocrates (470–360 BC) On the articulations. The genuine works of Hippocrates, translated from the Greek with a preliminary discourse and annotations (Adams F, tr, 1849). Sydenham Society, London, part 58

Holloszy J O 2000 The biology of aging. Mayo Clinic Proceedings 75 (Supplement):S3–S9

Huang Y, Macera C A, Blair S N et al 1998 Physical fitness, physical activity, and functional limitation in adults age 40 and older. Medicine and Science in Sports and Exercise 30:1430–1435

Humpel N, Owen N, Iverson D et al 2004 Perceived environmental attributes, residential location, and walking for particular purposes. American Journal of Preventive Medicine 26:119–125

Hunter G R, McCarthy J P, Bamman M M 2004 Effects of resistance training in older adults. Sports Medicine 34:329–348

Hyatt R H, Whitelaw M N, Bhat A et al 1990 Association of muscle strength with functional status of elderly people. Age and Ageing 19(5):330–336

Jette A M, Branch L G 1981 The Framingham Disability Study: II. Physical disability among the aging. American Journal of Public Health 71(11):1211–1216

Jette A M, Lachman M, Giorgetti M M et al 1999 Exercise – it's never too late: the strong-for-life program. American Journal of Public Health 89:66–72

Judge J O 2003 Balance training to maintain mobility and prevent disability. American Journal of Preventive Medicine 25(3Sii):150–156

Khan K M, Liu-Ambrose T, Donaldson M G et al 2001 Physical activity to prevent falls in older people: time to intervene in high risk groups using falls as an outcome. British Journal of Sports Medicine 35:144–145

King A C, Blair S N, Bild D E et al 1992 Determinants of physical activity and interventions in adults. Medicine and Science in Sports and Exercise 24(6 Suppl):S221–S236

King A C, Rejeski W J, Buchner D M 1998 Physical activity interventions targeting older adults. A critical review and recommendations. American Journal of Preventive Medicine 15:316–333

King A C, Castro C, Wilcox S et al 2000 Personal and environmental factors associated with physical inactivity among different racial-ethnic groups of US middle-aged and older-aged women. Health Psychology 19:354–364

King W C, Brach J S, Belle S et al 2003 The relationship between convenience of destinations and walking levels in older women. American Journal of Health Promotion 18:74–82

Klitgaard H, Mantoni M, Schiaffino S et al 1990 Function, morphology and protein expression of ageing skeletal muscle: a cross-sectional study of elderly men with different training backgrounds. Acta Physiologica Scandinavica 140(1):41–54

Kolt G S, Driver R P, Giles L C 2004 Why older Australians participate in exercise and sport. Journal of Aging and Physical Activity 12(2):185–198

Kutner N G, Barnhart H, Wolf S L et al 1997 Self-report benefits of Tai Chi practice by older adults. Journals of Gerontology Series B: Psychological Sciences and Social Sciences 52(5):P242–P246

Lakatta E G 1993 Cardiovascular regulatory mechanisms in advanced age. Physiological Reviews 73:413–469

Larsson L 1983 Histochemical characteristics of human skeletal muscle during aging. Acta Physiologica Scandinavica 117(3):469–471

Lee C 1993 Factors related to the adoption of exercise among older women. Journal of Behavioural Medicine 16:323–334

Lexell J 1995 Human aging, muscle mass, and fiber type composition. Journals of Gerontology Series A: Biological Sciences and Medical Sciences 50 Spec No: 11–16

Lindle R S, Metter E J, Lynch N A et al 1997 Age and gender comparisons of muscle strength in 654 women and men aged 20–93 yr. Journal of Applied Physiology 83(5):1581–1587

Lu Y, Genant H K, Shepherd J et al 2001 Classification of osteoporosis based on bone mineral densities. Journal of Bone Mineral Research 16:901–910

Lubitz J, Cai L, Kramarow E et al 2003 Health, life expectancy, and health care spending among the elderly. New England Journal of Medicine 349:1048–1055

Lupton D 1994 Medicine as culture: illness, disease and the body in western societies. Sage, London

Manderson L, Reid J C 1994 What's culture got to do with it? In: Waddell C, Peterson A (eds) Just health: inequality in illness care and prevention. Churchill Livingstone, Melbourne

Manson J E, Greenland P, LaCroix A Z et al 2002 Walking compared with vigorous exercise for the prevention of cardiovascular events in women. New England Journal of Medicine 347(10):716–725

Marshall D, Johnell O, Wedel H 1996 Meta-analysis of how well measures of bone mineral density predict occurrence of osteoporotic fractures. British Medical Journal 312:1254–1259

Melton L J 2000 Who has osteoporosis? A conflict between clinical and public health perspectives. Journal of Bone Mineral Research 15:2309–2314

Metter E J, Lynch N, Conwit R et al 1999 Muscle quality and age: cross-sectional and longitudinal comparisons. Journals of Gerontology Series A: Biological Sciences and Medical Sciences 54(5):B207-B218

Mor V, Wilcox V, Rakowski W et al 1994 Functional transitions among the elderly: patterns, predictors, and related hospital use. American Journal of Public Health 84:1274–1280

Nelson M E, Fiatarone M A, Morganti C M et al 1994 Effects of high-intensity strength training on multiple risk factors for osteoporotic fractures. A randomized controlled trial. Journal of the American Medical Association 272(24):1909–1914

O'Brien Cousins S 2000 'My heart couldn't take it': older women's beliefs about exercise benefits and risks. Journals of Gerontology 55B:283–294

O'Brien Cousins S, Keating N 1995 Life cycle patterns of physical activity among sedentary and active older women. Journal of Aging and Physical Activity 3:340–359

O'Brien S J, Vertinsky P A 1991 Unfit survivors: exercise as a resource for aging women. Gerontologist 31:347–357

Overend T J, Cunningham D A, Paterson D H et al 1992 Thigh composition in young and elderly men determined by computed tomography. Clinical Physiology 12(6):629–640

Paffenbarger R S, Lee I M 1996 Physical activity and fitness for health and longevity. Research Quarterly for Exercise and Sport 67(3) (Supplement):11–28

Paffenbarger R S, Hyde R T, Wing A L et al 1986 Physical activity, all-cause mortality and longevity of college alumni. New England Journal of Medicine 314:605–613

Parkkari J, Kannus P, Palvanen M et al 1999 Majority of hip fractures occur as a result of a fall and impact on the greater trochanter of the femur: a prospective controlled hip fracture study with 206 consecutive patients. Calcified Tissue International 65(3):183–187

Parsons P A 2003 From the stress theory of aging to energetic and evolutionary expectations for longevity. Biogerontology 4(2):63–73

Pate R R, Pratt M, Blair S N et al 1995 Physical activity and public health. A recommendation from the Centers for Disease Control and Prevention and the American College of Sports Medicine. Journal of the American Medical Association 273(5):402–407

Peck W A, Riggs B L, Bell N H et al 1988 Research directions in osteoporosis. American Journal of Medicine 84(2):275–282

Pekkanen J, Marti B, Nissinen A et al 1987 Reduction of premature mortality by high physical activity: a 20-year follow-up of middle-aged Finnish men. Lancet 1(8548):1473–1477

Pendergast D R, Fisher N M, Calkins E 1993 Cardiovascular, neuromuscular, and metabolic alterations with age leading to frailty. Journal of Gerontology 48:61–67

Penninx B W J H, Messier S P, Rejeski W J et al 2001a Physical exercise and the prevention of disability in activities of daily living in older persons with osteoarthritis. Archives of Internal Medicine 161:2309–2316

Penninx B W, Beekman A T, Honig A et al 2001b Depression and cardiac mortality: results from a community-based longitudinal study. Archives of General Psychiatry 58(3):221–227

Pereira M A, Kriska A M, Day R D et al 1998 A randomised walking trial in postmenopausal women: effects of physical activity and health 10 years later. Archives of Internal Medicine 158:1695–1701

Perusse L, Rankinen T, Rauramaa R et al 2003 The human gene map for performance and health-related fitness phenotypes: the 2002 update. Medicine and Science in Sports and Exercise 35(8):1248–1264

Reaven P D, McPhillips J B, Barrett-Connor E L et al 1990 Leisure time exercise and lipid and lipoprotein levels in an older population. Journal of the American Geriatrics Society 38(8):847–854

Resnick B 2000 A seven step approach to starting an exercise program for older adults. Patient Education and Counseling 39(2–3):243–252

Resnick B, Spellbring A M 2000 Understanding what motivates older adults to exercise. Journal of Gerontological Nursing 26(3):34–42

Rhodes R E, Martin A D, Taunton J E et al 1999 Factors associated with exercise adherence among older adults: an individual perspective. Sports Medicine 28:397–411

Robertson M C, Devlin N, Gardner M M et al 2001a Effectiveness and economic evaluation of a nurse delivered home exercise programme to prevent falls. 1: Randomised controlled trial. British Medical Journal 322(7288):697–701

Robertson M C, Gardner M M, Devlin N et al 2001b Effectiveness and economic evaluation of a nurse delivered home exercise programme to prevent falls. 2: Controlled trial in multiple centres. British Medical Journal 322(7288):701–704

Robinson J I, Rogers M A 1994 Adherence to exercise programmes: recommendations. Sports Medicine 17:39–52

Rose M 1999 Can human aging be postponed? Scientific American 281(6):106–111

Rose M R, Nusbaum T J 1994 Prospects for postponing human aging. Federation of American Societies Experimental Biology Journal 8:925–928

Roubenoff R, Hughes V A 2000 Sarcopenia: current concepts. Journals of Gerontology Series A: Biological Sciences and Medical Sciences 55(12):M716–724

Sallis J F, Hovell M F, Hofstetter R 1992 Predictors of adoption and maintenance of vigorous physical activity in men and women. Preventive Medicine 21:237–251

Salmon J, Owen N, Crawford D et al 2003 Physical activity and sedentary behaviour: a population-based study of barriers, enjoyment, and preference. Health Psychology 22:178–188

Sartorio A, Lafortuna C, Capodaglio P et al 2001 Effects of a 16-week progressive high-intensity strength training (HIST) on indexes of bone turnover in men over 65 years: a randomized controlled study. Journal of Endocrinological Investigation 24(11):882–886

Satariano W A, McAuley E 2003 Promoting physical activity among older adults: from ecology to individual. American Journal of Preventive Medicine 25 (3Sii):184–192

Schneider J K, Eveker A, Bronder D R et al 2003 Exercise training program for older adults. Incentives and disincentives for participation. Journal of Gerontological Nursing 29(9):21–31

Seguin R, Nelson M E 2003 The benefits of strength training in older adults. American Journal of Preventive Medicine 25(Sii):141–149

Shephard RJ 1996 Exercise and cancer: Links with obesity? Critical Reviews in Food Science and Nutrition 36:321–329

Sims J, Huang N, Pietsch J et al 2004 The Victorian Active Script Programme: promising signs for general practitioners, population health, and the promotion of physical activity. British Journal of Sports Medicine 38(1):19–25

Skelton D, Young A, Greig C et al 1995 Effects of resistance training on strength power, and selected functional abilities of women aged 75 and older. Journal of the American Geriatric Society 43:1081–1087

Skelton D, Young A, Walker A et al 1999 Physical activity in later life: further analysis of the Allied Dunbar National Fitness Survey and the Health Education Authority National Survey of Activity and Health. Health Education Authority, London

Spirduso W W, Cronin D L 2001 Exercise dose-response effects on quality of life and independent living in older adults. Medicine and Science in Sports and Exercise 33:S598–S608

Sports Council and Health Education Authority 1992 Allied Dunbar National Fitness Survey. Sports Council and Health Education Authority, London

Ståhl T, Rütten A, Nutbeam D et al 2001 The importance of the social environment for physically active lifestyle – results from an international study. Social Science and Medicine 52:1–10

Taaffe D R, Duret C, Wheeler S 1999 Once-weekly resistance exercise improves muscle strength and neuromuscular performance in older adults. Journal of the American Geriatrics Society 47(10):1208–1214

Taylor A H 2000 Physical activity, anxiety and stress: a review. In: Biddle S J H, Fox K R, Boutcher S H (eds) Physical activity and psychological well-being. Routledge, London, p 10–45

Taylor A H, Cable N T, Faulkner G et al 2004 Physical activity and older adults: a review of health benefits and the effectiveness of interventions. Journal of Sports Sciences 22:703–725

Thelen D G, Brockmiller C, Ashton-Miller J A et al 1998 Thresholds for sensing foot dorsi- and plantarflexion during upright stance: effects of age and velocity. Journals of Gerontology Series A: Biological Sciences and Medical Sciences 53:33–38

Topp R, Mikesky A, Wigglesworth J et al 1993 Effect of a 12-week dynamic resistance strength training program on gait velocity and balance of older adults. The Gerontologist 33:501–506

Topp R, Mikesky A, Dayhoff N E et al 1996 Effect of resistance training on strength, postural control, and gait velocity among older adults. Clinical Nursing Research 5(4):407–427

United Nations Population Division of Economic and Social Affairs (DESA) 2004 World population Trends. Online. Available: http://www.un.org/popin/wdtrends.htm December 2004

USDHHS 1996 Physical activity and health: A report of the Surgeon General, US Department of Health and Human Services, Center for Disease Control and Prevention, National Center for Chronic Disease Prevention and Health Promotion. USDHHS, Atlanta, GA

van der Bij A K, Laurant M G, Wensing M 2002 Effectiveness of physical activity interventions for older adults: a review. American Journal of Preventive Medicine 22(2):120–133

Vina J, Sastre J, Pallardo F et al 2003 Mitochondrial theory of aging: importance to explain why females live longer than males. Antioxidants and Redox Signalling 5(5):549–556

Vincent K R, Braith R W, Feldman R A et al 2002 Resistance exercise and physical performance in adults aged 60 to 83. Journal of the American Geriatrics Society 50(6):1100–1107

Wenger N K 1996 Physical inactivity and coronary heart disease in elderly patients. Clinics in Geriatric Medicine 12(1):79–88

WHO (World Health Organization) 1994 The WHO study group on osteoporosis. Assessment of fracture risk and its application to screening for post-menopausal osteoporosis. WHO, Geneva

WHO 1997 The Heidelberg guidelines for promoting physical activity among older persons. Journal of Aging and Physical Activity 5:1–8

Wolf S L, Sattin R W, Kutner M et al 2003 Intense tai chi exercise training and fall occurrences in older, transitionally frail adults: a randomized, controlled trial. Journal of the American Geriatrics Society 51(12):1693–1701

Wood RH, Reyes R, Welsch MA, Favaloro-Sabatier J, Sabatier M, Matthew Lee C, Johnson LG, Hooper PF 2001 Concurrent cardiovascular resistance training in healthy older adults. Medicine and Science in Sports and Exercise 33(10):1751-8

Young A, Skelton D A 1994 Applied physiology of strength and power in old age. International Journal of Sports Medicine 15(3):149–151

CHAPTER 14

Therapeutic medications: influences with regard to physical activity and exercise

CHAPTER CONTENTS

Introduction 219
Definitions 220
Drug administration, distribution and excretion 220
Flow and capacity limited drugs 221
    Flow limited 221
        Flow limited drugs and physical activity/exercise 221
    Capacity limited 221
        Capacity limited drugs and physical activity/exercise 221
Pharmacokinetics, pharmacodynamics and physical activity and exercise 221
    Internal factors 221
    External factors 222
Physical activity and exercise 222
    Haemodynamics 222
    Body temperature and pH 222
    Timing of drug administration 223
    Drug absorption 223
    Physical training 223
Therapeutic medications: influence on functional ability 223
    Cardiovascular drugs 223
        Angiotensin-converting enzyme inhibitors 223
        Beta-blockers 225
        Alpha-blockers 226
        Calcium channel blockers 226
        Diuretics 226
        Inotropic drugs 226
        Anti-arrhythmia drugs 226

        Nitrates 226
Lipid-lowering medications 226
Medications for the control of blood glucose 227
Anti-clotting medication 227
    Warfarin 228
    Heparin 228
    Aspirin 228
    Clopidogrel 228
    Streptokinase 228
Medication for treatment of obesity 229
Respiratory medication 229
    Bronchodilators 229
    Anti-inflammatories 230
    Antibiotics 230
    Mucolytic agents 230
Arthritis 230
    Non-steroidal anti-inflammatory drugs 230
    Disease-modifying anti-rheumatic drugs 231
Osteoporosis 231
    Parathyroid hormone and vitamin D 231
    Bisphosphonates 231
    Calcitonin 231
    Oestrogen 231
    Selective oestrogen-receptor modulators 231
Cancer 231
    Chemotherapy 231
    Hormone therapy 232
Summary 232
Suggested readings, references and bibliography 232

INTRODUCTION

The beneficial health effects of physical activity (PA)/exercise are now well recognized, and increasingly research is being conducted to determine appropriate PA/exercise prescription for symptomatic individuals.

However, although the vast majority of these individuals will be performing PA/exercise whilst taking medication, relatively little is known regarding the interaction between PA/exercise and these therapeutic medications, or the potential limiting effect of these drugs upon PA/exercise performance or functional ability.

The objective of this chapter is to provide a simplified general background to the metabolism and pharmacokinetics of drugs, outlining the possible influence that PA/exercise might have. This will be followed by a look at current research regarding the effect of these therapeutic medications, most commonly used to treat the diseases and conditions described in previous chapters, upon functional ability. The aim therefore is to assist the exercise practitioner in understanding the possible effects that a person's medications may have on functional ability, and how PA/exercise may influence the medication that a client/patient is currently taking. This should enable the practitioner to tailor the PA/exercise programme more specifically to the individual client/patient.

DEFINITIONS

A *drug* may be described as any substance that when introduced into the body alters the body's function by interaction at a subcellular level. The *pharmacodynamics* of a drug describes the effect of the drug upon the body, more specifically, the drug-receptor binding characteristics and dose–response relationship; the *pharmacokinetics* of a drug relates to the manner in which the body manages the drug once it enters the body, or how the drug is absorbed, distributed, metabolized and eliminated.

DRUG ADMINISTRATION, DISTRIBUTION AND EXCRETION

Drugs may be administered through various routes, such as orally, topically/transdermally through patches, creams or gels, intramuscular injection or intravenously. The majority of drugs need to be absorbed into the systemic circulation for transportation and distribution to organs and receptor sites, where the action, reaction and/or interaction can occur. Some drugs, for instance, bind to plasma proteins, mainly albumin (only the unbound part of the drug is pharmacologically active) (Somani 1981). The majority of drugs act at a subcellular level through tissue macromolecules. These macromolecules are relatively large chemical substances, and take the form of proteins, carbohydrate protein structures, lipid protein structures and/or a nucleic acid drug (drugs that interact with DNA and may take the form of an enzyme). The main determinant of the rate and extent of drug entry into the body is the formation of the drug (i.e. in tablet form, capsule, ointment or powder), as well as certain physiochemical properties of the drug, such as its molecular size, lipophilicity (affinity to fat) and acid–base characteristics (pH) (Somani & Kamimori 1996).

Drugs are transported across cell lipid membranes by four main mechanisms: diffusion, filtration, active transport and endocytosis. The most common of these

Table 14.1 Main mechanisms of drug transportation across the cell membrane

Mechanism	Description
Diffusion	The movement of molecules from a region of high concentration to one of a lower concentration
Filtration	The passing of a plasma liquid through a filter or filtration medium, accomplished by gravity, pressure or vacuum (suction)
Active transport	Transport of ions, nutrients or molecules into a cell against a concentration gradient; requires the expenditure of energy through ATP hydrolysis
Endocytosis	A cell may take up a molecule by invagination of the cell's plasma membrane (see Fig. 3.6)

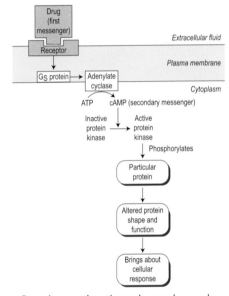

Figure 14.1   Drug interaction through membrane, bound receptors and secondary messengers (adapted from Vander et al 1990).

mechanisms is diffusion (Table 14.1). Once the drug reaches the systemic circulation it binds to plasma proteins, and since the protein albumin makes up to 70% of plasma proteins, it is albumin that is the major site of drug binding. Once the drug is in systemic circulation the drug molecules are either bound or unbound to organs and tissues. The ability of the organ to extract the drug is altogether dependent upon the characteristics of the drug and organ in question. Drug interactions usually occur through the cell membrane, bound receptor and/or through structures within the target cell. However, the binding of a drug to a 'secondary messenger' molecule is generally not permanent and is often reversible (Somani & Kamimori 1996) (Fig. 14.1). Any changes in drug binding may affect toxicity. For instance, the fraction of the bound drug is considered pharmacologically inactive and

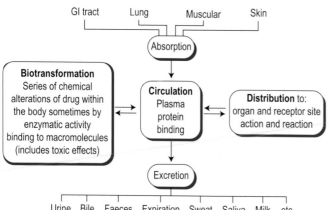

Figure 14.2 General representation of drug absorption, distribution, metabolism and excretion (adapted from Somani 1996).

Table 14.2 Percentage distribution of cardiac output during rest, light, moderate and vigorous exercise (adapted from Anderson 1968)

Tissue	Rest	Light	Moderate	Vigorous
Splanchnic	27	12	3	1
Renal	22	10	3	1
Cerebral	14	8	4	3
Coronary	4	4	4	4
Muscle	20	47	71	88
Skin	6	15	12	2
Other	7	4	3	1

non-toxic, but when a strongly bound drug is displaced, this may cause toxicity (Somani & Kamimori 1996). The body may excrete the metabolites of drugs through a variety of pathways, such as through the urine, faeces, bile, sweat, saliva, tears, milk and/or breath (Fig. 14.2).

FLOW AND CAPACITY LIMITED DRUGS

Drugs are generally categorized into two types. Those that are *flow limited* and those that are *capacity limited*. However, determining whether a drug is a flow or capacity limited drug is not always easy. Somani & Kamimori (1996) have categorized a short list of drugs, which can be found in Somani (1996, pp. 14–15).

FLOW LIMITED

Flow limited drugs are not limited by binding to other macromolecules but by blood flow. These types of drugs tend to have a high clearance rate, high extraction ratio and high intrinsic clearance. For example, most of the drug propranolol (beta-blocker) is extracted before being bound to macromolecules. Therefore, even if binding is changed, extraction and metabolism of the drug may not alter (Somani & Kamimori 1996).

Flow limited drugs and physical activity/exercise

Physical activity/exercise can alter the time course of some flow limited drugs, affecting the distribution and kinetics of the drugs, by delivering more blood to active muscle (Table 14.2) and consequently more of the drug to these muscles (Somani & Kamimori 1996).

CAPACITY LIMITED

Capacity limited drugs are strongly bound to macromolecules, and a high proportion of these drugs will be bound to plasma after administration, and are thus poorly extracted. The anticoagulant drug warfarin is a capacity limited drug and is extracted by the liver. Its function therefore depends upon the fraction of unbound drug that exists in the blood (Somani & Kamimori 1996).

Capacity limited drugs and physical activity/exercise

During PA/exercise a change in blood flow to certain areas of the body may increase the extraction ratio of capacity limited drugs in those tissues with increased blood flow (Table 14.2). Since removal of certain drugs requires time to complete, a reduction of blood flow to a particular tissue or organ may result in the drug staying in contact with these tissues for a longer time leading to greater extraction of the drug from the plasma. However, this potential problem is not highly researched and the effect of PA/exercise on many capacity limited drugs is still unknown (Somani & Kamimori 1996).

PHARMACOKINETICS, PHARMACODYNAMICS AND PHYSICAL ACTIVITY AND EXERCISE

The rate of metabolism and excretion of drugs generally determines their duration and action. The main rate-limiting factors for drug metabolism and elimination are the delivery of the drug to the site of metabolism and/or the ability of the enzyme systems to handle drug metabolism. Thus, blood flow and enzyme activity are important factors in pharmacokinetics and pharmacodynamics. Pharmacokinetics can also be modified by internal and external factors that have the capacity to affect drug absorption, distribution, metabolism and elimination (Sweeney 1981, Buckenmeyer & Somani 1996).

INTERNAL FACTORS

Internal factors such as plasma protein binding, pH, metabolic disease and drug-to-drug interaction may influence the pharmacokinetics and dynamics of a drug (Somani 1996).

EXTERNAL FACTORS

External factors such as temperature, humidity, altitude, hypoxia, posture and age have all been cited as factors that potentially influence drug pharmacokinetics and dynamics (Somani & Kamimori 1996).

PHYSICAL ACTIVITY AND EXERCISE

The effect of PA/exercise on the pharmacokinetics and pharmacodynamics of the wide variety of therapeutic medications is scantly researched. Thus, only a brief discussion of the currently known effect of PA/exercise on these factors is provided.

Physical activity/exercise affects blood flow (haemodynamics) (Table 14.2) and pH and increases body heat, which may affect drug pharmacokinetics and pharmacodynamics. Other potential effects of PA/exercise upon pharmacokinetics are its influence on plasma protein binding and diffusion of a drug across the cell membranes, and on hepatic clearance of drugs, as there is an increase in bile flow and excretion during PA/exercise, which may have possible clinical implications. If a drug is removed more rapidly from the system, then the normal dosing schedules may be inadequate, due to either a decrease in drug residence time or inadequate drug concentration. Conversely, a decrease in drug clearance, with no modifications to drug dosing schedules, may lead to an increase in drug concentration, and greater potential for toxicity (Somani & Kamimori 1996). For instance, drugs such as digoxin (cardiac glycoside) (Orlov et al 1990) and oxprenolol (beta-blocker) require maintenance within a therapeutic concentration range (Lemmer 1982, Louis et al 1982), and may be affected by PA/exercise (Somani & Kamimori 1996). In a study looking to determine whether exercise affected the distribution and renal excretion of digoxin (an inotropic and flow limited drug prescribed for cardiac arrhythmia), compared to resting conditions, 0.50 mg was intravenously injected into 12 healthy male volunteers prior to 8 hours of intermittent cycle ergometry (80 watts for the first 2 hours, then 45 minutes at 4, 6 and 8 hours after first intake of drug). At 30 and 45 minutes after intake of digoxin, serum concentration was significantly higher during exercise compared to rest, indicating increased absorption rate during exercise. However, at 2 and 4 hours after intake, serum digoxin was significantly lower than during the exercise. The exercise also decreased renal excretion. The researchers concluded that these changes in pharmacokinetics were probably due to increased binding of digoxin to the exercising muscles, and that any variation in daily PA/exercise in digoxin-treated individuals may cause variations in the effect of the drug (Jogestrand & Andersson 1989). Additionally, a study carried out on horses found drugs that displayed effective hepatic extraction at rest showed decreased hepatic clearance when the horses exercised at 40%, 60% and 80% of maximal aerobic capacity, for 15 minutes at each intensity (drugs were administered over a period of 45 to 60 seconds during the first minute of treadmill exercise) (Dyke et al 1998).

HAEMODYNAMICS

The profound alterations in haemodynamics during PA/exercise and changes in tissue blood flow have been identified as major factors affecting pharmacokinetics. During an acute bout of PA/exercise, blood flow to the liver is reduced. For instance, during intense PA/exercise cardiac output may increase five to six times that of rest. Hence there will be an increase in the plasma concentration of those drugs that have a high clearance rate, such as flow limited drugs. High clearance drugs generally involve the liver or other organs, taking the drug out of the blood quickly. If the blood flow to these organs is decreased, then clearance with be hindered, and the drug may stay in the blood longer, resulting in a possible increase in toxicity. Furthermore, blood flow is shunted away from the gastrointestinal tract, potentially affecting absorption of oral drugs taken just prior to PA/exercise (Somani & Kamimori 1996).

BODY TEMPERATURE AND PH

Increases in body heat can affect changes in enzyme activity, and potentially affect the pharmacokinetics of certain drugs. For instance, an increase in enzyme activity may lead to an increase in metabolic clearance of a drug. Furthermore, an increase in body temperature could affect the ability of the drug to bind to plasma protein, which may lead to an increase in the free fraction of the drug. However, the research regarding this is conflicting (Somani & Kamimori 1996) and may be dependent upon many factors, such as the drug in question, extent of increase and duration of the increase in temperature.

Physical activity/exercise may be accompanied by an increase in the acidity of the blood, particularly during intense PA/exercise where the body relies more heavily upon anaerobic glycolysis for energy, which increases the release of hydrogen ions into the blood. With an increase in acidosis there is a drop in pH, which could lead to changes in drug ionization and polarity. This in turn may either increase or decrease drug absorption depending on the molecular structure of the drug (Somani & Kamimori 1996).

TIMING OF DRUG ADMINISTRATION

Jogestrand & Andersson (1989) have demonstrated that timing of PA/exercise in relation to drug administration, or vice versa, can significantly modify drug pharmacokinetics, potentially affecting the therapeutic value of the drug. It appears that PA/exercise has the greatest effect on drugs that have a relatively short half-life (Somani & Kamimori 1996). Thus it has been suggested that it may be better to administer a drug after exercise or several hours before, depending on the time course of the drug (Somani 1996). Although there is little research to support this, it is also fair to assume that the intensity of PA/exercise performed has implications for the timing of drug administration.

Kamimori et al (1990) examined the pharmacokinetics of atropine, a potent vasodilator and flow limited drug that can be used in acute situations to treat cardiac patients and for organophosphate poisoning. In their study, atropine was administered intramuscularly into the quadriceps of seven healthy young males (19 to 32 years) after cycle ergometry at 40% of aerobic capacity (intermittent cycling for 90 minutes, 25 minutes' cycling with 5 minutes' rest). When the drug was administered post-exercise, they found an increase in the rate and peak serum concentration, when compared to resting conditions, which was concluded to be the result of the increase in muscle blood flow. When administered pre-exercise, there was no change in absorption rate, though there was a significant decrease in the distribution of the drug, in addition to an increase in serum concentration. Thus, it would appear that in this instance, prior administration caused only a minimal effect on absorption but a greater effect on distribution, demonstrating that the timing of drug administration, in relation to a bout of PA/exercise, is important for drug pharmacokinetics and dynamics. However, much work still needs to be done in this area, to fully determine the effect/s of timing of drug administration with regard to PA/exercise upon drug absorption and distribution (Somani & Kamimori 1996).

DRUG ABSORPTION

The way in which a drug is administered may affect its absorption. For example, during an acute bout of PA/exercise, blood flow to the active muscle is enhanced. This tends to increase absorption of a drug that is injected into the active muscle just prior to or during PA/exercise. Additionally, the active muscle can enhance the uptake of drugs, such as insulin, employed to treat insulin-dependent diabetes mellitus (Sweeney 1981, Burr & Dinesh 1999, Patel 1999) (Ch. 4, p.72). Low-intensity PA/exercise (Ciccone 1995) has also been found to increase absorption of transdermally administered drugs, such as ointments or patches applied to the skin. In addition, since blood flow is shunted away from the gastrointestinal tract, there is the potential for this to affect drug absorption of oral medication/s taken just prior to PA/exercise (Somani & Kamimori 1996).

PHYSICAL TRAINING

It is clear that little research has been performed looking into the acute effects of PA/exercise on the pharmacokinetics and dynamics of therapeutic medications. However, even less research has been carried out looking into the effect that physical training might have. From the few studies that have been carried out, evidence suggests that habitual PA/exercise enhances metabolic efficiency and activity, thus potentially affecting drug metabolism. It appears that in young and physically trained people, there is an elevation in the rate of drug metabolism when compared to untrained individuals, which has been termed 'endogenous enzyme induction' (Vesell 1984). Yet, with regard to factors that influence drug metabolism, aerobic fitness does not appear to have been accounted for (Breimer 1983, Somani & Kamimori 1996). A more recent review of research shows that physical training can affect drug absorption by increasing collateral blood flow and changes in gastrointestinal transit times. Additionally, habitual PA/exercise may affect volume distribution of drugs, since physical training can increase lean body mass, plasma protein and volume, and decrease fat mass. The changes in hepatic clearance of drugs may also explanain the differences in systemic clearance observed between physically trained and sedentary individuals. Research is, however, contradictory as to whether physical training causes any change in hepatic enzymes (Persky et al 2003).

THERAPEUTIC MEDICATIONS: INFLUENCE ON FUNCTIONAL ABILITY

The influence of therapeutic medication on functional ability is not widely researched. Nonetheless, outlined below are some of the known effects of commonly employed drugs, used to treat the diseases and conditions mentioned in previous chapters, and their effect on functional ability and related parameters.

CARDIOVASCULAR DRUGS

The functions of cardiovascular medications are described elsewhere (Ch. 2), and compared to other medications, cardiovascular drugs have received relatively more attention with regard to their potential effect on an individual's functional ability (Table 14.3).

Angiotensin–converting enzyme inhibitors

Studies on the effect of angiotensin-converting enzyme (ACE) inhibitors on functional ability have shown varying

Table 14.3 Cardiovascular drugs: implications and considerations for physical activity/exercise (adapted from Frank 1996, BACR 2002)

Type of drug	Prescribed for	Positive effects	Considerations
ACE inhibitor	Hypertension Heart failure Left ventricular (LV) function in post MI patients	Enhances PA/exercise tolerance Enhances PA/exercise capacity, in chronic heart failure patients Enhances PA/exercise endurance Reduces systolic and diastolic blood pressure (SBP and DBP) Increases blood flow to active muscles Enhances oxygen uptake ($\dot{V}o_2$)	Reduced heart rate and blood pressure response
Beta-blocker	Hypertension Angina Tachycardia/arrhythmias	Reduces SBP and DBP Reduces heart rate Improves PA/exercise tolerance in angina Reduces silent myocardial ischaemia Reduces PA/exercise-induced arrhythmias Reduces platelet aggregability	Reduced PA/exercise tolerance Can increase peripheral resistance Can reduce PA/exercise capacity Increases fall in blood glucose Slows heart rate Hypotension Fatigue, lethargy Dizziness Airway constriction Cold fingers/toes Thermoregulation
Alpha-blocker	Hypertension, when not controlled by other medication		Postural hypotension Headache
Calcium channel blocker	Hypertension Angina Control of arrhythmias	Enhances PA/exercise endurance in sufferers of angina Enhances metabolic equivalent (MET) scores Reduces abnormalities in the ST segment of ECG Reduces number of angina attacks Reduces need for nitroglycerine Reduces SBP and DBP Enhances workload ability	Possible reduction in heart rate response in PA/exercise Postural hypotension Headache Dizziness Nausea
Diuretic	Acute heart failure Short-term use for mild heart failure Hypertension	May prolong submaximal PA/exercise duration	Reduced PA/exercise capacity Possible potassium loss with some diuretics Tiredness Muscle weakness and cramps Ventricular arrhythmias Diabetes Dehydration in hot weather
Inotropic	Supraventricular tachycardia Atrial fibrillation Occasionally for heart failure	Enhances exercise capacity Enhances endurance	Possible reduction in exercise capacity Nausea Vomiting Fatigue Slow heart rate

Table 14.3   Cardiovascular drugs: implications and considerations for physical activity/exercise (adapted from Frank 1996, BACR 2002)—*continued*

Type of drug	Prescribed for	Positive effects	Considerations
Anti-arrhythmia	Atrial fibrillation or flutter	Enhances maximal PA/exercise tolerance	Nausea Vomiting Fatigue Slow resting heart rate
Nitrate	Relief and prevention of angina Heart failure	Increases PA/exercise tolerance	Postural hypotension Headache Dizziness Nausea

results, which appear to be dependent on the ACE inhibitor administered and the type of cardiovascular condition being treated. A study looking into the effects of captopril found no significant effect upon exercise capacity in untrained individuals (Aldigier et al 1993). Yet, in another study on heart failure patients, quinapril enhanced exercise capacity (Northridge & Dargie 1990), which is thought to be the same for most ACE inhibitors (Buckenmeyer & Somani 1996), since ACE inhibitors work in similar ways although far from all ACE inhibitors have been researched with regard to their effect upon functional ability. The ACE inhibitor fosinopril has, however, been found to lower systolic and diastolic blood pressure during exercise, showing a slight increase in exercise endurance (Fortini et al 1994). On the other hand, temocapril was found to produce no change in haemodynamics during exercise in a group of mild hypertensives (Artia et al 1994).

In the treatment of chronic heart failure patients, long-term treatment with ACE inhibitors tends to increase blood flow to the working muscles, thus improving oxygen uptake. This is thought to be due to the inhibition of the renin–angiotensin system, and beneficial alterations in the vasculature (Munzel et al 1993, Buckenmeyer & Somani 1996), which potentially enhance functional ability.

Beta-blockers

The extent to which beta-blockers affect functional ability is dependent upon sympathetic tone, systolic and diastolic function of the patient, and the type of beta-blocker taken. Since beta-blockers slow the heart rate and lower blood pressure, they generally show a decreasing maximal exercise tolerance (Buckenmeyer & Somani 1996), but do not appear to affect submaximal oxygen uptake (Woolf-May & Bird 2005). Initially most beta-blockers cause

vasoconstriction, which tends to diminish over time, and may limit blood flow to the working muscles, and affect functional ability. Nonetheless, the degree to which the increase in local metabolites, which increase with onset of exercise and cause vasodilation of the exercising muscles, may override this is not totally clear.

For hypertensives taking diuretics who wish to participate in PA/exercise, beta-blockers are not recommended as the first choice of drug (Chick et al 1988, Houston 1992), partly due to increased risk of postural hypotension with this combination. Nonetheless, β_1 selective beta-blockers may be more advantageous to those with systolic hypertension and myocardial ischaemia during PA/exercise, as they reduce systolic blood pressure and heart rate. Beta-blockers can, however, restrict bronchodilation, which may increase breathlessness in some chronic heart failure patients (Witte et al 2003). Research is also conflicting as to whether beta-blockers are contraindicated in those with asthma and chronic obstructive pulmonary disease (COPD), though this may depend upon the beta-blocker being used (Salpeter et al 2003, Covar et al 2005).

In general, beta-blockers display no advantage during PA/exercise, though increases in aerobic fitness can be achieved irrespective of the drug. The reduction in exercise capacity is thought to be partly due to the effect of the beta-adrenoreceptor blockers inhibiting lipolysis of adipose tissue, shifting from fat to carbohydrate metabolism and increasing the uptake of blood glucose. For this reason, it has been suggested that β_1-blocking drugs may be advantageous to type I diabetics (Frank 1996). Furthermore, beta-blockers may interfere with thermoregulation during prolonged PA/exercise, by blocking the physiological mechanisms in response to physical exertion or stress that lead to an increase in body temperature (Van Baak 1988, Mayfield et al 1999).

It is important that any assessment of the client/patient prior to PA/exercise prescription is done when they are taking their medication, so that a clearer indication of their functional ability can be determined (Frank 1996), since their heart rate responses during PA/exercise will be blunted (Wenisch et al 2003, Woolf-May & Bird 2005). Wenisch et al (2003), for example, showed a mean reduction in heart rate of 19 beats per minute at aerobic threshold and 22 beats per minute at anaerobic threshold, in ten healthy males when taking beta-blocking medication.

Alpha-blockers

Alpha-blockers as a means of controlling blood pressure are more suitable than beta-blockers for hypertensive individuals who wish to perform PA/exercise (Houston 1992) though they may cause postural hypotension. They have, however, been found to reduce the effect of exercise-induced vasoconstriction in stenotic coronary artery disease (Julius et al 1999). However, for those with chronic heart failure alpha-blockers may affect ventilatory response to PA/exercise, thus causing an increase in breathlessness (Witte et al 2003). They do not appear to be contraindicated for those with respiratory disease (Reid 1993), though the role of alpha-receptors in asthma, for example, is unclear (Barnes 1986).

Calcium channel blockers

Calcium channel blockers work through various different mechanisms, and how they interact with PA/exercise will depend on the type of calcium channel blocker taken. Their general effects, in those with chronic stable angina, include an increase in exercise endurance (Navarro Estrada et al 1993) and enhanced coronary vasodilation during exercise in patients with coronary stenotic lesions (Kaufmann et al 1998). Calcium channel blockers have also been found to significantly delay the onset of 1 mm ST-segment depression (an electrocardiographic (ECG) indication of ischaemia, p. 245) during cycle ergometry in 335 subjects with exercise-induced angina (Cleophas et al 1999).

Diuretics

The effect of diuretics on functional ability is minimal. Nonetheless, for those with congestive heart failure, diuretics have been shown to enhance exercise tolerance (Mathur et al 1984) and, during PA/exercise, reduce symptoms of breathlessness (Follath 1998). Depending on the type and dose of diuretic taken, diuretics can lead to muscle weakness, which may affect functional ability, and during prolonged PA/exercise there is a risk of dehydration, especially in humid and hot weather. As with the vast majority of therapeutic drugs, there is a lack of research into the long-term effect of diuretics upon functional ability (Frank 1996).

Inotropic drugs

Inotropic drugs have generally been shown to improve haemodynamics, though not all studies have found them to enhance oxygen uptake (Munzel et al 1993). Notwithstanding this, digoxin, has been shown to improve exercise capacity and cardiac haemodynamics, increase ejection fraction and prevent congestive heart failure (Beaune 1989). Other inotropic drugs have been found to increase exercise endurance and performance (Frank 1996).

Anti-arrhythmia drugs

Amiodarone, a commonly prescribed drug to control arrhythmias, has been shown to increase exercise tolerance in patients with congestive heart failure (Hamer et al 1989).

Nitrates

Organic nitrates are effective in the treatment of angina pectoris. They considerably reduce the onset of symptoms and improve PA/exercise duration. However, they do not enhance exercise tolerance in those with mild to moderate heart failure (Frank 1996).

Table 14.4 Lipid-lowering drugs: implications and considerations for physical activity/exercise

Type of drug	Prescribed for	Effect on functional ability	Considerations
Bile-acid binders	Reduction of low-density lipoprotein cholesterol (LDL-C)	No known research in this area	Gastrointestinal (GI) problems
Fibrates	Reduction of triglycerides (TG) and LDL-C Increase of high-density lipoprotein cholesterol (HDL-C)	May result in premature fatigue during prolonged moderate intensity PA/exercise	Aching legs GI upset Muscle pain
Statins	Reduction of LDL-C Moderate reduction of TG and increased HDL-C	No known research in this area	GI upset

LIPID-LOWERING MEDICATIONS

There is very little research into the effect that lipid-lowering medications have on functional ability (Table 14.4). One of the few studies that have been carried out examined the interaction between aerobic exercise and lipid-lowering drugs in a randomized crossover study. Sixteen healthy subjects underwent 21 days of treatment with bezafibrate (a fibrate, 400 mg dose), fluvastatin (a statin, 40 mg dose) or placebo. The findings revealed that the statin and fibrate treatments independently reduced pre-exercise total cholesterol (TC), low-density lipoprotein cholesterol (LDL-C) and plasma triglycerides (TG) compared to pre-treatment values (Table 14.4). During exercise, the medications each caused a reduction in fat oxidation and plasma free fatty acid (FFA). After 90 minutes of moderate-intensity exercise, the statin had no effect on fat metabolism, compared to the placebo, but there was a reduced FFA concentration and lower fat oxidation. The possibility that fibrates might impair fat metabolism suggests that the use of fibrates could result in premature fatigue during prolonged exercise of moderate intensity (Eagles et al 1996).

It is known that high doses of statin medication can lead to myopathy (p. 256), which may affect functional ability, and when combined with fibrate medication may increase the risk of muscle damage. Although statins can lead to myopathy, niacin, which suppresses very LDL synthesis by the liver and is a vasodilator, does not appear to affect functional ability. Though it can reduce blood pressure and increase risk of postural hypotension, it may help reduce the risk of myopathy when given in combination with a statin rather than a fibrate (Shek & Ferril 2001). However, mild myopathy is reversible after statin withdrawal (Riesco-Eizaguirre et al 2003), and statin medication has been shown to improve symptoms associated with claudication (Hiatt 2004), and thus may enhance functional ability.

MEDICATIONS FOR THE CONTROL OF BLOOD GLUCOSE

Medications for the control of blood glucose levels are prescribed to type I and II diabetics (Ch. 4). Poorly controlled diabetes is detrimental to functional ability, and any of the drugs prescribed that assist in control of blood glucose levels will ultimately assist functional ability.

Insulin is the major drug for control of blood glucose in type I diabetics and the timing and administration of insulin during PA/exercise are extremely important (see p. 73, Table 4.12). The effects of other commonly prescribed diabetic medications, such as sulphonylureas, biguanides (metformin), thiazolidinediones and alpha-glycosidase inhibitors (acarbose) (see Table 4.10) have not received such comprehensive investigation as insulin with regard to their effect upon functional ability. Although there is research looking into the combined effect of both acute and chronic PA/exercise and these drugs, and their effect upon blood glucose levels, the research shows conflicting results; hence, no clear outcome as to their effect upon functional ability can be drawn.

Thiazolidinediones appear to improve flow-mediated vasodilation, decrease macrophage and smooth muscle cell activation, proliferation and migration, and decrease plaque formation. Thus, their multifaceted effect helps to restore vascular physiology to a healthier state. Hence, although they may not have any acute effect upon functional ability, in the long term they may assist in the enhancement of overall aerobic capacity (Reusch et al 2003). Biguanides, on the other hand, have been found to induce elevations in blood serum lactic acid (Irsigler et al 1978), which may remain after an acute bout of submaximal exercise in diabetic patients (Pilger et al 1979). In a more recent study, Blogosklonnaia et al (1990) observed no increase in blood serum levels in 232 diabetics after an exercise test, which has been supported by the findings of Fletcher et al (1986) from 103 type II diabetics taking biguanides after a 3-minute cycle ergometry test.

ANTI-CLOTTING MEDICATION

Medications most commonly employed to prevent or reverse blood coagulation are warfarin (Coumadin), heparin, aspirin, clopidogrel and streptokinase. Warfarin and heparin are used to treat those who are prone to thrombosis, heart failure or have an abnormal heart rhythm. Antiplatelet drugs such as aspirin and clopidogrel are often used in low doses to reduce risk of thrombosis, helping to

Table 14.5 Anti-clotting medication: implications and considerations for physical activity/exercise

Type of drug	Considerations
Warfarin (Coumadin)	Predisposes to nosebleeds, especially with high-intensity PA/exercise; low to moderate intensity PA/exercise preferred Bruising in exercising muscle has been reported Perform PA/exercise at similar time and intensity each day
Heparin	Enhances PA/exercise duration in angina patients Possible increase in PA/exercise heart rate, blood pressure and rate pressure product (RPP)
Aspirin	Possible increase in systolic blood pressure with PA/exercise Possible modification in blood flow during PA/exercise
Clopidogrel	High-intensity PA/exercise may counteract platelet-stabilizing action of this drug

protect against stroke or heart attack. Plasminogen activator, streptokinase, is also employed for controlling coagulation, but is especially useful at restoring the patency of coronary arteries following thrombosis, and particularly in the short period immediately following myocardial infarction (Table 14.5).

Warfarin

Those taking warfarin (Coumadin) require specialized dosing and monitoring to individualize therapy, maximize effectiveness, and decrease incidence of associated haemorrhage and thromboembolic complications. Therefore, regular monitoring of warfarin blood levels is required, and an understanding of the interaction of factors such as other drugs, food, disease (Chaffman & Pharm 2001) and PA/exercise is essential (Lenz et al 2004). Thus, it may be important for those taking this type of medication who wish to be physically active to perform their PA/exercise at a similar time and intensity each day, so that appropriate blood levels of warfarin can be more accurately determined. For those taking warfarin, a regular lifestyle is recommended.

There are no known reports regarding the effect of warfarin on functional ability. However, there are some considerations that the exercise practitioner should be aware of when prescribing PA/exercise to those taking this drug. For instance, nosebleeds are fairly common in those taking this type of medication (Verrier et al 1986, Glueck et al 1998), hence any rise in blood pressure due to PA/exercise may predispose the individual to nosebleeds. It is therefore advisable for PA/exercise intensity to be kept at low to moderate levels. Furthermore, it is important to note that isokinetic leg exercise has also been shown to produce extensive bruising in the posterior thigh of an older individual taking warfarin (Richter 1992), indicating the need for appropriate regulation of warfarin blood levels in physically active individuals.

Heparin

Heparin is used to prevent blood clotting, by inhibiting the coagulation cascade (p. 114). However, it has been reported to have other physiological effects that may have an influence upon functional ability. For instance, heparin has been shown to produce marked elevations in plasma FFA (Fragasso et al 2000). A study carried out by Ahlborg & Hagenfeld (1977) found, from six healthy male subjects after cycle exercise for 90 minutes, that while prior heparin administration did not result in an increase in plasma FFA levels, FFA uptake was augmented in the exercising legs. This suggests that heparin may increase FFA availability and potentially enhance PA/exercise duration. This is demonstrated by a study carried out by Fujita et al (1988), who found an increase in total exercise duration (from 6.3 ± 1.9 (SD) minutes to 9.1 ± 2.2 minutes) in 10 stable angina patients, whilst performing a standard Bruce protocol

treadmill test, after prior intravenous administration of heparin (5000 IU). Similar results have also been found from other studies using patients with effort-induced angina (Fujita et al 1991, Ejiri et al 1993). Ejiri et al (1993), for example, observed an increase in exercise duration from 6.6 ± 1.6 minutes to 9.4 ± 1.9 minutes, for 16 angina patients after administration of heparin (5000 IU) prior to a Bruce protocol treadmill test. Yet administration of heparin prior to PA/exercise may increase maximal rate pressure product (RPP) (p. 88) and RPP at onset of angina by a mean of about 32% (Ejiri et al 1993), indicating simultaneous increases in exercise heart rate and blood pressure, which may be contraindicated for some cardiac patients. This effect may possibly be due to heparin-induced reduction of endothelial nitric oxide (a vasodilator). Yet conversely, a more recent study found heparin to lower RRP at onset of ischaemia, as determined by onset of 1 mm ST-segment depression (p. 245) (Fragasso et al 2000).

Furthermore, heparin administration over time has also been found to accelerate exercise-induced coronary collateral development by promoting angiogenesis (Fujita et al 1988), which potentially would aid functional ability. It is thought that during hypoxic conditions, such as those induced during PA/exercise, repeated ischaemia or coronary occlusion, the presence of heparin may facilitate angiogenesis through interaction with polypeptide growth factor mitogens, which stimulate endothelial cell proliferation (Bombardini & Picano 1997). However, in the animal model, heparin has not been found to accelerate coronary collateral development in dogs with coronary obstructive disease (Cohen et al 1993).

Aspirin

Recent studies indicate that aspirin does not affect functional ability in those with chronic heart failure (Witte & Clark 2004) or affect exercise-induced angina in men with coronary artery disease (Davis et al 1978). However, when combined with ACE inhibitors aspirin does appear to reduce exercise performance and ventilation efficiency (Guazzi et al 1999). Additionally, aspirin has been shown to cause an increase in systolic blood pressure during exercise (Cowley et al 1985), and in healthy individuals, to cause changes in blood flow during upright exercise (Cowley et al 1984). It is thought that aspirin inhibits prostacyclin, which has vasodilatory properties, and may thus modify circulation (Cowley et al 1984, 1985).

Clopidogrel

Clopidogrel attenuates platelet activity at rest, and there is little research to determine whether clopidogrel has any influence upon functional ability. However, exhaustive exercise has been shown to increase platelet aggregation, and appears to counteract the platelet stabilizing effect of clopidogrel (Perneby et al 2004). Therefore, exhaustive PA/exercise is not recommended for those taking this drug.

Streptokinase

Whilst treatment with streptokinase has been shown to reduce the number of positive exercise stress tests in cardiac patients (i.e. onset of 1 mm ST–segment depression or elevation from ECG, p. 245) (Weiss et al 1989, Hamouratidis et al 1991), it has not been found to directly affect functional ability.

MEDICATION FOR TREATMENT OF OBESITY

The most commonly employed drugs for the treatment of obesity are sibutramine and orlistat (Cunill & Jimenez 2005). Sibutramine inhibits the reuptake of serotonin, potentially suppressing the appetite, and is structurally related to amphetamines. Hence, this type of drug raises heart rate and blood pressure, and for this reason some healthcare professionals do not like to use this drug in the management of obesity. Nevertheless, if an obese client/patient is taking this type of medication, great care is needed to ensure that blood pressure does not exceed the recommended levels (p. 82) and the client/patient should be carefully monitored. On the other hand, orlistat, which is a lipase inhibitor, reduces the absorption of dietary fat and does not appear to have any effect upon functional ability.

RESPIRATORY MEDICATION

Asthma (Ch. 8) and COPD (Ch. 9) may be treated with similar medication, though their responses to these medications may differ (Table 14.6).

Bronchodilators

Bronchodilators such as beta agonists, methylxanthines and anticholinergics are prescribed to treat both asthma and COPD. Bronchodilators work by relaxing the smooth muscle of the airways. However, the response from these drugs may be different between the two disorders.

Asthma

For the asthmatic the prevention of bronchoconstriction will undoubtedly enhance functional ability. Short-acting inhaled β_2 agonists taken prior to (10 to 60 minutes) PA/exercise are the most effective (Spooner et al 2003) treatment for the prevention of exercise-induced asthma/bronchoconstriction (Gotshall 2002, Spooner et al 2003). Whilst methylxanthines have been shown to attenuate exercise-induced bronchoconstriction (Magnussen et al 1988), they appear to be less effective than β_2 agonists (Anderson 1981). Additionally, whereas long-acting beta agonists improve lung function, they do not appear to affect exercise capacity in asthmatic individuals (Robertson et al 1994, Revill & Morgan 1998).

Table 14.6 Respiratory medication: implications and considerations for physical activity/exercise

Type of drug	Prescribed for	Physical effects and considerations
Bronchodilators	Asthma	Prevention of exercise induced asthma (EIA) Methylxanthines, i.e. caffeine, do not appear to effect exercise capacity in asthmatics
	COPD	In some patients with COPD, can reduce dyspnoea and improve exercise capacity Anticholinergic agents most effective bronchodilator during steady-state exercise, dose–response relationship Methylxanthines generally improve exercise capacity and endurance, probably not related to bronchodilation
Glucocorticoids and corticosteroids	Asthma and COPD	Increased breakdown of muscle proteins Long-term use leads to muscle myopathy Acute use prolongs PA/exercise endurance
Leukotriene modulators	Asthma	Reduce EIA
Nedocromil and cromolyn (cromoglicate)	Asthma	Reduce severity and duration of EIA
Antibiotics	Asthma and COPD	May induce feelings of fatigue and decrease physical performance Do not appear to affect aerobic capacity and muscle strength

Chronic obstructive pulmonary disease

Although the use of bronchodilators just prior to PA/exercise may help to reduce dyspnoea and improve exercise capacity in individuals with COPD, this may not be seen in all COPD patients. A systemic review of 33 studies found that in only around half of the studies bronchodilator therapy had a significant effect on exercise capacity. Anticholinergic agents were, however, found to have a significant beneficial effect in the majority of studies, particularly when measured during steady-state exercise; with higher doses appearing to be more effective than low-dose anticholinergic agents. Short-acting β_2 antagonists were also found to have a favourable effect in nearly two-thirds of studies, although the effect of long-acting β_2 antagonists was more equivocal (Liesker et al 2002), which is contrary to other studies that have found long-acting agents to have a more significant impact than short-acting agents (Campos & Wanner 2005). However, most studies showed an improvement in dyspnoea, even in the absence of improved exercise capacity (Liesker et al 2002). In addition, methylxanthines, such as caffeine, may improve exercise capacity (Lam & Newhouse 1990) and endurance (Graham et al 1994) in some COPD patients, though this may not be related to bronchodilation (Lam & Newhouse 1990).

Anti-inflammatories

Glucocorticoids, leukotriene modulators, nedocromil and cromolyn are anti-inflammatory medications prescribed to inhibit the release of chemical mediators associated with the inflammatory response in asthma, but may also be prescribed for those with COPD. Since the mechanism for lung inflammation is different between asthma and COPD, COPD patients are often prescribed corticosteroids, which may not be considered suitable for asthmatics, as they increase eosinophils, which are primarily involved in lung inflammation in asthmatic individuals.

Glucocorticoids/corticosteroids

Glucocorticoids have not only an anti-inflammatory effect but also catabolic properties. Glucocorticoids increase the net protein degradation in muscle and are thus associated with an increase in the breakdown of muscle protein (Block & Buse 1990). In the animal model, both acute and chronic glucocorticoid treatment has been found to increase rat muscle cell enzymes (Block & Buse 1990), with increases in myofibrillar protease activity being found in both types of muscle fibres with exhaustive exercise. However, in rats, moderate-intensity PA/exercise has been shown, to a certain extent, to minimize the catabolic effect of synthetic glucocorticoids (Seene & Viru 1982).

Glucocorticoids accelerate catabolism and increase protein production for gluconeogenesis and provision of adenosine triphosphate for muscle work (Block & Buse 1990). In the short term this might enhance functional ability by increasing available 'fuel' for the working muscles. However, long-term use in animals has been shown to result in muscle atrophy (Eason et al 2003), which would be detrimental to functional ability.

Corticosteroids have similar effects to those of glucocorticoids, and have been found to regulate hepatic glycogen and peripheral glucose utilization during exercise, and control glycogenolysis in muscles, thus potentially influencing acute functional ability (Viru et al 1994). They have also been reported to prolong PA/exercise duration (Viru et al 1996).

Glucocorticoids can lead over time to muscle myopathy (Hickson et al 1990, BMA, RPS GB 2002), which may have a detrimental effect on functional ability. Furthermore, their long-term use can increase risk of osteoporosis. Thus low-impact, non-contact PA/exercise is deemed most appropriate (Maquirriain 2001).

Leukotriene modulators

Leukotrienes play an important biological role in the pathogenesis of asthma, and medications to block these deleterious effects can be prescribed (Devillier et al 1999). The use of these drugs has been found to be effective at reducing exercise-induced asthma in both children (Selvadurai & Mellis 2000, Moraes & Salvadurai 2004) and adults (Spahr & Krawiec 2004).

Nedocromil and cromolyn

Nedocromil and cromolyn (cromoglicate) are mast-cell stabilizing agents, and are used as prophylactic treatments in exercise-induced asthma. Nedocromil has been shown to be effective at reducing the severity and duration of exercise-induced asthma in both adults and children with asthma (Spooner et al 2005), and its effect appears to be dose-dependent (Todaro et al 1993). Similarly, cromolyn reduces exercise-induced bronchoconstriction in both children (Pollock et al 1977) and adults (Schwank et al 1978, Weiner et al 1984).

Antibiotics

Antibiotics have been reported to induce sensations of fatigue and decrease physical performance. However, no differences in aerobic capacity and muscle strength or perceived exertion were found when 50 healthy males (aged 18 to 25 years) were randomly assigned into placebo or antibiotic treatment (tetracycline, ampicillin or trimethoprim/sulfamethoxazole) for 3 days (Burstein et al 1993). Nonetheless, far more research is required to fully determine the effect of antibiotics on functional ability and any interaction effect with other medications.

Mucolytic agents

There is little or no current research to suggest that mucolytic agents have any effect on functional ability.

ARTHRITIS

There are three main categories of drug therapies used in the treatment of arthritis. Generally sufferers are initially prescribed non-steroidal anti-inflammatory drugs (NSAIDs) (Table 14.7), which may be followed by the use of glucocorticoid steroids, which are very effective in relieving joint pain and stiffness. For those with rheumatoid arthritis, disease-modifying anti-rheumatic drugs (DMARDs) may be prescribed (p. 231).

Table 14.7   Musculoskeletal drugs: implications and considerations for physical activity/exercise

Type of drug	Prescribed for	Physical effects and considerations
NSAIDs	Arthritis	Aid recovery from muscular injury; however, may mask pain and thus overuse of injured muscle, thus leading to exercise-induced injury
		Possible increase in toxicity and gastric problems with prolonged PA/exercise
Bisphosphonates	Osteoporosis	May cause musculoskeletal pain
Oestrogen	Osteoporosis	May have a protective role against musculoskeletal damage with PA/exercise

Non-steroidal anti-inflammatory drugs

Aspirin and ibuprofen are the most commonly prescribed NSAIDs for pain relief from arthritis; however, their effect upon functional ability is still not clear. Nonetheless, they have been found to be beneficial for short-term recovery of muscle function in exercise-induced muscle injury (Lanier 2003). But caution is needed, as a reduction in pain may allow continued use of the injured muscle, increasing exercise-related muscle injury (Hung et al 2002). Furthermore, NSAIDs may lead to increased toxicity (Hodde 2002), or gastrointestinal problems during prolonged exercise, though the latter may be a symptom of prolonged exercise. Thus, the precise effect is difficult to determine (Smetanka et al 1999).

Disease-modifying anti-rheumatic drugs

Disease-modifying anti-rheumatic drugs directly affect the immunopathological processes that contribute towards rheumatoid arthritis. There are, however, no known data regarding the effect of these drugs on functional ability.

OSTEOPOROSIS

A variety of drugs are prescribed for the treatment and prevention of osteoporosis: parathyroid hormone and vitamin D, bisphosphonates, calcitonin, oestrogen and selective oestrogen-receptor modulators.

Parathyroid hormone and vitamin D

Although parathyroid hormone and vitamin D promote bone formation they do not appear to have any effect upon functional ability.

Bisphosphonates

Bisphosphonates are anti-resorptive medications and are effective at reducing bone loss and increasing bone density, and although they do not appear to affect PA/ability a common side effect can be musculoskeletal pain, which may have an adverse effect (Table 14.7).

Calcitonin

Calcitonin is a naturally occurring non-sex hormone involved in calcium regulation and bone metabolism. Its effect upon functional ability has not been fully investigated.

Oestrogen

Oestrogen treatment is an anti-resorptive therapy that is effective at reducing bone loss and increasing bone mineral density. Oestrogen does not appear to have any significant effect upon functional ability. However, there is research to indicate that oestrogen may have a protective role against skeletal muscle damage (Kendall & Eston 2002); and a study using downhill running, in 15 women taking oral contraceptives and 10 eumenorrhoeic women (mean age 24 years), found a trend in the data that potentially would support these findings (Styers 1999) (Table 14.7).

Selective oestrogen-receptor modulators

There are no known data regarding the effects of selective oestrogen-receptor modulators on PA/exercise ability.

Table 14.8   Treatments for cancer: implications and considerations for physical activity/exercise

Type of treatment	Physical effect
Chemotherapy	Peripheral nerve damage
	Cardiomyopathy
	Pulmonary fibrosis
	Anaemia
	Increased fatigue
	Decrease in functional ability and peak oxygen uptake
Hormone therapy	Muscle weakness
	Fatigue

CANCER

Treatments prescribed for cancer can include chemotherapy, endocrine/hormone therapy and biological/immunotherapy (Table 14.8).

Chemotherapy

Chemotherapy is given in repeated courses over a 3- to 6-month period and produces side effects that can affect the individual's functional ability. These include peripheral nerve damage, cardiomyopathy, pulmonary fibrosis and anaemia, the outcome being an increase in fatigue and decrease in functional ability. For example, a study on 9 female cancer patients found a significant decrease in peak oxygen uptake at the end of chemotherapy (pre-treatment 28.3 ± 5.5 versus post-treatment 24.5 ± 6.1 ml kg^{-1} min^{-1}) (Wiley 2000), though this may have been due to an overall decrease in physical activity over this period.

Hormone therapy

Hormone therapy, to block the effect of oestrogen (p. 194, 196) and progesterone, is used for the treatment of breast cancer. These drugs can cause an increase in body weight, decrease muscle mass, and increase proximal muscle weakness and fatigue. Additionally, hormone therapy to block testosterone in men with prostate cancer may also cause muscle weakness and fatigue, potentially affecting functional ability.

SUMMARY

- Relatively little is known regarding the interaction between PA/exercise and therapeutic medications or the potential limiting effect of these drugs upon PA/exercise performance or functional ability.
- The majority of drugs need to be absorbed into systemic circulation for transportation and distribution to organs and receptor sites, where the action, reaction and/or interaction can occur.
- Drugs are generally categorized into two types, that of *flow* or *capacity* limited drugs. An acute bout of PA/exercise may have differing effects upon these types of drugs.
- The main rate-limiting factors for drug metabolism and elimination are the delivery of the drug to the site of metabolism and/or the ability of the enzyme systems to handle drug metabolism.
- Blood flow and enzyme activity are important factors in pharmacokinetics and pharmacodynamics.
- Internal and external factors have the capacity to affect drug absorption, distribution, metabolism and elimination.
- The effect of PA/exercise on the pharmacokinetics and pharmacodynamics of therapeutic medications has not been extensively researched.
- Physical activity/exercise affects blood flow (haemodynamics) and pH and increases body heat, which may affect pharmacokinetics and dynamics.
- The timing of PA/exercise in relation to drug administration, or vice versa, can significantly modify drug pharmacokinetics, potentially affecting the therapeutic value of the drug.
- Enhanced blood flow to the active muscle tends to increase absorption of transdermally administered drugs or drugs injected into the active muscle just prior to or during PA/exercise.
- Physically trained individuals have been shown to display an elevation in the rate of drug metabolism, termed 'endogenous enzyme induction'.
- The effect of therapeutic medications on functional ability and considerations for PA/exercise are listed in Tables 14.3 to 14.8.

Suggested readings, references and bibliography

Suggested reading

Somani S M 1996 Pharmacology in exercise and sports. CRC Press, Boca Raton, FL

Sweeney G D 1981 Drugs – some basic concepts. Medicine and Science in Sports and Exercise 13(4):247–251

References and bibliography

Ahlborg G, Hagenfeld L 1977 Effect of heparin in the substrate utilization during prolonged exercise. Scandinavian Journal of Clinical and Laboratory Investigation 37(7):619–624

Aldigier J C, Huang H, Dalmay F et al 1993 Angiotensin-converting enzyme inhibition does not suppress plasma angiotensin II increase during exercise in humans. Journal of Cardiovascular Pharmacology 21(2):289–295

Anderson K L 1968 Exercise physiology. Academic Press, New York

Anderson S D 1981 Drugs affecting the respiratory system with particular reference to asthma. Medicine and Science in Sports and Exercise 13(4):259–265

Artia M, Ueno Y, Nakamura C et al 1994 Effect of temocapril on haemodynamics and humoral responses to exercise in patients with mild essential hypertension. Clinical and Experimental Pharmacology and Physiology 21(3):195–200

BACR (British Association of Cardiac Rehabilitation) 2002 British Association of Cardiac Rehabilitation Phase IV training module, 3rd edn. Human Kinetics, Leeds

Barnes P J 1986 Airway inflammation and autonomic control. European Journal of Respiratory Diseases 147:80–87

Beaune J 1989 Comparison of enalapril vs digoxin for congestive heart failure. American Journal of Cardiology 63:22D–25D

Block K P, Buse M G 1990 Glucocorticoid regulation of muscle branched-chain amino acid metabolism. Medicine and Science in Sports and Exercise 22(3):316–324

Blogosklonnaia La V, Krasil'nikova E I, Zaied N et al 1990 Effect of biguanides on the indicators of thromblestography and the level of lactic acid in diabetes mellitus. Sovetskaia Meditsina (12):17–20

BMA, RPS GB (British Medical Association & Royal Pharmaceutical Society of Great Britain) 2002 British National Formulary. Pharmaceutical Press, London

Bombardini T, Picano E 1997 The coronary angiogenetic effect of heparin: experimental basis and clinical evidence. Angiology 48(11):969–976

Breimer D D 1983 Variability in human drug metabolism and its implications. International Journal of Clinical Pharmacology Research 3(6):399–413

Buckenmeyer P J, Somani S M 1996 Exercise and pharmacodynamics of drugs. In: Somani S M Pharmacology in exercise and sports. CRC Press, Boca Raton, FL

Burr B, Dinesh N (eds) 1999 Exercise and sport diabetes. John Wiley, Chichester

Burstein R, Hourvitz A, Epstein Y et al 1993 The relationship between short-term antibiotic treatments and fatigue in healthy individuals. European Journal of Applied Physiology and Occupational Physiology 66(4):372–375

Campos M A, Wanner A 2005 The rationale for pharmacological therapy in stable chronic obstructive pulmonary disease. American Journal of the Medical Sciences 329(4):181–189

Chaffman M O, Pharm D 2001 Anticoagulation in the ambulatory patient: basic principles and current concepts in warfarin therapy. Topics in Geriatric Rehabilitation 17(2):18–37

Chick T W, Halperin A K, Gacek E M 1988 The effect of antihypertensive medication on exercise performance: a review. Medicine and Science in Sports and Exercise 20(5):447–454

Ciccone C D 1995 Basic pharmacokinetics and the potential effect of physical therapy interventions on pharmacokinetic variables. Physical Therapy 75(5):343–351

Cleophas T J, van der Sluijs J, van de Vring J A et al 1999 Combination of calcium channel blockers and beta-blockers for patients with exercise-induced angina pectoris: beneficial effects of calcium channel blockers largely determined by their effect on heart rate. Journal of Clinical Pharmacology 39(7):738–746

Cohen M V, Chukwuogo N, Yarlagadda A 1993 Heparin does not stimulate coronary-collateral growth in a canine model of progressive coronary-artery narrowing and occlusion. American Journal of the Medical Sciences 306(2):75–81

Covar R M, Macomber B A, Szefler S J 2005 Medications as asthma triggers. Immunology and Allergy Clinics of North America 25(1):169–190

Cowley A J, Stainer K, Rowley J M et al 1984 The effect of aspirin on peripheral haemodynamic changes following submaximal exercise in normal volunteers. Cardiovascular Research 18(8):511–513

Cowley A J, Stainer K, Rowley J M et al 1985 The effect of aspirin and indomethacin on exercise-induced changes in blood pressure and limb blood flow. Cardiovascular Research 19(3):177–180

Cunill P J, Jimenez A R 2005 Obesity pharmacological treatment. Revista Clinica Espanola 205(4):175–177

Davis J W, Lewis H D Jr, Phillips P E et al 1978 Effect of aspirin on exercise-induced angina. Clinical Pharmacology and Therapeutics 23(3):505–510

Devillier P, Baccard N, Advenier C 1999 Leukotrienes, leukotriene receptor antagonists and leukotriene synthesis inhibitors in asthma: an update. Part II: clinical studies with leukotriene receptor antagonists and leukotriene synthesis inhibitors in asthma. Pharmacological Research 40(1):15–29

Dyke T M, Sams R A, Hinchcliff K W 1998 Intensity-dependent effects of submaximal exercise on the pharmacokinetics of bromsulphalein in horses. American Journal of Veterinary Research 59(11):1481–1487

Eagles C J, Kendall M J, Maxwell S 1996 A comparison of the effects of fluvastatin and bezafibrate on exercise metabolism: a placebo-controlled study on healthy normolipidaemic subjects. British Journal of Clinical Pharmacology 41(5):381–387

Eason J M, Dodd S L, Powers S K 2003 Use of anabolic steroids to attenuate the effects of glucocorticoids on the rat diaphragm. Physical Therapy 83(1):29–36

Ejiri M, Fujita M, Hirai T et al 1993 Determinants of beneficial effect of heparin exercise treatment on treadmill capacity and long-term efficacy of the therapy in patients with chronic effort angina. Japanese Circulation Journal 57(8):769–774

Fletcher P, Hirji M R, Kuhn S et al 1986 The effects of diabetes mellitus, exercise and single doses of biguanides upon lactate metabolism in man. British Journal of Clinical Pharmacology 21(6):691–699

Follath F 1998 Do diuretics differ in terms of clinical outcome in congestive heart failure? European Heart Journal 19(suppl P):P5–P8

Fortini A, Cappelletti C, Cecchi L et al 1994 Fosinopril in the treatment of hypertension: effects on 24 h ambulatory blood pressure and on blood pressure response to exercise. Journal of Human Hypertension 8(6):469–474

Fragasso G, Leonardo F, Piatti P et al 2000 Detrimental effects of acute heparin administration on ischaemic threshold in patients with coronary artery disease. Italian Heart Journal 1(6):407–411

Frank S 1996 Exercise, drugs, and the cardiovascular system. In: Omani S M Pharmacology in exercise and sports. CRC Press, Boca Raton, FL

Fujita M, Sasayama S, Asanoi H et al 1988 Improvement of treadmill capacity and collateral circulation as a result of exercise with heparin pretreatment in patients with effort angina. Circulation 77(5):1022–1029

Fujita M, Yamanishi K, Hirai T et al 1991 Comparative effect of heparin treatment with and without strenuous exercise on treadmill capacity in patients with stable effort angina. American Heart Journal 122(2):453–457

Glueck C J, McMahon R E, Bouquot J E et al 1998 A preliminary pilot study of treatment of thrombophilia and hypofibrinolysis and amelioration of the pain of osteonecrosis of the jaws. Oral surgery, Oral Medicine, Oral Pathology, Oral Radiology and Endodontics 85(1):64–73

Gotshall R W 2002 Exercise-induced bronchoconstriction. Drugs 62(12):1725–1739

Graham T E, Rush J W E, van Soeren M H 1994 Caffeine and exercise: metabolism and performance. Canadian Journal of Applied Physiology 19(2):111–138

Guazzi M, Pontone G, Agostoni P 1999 Aspirin worsens exercise performance and pulmonary gas exchange in patients with heart failure who are taking angiotensin-converting enzyme inhibitors. American Heart Journal 138(2 Pt 1):254–260

Hamer A W, Arkles L B, Johns J A 1989 Beneficial effects of low dose amiodarone in patients with congestive cardiac failure: a placebo-controlled trial. Journal of the American College of Cardiology 14(7):1768–1774

Hamouratidis N, Katsaliakis N, Manoudis F et al 1991 Early exercise test in acute myocardial infarction treated with intravenous streptokinase. Angiology 42(9):696–702

Hiatt W R 2004 Treatment of disability in peripheral arterial disease: new drugs. Current Drug Targets – Cardiovascular and Haemotological Disorders 4(3):227–231

Hickson R C, Czerwomslo S M, Falduto M T et al 1990 Glucocorticoid antagonism by exercise and androgenic-anabolic steroids. Medicine and Science in Sports and Exercise 22(3):331–340

Hodde J 2002 NSAIDs and ultras: a dangerous combination? UltraRunning 22(7):12–13

Houston M C 1992 Exercise and hypertension. Maximizing the benefits in patients receiving drug therapy. Postgraduate Medicine 92(6):139–144

Hung M C, Chen F A, Hsu C H et al 2002 The effects of non-steroidal anti-inflammatory drugs on skeletal muscles. The Sport Journal. Online Available: http://www.thesportjournal.org/2002journal/vol5-no2/NSAID.htm March 2006

Irsigler K, Kirtz H, Regal H et al 1978 The risk of lactate acidosis: a comparison of 3 biguanides in treatment of diabetes. Wiener Klinische Wochenschrift 90(10):332–337

Jogestrand T, Andersson K 1989 Effect of physical exercise on the pharmacokinetics of digoxin during maintenance treatment. Journal of Cardiovascular Pharmacology 14(1):73–72336

Julius B K, Vassalli G, Mandinov L et al 1999 Alpha-adrenoceptor blockade prevents exercise-induced vasoconstriction of stenotic coronary arteries. Journal of the American College of Cardiology 33(6):1499–1505

Kamimori G H, Smallridge R C, Redmond D P et al 1990 The effect of exercise on atropine pharmacokinetics. European Journal of Clinical Pharmacology 39:395–397

Kaufmann P A, Frielingsdorf J, Mandinov L et al 1998 Reversal of abnormal coronary vasomotion by calcium antagonists in patients with hypercholesterolemia. Circulation 97(14):1348–1354

Kendall B, Eston R 2002 Exercise-induced muscle damage and the potential protective role of estrogen. Sports Medicine 32(2):103–123

Lam A, Newhouse M T 1990 Management of asthma and chronic airflow limitation: Are methylxanthines obsolete? Chest 98(1):44–52

Lanier A B 2003 Use of nonsteroidal anti-inflammatory drugs following exercise-induced muscle injury. Sports Medicine 33(3):177–185

Lemmer B 1982 Pharmacological basis for the therapy of cardiovascular disease with beta-adrenoceptor blocking drugs. Herz 7(3):168–178

Lenz T, Lenz N J, Faulkner M A 2004 Potential interactions between exercise and drug therapy. Sports Medicine 34(5):293–306

Liesker J J, Wijkstra P J, Ten Hacken N H et al 2002 A systemic review of the effect of bronchodilators on exercise capacity in patients with COPD. Chest 121(2):597–608

Louis W T, Taylor H, McNeil J J et al 1982 Clinical pharmacology of adrenergic-adrenoceptor-blocking drugs. American Heart Journal 104(2 Pt 2):407–412

Magnussen H, Reuss G, Jone R 1988 Methylxanthines inhibit exercise-induced bronchoconstriction at low serum theophylline concentration and in a dose-dependent fashion. Journal of Allergy and Clinical Immunology 81(3):531–537

Maquirriain J 2001 Fracture in active patients with transplant organs: treatment and exercise recommendations. Physician and Sportsmedicine 29(1):37–40

Mathur P N, Pugsley S O, Powles A C et al 1984 Effect of diuretics on cardiopulmonary performance in severe chronic airflow obstruction. A controlled clinical trial. Archives of Internal Medicine 144(11):2154–2157

Mayfield K P, Soszynski D, Kozak W et al 1999 Beta-adrenergic receptor subtype effects on stress fever and thermoregulation. Neuroimmunomodulation 6(4):305–317

Moraes T J, Salvadurai H 2004 Management of exercise-induced bronchospasm in children: the role of leukotriene antagonists. Treatments in Respiratory Medicine 3(1):9–15

Munzel T, Kurz S, Drexler et al 1993 Are alterations of skeletal muscle ultrastructure in patients with heart failure reversible under treatment with ACE-inhibitors? Herz 18(suppl 1):400–405

Navarro Estrada J L, Oliveri R 1993 Long-term efficacy of amlodipine in patients with severe coronary artery disease. Journal of Cardiovascular Pharmacology 22(suppl A):S24–S28

Northridge D B, Dargie H J 1990 Quinapril in chronic heart failure. American Journal of Hypertension 3(11):283S–287S

Orlov V A, Zavolovskaia I I, Barhnova A G et al 1990 The efficacy of lanikor in treating patients with chronic cor pulmonale. Klinicheskaia Meditsina 68(10):64–65

Patel A 1999 Diabetes in focus. Pharmaceutical Press, London

Perneby C, Wallen N H, Hu H et al 2004 Prothrombotic responses to exercise are little influenced by clopidogrel treatment. Thrombosis Research 114(4):235–243

Persky A M, Eddington N D, Derendorf H 2003 A review of the effects of chronic exercise and physical fitness level on resting pharmacokinetics. International Journal of Clinical Pharmacology and Therapeutics 41(11):504–506

Pilger E, Schmid P, Goebel R 1979 Effect of biguanides on the lactate metabolism. Studies in diabetics in submaximal ergometric exercise. Medizinische Klinik 74(22):859–865

Pollock J, Kiechel F, Cooper D et al 1977 Relationship of serum theophylline concentration to inhibition of exercise-induced bronchospasm and comparison with cromolyn. Paediatrics 60(6):840–844

Reid J C 1993 The place of alpha blockers in the treatment of hypertension. Clinical and Experimental Hypertension 15(6):1291–1297

Reusch J E, Regansteiner J G, Watson P A 2003 Novel actions of thiazolidinediones on vascular function and exercise capacity. American Journal of Medicine 115(suppl 8A):69S–74S

Revill S M, Morgan M D 1998 The cardiorespiratory response to submaximal exercise in subjects with asthma following pre-treatment with controlled release oral salbutamol and high-dose inhaled salmeterol. Respiratory Medicine 92(8):1053–1058

Richter K J 1992 Subcutaneous haemorrhage in patient on Coumadin: an isokinetic exercise complication. Journal of Sport Rehabilitation 1(3):264–266

Riesco-Eizaguirre G, Arpa-Gutierrez F J, Gutierrez M et al 2003 Severe polymyositis with simvastatin use. Revista de Neurologia 37(10):934–936

Robertson W, Simkins J, O'Hickey S P et al 1994 Does single dose salmeterol affect exercise capacity in asthmatic men? European Respiratory Journal 7(11):1978–1984

Salpeter S R, Ormiston T M, Salpeter E E et al 2003 Cardioselective beta-blockers for chronic obstructive pulmonary disease: a meta-analysis. Respiratory Medicine 97(10):1094–1101

Schwank S, Kyd K, Scherrer M 1978 Exercise-induced asthma and placebos. Schweizerische Medizinische Wochenschrift. Journal Suisse de Medecine 108(7):225–228

Seene T, Viru A 1982 The catabolic effect of glucocorticoids on different types of skeletal muscle fibres and its dependence upon muscle activity and interaction with anabolic steroids. Journal of Steroid Biochemistry 16(2):349–352

Selvadurai H, Mellis C 2000 Antileukotriene drugs in childhood asthma: what is their place in therapy? Paediatric Drugs 2(5):367–372

Shek A, Ferril M J 2001 Statin-fibrate combination therapy. Annals of Pharmacology 35(7):908–917

Smetanka R D, Lambert G P, Murray R et al 1999 Intestinal permeability in runners in the 1996 Chicago Marathon. International Journal of Sports Medicine 9(4):426–433

Somani S M 1981 Metabolism and disposition of chemicals in relation to toxicity. In: Somani S M, Cavender F L (eds) Environmental toxicology: principles and policies. Charles C Thomas, Springfield, IL, p 11–28

Somani S M 1996 Pharmacology in Exercise and Sports. CRC Press, Boca Raton, FL

Somani S M, Kamimori G H 1996 The effects of exercise on absorption, distribution, metabolism, excretion and pharmacokinetics of drugs. In: Somani S M Pharmacology in exercise and sports. CRC Press, Boca Raton, FL

Spahr J E, Krawiec M E 2004 Leukotriene receptor antagonists – risk and benefits for use in paediatric asthma. Expert Opinion on Drug Safety 3(3):173–185

Spooner C H, Spooner G R, Rowe B H 2003 Mast-cell stabilising agents to prevent exercise-induced bronchoconstriction. Cochrane Database of Systemic Reviews (4):CD002307

Spooner C H, Saunders L D, Rowe B H 2005 Nedocromil sodium for preventing exercise-induced bronchoconstriction. Cochrane Database of Systemic Reviews (1):CD001183

Styers A 1999 The effect of estrogen status on muscle tissue damage in women following an eccentric exercise bout. University of Oregon 1 microfiche (71Fr)

Sweeney G D 1981 Drugs – some basic concepts. Medicine and Science in Sports and Exercise 13(4):247–251

Todaro A, Faina M, Alippi et al 1993 Nedocromil sodium in the prevention of exercise-induced bronchospasm in athletes with asthma. Journal of Sports Medicine and Physical Fitness 33(2):137–145

Van Baak M A 1988 Beta-adrenoceptor blockade and exercise. Sports Medicine 5(4):209–225

Vander A J, Sherman J H, Luciano D S 1990 Human physiology, 5th edn. McGraw-Hill, New York

Verrier E D, Tranbaugh R F, Soifer S J et al 1986 Aspirin anticoagulation in children with mechanical aortic valves. Journal of Thoracic and Cardiovascular Surgery 92(6):1013–1020

Vesell E S 1984 Complex effects of diet on drug disposition. Clinical Pharmacology and Therapeutics 36(3):285–296

Viru M, Liitvinova L, Smirnova T et al 1994 Glucocorticoids in metabolic control during exercise: glycogen metabolism. Journal of Sports Medicine and Physical Fitness 34(4):377–382

Viru A, Smirnova T, Viru M 1996 Significance of hormonal metabolic control in sports performance. Acta Kinesologiae Universitatis Tartuensis 1:23–40

Weiner P, Greif J, Fireman E et al 1984 Bronchodilating effect of cromolyn sodium in asthmatic patients at rest and following exercise. Annals of Allergy 53(2):186–188

Weiss A T, Maddahi J, Shah P K et al 1989 Exercise-induced ischemia in the streptokinase-reperfused myocardium: relationship to extent of salvaged myocardium and degree of residual coronary stenosis. American Heart Journal 118(1):9–16

Wenisch M, Hofmann P, Fruhwald F M et al 2003 Influence of beta-blocker use on percentage of target heart rate exercise prescription. European Journal of Cardiovascular Prevention and Rehabilitation 10(4):296–301

Wiley L D 2000 Evaluation of exercise tolerance in women receiving surgery and chemotherapy as treatment for stage II breast cancer. University of Oregon 1 microfiche (78 Fr)

Witte K K, Clark A L 2004 The effect of aspirin on the ventilatory response to exercise in chronic heart failure. European Journal of Heart Failure 6(6):745–748

Witte K K, Thackray S D, Nikitin N P et al 2003 The effects of alpha and beta blockade on ventilatory responses to exercise in chronic heart failure. Heart 89(10):1169–1173

Woolf-May K, Bird S 2005 Physical activity levels during phase IV cardiac rehabilitation in a group of male myocardial infarction patients. British Journal of Sports Medicine Mar 39(3):e12

Appendix A

Screening and assessment for prescription of physical activity and exercise

PRE-PHYSICAL ACTIVITY/EXERCISE SCREENING AND EVALUATION

The major purpose of physical activity (PA)/exercise screening is to identify individuals with known health problems and determine their current PA/exercise status. Without pre-exercise screening, it is impossible to determine whether an individual may be at risk during PA/exercise. Therefore, even for those who present with a known injury, disease or condition, pre-screening is still important.

Effective screening will identify those with special needs, who should begin their regimen within a supervised programme, or who should not at present participate in PA or exercise (ACSM 1991, Fletcher et al 1996). Moreover, pre-screening is important for educating those new to regular PA and exercise about the signs and symptoms of the adverse effects of PA/exercise. For instance, increasing awareness might help individuals terminate PA/exercise before a cardiac event occurs (Libonati et al 2002). Pre-screening will also help determine the appropriate methods of assessment and PA/exercise prescription.

SCREENING QUESTIONNAIRES

There are a range of screening questionnaires that vary in complexity, and can take the form of a simple self-administered health questionnaire, such as the physical activity readiness questionnaire (PAR-Q) (Public Health Agency of Canada 1975) (Fig. A.1) or more comprehensive questionnaires that may need to be completed with an exercise practitioner.

Although, the PAR-Q is simple, it is effective at identifying those with health problems who may need more comprehensive screening. The American Heart Association (AHA) and the American College of Sports Medicine (ACSM) pre-exercise screening questionnaire is rather more complex than the PAR-Q (Balady et al 1998) and adapted versions have been developed and are employed to suit the needs of different organizations (Fig. A.2). Screening may

> 1. Has your doctor ever said you have heart trouble?
> 2. Do you frequently suffer from pains in your chest?
> 3. Do you often feel faint or have spells of severe dizziness?
> 4. Has a doctor ever said your blood pressure was too high?
> 5. Has a doctor ever told you that you have a bone or joint problem such as arthritis that has been aggravated by exercise, or might be made worse with exercise?
> 6. Is there a good physical reason not mentioned here why you should not follow an activity programme even if you wanted to?
> 7. Are you over 65 and not accustomed to vigorous exercise?

Figure A.1 Questions asked in the physical activity readiness questionnaire (PAR-Q). (Source: Physical activity readiness questionnaire (PAR-Q) validation report. Public Health Agency of Canada, 1975. Reproduced with the permission of the Minister of Public Works and Government Services Canada, 2006.

also help determine the appropriate method of pre-PA/exercise programme assessment (p. 243).

There are occasions when it is not recommended or appropriate for an individual to undertake PA/exercise and these are listed in Table A.1.

RISK STRATIFICATION

Risk stratifying an individual for participation in PA/exercise is extremely important so that an appropriate prescription can be made. Individuals can be classified into there categories (ACSM 1991).

- *Apparently healthy individuals.* Those who are asymptomatic and apparently healthy with no more than one major coronary risk factor (p. 10).
- *Individuals at higher risk.* Those who have symptoms suggestive of possible cardiopulmonary or metabolic disease and/or two or more major coronary risk factors.
- *Individuals with disease.* Those with known cardiac, pulmonary (p. 8,9) or metabolic diseases (diabetes & obesity, pp. 57 and 95, respectively).

Risk stratification for different diseases may have specific criteria.

ACTIVITY FOR HEALTH

PRE-SCREENING HEALTH QUESTIONNAIRE
Strictly Confidential

PART 1.   Personal Details

Full Name: _____ Age: _____ D.O.B: _____

Address: _____

_____

_____

_____

e-mail _____

Telephone No: (Home)   _____

(Work)   _____

(Mobile)   _____

GPs Name: _____

Address: _____

_____

_____

_____

Telephone No: _____

Emergency Contact Name: _____

Telephone No: _____

FOR OFFICIAL USE ONLY:			
Medical Conditions _____			
Medications	For	Amount	× day

Figure A.2   An example of a medical screening and physical activity questionnaire that has been adapted from the AHA and ACSM questionnaire, and used by the charity Activity for Health.

Figure A.2
Continued

PART 2.   **Medical History**

1.   Circle any of the relatives below who died of a heart attack before age 50 *(RF)*:

Father   Mother   Brother   Sister   Grandparent

2.   Date of last medical exam by your GP _____ (year)

Date of last physical fitness test   _____ (year)

3.   Circle operations you have had: (please put approximate date)

Back*(SLA)* _____Heart*(MC)* _____ Kidney*(SLA)* _____ Eyes*(SLA)* _____

Joint*(SLA)* _____Neck*(SLA)*_____ Ears*(SLA)* _____ Hernia*(SLA)*_____

Lung*(SLA)* _____ Other _____

Details: _____

_____

4.   Please circle any of the following for which you have been diagnosed or treated by a GP or other health professional (please put approximate date)

Alcoholism*(SEP)*	Diabetes*(SEP)*	Kidney problems*(MC)*
Anaemia, sickle cell*(SEP)*	Emphysema*(SEP)*	Mental illness*(SEP)*
Anaemia, other*(SEP)*	Epilepsy*(SEP)*	Neck strain*(SLA)*
Asthma*(SEP)*	Eye problems*(SLA)*	Obesity*(RF)*
Back strain*(SLA)*	Gout*(SLA)*	Osteoarthritis*(SLA)*
Hearing loss*(SLA)*	Rheumatoid arthritis*(SLA)*	Phlebitis*(MC)*
Bronchitis*(SEP)*	Heart problems*(MC)*	Stroke*(MC)*
Cancer*(SEP)*	High blood pressure*(RF)*	Thyroid problems*(SEP)*
Cirrhosis, liver*(MC)*	Low blood sugar*(SEP)*	Ulcer*(SEP)*
Concussion*(MC)*	High cholesterol*(RF)*	TB*(MC)*

Osteoporosis*(SLA)*

Other _____

Further Details _____

Figure A.2
Continued

5.   Medications

Please list below **all** the medications that you are currently taking. This includes any vitamins, minerals and/or food supplements.

Name of medication	For	Amount and how many times per day

6.   Any of the health symptoms listed below that occur frequently are the basis for medical attention. Circle the number indicating how often you have each of the following

1	2	3	4	5
Practically never	Infrequently	Sometimes	Fairly Often	Very Often

a. **Cough up blood***(MC)*
    1 2 3 4 5

b. **Abdominal pain***(MC)*
    1 2 3 4 5

c. **Low-back pain***(MC)*
    1 2 3 4 5

d. **Leg Pain***(MC)*
    1 2 3 4 5

e. **Arm or shoulder pain***(MC)*
    1 2 3 4 5

f. **Chest pain***(MC)*
    1 2 3 4 5

g. **Swollen joints***(MC)*
    1 2 3 4 5

h. **Feel faint***(MC)*
    1 2 3 4 5

i. **Dizziness***(MC)*
    1 2 3 4 5

j. **Breathless with slight exertion***(MC)*
    1 2 3 4 5

k. **Palpitation or fast heart beat***(MC)*
    1 2 3 4 5

l. **Unusual fatigue with normal activity***(MC)*
    1 2 3 4 5

Further Details _____

Figure A.2
Continued

PART 3:   Health Related Behaviour

7. **Do you smoke***(RF)***?**   Yes   No

8. **If so, how many do you smoke a day:**

    Cigarettes: 40 or more   20–39   10–19   1–9
    Cigars or pipes only: 5 or more or any inhaled   Less than 5, none inhaled

9. **How many units of alcohol do you consume each week? (1 unit = 1 pint or 1 wine glass)**

    21 or more   14–21   7–14   1–7   None

10. **Do you exercise regularly?**   Yes   No

    If yes, please give details_____

11. **How many days a week do you accumulate 30 minutes of moderate activity?**
    (activity which makes you slightly breathless)

    0   1   2   3   4   5   6   7   days per week

12. **How many days per week do you normally spend at least 20 minutes of vigorous exercise (activity**
    which makes you hot, sweaty and out of breath)

    0   1   2   3   4   5   6   7   days per week

13. **Can you walk 4 miles briskly without fatigue?**   Yes   No

14. **Weight now:_____   One year ago _____   Age 21_____**

PART 4:   Health Related Attitudes

15. **Do you consider yourself:**

    Impatient, time-conscious, and competitive. (Circle the number below that corresponds to how you feel)

    6   Strongly agree
    5   Moderately agree
    4   Slightly agree
    3   Slightly disagree
    2   Moderately disagree
    1   Strongly disagree

16. **Do you have any other physical condition or injury that is not covered by the above questions?**
                                        Yes   No

    If yes, please give details: _____

Figure A.2
Continued

17.   **How did you hear about the 'Active For Life' classes?** _____

I HAVE READ, UNDERSTOOD AND COMPLETED THIS QUESTIONNAIRE. ALL QUESTIONS HAVE BEEN ANSWERED TO THE BEST OF MY KNOWLEDGE.

Signature _____   Date _____

Signature of Instructor _____   Date _____

This information will be kept on a confidential computerised database (in accordance with the Data Protection Act 1998) and information on it may be used for NHS auditing purposes. If you do not wish this information to be recorded please tick the box. ☐

FOR OFFICE USE ONLY:

EI –   Emergency Information – must be readily available
MC –   Medical Clearance needed – do not allow exercise without GP permission
SEP –   Special Emergency Procedures needed – do not allow participant to exercise alone; make sure exercise partner knows what to do in case of an emergency
RF –   Risk Factor for CHD (Educational materials and information needed for client)
SLA –   Special or Limited Activities may be needed – you may need to include or exclude specific exercises

Accepted _____   Date Started _____   Referred back to GP _____

Table A.1 Absolute contraindications for physical activity and exercise (adapted from ACSM 1993)

Unstable angina
Resting systolic blood pressure (BP) >200 mmHg or resting diastolic BP >115 mmHg
Orthostastic BP drop ≥20 mmHg
Moderate to severe aortic stenosis
Acute illness or fever
Uncontrolled atrial or ventricular dysrhythmias
Uncontrolled sinus tachycardia (≥120 beats per minute)
Uncontrolled congestive heart failure
3° A-V heart block
Active pericarditis or myocarditis
Recent embolism
Thrombophlebitis
Resting ST displacement (>3 mm)
Uncontrolled diabetes
Orthopaedic problems that would prohibit exercise

INFORMED CONSENT

Prior to any physical assessment or entry into any PA/exercise programme it is important that the participating individual is fully aware of the test protocol and/or what is involved in the programme; and that they read and sign an informed consent form (Fig. A.3).

ASSESSMENTS

The type of pre-PA/exercise programme assessment used to assist in designing an appropriate PA/exercise programme will depend upon the setting, available equipment and the individual patient/client's physical status. Below are outlined some of the most common types of tests that can be employed in relation to health related

---

ACTIVITY FOR HEALTH

INFORMED CONSENT FORM FOR PARTICIPANTS

The benefits of exercise are well known; it improves your general good health and maintains and improves your ability to deal with the demands of everyday life.

As well as improving the quality of your life, increasing the amount of physical activity you do can reduce the risk and severity of many disorders such as coronary heart disease, diabetes, asthma, osteoporosis, obesity, etc. However, as with any physical exertion there is the increased risk of a cardiac event. Participating in an 'Active For Life' class such as that at Wesley Sports Centre is a relatively safe way of increasing your level of physical activity whilst being monitored by qualified instructors.

A typical 'Active For Life' class will run as follows:

You will be asked your pre-exercise heart rate which will be recorded on your own exercise record card. Everyone will then take part in a 15 minute warm-up run by the instructor; this will include some simple mobility and stretching exercises. After the warm-up you will then follow your own programme of exercises which have been prescribed by the instructor at an appropriate level for you. You will perform the exercises on a selection of equipment arranged around the room, you will be asked to move around the equipment in a certain order and to perform the exercises for a specific amount of time. Once you have completed one circuit of the room, you will report back to the instructor, and depending on how you feel the next circuit will be adjusted accordingly. At the end of the class, which may consist of 1, 2 or 3 circuits you will again be asked to record your heart rate and then will be asked to complete a 10 minute cool-down consisting of walking around the room followed by some stretching exercises.

Taking part in exercise at an *inappropriate* level can carry certain health risks. The reason you have been asked to complete the pre-screening questionnaire is to enable us to prescribe the appropriate level of exercise for *you*. This level of exercise prescribed for you should convey health benefits without incurring major risks. It is therefore important that you have answered the questionnaire as fully and honestly as you can.

Could you please confirm you have read and understood the information given on this sheet by signing below.

Signature _____ Date _____

Figure A.3 Example of pre-physical assessment informed consent.

PA/exercise. There are, however, a vast variety of assessments and protocols and for more comprehensive descriptions refer to ACSM (1991, 1997).

AEROBIC CAPACITY

It is extremely useful in the prescribing of PA/exercise to gain at the least some indication of the client/patient's aerobic capacity. Whilst this is generally not a problem for the vast majority of asymptomatic individuals, for those with existing diseases and conditions this may not always be appropriate. Determining whether it is appropriate to test an individual will usually become apparent after the pre-screening. However, in some instances this may not become clear until the assessment has begun, in which case the test may need to cease or be altered to suit the individual.

There are a wide variety of tests employing different modes, such as walking, running, stepping, rowing or cycle ergometry. Regardless of the mode, generally the principles for testing are similar (refer to ACSM 1991).

Tests of aerobic capacity usually involve direct or predicted measures of oxygen uptake ($\dot{V}O_2$), which can be expressed in absolute (litres per minute) or relative terms (ml kg^{-1} min^{-1}). However, absolute measures of $\dot{V}O_2$ do not account for body mass, whereas relative measures do. Therefore whilst absolute measures will provide an indication of an individual's ability to perform external work, relative measures will provide an indication of the body's ability to work aerobically.

Graded tests, such as the Bruce protocol (Bruce 1977) (Table A.2) or 10-metre shuttle walking test (Singh et al 1992) (Table A.3), where the heart rate $\dot{V}O_2$ relationship is determined, are generally more accurate than endurance tests. The end point may be either at the point of exhaustion, peak, ischaemic threshold, or a set point. When a set point is used, the $\dot{V}O_2$max may be predicted by extrapolating the heart rate $\dot{V}O_2$ relationship to the age-

Table A.2 Bruce protocol: treadmill protocol for the assessment of aerobic fitness

Stage	Miles per hour	Grade	Minutes
1	1.7	10	1–3
2	2.5	12	4–6
3	3.4	14	7–9
4	4.2	16	10–12
5	5.0	18	13–15

predicted heart rate maximum (HRmax) (refer to McArdle et al 2000, p. 199). However, this may only be applicable for those individuals whose heart rate is not affected, by medication for example.

Endurance tests

Endurance tests, such as the 6- or 12-minute, where the individual for example, walks, cycles or rows as far as they can in the time allocated, measure the ability of an individual to sustain a submaximal aerobic exercise (ACSM 1997). Whilst these tests are fairly good at showing changes pre- and post-PA/exercise intervention, they are not best for determining an individual's $\dot{V}O_2$max or metabolic equivalent (MET) value (p. 247).

Ischaemic threshold

Those with cardiac conditions invariably undergo what is termed an *exercise stress test* (often using the Bruce protocol). This type of test is to determine the ischaemic threshold, which is the point where the metabolic or oxygen demands of the exercise cannot be met as a result of occluded blood flow. During the test the patient wears a 12-lead electrocardiograph (ECG) (refer to ACSM 1991, pp. 74–83, and Lilly 1997, pp. 133–136) and the point of ischaemia is determined by a minimum of 1mm elevation or depression in the ST segment (Fig. A.4).

Table A.3 Protocol for 10-metre shuttle walking test (Singh et al 1992)

Level	Speed (miles per hour)	Number of shuttles
1	1.12	1 2 3
2	1.50	4 5 6 7
3	1.88	8 9 10 11 12
4	2.26	13 14 15 16 17 18
5	2.64	19 20 21 22 23 24 25
6	3.02	26 27 28 29 30 31 32 33
7	3.40	34 35 36 37 38 39 40 41 42
8	3.78	43 44 45 46 47 48 49 50 51 52
9	4.16	53 54 55 56 57 58 59 60 61 62 63
10	4.54	64 65 66 67 68 69 70 71 72 73 74 75
11	4.92	76 77 78 79 80 81 82 83 84 85 86 87 88
12	5.30	89 90 91 92 93 94 95 96 97 98 99 100 101 102

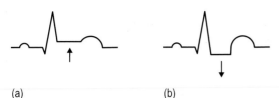

(a)   (b)

Figure A.4   Examples of ECG ST-segment elevation (a) and depression (b). (From Hampton 2003.)

STRENGTH

An individual's suitability to perform a test to determine their strength should become apparent from the pre-screening. Strength tests measure the ability of an individual to do unsustained work against a high resistance, such as the maximum voluntary contraction, or 1 repetition maximum. The latter, for example, is where the initial weight is just below a weight of maximal lifting capacity for the particular muscle or muscle group being tested, where only one repetition can be achieved (refer to McArdle et al 2000, p. 392).

FLEXIBILITY AND MOBILITY

Tests for the measure of flexibility/mobility assess the ability to move joints through a prescribed range of motion. The sit and reach test, for example, is easily employed and cost effective. A goniometer measures the range of motion and is useful for testing older and arthritic individuals (ACSM 1997).

BLOOD GASES

Oxygen (O_2) is carried to the tissues through the blood, where it is required for basic metabolic processes. The by-product of some of these processes is carbon dioxide (CO_2), which is also carried by the blood to be processed or excreted by the lungs, liver or kidneys. Many diseases and conditions can affect blood flow and affect blood gases. The measure of blood gases can indicate, for example, acidosis, lung, liver and kidney problems (Table A.4), and is determined by the measure of arterial as opposed to venous blood. This measure can provide clues to underlying

Table A.4   Measures of blood gases (adapted from Jenkins 2005)

Component	Normal range (approximate)	Meaning
pH	7.36–7.44	Measure of acidity
P_{CO_2}	4.6–5.9 kPa (kilopascal =7.500638 mmHg)	Measures ventilatory component of lung function only
P_{O_2}	11–13 kPa	
HCO_3 (bicarbonate)	22–26 mmol/litre	High – in compensated respiratory acidosis and in metabolic alkalosis Low – in compensated respiratory alkalosis and in metabolic acidosis
O_2 saturation	95–97%	Low – perfusion or ventilation disorders

disease and check whether oxygen therapy is effective or needs altering (sBMJ 2005, Jenkins 2005).

PULSE OXIMETRY

Pulse oximetry is a simple non-invasive method of monitoring the percentage of haemoglobin (Hb) which is saturated with oxygen. A small probe may be attached to a fingertip or ear lobe, and two wavelengths of light emanate from the probe and pass through. The light is partly absorbed by the Hb by amounts that differ depending on whether the Hb is saturated or desaturation with oxygen. Thus oxygen saturation can be calculated. Oxygen saturation less than 90% represents serious hypoxia. However, most oximeters cannot distinguish between different forms of Hb, and give no indication about the level of carbon dioxide (Fearnley 1995).

LUNG FUNCTION

Tests for the measurement of lung function are described in Chapter 9 (p. 147).

Suggested readings, references and bibliography

Suggested Reading

ACSM (American College of Sports Medicine) 1991 Guidelines for exercise testing and prescription. Lea and Febiger, Philadelphia

Balady G J, Chaitman B, Driscoll D et al 1998 Recommendations for cardiovascular screening, staffing and emergency policies at health/fitness facilities. Circulation 97(22):2283–2293

Libonati J R, Glassberg H L, Thompson P D 2002 Exercise and coronary artery disease: assessing causes and managing risks. The Physician and Sportsmedicine 30(11):23–29

McArdle W D, Katch F I, Katch V L 2000 Essentials of exercise physiology, 2nd edn. Lippincott William & Wilkins, Philadelphia

References and bibliography

ACSM (American College of Sports Medicine) 1991 Guidelines for exercise testing and prescription. Lea and Febiger, Philadelphia

ACSM 1993 ACSM position stand: PA, physical fitness, and hypertension. Medicine and Science in Sports and Exercise 25(10):i–x

ACSM 1997 ACSM's exercise management for persons with chronic diseases and disabilities. Human Kinetics, Champaign, IL

Balady G J, Chaitman B, Driscoll D et al 1998 Recommendations for cardiovascular screening, staffing and emergency policies at health/fitness facilities. Circulation 97(22):2283–2293

Bruce R A 1977 Exercise testing for ventricular function. New England Journal of Medicine 296:671–675

Fearnley S J 1995 Pulse oximetry. Update in Anaesthesia 5(2):1–3

Fletcher G F, Balady G, Blair S N et al 1996 Statement on exercise: benefits and recommendations for physical activity programs for all Americans: a statement for health professionals by the committee on exercise and cardiac rehabilitation of the council in clinical cardiology, American Heart Association. Circulation 94(4):857–862

Jenkins G 2005 Your health: blood gases. Online. Available: http://www.bbc.co.uk/health/talking/tests/blood_gases.shtml July 2005

Hampton J R The ECG made easy, 6th edn. Churchill Livingstone, Edinburgh

Libonati J R, Glassberg H L, Thompson P D 2002 Exercise and coronary artery disease: assessing causes and managing risks. The Physician and Sportsmedicine 30(11):23–29

Lilly L S 1997 Pathophysiology of heart disease, 2nd edn. Lippincott Williams & Wilkins, Philadelphia

McArdle W D, Katch F I, Katch V L 2000 Essentials of exercise physiology, 2nd edn. Lippincott William & Wilkins, Philadelphia

Public Health Agency of Canada 1975 Physical activity readiness questionnaire (PAR-Q) validation report.Public health Agency of Canada

sBMJ 2005 Acute care: arterial blood gases. Online. Available: http://www.studentbmj.com July 2005

Singh SJ, Morgan MD, Scott S et al 1992 Development of a shuttle walking test of disability in patients with chronic airways obstruction. Thorax 47(12):1019–1024

Appendix B

Physical activity and exercise: intensity, endurance and progression

PHYSICAL ACTIVITY AND EXERCISE INTENSITY

In order to achieve a training effect (Ch. 1, p. 3) that will be sufficient to enhance a health benefit, it is important to work physically at an appropriate physical activity (PA)/exercise intensity. Physical activity/exercise intensity is usually prescribed as a percentage of an individual's maximal aerobic or anaerobic capacity, or strength, and there are several different methods for this purpose.

METABOLIC EQUIVALENTS (METS)

During supine rest, relative oxygen uptake ($\dot{V}O_2$) is estimated to be around 3.5 ml kg^{-1} min^{-1}, termed one metabolic equivalent (MET). Hence 2 METs would be twice the metabolic equivalent of rest. Considerable research has been carried out to determine the MET values of different types of physical activities and examples of these can be found in the ACSM guidelines (1991, pp. 285–300). When prescribing PA/exercise it is useful to know an individual's maximal aerobic capacity in terms of METs so that appropriate activities, at a percentage of this, can be prescribed. For example, an individual may have a $\dot{V}O_2$max of around 8 METs (~28 ml kg^{-1} min^{-1}), and is prescribed to exercise at around 75% of their maximum. According to ACSM (1991) guidelines, this would be about equivalent to walking up a 5% gradient at 2.1 kilometres per hour, which is equivalent to 5.9 METs, or an easy game of tennis, 4–9 METs. It should, however, be noted that MET values can be affected by various factors, such as the environment or clothing worn during the activity (ACSM 1995).

SCALES OR RATINGS OF PERCEIVED EXERTION (RPE)

Heart rate is often used as an indicator of PA/exercise intensity. However, it may not always be easily determined or be a reliable indicator of intensity, especially in those with heart conditions (Ch.2). Therefore, PA/exercise

intensity scales may be employed. Since Borg (1974) introduced the now commonly employed ratings of perceived exertion (RPE) scales, several different scales have been developed for use on different populations, such as scales of breathlessness (Table B.1), for those with chronic obstructive pulmonary disease or asthma, and the claudication ischaemia scale (Table B.2). These scales have been matched to percentage of maximum heart rate and $\dot{V}O_2$ (Table B.3). However, not all scales are validated; and care should be taken when using scales validated on healthy populations for those with various diseases and disorders. Additionally, RPE may remain similar with different heart rate responses to different activities (Buckley 2002). Thus it is important to be aware of the limitations of these scales. Nonetheless, they do allow the individual to give a subjective indication of how they are feeling and can be

Table B.1 The Medical Research Council dyspnoea scale (adapted from Crockett 2000)

Level	Degree of breathlessness
0	Only breathless on strenuous exercise
1	Breathless on mild exertion
2	Breathless even when walking on the level, has to frequently stop for breath
3	Has to stop for breath after 100 yards or a few minutes on the level
4	Breathless on dressing, too breathless to leave house

Table B.2 The claudication ischaemia scale (adapted from Leutholtz & Ripoll 1999)

Level	Degree of pain
1	Light, barely noticeable
2	Moderate, bothersome
3	Severe, very uncomfortable
4	Severe discomfort, cannot continue

Table B.3 Comparative percentage exercise intensity, in relation to aerobic capacity ($\dot{V}O_2max$), maximum heart rate (HRmax) and ratings of perceived exertion (RPE) (6–20 Borg scale) (adapted from US Department of Health and Human Services 1996)

	Very light (%)	Light (%)	Moderate (%)	Hard (%)	Very hard (%)	Maximal (%)
$\dot{V}O_2max$ (ml kg^{-1}min^{-1})	<20	20–30	40–59	60–84	>85	100
HRmax (beats per minute)	<35	35–54	55–69	70–89	>90	100
RPE	<10	10–11	12–13	14–16	17–19	20

extremely useful when other measures are unreliable or unattainable (refer to Borg 1998, Roberston 2004).

DURATION

The PA/exercise duration of each session is still very much under debate for both asymptomatic and symptomatic individuals. The initial session for aerobic activities may start at around 5–15 minutes, but depends very much on the individual. It is not advisable though to increase the duration by more than 10% per week. Exceeding this increment will not allow the individual time to adjust to the activity and may put them at an increased risk of injury. Once the individual can manage about 20 minutes of aerobic activity they may increase the intensity if appropriate. The activity may range between 15 and 90 minutes per session, with 3 to 7 sessions per week.

The initial duration of resistance and anaerobic activities will depend upon the individual and the physical activity.

PROGRESSION

Progression and progressive overload are important in all training programmes in order to stimulate ongoing fitness improvements, and the rate of progression will very much depend upon the individual. Initial PA/exercise sessions may include moderate intensity and for those for whom further progression is deemed appropriate after a number of sessions/weeks, moderate intensity PA/exercise may be interspersed with periods of more intense activity. The duration of these may commence at 10–30 seconds and be extended as fitness improves.

Suggested readings, references and bibliography

References and bibliography

ACSM (American College of Sports Medicine) 1991 Guidelines for exercise testing and prescription. Lea and Febiger, Philadelphia

ACSM 1995 ACSM's guidelines for exercise testing and prescription, 5th edn. Williams & Wilkins, Baltimore

Borg G A 1974 Perceived exertion. Exercise and Sports Sciences Reviews 2:131–153

Borg G A V 1998 Borg's perceived exertion and pain scales. Human Kinetics, Champaign, IL

Buckley J 2002 How hard is hard? SportEX Health 11:19–22

Crockett A 2000 Managing chronic obstructive pulmonary disease in primary care. Blackwell Science, Oxford

Leutholtz B C, Ripoll L 1999 Exercise and disease management. CRC Press, Boca Raton, FL

Roberston R J 2004 Perceived exertion for practitioners: ratings effort with the OMNI picture system. Human Kinetics, Champaign, IL

US Department of Health and Human Services 1996 Physical activity and health: A report of the surgeon general. Centers for Disease Control and Prevention, National Center for Chronic Disease Prevention and Health Promotion, Government Printing Office, Washington DC

Glossary of terms

Acetylcholine   A neurotransmitter that influences parasympathetic, somatic and some central nervous system (CNS) neurons. A stimulant of the parasympathetic nervous system, and vasodilator and cardiopressor.

Acetyl-CoA (acetyl coenzyme A)   A biomolecule that carries 2-carbon acetyl units. Important in metabolic processes. Its formation is critical in the step between anaerobic glycolysis and the citric acid (Kreb) cycle.

Acidosis   Any situation in which acidity (hydrogen ions, H^+) are elevated.

Acyl   A monovalent radical (CH_3CO), that is capable of combining with or being substituted for one hydrogen atom.

Adenosine   A compound derived from nucleic acids.

Adenosine diphosphate (ADP)   Two-phosphate product in the breakdown of ATP.

Adipocytes   Fat cells, mainly consisting of triglyceride.

Adrenal cortex   Endocrine gland that forms outer shell of each adrenal gland; secretes mainly cortisol, aldosterone and androgenic steroids.

Adrenaline (epinephrine)   A catecholamine hormone secreted by the adrenal medulla that is the most potent stimulant of the sympathetic nervous system, resulting in increased heart rate and force of contraction, vasoconstriction or vasodilation, relaxation of bronchiolar and intestinal smooth muscle, glycogenolysis, lipolysis, and other metabolic effects.

Adrenocortical steroids   Steroids secreted from the outer portion of the adrenal gland.

Afterload   The tension produced by the heart muscle after contraction.

Aldosterone   Corticosteroid produced by the adrenal cortex, which causes the renal tubule to retain sodium, conserve water by resorption and increase potassium excretion.

All-cause mortality   Mortality rates from all causes.

Amenorrhoea   Absence of menstruation.

Aminoacetic acid   Glycerine.

Amphipathic   A molecule having two sides with characteristically different properties.

Anaerobic   In the absence of oxygen.

Anaplasia   A change in the structure or the orientation of cells, characteristic of malignancy.

Androgen   Any steroid hormone that increases male characteristics.

Aneurysm   Localized dilation of the wall of a blood vessel.

Angina (pectoris)   A spasmodic cramp-like choking feeling; a heart condition marked by paroxysms of chest pain due to reduced oxygen to the heart.

Angiogenesis   The ability to evoke blood vessel formation. Vascular growth. A common property of malignant tissue.

Angioplasty   The reconstruction of blood vessels damaged by injury or disease (*see* Percutaneous transluminal coronary angioplasty).

Angiotensin   A renin substrate released from the liver and cleaved in circulation to form biologically inactive angiotensin I.

Angiotensin I   Polypeptide in the blood that is rapidly hydrolyzed to form the active component angiotensin II.

Angiotensin II   Circulates in the blood and causes profound vasoconstriction, resulting in increased blood pressure.

Angiotensinogen   Serum glycoprotein produced in the liver, precursor to angiotensin.

Anti-angiogenic   Able to halt the process of angiogenesis.

Antidiuretic hormone (ADH) (vasopressin)   Peptide hormone synthesized by the hypothalamus, released by posterior pituitary, increases water permeability of the kidneys' collection ducts.

Antigen   Substance, usually a protein, that the body recognizes as foreign, and can evoke an immune response.

Antilipolytic   The halting or retardation of the chemical breakdown of fat.

Antineoplastic   Inhibiting or preventing the development or maturation of cells.

Antioxide   A chemical or agent that inhibits or retards oxidation of a substance to which it is added.

Aortic regurgitation   The flow of blood from the aorta back into the left ventricle during diastole, resulting from failure of the aortic valve to close completely.

Aortic stenosis   Narrowing of structure of the aortic valve.

Apnoea   The absence of spontaneous respiration.

Apolipoprotein   The protein component of lipoprotein complexes.

Apoptosis   A type of cell death in which the cell uses specialized cellular machinery to kill itself.

Arrhythmia   Any deviation from the normal pattern of heartbeat.

Arteriogenesis   Enlargement of conduit blood vessels.

Aspiration pneumonia   The inappropriate passage of food, water, stomach acid, vomit or foreign material into the lungs.

Asymptomatic   Without obvious signs or symptoms of disease.

Atherectomy   The surgical removal of atherosclerotic plaques (atheroma).

Atherogenesis   The formation of subintimal plaques in the lining of arteries.

Atherosclerosis   The progressive narrowing and hardening of the arteries over time.

Atrial fibrillation   The disorganized electrical conduction of the atria, resulting in ineffective pumping of blood into the ventricle.

Autoimmune   An immune response to one's own tissues, resulting in the production of antibodies against the body's own cells, which act against the body's cells to cause localized and systemic reactions.

Autonomic nervous system   Neurons that are not under conscious control, comprising two antagonistic components, the sympathetic and parasympathetic nervous systems.

Baroreceptor   Pressure receptor in the wall of the atrium of the heart, vena cava, aortic arch and carotid sinus which is sensitive to stretching of the wall that occurs with an increase in pressure.

B cell   A type of white blood cell, which can produce antibody proteins necessary to fight off infections, such as viruses.

Benign   Something that does not metastasize with treatment or removal, is curative and of no danger to health.

Beta (β)-adrenergic receptors   Adrenergic receptors in effector tissues that are capable of selective activation and blockade by drugs.

Beta-hydroxybutyrate   A ketone body produced from acetyl-CoA, used as an alternative form of fuel.

Beta-oxidation   The oxidative breakdown of fatty acids into acetyl-CoA, by repeated oxidation at the beta-carbon atom.

Biliary   Relating or belonging to bile.

Blood pressure   The force that the circulating blood exerts on the walls of the arteries. This measurement is divided into systolic (pressure during contraction of the heart) and diastolic (pressure during relaxation phase of the heart).

Bradykinin   A biologically active polypeptide, consisting of nine amino acids, that forms from a blood plasma globulin; it acts on endothelial cells and mediates the inflammatory response, increases vasodilation, and causes contraction of smooth muscle.

Carcinogen   Substance that increases the risk of neoplasms, such as in cancer.

Carcinogenesis   The generation of cancer from normal cells.

Cardiac output ($\dot{Q}$)   A measurement of the blood flow through the heart to the systemic (and pulmonary) circulation. Expressed as volume of blood per unit time, generally measured in litres per minute.

Cardiogenic shock   Inadequate delivery of oxygen to the tissues that occurs secondary to the weakened pumping function of the heart. May be precipitated by myocardial infarction (heart attack) or cardiomyopathy.

Cardiomyopathy A general diagnostic term designating primary myocardial disease, often of obscure or unknown aetiology.

Cardiovascular disease (CVD) Disease of the heart together with the network of blood vessels.

Carotid sinus A slight dilation in the carotid artery at its bifurcation into the external carotid arteries. It contains baroreceptors (pressure sensors) that when stimulated will cause a reflex of slowing of the heart, vasodilation and a fall in blood pressure.

Catabolism Any destructive metabolic process by which organisms convert substances into excreted compounds.

Catecholamines These include adrenaline, noradrenaline and dopamine, with roles as hormones and neurotransmitters.

Central adaptations Adaptations to physical training that are central to the body, such as cardiovascular changes, as opposed to peripheral adaptations. However, both central and peripheral adaptations are inextricably linked.

Cholangiocarcinoma A relatively rare cancer that arises from the cells of the bile ducts.

Cholesterol A white crystalline substance, $C_{27}H_{45}OH$ (fat-like steroid alcohol crystallizing in the form of dilute alcohol), found in animal tissues and various foods, that is normally synthesized by the liver and is important as a constituent of cell membranes and a precursor to steroid hormones. Its level in the bloodstream can influence the pathogenesis of certain conditions, such as the development of atherosclerotic plaque and coronary artery disease.

Cholesteryl ester Cholesterol produced by combining an acid with an alcohol.

Chronotropic Affecting the time or rate, such as the rate of contraction of the heart.

Cirrhosis Liver disease characterized by loss of normal architecture.

Claudication Cramp-like pains in the calf caused by poor circulation of blood in the leg muscles, commonly associated with arteriosclerosis.

Cleavage The cut-off process or splitting, primarily from a more complex molecule into two or more simple molecules.

Coagulation The process of clot formation.

Coeliac disease A chronic nutritional disturbance, usually of young children, characterized by the inability to metabolize peptides containing gluten, which results in malnutrition, a distended abdomen, muscle wasting, and the passage of stools having a high fat content.

Cofactor Inorganic complement of an enzyme reaction.

Cold pressor response Circulatory challenge, conventionally performed by immersing the hand or face in ice cold water for two or more minutes, to acutely raise blood pressure. Causes resistance to ejection of blood from the left ventricle into the systemic arterial system, thus acutely increasing afterload (see diving reflex).

Collagen The protein substance of the white collagenous fibres of the skin, tendon, bone, cartilage and all other connective tissue.

Co-morbidities The presence of coexisting or additional diseases with reference to an initial diagnosis.

Concentric hypertrophy Thickening of the walls of the heart or any cavity with apparent diminution of the capacity of the cavity.

Congestive heart failure Ineffective pumping of the heart leading to accumulation of fluid in the lungs. Symptoms include shortness of breath with exertion, breathing difficulties when lying flat, leg and ankle swelling. Caused by chronic hypertension, cardiomyopathy and myocardial infarction.

Contact inhibition The inhibition or continued growth and division of a cell or colony due to physical contact with other cells or colonies. Stopping of continued growth when a certain density of cells has been reached.

Controlled crossover study A study that compares two or more interventions including a controlled situation of no intervention. The subjects upon completion of one of the conditions will cross over and undergo the other condition.

Coronary artery bypass graft A surgical procedure which involves replacing diseased or narrowedzcoronary arteries with veins obtained from the patient's extremities.

Coronary artery disease (CAD) Term used to describe the more specific disease of the arteries that supply blood to the heart.

Coronary heart disease (CHD) Describes the malfunction of the heart, often caused by blockage of one or more of the coronary arteries.

Corticosteroid Any one of a number of natural or synthetic hormones that influence or control key processes of the body. One of their functions is to increase the number of eosinophils.

Cortisol The major adrenal glucocorticoid; stimulates conversion of proteins to carbohydrates, raises blood sugar levels and promotes glycogen storage in the liver.

Crohn's disease Chronic inflammatory bowel disease of unknown origin; presents with thickening of the soft tissue, with fat infiltration, inflammation, abscess and fistula development.

Cross-sectional study Study in which the presence or absence of disease or other health-related variables are determined in each member of the study population, or in a representative sample at one particular time.

Cyclic GMP (cyclic 3′,5′-guanosine monophosphate) A secondary messenger that acts at the cellular level to regulate various metabolic processes and mediate the action of certain hormones, possibly as an antagonist to cyclic AMP.

Cystic fibrosis Disease where there is widespread dysfunction of the exocrine glands, characterized by chronic pulmonary disease, pancreatic deficiency, high levels of electrolytes in the sweat, and ineffective immune defence against bacteria in the lungs.

Cytokines Protein messengers secreted by macrophages or monocytes, involved in cell-to-cell communication.

Cytoplasmic Related to cytoplasm; the protoplasm of the cell exclusive of the nucleus. Consists of continuous aqueous solution (cytosol) and organelles. The site of most chemical activities of the cell.

Cytoplasmic vesicle Membrane shell of the cytosol, important in intracellular transport process.

Cytoskeleton The part of the cytoplasm that remains when organelles and internal membrane system are removed.

Cytotoxic Lymphocyte (type of white blood cell) that when activated by an antigen will attack a cell bearing that antigen; a major killer of virus-infected and tumour cells.

Cytotoxin Substance that has a toxic effect on certain cells. An antibody may act as a cytotoxin, having a cytotoxic effect.

Deoxyribonucleic acid (DNA) The molecule that encodes genetic information in the nucleus of cells. It determines the structure, function and behaviour of the cell.

Developmental stretch A stretch that is held for long enough and frequently enough to induce physical development in complex anatomical structures, with the aim of increasing flexibility.

Diastolic Time between ventricular contractions (systole) when ventricular filling occurs.

Differentiate Process that cells undergo as they mature into normal cells.

Diffusion The process of becoming diffused or widely spread. Spontaneous movement of molecules that require no additional energy; where a solution reaches a uniform concentration.

Dilated cardiomyopathy A group of disorders where the heart muscle is weakened and cannot pump effectively. Net result is dilation of the cardiac chambers or cardiac enlargement; can result in congestive heart failure.

Diuresis Increased excretion of urine. In diabetes can be due to increased blood glucose levels causing water to be lost in the urine.

Diving reflex A reflexive response to diving in many aquatic mammals and birds, characterized by physiological changes that decrease oxygen consumption, such as slowed heart rate and decreased blood flow to the abdominal organs and muscles, until breathing resumes. Though less pronounced, the reflex also occurs in certain non-aquatic animals, including humans, upon submersion in water.

Dizygous Twins who share a common uterine environment; fertilization of two different ova by different sperm.

Dyslipidaemia Abnormality in or abnormal amount of lipids and lipoproteins in the blood.

Dysplasia Abnormality of development in the size and shape and organization of adult cells.

Dyspnoea Shortness of breath, difficult or laboured breathing.

Echocardiography A diagnostic test using ultrasound waves that produce images of the heart chamber, valves and surrounding structures. Can be used to detect abnormality in anatomy or infections of the heart valves; measures cardiac output.

Effusion Loss or leakage of fluid.

Ejection fraction The portion of blood pumped out with each beat. Normal resting values are about $62 \pm 6\%$.

Elastin Glycoprotein randomly coiled and cross-linked to form elastic fibres that are found in connective tissue.

Electrocardiograph A recording of the electrical activity of the heart; detects and records electrical potential of the heart during cardiac cycle.

Electrolyte Substance that dissociates into ions in solution and is capable of conducting electricity.

Embolism The sudden blocking of an artery by a clot or

foreign material, which has been brought to its site of lodgement by the blood current.

Emphysema Destruction of the gas-exchanging surface of the lung alveoli, resulting in a pathological accumulation of air in tissues and organs.

Endocytosis Uptake of material into a cell by the formation of a membrane-bound vesicle.

Endogenous Developing or originating within the organism, or arising from causes within the organism.

Endometrium The tissue lining the uterus.

Endothelin Group of potent vasoconstrictor peptide hormones released by the endothelial cells.

Endothelium-derived hyperpolarizing factor A vasodilator.

Eosinophils Leukocytes that are larger than neutrophils and constitute 1–3% of white blood cells; they increase in number with allergy.

Epidemiology The study of the distribution and determinants of health-related states and events in a population. The study of epidemic disease.

Epileptic One affected by epilepsy.

Erythrocyte A red blood cell.

Exercise Structured bouts of physical activity over and above those of normal daily activities. Bodily exertion for the sake of keeping the organs and functions in a healthy state.

Exercise hypotension Abnormally low blood pressure, generally caused when moving from a low to a more upright position (orthostatic hypotension).

Exercise stress test A physical cardiac challenge test, generally used to determine the point of abnormal cardiac function.

Exogenous Developed or originating from outside the organism.

False-positive An erroneous or mistakenly positive response.

Fatty acids Organic, monobasic acids, derived from hydrocarbons by the equivalent of oxidation of a methyl group to an alcohol, aldehyde and then acid. Fatty acids are saturated and unsaturated.

Fibrillation A small local involuntary contraction of muscle, resulting in spontaneous activation of a single muscle cell or muscle fibres.

Fibrinogen Soluble plasma protein found in the blood plasma that is essential for the coagulation of blood

and is converted to fibrin by the action of thrombin in the presence of ionized calcium.

Fibrinolysis Solubilization of fibrin in blood clots, chiefly by the proteolytic action of plasmin.

Fibrosis The formation of fibrous tissue.

Foam cells Lipid-laden macrophages originating from monocytes or from smooth muscle cells.

Follicular Affecting the follicles.

Free fatty acid (FFA) A metabolic by-product from the breakdown of fats. FFAs are present in living tissues in low concentrations. The esterified forms are important both as energy storage molecules and as structural molecules. Non-esterified FFAs are released by the hydrolysis of triglyceride in adipose tissue.

Free radicals Highly reactive molecules, which are produced in both normal and pathological processes. They are proven or suspected agents of tissue damage in a wide variety of circumstances.

Functional residual capacity (FRC) The volume of air remaining in the lungs at the end of a normal, quiet expiration. The sum of residual volume and the expiratory reserve volume.

Gestational hypertension High blood pressure during pregnancy; often abates postpartum.

Glomeruli Network of tiny blood vessels in the kidneys where the blood is filtered and waste products are removed.

Glucagon Peptide hormone secreted by the cells of the islets of Langerhans in the pancreas in response to a fall in blood sugar. Induces hyperglycaemia.

Glucocorticoid Adrenocortical steroid hormone that increases gluconeogenesis and exerts an anti-inflammatory effect. Also influences many body functions.

Glucose-6-phosphatase An intermediate of the glycolytic pathway, but also readily converted to glycogen.

Glycation The uncontrolled non-enzymatic reaction of sugars with proteins. Chemical glycation is important in the damage done to diabetics when their sugar levels rise above normal, and in damage done to critical proteins of nerve cells in ageing.

Glyceryl trinitrate (GTN) Nitroglycerine, a potent coronary vasodilator.

Glycogen synthase An enzyme that catalyzes the uptake of glucose into the cell.

Glycolysis The conversion of monosaccharide (generally

glucose) to pyruvate via the glycolytic pathway in the cytosol.

Glycoproteins Proteins containing one or more covalently linked carbohydrate residues. Term often used generically to include the mucoproteins and proteoglycans.

Gonadotropic Describing or relating to the actions of gonadotropin.

Gonadotropin Hormone capable of promoting gonadal growth and function, acting on or stimulating the testes or ovaries.

Guanylic acid (GMP) A major component of ribonucleic acids.

Haematopoietic Cell that give rise to distinct daughter cells, one that will further proliferate and differentiate into a mature blood cell.

Haemostasis The arrest of bleeding.

Half–life The period over which the concentration of a specific chemical or drug falls to half its original concentration in a specific fluid or blood.

Heart block Conduction disturbance that results in inappropriate delay (or complete inability) of an electrical impulse generated in the atria to reach the ventricle, via the atrioventricular node.

Heart rate (HR) The number of heartbeats per minute.

Helicobacter pylori A bacteria that has been implicated in the development of duodenal and gastric ulcers.

Hepatic Pertaining to the liver.

Hepatic lipase Enzyme of the liver that catalyzes the hydrolysis of fats.

Hepatitis Inflammation of the liver.

Hepatitis B and C Forms of viral hepatitis; B is more serious than type C.

Hexokinase A transferase enzyme that catalyzes the transfer of phosphate from ATP to glucose to form glucose 6-phosphate, the first reaction in the metabolism of glucose via the glycolytic pathway.

Histamine A compound found in most cells. It is released in allergic inflammatory reactions and causes dilation of capillaries, a decrease in blood pressure, an increase in secretion of gastric juices and constriction of smooth muscles of the bronchi and uterus.

Histology The study of cells and tissue on the microscopic level.

Hydrocarbonate (HCO$_3$) A hydrous (pertaining to water) carbonate (a salt of carbonic acid).

Hydrolysis The chemical alteration or decomposition of a compound with water.

Hydrolyze To bring about hydrolysis.

Hydrophobic Not readily absorbing water, or being adversely affected by water.

Hydroxyestrones Estrone derivatives substituted with one or more hydroxyl groups. Important metabolites of oestrogens.

Hydroxyl A compound or unsaturated group, consisting of one atom of hydrogen and one of oxygen. A characteristic part of the alcohols, oxygen acids.

Hydroxylation To introduce hydroxyl; usually replacement of hydrogen.

Hyperglycaemia Too high levels of blood glucose, indicative of out of control diabetes.

Hyperinsulinaemia High blood insulin levels.

Hyperplasia The abnormal multiplication or increase in the number of normal cells in normal arrangement in a tissue.

Hypertensive Individual with high blood pressure.

Hyperthyroidism Excessive functional activity of the thyroid gland.

Hypertriglyceridaemia Elevated triglyceride levels in the blood.

Hypertrophic Relating to characteristics of hypertrophy.

Hypertrophic cardiomyopathy Congenital heart disease that results in abnormal thickening of the ventricular septum and left ventricular wall.

Hypertrophy The enlargement or overgrowth of an organ, or part, due to an increase in size of its constituent cells.

Hyperventilation A state in which there is an increased amount of air entering the pulmonary alveoli, resulting in reduction of carbon dioxide tension, eventually leading to alkalosis.

Hypotension Abnormally low blood pressure.

Hypoventilation A state in which there is a reduced amount of air entering the pulmonary alveoli.

Hypoxaemia Below normal oxygen content of arterial blood, due to deficient oxygenation of the blood, resulting in hypoxia.

Hypoxia Reduction of oxygen supply to tissue below physiological levels, despite adequate perfusion of the tissue by the blood.

Immunogen Any agent or substance capable of provoking an immune response, or producing immunity.

Immunoglobulin A specific protein that is produced in the plasma cells to aid in fighting infection. Takes part in various responses of the body to bacteria or foreign substances (allergen, tumour or transplant tissue). There are five main classes – IgM, IgG, IgA, IgD and IgE.

Inotropic Affecting the force or energy of muscular contractions.

Insulin A polypeptide hormone, secreted by the cells of the pancreas in response to high blood sugar levels, and induces hypoglycaemia. Defective secretion in diabetes mellitus.

Insulinogenic Related to production of insulin.

Insulin shock A condition caused by an overdose of insulin, decreased food intake or excessive exercise. Characterized by sweating, trembling, chilliness, nervousness, irritability, hunger, hallucination, numbness and pallor.

Interleukin-1 (IL-1) A protein with numerous immune system functions. These include activation of resting T cells (T lymphocytes), endothelial cells, macrophages and mediation of inflammation. IL-1 can induce fever, sleep, adrenocortical hormone release, and non-specific resistance to infection.

Intermittent claudication A symptom complex, characterized by leg pain and weakness, brought on by walking; symptoms subside with brief rest.

Interstitial fluid The fluid in spaces between the tissue cells, constituting about 16% of the weight of the body. Similar in composition to lymph.

In vitro Within a glass, observable in a test tube, in an artificial environment.

In vivo Within the body.

Ischaemia A low oxygen state usually due to obstruction of the arterial blood supply or inadequate blood flow leading to hypoxia in the tissue.

Ischaemic Affected by ischaemia.

Isokinetic Physical movement or exercise with maximal resistance of which the muscle is capable throughout the range of movement.

Ketoacidosis Acidosis accompanied by the accumulation of ketone bodies (ketosis) in the body tissues and fluids, as in diabetic acidosis.

Ketones A by-product of fat metabolism. An overabundance of ketones in the bloodstream is seen in a severe metabolic derangement known as diabetic ketoacidosis.

Kinins Inflammatory mediators that cause dilation of blood vessels and vascular permeability.

Kyphosis An abnormal condition of the vertebral column, characterized by increased convexity in the curvature of the thoracic spine as viewed from the side (see Fig. 11.2).

L-arginine See nitric oxide (NO).

Lecithin–cholesterol acyltransferase An enzyme that reversibly transfers an acyl residue from a lecithin to cholesterol; main enzyme involved in reverse cholesterol transport.

Left ventricular hypertrophy (LVH) Enlargement of the left ventricle.

Leukocyte (white blood cell, white corpuscle) Any of various blood cells that have a nucleus and cytoplasm, separate into a thin white layer when whole blood is centrifuged, and help protect the body from infection and disease. White blood cells include neutrophils, eosinophils, basophils, lymphocytes and monocytes.

Lipaemia Presence of an abnormally high amount of lipid in the bloodstream.

Lipogenesis The production of fat, either fatty degeneration or fatty infiltration; also applied to the normal deposition of fat or the conversion of protein to fat.

Lipolysis The breakdown or destruction of fat.

Lipolytic Related to the breakdown of fats.

Lipophilicity Affinity to fat.

Lipoprotein lipase (LPL) The enzyme hydrolyzes triglyceride in chylomicrons, very low-density lipoproteins, low-density lipoprotein. Occurs in capillary endothelial surfaces.

Lithium The lightest alkali metal. Important as an antidepressant; reduces the efficiency of the phosphatidyl signalling pathways.

Liver fluke A parasitic trematode (worm). Affects humans in industrialized countries, usually acquired by eating freshwater fish containing the encysted larvae. The larvae are released into the duodenum, enter the common bile duct and migrate to other bile ducts, gall bladder and pancreas.

Lumen The cavity or channel within a tube or tubular organ.

Luteal Related to the cells of the corpus luteum of the ovary. Luteal cells secrete progesterone and oestrogen.

Lymphatic Pertaining to the lymph.

Lymphocyte Variety of near colourless cell found in

the blood, lymph and lymphoid tissues, constituting approximately 25% of white blood cells and including B cells, which function in humoral immunity, and T cells, which function in cellular immunity; can be divided into helper, killer or suppressor cells.

Lymphoedema   Swelling of the subcutaneous tissues causes by obstruction of the lymphatic drainage. Results from fluid accumulation and may arise from surgery, radiation or the presence of a tumour in the area of the lymph nodes.

Lysosome   A cytoplasmic membrane-bound particle that contains hydrolytic enzymes that function in intracellular digestive processes.

Macrophages   Macrophages from different sites have distinctly different properties. In response to foreign material they may become stimulated or activated. Play an important role in killing some bacteria and some cells, and release substances that stimulate other cells of the immune system.

Maximal heart rate reserve   The highest heart rate (beats per minute) that can be achieved.

Maximal voluntary contraction (MVC)   Maximal pulling force of a muscle or muscle group in a single voluntary contraction.

Mean arterial blood pressure   The mean of systolic and diastolic blood pressure.

Mesangial cells   The cellular network of the renal glomerulus that helps support the capillary loops.

Mesentery   The area between the intestine and the posterior abdominal wall.

Meta-analysis   A quantitative method of combining the results of independent studies and synthesizing summaries and conclusions.

Metabolic equivalents (METs)   The oxygen cost of energy expenditure measured at supine rest (1 MET = 3.5 ml O_2 per kg of body weight per minute). Multiples of MET are used to estimate the oxygen cost of physical activity.

Metabolic syndrome   A multi-component disorder characterized by excess of body fat, especially abdominal fat, leading to impaired glucose and lipid metabolism, and hyperinsulinaemia (a high blood insulin level, also known as insulin resistance). At its most severe, this leads to diabetes.

Metabolite   A substance produced by metabolic action or by taking part in a metabolic process.

Metastasis   The transfer of disease from one organ or part to another that is not directly connected with it.

Metastasize   To spread to another part of the body, usually through the blood vessels, lymph channel or spinal fluid.

Methoxyestradiol   Has multiple mechanisms of action, including inhibiting angiogenesis, disrupting microtubule (cell structure) formation and inducing apoptosis (cell death). Particularly relevant to the treatment of cancer involving inhibiting endothelial cell growth (anti-angiogenic activity) and killing tumour cells directly (pro-apoptotic activity). Additionally, pre-clinical models show that it has potential therapeutic applications in inflammatory diseases such as rheumatoid arthritis.

Microfilament   Any of the finest of the fibrous cellular filaments, found in the cytoplasm of most cells; primary function is as a supportive system.

Microorganism   A microscopic organism.

Mitochondria   Small intracellular organelle which is responsible for energy production and cellular respiration.

Mitogen   A substance that is able to induce mitosis.

Mitogenic   Causing mitosis.

Mitosis   A method of indirect division of cells, consisting of a complex of various processes.

Moiety   A part of a molecule that exhibits a particular set of chemical and pharmacological characteristics.

Monounsaturated fat   A fatty acid chain with at least two empty spaces.

Monozygous   Relating to identical twins originating from a single fertilized egg (a zygote).

Morbidity   Incidence of a disease or state within a population.

Mortality   Death rate, the ratio of the total number of deaths to the total population.

Motile   Capable of spontaneous but unconscious or involuntary movement.

Mucin   A chief ingredient of mucus. Mucin is the lubricant that protects body surfaces from friction or erosion.

Mutagenesis   The development of mutations.

Mutagenic   Inducing genetic mutation.

Myelinated sheath   An insulating layer surrounding vertebrate peripheral neurons that significantly increase the speed of contraction; is formed by specialized Schwann cells.

Myocardial infarction   Describes irreversible injury to the heart muscle, synonymous with heart attack.

Myocarditis Inflammation of the muscular walls of the heart.

Myoglobin Has a higher affinity for oxygen than haemoglobin at all partial pressures. In capillaries oxygen is efficiently removed from haemoglobin and diffused into muscle fibres where it binds to myoglobin which acts as an oxygen store.

Myopathy Any disease of the muscle.

Neoplasia New growth; usually refers to abnormally new growth, such as a tumour either benign or malignant.

Neoplasm New abnormal growth of tissue.

Nephritic syndrome A group of signs and symptoms of a urinary tract disorder, including hypertension, renal failure and haematuria (blood in urine).

Nephropathy Any disease of the kidneys.

Nephrosclerosis Hardening (sclerosis) of the kidney usually due to disease of the blood vessels from atherosclerosis.

Neurohormonal Hormones produced in neurosecretory cells such as adrenaline. When the hormone is not a true hormone, may be a cell product that induces the release of a tropic hormone, which then stimulates the endocrine gland to release a systemic hormone.

Neuropathy General term to denote functional disturbances and/or pathological changes in the peripheral nervous system.

Neuropeptide Any of various short-chain peptides found in brain tissue, such as endorphins. Released by neurons as intercellular messengers. Many are also hormones released by non-neuronal cells; can cause bronchoconstriction.

Neurotrophic Involved in the nutrition or maintenance of neural tissue, i.e. nerve growth factor.

Neutrophil White blood cells that remove and destroy bacteria, cellular debris and solid particles.

Nitrates A group of medications that are made from chemicals with nitrogen base, which relax smooth muscle, dilate veins and lower blood pressure and improve blood flow through the coronary arteries. Potent vasodilator.

Nitric oxide (NO) Compound produced from L-arginine by the enzyme nitric oxide synthase (NOS). A potent vasorelaxant and dilator through elevation of intracellular cGMP in vascular smooth muscle.

Noradrenaline (norepinephrine) Catecholamine neurohormone, the neurotransmitter of the sympathetic nervous system (adrenergic neurons); binds most strongly to adrenergic receptor. Stored and released from the adrenal medulla.

Normotensive Characterized by normal tone, tension and pressure. Normal blood pressure.

Nuclear radiography A branch of radiograph that uses radioactive materials in the diagnosis and treatment of health disorders.

Oestrogen (estrogen) Generic term oestrus. An endocrine hormone, producing steroid compounds such as the female sex hormones in humans. Formed in the ovary and possibly the adrenal cortex, testis and fetoplacental unit. Has various functions in both sexes.

Oncology The study of diseases that cause cancer.

Orthostatic Pertaining to an erect or standing position.

Osteocalcin A protein found in the extracellular matrix of bone and dentin, which is involved in regulating materialization in the bones and teeth.

Osteopenia A condition of bone in which decreased calcification, decreased density, or reduced mass occurs.

Osteoporotic Fragile, brittle bones as a result of a reduction in bone mineral density and mass.

Ovarian Pertaining to the ovaries.

Oxidize To combine or cause an element or radical to combine with oxygen or to lose electrons.

Oxygen pulse Oxygen uptake per heartbeat.

Oxygen tension The partial pressure of oxygen molecules dissolved in a liquid such as blood plasma.

Pa_{CO_2} Partial pressure of carbon dioxide.

Palliative care Treatment aimed at relieving symptoms and pain rather than effecting a cure.

Pancreatic Pertaining to the pancreas.

Papilloma virus A virus containing DNA, such as warts; some are associated with induction of carcinoma.

Parasympathetic nervous system (PNS) One of the two divisions of the vertebrate autonomic nervous system. Slows heart rate, increases intestinal peristalsis and activity, and relaxes sphincters.

Patency A state of being open.

Pathogen A microorganism capable of producing disease.

Peak aerobic capacity The highest measured oxygen uptake achieved during maximal or near maximal physical exertion. The ability to achieve maximal physical exertion may be limited by other factors.

Percutaneous transluminal coronary angioplasty An operation for enlarging a narrowed vascular lumen by inflating and withdrawing through the stenotic region a balloon on the tip of an angiographic catheter; may include the positioning of an intravascular stent (*see* Angioplasty).

Perfusion Liquid poured over or through an organ or tissue.

Pericarditis Inflammation of the pericardium.

Peripheral adaptation Adaptation of skeletal muscle to physical training.

Peripheral vascular disease Term describing the progressive occlusive disease of the arteries that supply the extremities. Risk factors include arteriosclerosis and diabetes.

Peristalsis A wave or contraction passing along the alimentary canal for variable distances.

Phagocyte A cell, such as a white blood cell, that engulfs and absorbs waste material, harmful microorganisms, or other foreign bodies in the bloodstream and tissues, and digests microorganisms and debris.

Pharmacokinetics The study of the action of drugs in the body, including mechanisms of absorption, distribution, metabolism and excretion.

Phenotype Observable characteristics of a group or organism, which include anatomical, physiological, biochemical and behavioural traits as determined by the interaction of genetic make-up and environmental factors.

Phosphofructokinase The pacemaker enzyme of glycolysis.

Phospholipid Lipid containing one or more phosphate groups. Polar lipids that are of great importance for the structure and function of cell membranes.

Phosphorylate To attach a phosphate group to a protein, sugar or other compound.

Phosphorylation The process of attaching a phosphate group to a protein, sugar or other compound.

Physical activity (PA) Any physical movement; generally, but not necessarily, refers to unstructured physical activities.

Pituitary An endocrine gland located at the base of the brain in the small recess of a bone. Certain sections of the pituitary each secrete important hormones including growth hormone and antidiuretic hormone (ADH).

Plasma Cellular fluid in which blood cells are suspended.

Plasmin Enzyme that is responsible for digesting fibrin in blood clots. Generated from plasminogen by the action of another protease, plasminogen activator.

Plasminogen The inactive precursor of plasmin.

Platelets Particles found in the bloodstream that bind fibrinogen at the site of a wound to begin the blood clotting process.

Polar Molecules that are hydrophilic, 'water-loving'.

Polarity A process where the neutral atom gains or loses electrons.

Polypeptide Long chain of amino acids jointed by peptide bonds. May be formed by partial hydrolysis of proteins or synthesized from free amino acids.

Polyunsaturated fat A fat that contains more than one carbon–carbon double bond.

Positive feedback system An increase in a function in response to a stimulus.

Postprandial Occurring after a meal.

Preload Tension in the heart muscle or chamber at the end of diastole and before contraction.

Progesterone Produced in the corpus luteum, as an antagonist of oestrogens. Promotes proliferation of uterine mucosa and the implantation of the blastocyst; prevents further follicular development.

Prophylaxis The prevention of disease, preventive treatment.

Proprioception The mechanism involved in the self-regulation of posture and movement through stimuli originating in the receptors embedded in the joints, tendons, muscles and labyrinth.

Prospective study A study where people are initially enrolled and then followed up subsequently.

Prostacyclin Unstable prostaglandin released by the mast cells and endothelium; a potent inhibitor of platelet aggregation, also causes vasodilation and increased vascular permeability. Release enhances bradykinin.

Prostaglandin A group of components that act by binding to specific cell surface receptors causing an increase in the level of the intracellular second messenger cyclic AMP (cAMP) (in some cases cyclic GMP, cGMP).

Proteinuria Too much protein in the urine. Possible sign of kidney damage.

Proteoglycans Glycoproteins which have a very high polysaccharide content and are one of several unsaturated fatty acids that act at exceedingly low concentrations on local target organs.

Proteolytic Ability to break down protein.

Prothrombinase (factor X) Glycoprotein blood coagulation factor than can be activated to factor Xa by both the intrinsic and extrinsic coagulation pathways.

Proximal Nearest to, closer to any point of reference, opposite to distal.

Pulmonary embolism (PE) The lodgement of a blood clot in the lumen of a pulmonary artery, causing severe dysfunction in respiratory function.

Rate-limiting factor The slowest step in the metabolic pathway or the step in an enzymatic reaction that requires the greatest amount of energy intake.

Rate pressure product (RPP) Method used to estimate the amount of work that the heart muscle has to do, calculated as peak systolic blood pressure times heart rate, divided by 100: $RPP = SBP \times HR/100$.

Renin A proteinase (enzyme) of high specificity that is released by the kidney and acts to raise blood pressure by activating angiotensin to generate angiotensin I.

Respiratory exchange ratio The ratio of the net output of carbon dioxide to the simultaneous net uptake of oxygen at a given site.

Respiratory failure A clinical syndrome that is defined either by the inability to rid the body of carbon dioxide or establish an adequate blood oxygen level (PaO_2).

Retinopathy Inflammation of the retina; or degenerative non-inflammatory condition of the retina.

Retrospective study A study where people are enrolled and then have, for example, their history or risk of infection measured or recorded.

Sarcomere Repeating subunit, from which the myofibrils of striated muscle are built.

Sarcopenia Reduction in muscle mass.

Saturated fat A fatty acid with all potential hydrogen binding sites filled. Holds the highest risk for the development of arteriosclerosis.

Schistosomiasis Disease caused by digenetic trematode worm of the genus *Schistosoma*. The adult worm lives in the urinary blood vessels. Eggs shed by the female worm pass to the outside in the urine or faeces, but also lodge in and obstruct the blood flow to the liver.

Schwann cells Neuroglial cells of the peripheral nervous system, which form the insulating myelin sheaths of peripheral axons.

Serotonin Neurotransmitter and hormone, synthesized from the amino acid tryptophan in the gut and bronchi.

Serum The clear liquid that separates from blood on clotting.

Shear stress Force in equilibrium that produces a shear (angular deformation without change in volume).

Sinoatrial (SA) Relating to the sinus venous and the right atrium of the heart.

Sinus atrial node The impulse-generating tissue (pacemaker) located in the right atrium under the epicardium. Specialized cardiac muscle fibres generate cardiac impulse.

Smooth muscle cells (SMCs) Muscle cells that line the walls of hollow organs, such as the stomach, intestine and blood vessels. Produce long slow contractions that are not under voluntary control.

Starling's law or mechanism A law which states that the stroke volume of the heart increases in response to an increase in the volume of blood filling the heart.

Stasis ulceration Common result of venous insufficiency of the legs.

Sterol A large subgroup of steroids. Sterols include cholesterol.

Stroke volume The amount of blood pumped out of one ventricle of the heart as the result of a single contraction. Is the sum of cardiac output (litres per minute) and heart rate (beats per minute).

ST segment displacement 1 mm ST segment depression or elevation electrocardiograph (ECG) indicator of cardiac ischaemia or infarction (see Appendix A, Fig. A.4).

Subcutaneous tissue The soft tissue immediately underlying the skin or epidermis.

Substrate A substance upon which an enzyme acts.

Supine Lying on back.

Supraventricular Situated or occurring above the ventricle, especially in an atrium or atrioventricular node.

Supraventricular tachycardia An elevated heartbeat coming from a situation above the ventricle, especially in an atrium or atrioventricular node.

Sympathetic nervous system One of two divisions of the autonomic nervous system. Most sympathetic neurons, but not all, use noradrenaline as a postganglionic neurotransmitter. Accelerates heart rate, constricts blood vessels, raises blood pressure.

Symptomatic   Exhibiting the symptoms of a particular disease.

Syncope   Temporary suspension of consciousness due to generalized cerebral ischaemia; faint.

Syndrome X   Angina pectoris or angina-like chest pain with normal coronary arteriogram and positive exercise test. Cause unknown. May also be used to refer to metabolic syndrome, which is different from that stated previously.

Synovitis   An inflammatory condition of the synovial membrane of a joint.

Systemic   Pertaining to or affecting the body as a whole.

Systolic   Indicating the maximum arterial pressure during contraction of the left ventricle of the heart.

Tachycardia   The excessive rapidity in the action of the heart, usually a resting heart rate above 100 beats per minute.

T cell (T lymphocyte)   A class of lymphocyte derived from the thymus. Involved primarily in controlling cell-mediated immune reaction and in the control of B cell development. There are three fundamental types of T cell: helper, killer and suppressor; each has subdivisions.

Testicular   Pertaining to testis.

Thermogenesis   The production of heat, specifically from physiological processes of the body.

Thrombin   Produced from prothrombin by the action of either the extrinsic (tissue factor plus phospholipid) or intrinsic (contact of blood with a foreign surface or connective tissue) coagulation systems. Both systems activate plasma factor X to factor Xa, which then, in conjunction with phospholipid (tissue derived platelet factor III) and factor C, catalyzes the conversion.

Thrombolytic   Dissolving or splitting a thrombus.

Thrombophlebitis   Inflammation of a vein associated with thrombus formation.

Thromboplastin   Traditional name for substance in plasma that converts prothrombin to thrombin.

Thromboxanes   Any of several compounds, originally derived from prostaglandin precursors in platelets, that stimulate aggregation of platelets and constriction of blood vessels.

Thrombus   The formation, development or presence of a blood clot.

Thyroid hormone   Iodine-containing compound secreted by the thyroid gland; thyroxine. These hormones increase rate of metabolism, and influence growth.

Thyroxine   Thyroid hormone; increases rate of metabolism, influences growth.

Tissue factor   Initiates blood clotting after binding factors VII or VIIa; sometimes referred to as factor III.

Torque   A force that produces a twist or rotary movement.

Total lung capacity   The volume of air contained in the lungs at the end of a maximal inspiration.

Total peripheral resistance (TPR)   The total resistance to flow of blood in the systemic circuit; the quotient produced by dividing the mean arterial pressure by the cardiac minute volume.

Toxins   Poisons produced by certain animals, plants or bacteria.

Training response   The physiological adaptations linked with physical training.

Trans fatty acid   An unsaturated fatty acid produced by the partial hydrogenation of vegetable oils and present in hardened vegetable oils, most margarines, commercial baked foods, and many fried foods. An excess of these fats in the diet is thought to raise the cholesterol level in the bloodstream.

Transmitral   Blood flow across the mitral valve of the heart.

Triglyceride (triacylglycerol)   Storage fat of animals' adipose tissue, composed largely of glycerol esters of saturated fatty acids.

Tumour necrosis factor (TNF)   A natural body protein with anticancer effects. Is produced by the body in response to the presence of toxic substances, such as bacterial toxins. May produce toxic shock and general ill health.

Vasoconstriction   The diminution of the calibre of vessels; constriction of arterioles leading to decreased blood flow to an area.

Vasodilation   A state of increased calibre of the blood vessels, enhancing blood flow to an area.

Vasopressin (ADH)   Peptide hormone released from the posterior pituitary lobe but synthesized in the hypothalamus. Has antidiuretic and vasopressor actions (stimulating contraction of the muscular tissue of the capillaries and arteries); used to treat diabetics.

Ventilation   The process of exchange of air between the lungs and the ambient air, measured in litres per minute; refers to total exchange. Alveolar ventilation refers to the effective ventilation of the alveoli in which gas exchange with the blood takes place.

Visceral   Pertaining to organs such as the brain, heart or stomach; applies to organs contained in the abdomen.

$\dot{V}O_2$ Symbol for oxygen consumption.

$\dot{V}O_2$**max**   Symbol for maximum oxygen consumption.

von Willebrand factor   Plasma factor involved in platelet adhesion through an interaction with factor VIII (a coagulation factor; deficiency in this factor leads to classic haemophilia).

White coat syndrome   Where an individual is being measured for blood pressure at rest, the blood pressure rises due to the situation, rather than the measure being a true indication of the blood pressure under normal resting conditions.

Bibliography

Anderson D M, Keith J, Novak P D et al (eds) 2002 Mosby's medical, nursing and allied health dictionary, 6th edn. Elsevier Science, Edinburgh

Centre for Cancer Education, University of Newcastle upon Tyne 2005 On-line medical dictionary. Online. Available: http://cancerweb.ncl.ac.uk July 2005

Kent M (ed) 1994 The Oxford dictionary of sports science and medicine. Oxford University Press, New York

Index

NOTE:

Notes: page numbers followed by 'f' and 't' refer to figures and tables respectively.
Abbreviations used: COPD = chronic obstructive pulmonary disease; PA = physical activity

A

abdominal fat
  cancer and, 197
  obesity diagnosis, 96
  regular physical activity/exercise effects, 104
acidity, changes in, 222
acidosis, 222
activated partial thromboplastin (tissue factor) time, 120
activities of daily living (ADL), limitations in older people, 205
adenosine-5'-diphosphate (ADP), 115
adhesion molecules, COPD, 144
adipocytes, 97
adipose tissue, 97
  glucose entry, 61
adrenaline (epinephrine)
  diabetes mellitus, 68
  hypertension, 84
  thrombosis risk, 119
adrenergic receptor blockers
  alpha-blockers, 13, 224t, 226
  beta-blockers *see* beta-blockers
adventitia, 12
aerobic activities
  adaptations, 3
  cardiovascular disease, 24
  COPD, 151, 152
  hyperlipidaemia, 49–50
  obesity, 107–108
  older adult, 210–211, 211
  osteoporosis, 184–185
  physical activity/exercise, 70–71
  rheumatoid arthritis, 167
aerobic capacity (Vo₂max), 2, 4–5
  age-adjusted mortality rates, 2f
  age-related changes, 211
  assessment/screening, 244
    in cardiovascular disease, 21, 23
  cardiovascular disease patients, 19, 21, 23
  cardiovascular health and, 211

exercise cardiac rehabilitation (ECR), 15
exercise intensity, 248t
  moderate, 5
genetic predisposition/background, 4
hypertension and, 90
obesity and, 101
physical work and, 4–5, 5f
aerobic fitness, 2
  see also aerobic capacity (Vo₂max)
age/ageing
  biological perspective, 204
  bone mineral density (BMD), 176
  hyperlipidaemia aetiology, 44
  hypertension, 84
  osteoporosis aetiology, 178–179
  physical activity/exercise, 204
    lipid changes due to, 47, 49
    thrombosis risk, 122
  socio-economic factors, 205–206
  thrombosis risk, 117–118, 122
  see also older adult, exercise and
airflow limitation, COPD, 145
  factors affecting, 145t
airway(s)
  branching of, 140f
  exercise-induced asthma, 130
  hyper-responsiveness, COPD, 143
  inflammation, physical activity/exercise, 150–151
airway rewarming theory, exercise-induced asthma, 130
albuminuria, diabetes mellitus, 63
alcohol consumption
  hyperlipidaemia aetiology, 43
  hypertension, 86
  osteoporosis aetiology, 181
aldosterone, 83
allergic asthma, 129
  antibody-mediated response, 132f
Allied Dunbar National Fitness Survey, 3
  older adult
    assessment, 211
    exercise effects, 206
alpha-1-antitrypsin, 142

genetics, 143
oxidative stress, 144
alpha-blockers
  cardiovascular disease, 13
  influence on functional ability, 224t, 226
alpha-glycosidase, influence on functional ability, 227
alveolar-capillary membrane, 141
amenorrhoea, physical activity/exercise and osteoporosis, 184
American College of Sports Medicine (ACSM)
  physical activity/exercise prescription guidelines, 23
  pre-exercise screening questionnaire, 237
  strength training in older adults, 209
American Heart Association (AHA), pre-exercise screening questionnaire, 237
amiodarone, cardiovascular disease, 14
AMP-activated protein kinase, 70
anabolic hormones, COPD, 149
anabolic process, osteoarthritis, 161
anaerobic threshold, obesity and, 101
anaplasia, 193
aneurysms, diabetes mellitus, 63
angina, 17
  during exercise, action plan for instructors, 22t
  physical activity/exercise prescription, 20
angiogenesis, heparin and, 228
angiotensin-converting enzyme (ACE), 83
  functional ability, 223, 224t, 225
  inhibitors, cardiovascular disease, 14
angiotensin II, thrombosis risk, 119
angiotensin receptor antagonists, cardiovascular disease, 14
aniline dyes, cancer aetiology, 192
ankle cuff weights, older adults, 209
anti-arrhythmia drugs
  cardiovascular disease, 14
  influence on functional ability, 225t, 226
antibiotics
  COPD, 148
  influence on functional ability, 230
antibodies, rheumatoid arthritis, 163, 164

antibody-mediated allergic response, asthma attack, 132f
anticholinergic agents, influence on functional ability, 229
anticoagulants, 117
    influence on functional ability, 227–229, 227t
    see also specific drugs
anticoagulation pathway, 116–117
anticonvulsants, obesity aetiology, 101
antidepressants, obesity aetiology, 101
antidiuretic hormone, catecholamines, 20
antigens, rheumatoid arthritis, 164
anti-inflammatories
    influence on functional ability, 230
    see also specific drugs
anti-obesity drugs, influence on functional ability, 229
anti-seizure medications, osteoporosis aetiology, 180
antithrombin III, 116
aorta, hypertension, 86
apo D, 41
apolipoprotein B, 40f
apolipoproteins (APOS), 38–39
    functions, 38, 38t, 40f
    structure, 35–41
appetite, physical activity/exercise, 104
arterial blood vessel(s)
    fibrous plaques, 12
    sheer stress, atheroprotective process, 15–16
    smooth muscle hypertrophy, diabetes mellitus, 64
    structure, 11, 12f
    thrombosis, 113
        risk factors, 114t
arthritis, 159–171
    definition, 159
    joint structure, 160, 160f
    obesity, 103
    physical activity/exercise, guidelines/considerations, 168t
    prevalence, 159–160
    treatment, influence on functional ability, 230–231
    see also osteoarthritis; rheumatoid arthritis (RA)
asbestos, cancer aetiology, 192
aspirin, 117
    glucose tests, 76–77
    influence on functional ability, 227, 228, 230–231
assessment/screening, 237–246
    absolute contraindications, 243t
    assessments, 243–244
    COPD, 147, 151
    informed consent, 243, 243f
    pre-screening/evaluation, 237
    questionnaires, 237, 238–242t
        risk stratification, 237
    see also specific tests
asthma, 127–137
    aetiology, 128–130
        allergic, 129, 132f
        childhood, 129

exercise-induced *see* exercise-induced asthma (EIA)
        intrinsic, 129
        nocturnal, 130
        occupational, 130
        steroid induced, 130
    attack, 130–132
        pathophysiology, 130–131
        severity, 132
    chemical/biological factors, 131t
    classification, 128–130, 128t
    COPD *vs.*, 143
    definition, 127–128
    diagnosis, 128
    non-pharmacological treatment, 132–133
        breathing techniques/aids, 132–133
        physical activity/exercise *see* asthma, physical activity/exercise and
        reducing risk, 133
    pharmacological treatment, 132
        influence on functional ability, 229
    symptoms, 128
asthma, physical activity/exercise and, 133
    adaptations to training, 133
    considerations, 134–135
        attack, what to do, 134
        contraindications, 134–136
        environment, 134
        medications, 134, 229
    participation, 133–134
    post, 135
    pre-PA/exercise participation, 134
    prescription, 134–135
    types, 134–135
    see also exercise-induced asthma (EIA)
atherosclerosis
    diabetes mellitus, 64
    exercise, 15–16
    pathophysiology, 11–13
        low-density lipoprotein (LDL), 39
        modified response-to-injury response, 12–13, 13f
Australia, asthma, 127
autoimmunity, rheumatoid arthritis, 164–166
autonomic neuropathy
    diabetes mellitus, 64
    physical activity/exercise, 76

B

balance training, older adults, 209
    strength training, 208
basal metabolic rate (BMR), body weight influence, 98
B cells, 195
    memory B cells, 195
    physical activity/exercise, 195
    rheumatoid arthritis, 164
benzene, cancer aetiology, 192
beta$_2$ agonists
    glucose tests, 77
    influence on functional ability, 229–230
beta-adrenergic receptor blockers *see* beta-blockers
beta-blockers

considerations/contraindications, 27
glucose tests, 77
heart/vascular disease, 13
hyperlipidaemia, 45
hypoglycaemia masking, 74
influence on functional ability, 224t, 225–226
beta-hydroxybutyric acid, 66
bezafibrate, influence on functional ability, 227
biguanides, influence on functional ability, 227
biochemical markers, osteoporosis assessment, 177
bisphosphonates, osteoporosis, 182, 186
blood coagulation *see* coagulation (haemostasis)
blood gases, assessment/screening, 245, 245t
blood glucose
    fasting plasma value, 60t
    homeostasis
        impaired, 59
        normal regulation, 60
        regular aerobic physical activity/exercise, 70–71
    negative feedback, 60f
    during physical activity/exercise, 72
    pre-physical activity/exercise, 72
    pre-physical activity/exercise levels, hyperglycaemia, 74–75
    storage, 60–61
    tests, drug interactions, 76–77
    tissue entry, 61
    tolerance, physical activity/exercise, 69
blood lipids, 33–55
    classifications, 34t
    healthy profile, 34
    mean serum levels, 37t
    metabolism, 35
    profile, 34–35
    structures, 35–41
    thrombosis risk, 118
    transport, 35–36
    see also hyperlipidaemia
blood pooling risk, failure to cool down, 26
blood pressure (BP), 81–93, 82
    classifications, 82t
    factors contributing, 83
    mechanisms controlling, 82–83
    physical activity/exercise
        changes during, 26
        mean reductions after, 89t
        resting values and, 91
        water-based activities, 25
    see also hypertension (HT)
blood volume, water immersion, 25
body composition, cancer, 197
body fat, classifications, 97t
body mass index (BMI)
    health risk, 97t
    normal values, 96t
    obesity classifications, 96t
    obesity diagnosis, 96–97
body temperature, drug interactions with physical activity/exercise, 222

bone(s)
  hypertrophy, 175
  mass
    increasing in older adult, 210
    mass/mineral density *see* bone mineral
      density (BMD)
  remodelling, 175–176
    factors influencing, 176t
  structure, 174–175, 175f
    cell types, 176t
bone health exercise, older adult, 210
bone mineral density (BMD), 175–176
  older adult, exercise and, 208, 210
  peak, 176–177
  physical activity/exercise during puberty,
    177
Borg scale, heart/vascular disease, 24
bradykinin, 115
breast cancer, hormones and, 196
  therapy, 194
breathing
  asthma
    pursed lip, 134
    techniques/aids, 132–133
  COPD
    mechanisms in emphysema, 141–142
    tidal breathing, 145, 146
  increased energy cost, 146f
breathlessness scale, exercise intensity, 247
bronchi, 140
bronchioles, 140–141
bronchitis, chronic, 143
bronchoconstriction
  asthma, 128, 131
  exercise-induced asthma, 130
bronchodilation
  drugs causing *see* bronchodilators
  restriction by beta-blockers, 225
bronchodilators
  asthma, 132, 229
  COPD, 148–149
    assessment and, 147
  influence on functional ability, 229–230,
    229t
bronchus, 140
Bruce protocol treadmill test, 244
  heparin effects, 228

C

caffeine, hypertension, 83, 87
calcitonin
  bone remodelling, 175–176
  influence on functional ability, 231t
  osteoporosis, 182, 186
calcium
  absorption, decline with ageing, 178–179
  bone remodelling, 175
  dietary, 179, 179t
  metabolism, cigarette smoking, 181
  osteoporosis aetiology, 179–180
  physical activity/exercise and, 180
calcium channel blockers
  cardiovascular disease, 14
  influence on functional ability, 224t, 226

calcium hydroxyapatite, bone structure,
  174–175
calories
  restriction, anti-cancer effects, 197
  weekly expenditure, 2
cancellate bone, 174–175
cancer, 191–201
  aetiology, 192–193
    age, 192–193
    physical inactivity, 193
  diabetes mellitus and, 65
  pathology, 193–194
  physical activity/exercise, 195–197
    body composition, 197
    considerations/contraindications, 199
    current guidelines, 198
    damage/repair, 196–197
    in debilitated individuals, 198
    hormones, 196
    immune system, 195–196
    insulin, 197
    newly diagnosed patients, 197
    in newly diagnosed patients, 197
    pre-prescription, 197–198
    prescription, 198
    survivors/patients undergoing
      treatment, 198
    treatment-related symptoms, 197
  stages, 194
  treatment, 194
    exercise during, 198
    influence on functional ability, 231–232
capacity limited drugs, 221
capillary base membrane, thickening, diabetes
  mellitus, 63
carbohydrates
  high-carbohydrate diet, 100
  hyperlipidaemia aetiology, 42
  ingestion, hypoglycaemia and physical
    activity/exercise, 73–74
  metabolism, 60–61
carbon dioxide (CO_2)
  blood gases, assessment/screening, 245
  COPD and, 143–144
    retention in physical activity/exercise,
      154–155
carbonic anhydrase inhibitors, heart/vascular
  disease, 14
cardiac arrest, during physical
  activity/exercise, 21
  action plan for instructors, 22t
cardiac arrhythmias
  drug treatment *see* anti-arrhythmia drugs
  during exercise, action plan for instructors,
    22t
cardiac glycosides, heart/vascular disease,
  14
cardiac muscle adaptations, physical
  activity/exercise, 3
cardiac output
  adaptation to physical activity/exercise, 4
  blood pressure, 82
  myocardial infarction, after, 16
  poor, chronic heart failure, 18
  water-based activities, 25
cardiac parameters, endurance athletes, 19

cardiac rehabilitation (CR), physical
  activity/exercise, 14–15
cardiorespiratory responses, myocardial
  infarction, after, 16
cardiovascular adaptations, physical
  activity/exercise, 3
cardiovascular changes, water immersion, 25t
cardiovascular disease, 9–31
  adverse cardiac events in exercise, 20–21
  action plan, 21–23t
  aetiology, 10–11
  atherosclerosis pathology, 11–13
  diabetes mellitus, 64, 75
  obesity and, 102
  physical activity/exercise *see*
    cardiovascular disease, physical
    activity/exercise and
  prevalence, 10
  risk factors, 10–11, 10t
    non-modifiable, 11
    primary, 10
    secondary, 11
  risk stratification, 21t
  thrombosis risk, 118
  treatments, 13–18
    pharmacological treatment, 13–14, 223,
      225–226
    physical activity/exercise *see*
      cardiovascular disease, physical
      activity/exercise and
    see also specific drugs/drug types
  vascular endothelium, function, 11
  see also specific conditions
cardiovascular disease, physical
  activity/exercise and, 14–18, 21–24
  adaptations to, 18–20
  aerobic activities, 24
  considerations/contraindications, 26–27,
    26t
  flexibility/stretching, 26
  physical intensity, 24
  pre-prescription, 21
  resistance/weight training, 24–25
  single bout, 18
  thrombosis risk, 122
  warming up/cooling down, 25–26
cardiovascular drugs, influence on functional
  ability, 223, 225–226
cardiovascular health, older adult, exercise
  and, 210–211, 214
cartilage, 160
cartilaginous joints, 160
catabolic process, osteoarthritis, 161
catecholamines
  cardiovascular disease, physical activity
    in, 19–20
  diabetes mellitus, 68
  hypertension, 84
  insulin, 64–65
cell damage, physical activity/exercise,
  196–197
central adaptations, 3
  in heart/vascular disease patients, 18–19
centrilobular emphysema, 142
cerebrovascular accidents, hypertension,
  85–86

chair-based exercise, osteoporosis, 185
chemicals
    cancer aetiology, 192
    COPD, 144
chemotherapy, 194
    influence on functional ability, 232
    physical activity/exercise and, 199
childhood asthma, 129
cholesterol, 12–13, 37–38
    aerobic activities, 50
    classification, 34t
    delivery/transport
        high-density lipoprotein (HDL), 40–41
        low-density lipoprotein receptors, 40
    hyperlipidaemia aetiology, 43
    see also hyperlipidaemia
cholesterol ester transfer protein (CETP),
    40–41
chronic heart failure (CHF), 18
chronic obstructive pulmonary disease see
    COPD
chylomicron remnants (IDL), 41
chylomicrons, 35, 39
    metabolism, 39
cigarette smoking
    cancer aetiology, 192
    cardiovascular disease, 10–11
    cessation, 149
    COPD, 143–144
    hyperlipidaemia aetiology, 43
    hypertension, 83
    osteoporosis aetiology, 181
    thrombosis risk, 118
ciliary dysfunction, COPD, 145
circuit training see resistance training
claudication ischaemia scale, 247t
clopidogrel, influence on functional ability,
    227, 228
clotting (haemostasis) see coagulation
    (haemostasis)
clotting factors, 115
    classification, 115t
coagulation (haemostasis), 113–125, 115
    anticoagulation medicine see
        anticoagulants
    anticoagulation pathway, 116–117
    physical activity/exercise and
        adverse cardiac event, 121
        considerations/contraindications,
            123
        medications, 123
        prescription, 122–123
        regular, 121
        single bout, 119–121, 120t
        thrombosis risk, 121–122
        types, 121
    system, 114–116
        clotting formation, 115
        extrinsic pathways, 114f, 116
        intrinsic pathways, 114f, 115–116
        phases, 114–115
        platelet plug formation, 114f, 115
    thrombosis risk, 117–119
        see also thrombosis
    vasoconstriction, 114f
coffee, hyperlipidaemia aetiology, 43

cognitive function, declines, older adult,
    exercise and, 212
cold air, exercise-induced asthma, 130
cold sensitivity, obesity, 101
collagen, 115
    fibres, ageing, 211
collapse, action plan for instructors, 23t
colon cancer, physical inactivity, 193
concentric hypertension, 84
contact inhibition, cancer, 193
continuous vs. interval physical activity/
    exercise in COPD, 151–152
cooling down
    arthritis, 168–169
    asthma, 135
    cardiovascular disease, 25–26
    diabetes mellitus, 76
    hypertension, 91
COPD, 139–158
    aetiology/risk factors, 142–147, 142t
        asthma, 143
        chronic bronchitis, 143
        emphysema, 142–143
        environmental exposure, 143–144
        host factors, 143
        inflammation, 144
        oxidative stress, 144
        respiratory infections, 144
    assessments, 147–148
        functional ability, 147–148
        lung function, 147, 147t
    breathing mechanisms, 141–142, 145, 146
    definition, 140
    pathophysiology, 144–147
        airflow limitation, 145
        gas exchange, 146
        mechanical changes, 146–147
        pulmonary hypertension, 145–146
        pulmonary vascular changes, 145
    physical activity/exercise see COPD,
        physical activity/exercise and
    prevalence, 140
    respiratory system in, 140–141, 140f
    severity, 146t
    symptoms, 147t
    terminology, 140t
    treatment, 148–149
        exercise prescription see COPD,
            physical activity/exercise and
        influence on functional ability, 229–230
        non-pharmacological, 149
        pharmacological, 148–149
COPD, physical activity/exercise and, 149–151
    considerations, 152–155, 153t
        contraindications, 153
        disease progression, 153
        limitations, 153–155
        lung sputum clearance/coughing, 153
        medication, 153
        progression, 153
    pre-prescription, 151
    prescription, 151–152
    types, 151–152
coronary arteries, 16f
    bypass graft, 17
    revascularization, 17f

coronary artery disease (CAD)
    aerobic activities, 50
    aetiology, 10
    energy expenditure, 2
    hypertension, 85
coronary heart disease (CHD)
    aerobic fitness, 2
    aetiology, 10
    apolipoproteins (APOS), 38–39
    calories expended, reduced risk, 2
    hypertension, 82
    physical activity, 1
    see also coronary artery disease (CAD);
        coronary vascular disease (CVD)
coronary vascular disease (CVD)
    aetiology, 10
    hyperlipidaemia and, 34
cor pulmonale, COPD, 146
cortical bone, 174
corticosteroid(s)
    asthma induction, 130
    COPD, 148
    influence on functional ability, 230
    thrombosis risk, 119
cortisol, thrombosis risk, 119
cough/coughing, COPD, 145, 153
cromolyn, influence on functional ability, 230
Cushing's syndrome, obesity aetiology, 100
cycling
    COPD assessment, 148
    ergometry, rheumatoid arthritis, 167
cytokines, osteoarthritis, 162

D

daily physical activities
    obesity, 107–108
    recommended amount, 3
dance, social, older adults, 209–210
day-to-day variation, hyperlipidaemia
    aetiology, 45
deep vein thrombosis (DVT), 113
dehydration, hyperglycaemia, 67, 74
deoxyribonucleic acid (DNA) mutations,
    cancer aetiology, 192
depression
    eating patterns, 100
    older adult, exercise and, 212
diabetes mellitus, 57–79
    aetiology, 58–59
    cardiovascular disease and, 11, 75
    diuresis, 67–68
    gestational, 59
    hyperglycaemia, 67
    hyperlipidaemia aetiology, 44
    hypoglycaemia, 66–67
    insulin-treated, physical activity/exercise,
        72–73
    ketoacidosis, 65–66
    macrovascular complications, 64–65
    microvascular complications, 63–64
    pathology, 61
    physical activity/exercise, 69–71
        blood glucose level recommendations,
        75t

considerations, 71–77
medications, 76–77
pre-exercise prescription, 71
prescription, 71
regular aerobic, 70–71
single bouts, 70
thrombosis risk, 122
prevalence, 58
risk factors, signs, symptoms, 71t
sympathetic nervous system, 68
thrombosis risk, 118
treatment, 68–69, 69t
type 1 (insulin-dependent)
aetiology, 58
physical activity/exercise, 70, 72
treatment, 68
see also insulin therapy
type 2 (non-insulin-dependent)
aetiology, 58–59
non-obese, 59
obese, 59
physical activity/exercise, 72
treatment, 68–69
diabetic diuresis, 67
diabetic foot, 64
physical activity/exercise, 76
diaphragm, 141–142
diastolic dysfunction, hypertension, 85
diet
cancer aetiology, 192
energy-restricted, obesity treatment, 104
hyperlipidaemia aetiology, 13, 42–43
obesity aetiology, 99–100, 99t
obesity treatment, 104, 106
physical activity/exercise and, 106
type 2 diabetes mellitus, 68
diffuse intercapillary glomerulosclerosis,
diabetes mellitus, 63
disease see illness/disease
disease modifying anti-rheumatic drugs
(DMARDs), 166
influence on functional ability, 231
diuresis/diuretics, 67–68
cardiovascular disease, 14
hyperlipidaemia, 45–46
influence on functional ability, 224t, 226
DNA mutations, cancer aetiology, 192
drug(s), 220–222
administration, 220–221, 221f
asthma treatment, 132
cancer treatment, 194
cardiovascular disease treatment, 13–14
considerations/contraindications,
PA/exercise prescription, 27
COPD management, 148–149
definition, 220
distribution, 220–221, 221f
excretion, 220–221, 221f
flow/capacity limited, 221
metabolism, elevation in physical
activity/exercise, 223
obesity
aetiology, 101
treatment, 103
osteoporosis
aetiology, 180

treatment, 182
physical activity/exercise and see drug
interactions with physical
activity/exercise
rheumatoid arthritis treatment, 166
transport, 220, 220t
see also specific drugs/drug types
drug interactions with physical
activity/exercise, 219–235, 220, 220f
body temperature and, 222
drug absorption and, 223
drug administration timing, 223
haemodynamics, 222
influence on functional ability, 223,
225–232
anti-clotting drugs, 227–229
anti-inflammatories, 230
anti-obesity drugs, 229
arthritis treatment, 230–231
cancer treatment, 231–232
cardiovascular, 223, 225–226
control of blood glucose, 227
lipid-lowering drugs, 226–227
musculoskeletal drugs, 231t
osteoporosis treatment, 231
respiratory medicine, 229–230, 229t
pH, 222
physical activity/exercise, diabetes
mellitus, 76–77
physical training, 223
see also specific drugs/drug types
dual energy X-ray absorptiometry (DXA),
osteoporosis assessment, 177
duration of physical activity/exercise, 248t
arthritis, 168
coagulation/fibrinolytic parameters,
120–121
hyperlipidaemia, 47
single bout PA/exercise, 47
hypertension, 90
obesity, 107
osteoporosis, 184
dusts, occupational, COPD, 144
dyslipidaemia, 47
see also hyperlipidaemia

E

eating patterns, obesity aetiology, 99–100
eccentric exercise, COPD, 152
economic costs, osteoporosis, 174
elastase
emphysema, 142
genetic factors, 143
elasticated bands (Theraband), older adult,
strength training, 207
elderly patients see older adult, exercise and
electrocardiograph (ECG), 244, 245f
embarrassment/humiliation, physical
activity/exercise in obesity, 106
emotional eating, obesity aetiology, 100
emphysema, 142–143
breathing mechanisms, 141–142
see also COPD
employment, sedentary, 1

endocrine gland cells, 59
endocrine system, 59
rheumatoid arthritis, 166
see also hormone(s)
endothelium, 11–12
cell modification response-to-injury theory,
12–13
exercise, 15–16
functional/dysfunction, 15f
physical activity/exercise, regular, 121
T-cell relationship, 16
endurance athletes, cardiac parameters, 19
endurance test, assessment/screening for
prescription, 244
endurance training, 19
adaptations, 3
COPD, 151
hypertension, 88
older adult, 210–211, 211
osteoporosis, 183
energy balance, obesity aetiology, 98
energy expenditure, 2
for changes to hyperlipidaemia, 47, 49
diabetes mellitus, 69
energy-restricted diet, obesity treatment, 104
environmental factors
asthma, 127
COPD, 143–144
motivators to exercise, older adult, 213
enzymes, changes in physical activity/
exercise, 4, 222
eosinophils, asthma, 131
epidemiological evidence, 2–3
aerobic fitness, 3
energy expenditure, 3
guidelines, 3
intensity, 3
epinephrine see adrenaline (epinephrine)
epithelial surfaces, 141
esterification, 38
ethno-cultural groups, motivators to exercise,
older adult, exercise and, 213
Europe, blood pressure classifications, 82
exercise see physical activity/exercise
exercise cardiac rehabilitation (ECR), 15
exercise-induced asthma (EIA), 129–130
assessment, 129–130
pathophysiology, 130
reducing risk, 133
severity, 132t
see also asthma, physical activity/exercise
and
exercise-induced coronary collateral, 228
exocrine gland cells, 59
expiration, 141
expired air, 141

F

fall(s)
fear of, in osteoporosis, 186
prevention
older adults, 209, 213–214
in osteoporosis, 183
risk in older adult, 206

fat(s)
  high-fat diet, 99–100
  hyperlipidaemia aetiology, 43
  insulin and, 61
  mass, osteoporosis aetiology, 178
  metabolism, fluvastatin, 227
  see also fatty acids (FA); lipid(s)
fat-free mass (FFM), physical
    activity/exercise, 105
fatty acids (FA)
  content, triglyceride, 36
  synthesis, insulin, 61
fertility, cancer, 196
fibre, hyperlipidaemia aetiology, 43
fibrin clot, formation, 115
fibrin, liquefaction, 117
fibrinogen, 115
fibrinolysis, 113–125, 117
  physical activity/exercise and
    regular, 121
    single bout, 119–121, 120t
fibrinolytic system, 117, 117f
fibrous joint, 160
fitness *see* physical fitness
flexibility
  assessment/screening, 245
  cardiovascular disease, 26
  exercises, dose-response effects, 211
  increased, strength training in older adult,
    208
  older adult, exercise and, 211–212, 214
flow limited drugs, 221
fluid oedema, asthma, 128
fluvastatin, influence on functional ability, 227
foam cells, modified response-to-injury
    theory, 13
food ingestion
  diabetes mellitus, physical
    activity/exercise and, 72–73
  hyperlipidaemia aetiology, 13, 42–43
  hypoglycaemia and physical activity/
    exercise, 73–74
  obesity aetiology, 99–100, 99t
  see also diet
forced expiratory volume (FEV₁), 141
  asthma, 128
  COPD assessment, 147
fosinopril, influence on functional ability,
    225
fractures
  hip, 209–210
  older adult, exercise and, 210
  rate, osteoporosis assessment, 177
Framingham study, older adult, 206
free fatty acids (FFA), 35, 36
  mobilization in obesity, 101
  structure, 36f
frequency of physical activity/exercise
  arthritis and, 168
  hyperlipidaemia treatment, 47
  obesity and, 107
  osteoporosis and, 184
  strength training in older adult, 208
functional capacity
  aerobic *see* aerobic capacity (Vo₂max)
  difficulties assessing, 205

drug effects *see* drug interactions with
    physical activity/exercise
  resistance/weight training, 24
FXIII, 115

G

gait velocity, older adult, strength training,
    208
gallstones, obesity, 103
gas exchange, 141
  COPD, 146
  factors affecting, 141
gender
  adipose tissue, 97
  bone mineral density (BMD), 176
  hyperlipidaemia aetiology, 44–45
  lipid for changes due to PA/exercise,
    47–48
    single bout, 49
  osteoporosis aetiology, 178
genetic factors
  aerobic capacity, 4
  ageing, 204
  bone mineral density (BMD), 176
  cancer aetiology, 192
  COPD, 143
  diabetes mellitus, 59
  heart/vascular disease, 11
  obesity aetiology, 100
  osteoporosis aetiology, 179
  rheumatoid arthritis, 165
genotype, ageing, 204
globulin, osteoporosis aetiology, 179
glomerulosclerosis, diabetes mellitus, 63
glucagon, 60
  physical activity/exercise, 72
  thrombosis risk, 119
glucocorticoids
  influence on functional ability, 230
  osteoporosis aetiology, 180
gluconeogenesis, 60
glucose levels *see* blood glucose
GLUT 1 glucose transporters, 61
GLUT 2 glucose transporters, 61
GLUT 4 glucose transporters, 61
  physical activity/exercise, 70
glycaemic control, 68
  see also blood glucose
glycosylated haemoglobin, 67
Gough–Wentworth paper mounted whole
    lung section, 142f
granules, 115
growth factors
  cancer, 193
  modified response-to-injury theory, 13

H

haemodynamic responses
  drug interactions, 222
  myocardial infarction, after, 16
  water immersion, 25

haversian canals, 174
health, 1–7
Health Survey of England, 211
heart
  enlarged, 18–19
  failure, 18
  obesity, 102
  see also entries beginning cardio-/cardiac
heart rate (HR)
  blood pressure, 82
  scale in exercise intensity, 247, 248t
  water-based activities, 25
heat
  drug interactions with physical
    activity/exercise, 222
  illness, PA/exercise prescription, 27
  during physical exertion, 26
  production, obesity, 101
Helicobacter pylori, cancer aetiology, 192
heparin, 116
  influence on functional ability, 227, 228
hepatitis B, cancer aetiology, 192
hepatitis C, cancer aetiology, 192
hereditary factors *see* genetic factors
hexokinase activity, 71
high-carbohydrate diet, obesity aetiology, 100
high-density lipoprotein (HDL), 40
  increases
    aerobic activities and, 49–50
    effect of regular physical
      activity/exercise, 45
    resistance/weight training, 50
  reverse cholesterol transport, 40–41
high-fat diet, obesity aetiology, 99–100
high-impact exercise
  older adults, 210
  osteoarthritis, 163
hip fractures, falls, 209–210
HMG CoA reductase (β-hydroxy-β-
    methylglutaryl-coenzyme A reductase),
    38, 40
home-based programmes, older adults, 214
hormone(s)
  anabolic, COPD, 149
  bone mineral density, 175
  physical activity/exercise, 196
  thrombosis risk, 119
  see also specific hormones
hormone replacement therapy (HRT)
  hyperlipidaemia aetiology, 44
  thrombosis risk, 119
hormone therapy
  cancer, 194, 199
  influence on functional ability, 232
humidity, during physical exertion, 26
hydrogen peroxide, oxidative stress, 144
hypercapnia, COPD in physical
    activity/exercise, 153
hypercholesterolaemia, diet-induced, 13
hypercoagulation, diabetes mellitus, 65
hyperglycaemia, 60, 67
  consequences, 67t
  physical activity/exercise, 74–75
hyperinsulinaemia
  diabetes mellitus, 64
  hypertension, 84

leptin, 98
obesity, 102–103
hyperlipidaemia, 33–55
    aetiology, 41–46
        familial, 42
        secondary, 42–45
    day-to-day variation, 45
    diabetes mellitus, 65
    hyperglycaemia, 67
    medication, secondary, 45–46
    obesity, 101
    physical activity/exercise
        considerations/contraindications,
            50–51
        pre-exercise prescription, 49
        prescription, 49–50
        see also individual considerations
        regular, 45–48
        single bout, 48–49
    prevalence, 33
        see also blood lipids
    secondary, medication, 45–46
    treatment, 45–49
        pharmacological, 45
        physical activity/exercise see above
hyperosmolar non-ketotic coma, 66
hyperosmolar theory, exercise-induced
    asthma, 130
hyperplasia, 97
hypertension (HT), 81–93
    definition, 82
    diabetes mellitus, 64–65
    lifestyle modifications, 86t
    orthostatic/postural, 85
    pathophysiology, 85–86
    physical activity/exercise, 87
        aerobic types, 88–89
        category A/B stage 1, 89–90
        category C stages ll and lll, 90
        considerations/contraindications, 26,
            27, 91
        during, action plan for instructors, 22t
        prescription, 89–91
        regular, 87–88
        resistance/weight training, 24, 27
        single bout, 87
    prevalence, 81
    primary, 83–84
        risk factors, 83–84
    screening, 82
    secondary, 84–85
    treatment, 86–87
        non-pharmacological, 86–87
        pharmacological, 86
    uncontrolled, 26
hypoglycaemia, 60, 66–67
    physical activity/exercise, 72–74, 73t
        carbohydrate/meal ingestion,
            73–74
        insulin-treated diabetes, 72–73
        masking, 74
        non-insulin-dependent diabetes, 73
        pre-physical activity/exercise, 72
        time of day, 74
    post-physical activity/exercise/delayed,
        74

symptoms, 66ft
hypoglycaemic agents, hyperlipidaemia, 46
hypotension
    cool down importance, 26
    during exercise, action plan for instructors,
        22t
hypothalamus
    body weight influence, 97–98
    physical activity/exercise, effect on, 105
hypothyroidism
    leptin, 98
    obesity aetiology, 100–101
hypoxaemia
    COPD, 146
    exercise-induced, chronic obstructive
        pulmonary disease assessment, 147
hypoxic-reperfusion injury, 166

I

ibuprofen, influence on functional ability,
    230–231
illness/disease
    hyperlipidaemia aetiology and, 43–44
    obesity aetiology and, 100–101
    see also specific conditions
immune response
    antigen, 195f
    cells mediating, 165t
    physical activity/exercise, 166
        regular, 195
        single bout, 195–196
immune system, rheumatoid arthritis, 164
immunogens, 195
    rheumatoid arthritis, 164
immunoglobulin E (IgE), asthma, 128
immunoglobulin G (IgG), rheumatoid
    arthritis, 165
inactivity, 3
infarct sites, common, 16, 16f
infectious agents, cancer aetiology, 192
inflammation
    asthma, 131
    COPD, 144
    osteoarthritis, 161
informed consent, assessment/screening,
    243, 243f
inotropic drugs, influence on functional
    ability, 225t, 226
inspiration, 141–142
inspired air, 141
instructors
    action plan for cardiac incidents, 22–23t
    empathy for obese patients, 106
insulin, 60–62
    absence and/or resistance, 61
    cancer, 197
    carbohydrate metabolism, 60–61
    enhanced sensitivity, physical
        activity/exercise, 69
    glucose storage, 61
    hypoglycaemia, 67
    influence on functional ability, 227
    lipid metabolism, 61
    physical activity/exercise, 72

cancer, 197
    hypertension, 88
    medications: interactions, 223
    proteins/minerals, 61
    receptor/mechanism action, 61–63
        glucose entry into tissues, 61
    sensitivity
        regular aerobic physical
            activity/exercise, 70–71
        single physical activity/exercise, 70
    therapy see insulin therapy
insulin resistance/insensitivity, 57–79
    hypertension, 84
    obesity, 102–103
    physical activity/exercise, 69, 105, 106
insulin therapy
    obesity aetiology, 101
    physical activity/exercise and, 72–73
        interactions, 223
    type 2 diabetes mellitus, 68
intensity of physical activity/exercise, 2, 49,
    247–248
    arthritis, 168
    asthma, 134
    cardiovascular disease, 24
    COPD, 152
    diabetes mellitus, 69
    health benefits, vigorous, 3
    high, cardiovascular disease patients,
        19
    hyperlipidaemia management, 47
        single bout PA/exercise, 47
    hypertension, 90
    low (sedentary), 84
    moderate, 5
        heart/vascular disease patients, 19
    obesity, 106–107
    osteoporosis, 184
    single-bout, coagulation/fibrinolytic
        parameters, 120
    strength training in older adult,
        208–209
interleukins, asthma, 128
intermediate-density lipoprotein (IDL)
    (remnant particle), 39
intermittent claudication, 17
intermittent physical activity/exercise,
    asthma, 134–135
interval training
    continuous vs., COPD, 151–152
    heart/vascular disease, 25
    hyperlipidemia, 50
intima, 12
intrinsic asthma, 129
ionizing radiation, cancer aetiology, 192
irritants, lung, 142
ischaemia/scarring, myocardial infarction,
    after, 16
ischaemic threshold, assessment/screening,
    244

J

joint pain, rheumatoid arthritis, 164
joint structure, 160, 160f

K

ketoacidosis, 65–66
  physical activity/exercise, 75
ketone bodies, 66
ketosis, 65
kidney(s)
  blood pressure and, 82–83
  diabetes mellitus, 63
  disease
    hyperlipidaemia aetiology, 44
    nephropathy, 63, 75–76, 86
  normal functional values, 63f
kilocalories, hyperlipidaemia aetiology, 42
kininogen, 115
kyphosis of spine, 174, 174f
  physical activity/exercise in osteoporosis, 185–186

L

lactate
  accumulation in chronic heart failure, 18
  acidosis, 66
  COPD assessment, 147
lactic acidosis, 66
laminae, 12
lean body mass, osteoporosis aetiology, 178
lecithin:cholesterol acyltransferase (LCAT), 38
  conversion of free cholesterol, 40
  physical activity/exercise mechanism, 46–47
left ventricle
  deterioration during exercise, action plan for instructors, 23t
  ejection fraction reduction, failure to warm up, 26
  hypertrophy (LVH), hypertension and, 85
leg weakness, older adult, 206
leptin
  body weight influence, 98
  physical activity/exercise, 105
leukotriene modulators, influence on functional ability, 230
lifestyle changes
  hypertension, 86t
  type 2 diabetes mellitus, 68
linoleic oil, obesity aetiology, 99
lipid(s)
  accumulation, 12
  blood see blood lipids
  lowering drugs, influence on functional ability, 226–227
  membranes, drug transport, 220, 220t
  metabolism, 36
    insulin, 61, 65
    intravascular, 41
    obesity, 101
  see also fat(s); hyperlipidaemia
lipid-lowering drugs, influence on functional ability, 226–227, 226t

lipolysis, 36
lipoprotein(s)
  constituents, 35f
  lipid composition, 35t
  metabolism defects, 42
  physical activity/exercise mechanism, 47
  structure, 35–41
  see also specific lipoproteins
lipoprotein A (LPA), 41
lipoprotein lipase (LPL), 36
  activity, physical activity/exercise, 105
  chylomicrons metabolism, 39
  very low-density lipoproteins metabolism, 39
lithium, obesity aetiology, 101
liver
  disease, hyperlipidaemia aetiology, 44
  insulin, fatty acid synthesis, 61
  triglyceride, 36
loop diuretics, heart/vascular disease, 14
low-density lipoprotein (LDL), 12–13
  cholesterol, exercise prescription, 49
  increase in trained muscle, 45
  receptors
    cholesterol delivery, 40
    endocytosis, 40f
    impaired, 42
  reduction, resistance/weight training, 50
  structure, 39
  transport, 35
lung(s)
  asthma attacks and, 132f
  capacity in obesity, 103
  growth, COPD, 143
  hyperinflation in COPD, 146
    physical activity/exercise and, 154–155
  inflammation, factors influencing, 142f
  irritants, 142
  physical activity/exercise, 150
  see also entries beginning pulmonary
lung function
  assessments, 147, 147t
  assessment/screening for prescription of physical activity/exercise, 245
  obesity, 103
  physical activity/exercise, 150
  reduction surgery and, 149
lung reduction surgery, COPD, 149
lung sputum clearance, COPD, 153
lung surface area, destruction, 146

M

macrophages
  asthma, 131
  COPD, 144
  modified response-to-injury theory, 13
  rheumatoid arthritis, 165–166
mast cells, asthma, 131
meals see food ingestion
media, 12
Medical Research Council, dyspnoea scale, 247t
medications see drug(s)
menarche, timing/breast cancer, 196

men, hyperlipidaemia aetiology, 44–45
menopause
  hyperlipidaemia aetiology, 44
  osteoporosis aetiology, 178, 179
menstrual function, cancer, 196
mental health, older adult, exercise and, 212, 214
metabolic dysfunction, diabetes mellitus, 63
metabolic equivalents (METS), exercise intensity, 247
metabolic profile, improvement with physical activity/exercise, 106
metabolic rate
  body weight influence, 98
  genetics, 100
metabolic syndrome, 10, 58
  obesity, 96
    aetiology, 100
metabolites
  build up during warm up, 26
  hypertension and, 88
metalloproteinases (MMP), osteoarthritis, 162
metastasis, 193–194, 194f
methylxanthines, influence on functional ability, 229
microvascular complications, diabetes mellitus, 63–64
minerals, insulin, 61
mitochondria, adaptation to physical activity/exercise, 4
mobility
  assessment/screening for prescription, 245
  older adult, 206
mononuclear cells, osteoarthritis, 162
motivators to exercise, older adults, 212
mucolytic agents
  COPD, 148
  influence on functional ability, 230
mucous glands, 141
mucus-clearing treatments, COPD, 148
Multiple Risk Factor Trial, hyperlipidaemia, 34
muscle(s)
  adaptation to physical activity/exercise, 4
  contraction, BMD enhancement, 175
  glucose entry, 61
  mass changes, older adult, 206
  myopathy, COPD in physical activity/exercise, 154
  strength declines, older adult, 206
muscle myoglobin, 4
musculoskeletal conditions
  definition, 159
  obesity and, 103
musculoskeletal drugs, influence on functional ability, 231t
myocardial adaptations, 19
myocardial infarction (MI), 16–17
  exercise cardiac rehabilitation (ECR), 15
  exercise-induced, 20–21
  hypertension, 82
  infarct sites, 16
  physical activity/exercise prescription, during
    action plan for instructors, 23t
    physically unfit, 121–122

risk, tar consumption, 10
sites, 16f
thrombosis, 113–114
myocardial oxygen, water-based activities, 25

N

natural killer cells, physical activity/exercise,
     195
nedocromil, influence on functional ability,
     230
neoplasia, 193
     see also cancer
nephropathy
     diabetes mellitus, 63
     hypertension, 86
     physical activity/exercise, 75–76
neurohormonal stimulation, in heart/vascular
     disease patients, 19–20
neuropathy
     diabetes mellitus, 63–64
     physical activity/exercise, 76
neutrophils
     asthma, 131
     COPD, 144
     physical activity/exercise, 150
New Zealand, asthma, 127
NHANES survey, obesity, 95–96
nicotine, hypertension, 83, 87
nitrates
     heart/vascular disease, 13–14
     influence on functional ability, 225t, 226
     physical activity/exercise prescription
          and, 27
nitric oxide (NO)
     arterial sheer stress effects, 16
     oxidative stress, 144
     vasodilation, 11
nocturnal asthma, 130
nocturnal hypoglycaemia, 74
non-steroid anti-inflammatory drugs
          (NSAIDs)
     influence on functional ability, 230–231
     osteoarthritis, 162
     rheumatoid arthritis, 166
noradrenaline (norepinephrine)
     diabetes mellitus, 68
     heart/vascular disease patients, 19
     hypertension, 84

O

obesity, 95–111
     aetiology, 98–101
     cancer and, 197
     cardiovascular disease, 11
     diabetes mellitus, 65
     diagnosis, 96–97
     hyperlipidaemia aetiology, 42
     hypertension, 83–84
     influences on body weight, 97–98
     medication, physical activity/exercise, 108
     osteoarthritis, 163
     physical activity/exercise, 104–106

abdominal fat, 104
appetite, 104
considerations/contraindications, 108
diet and, 106
fat-free mass, 105
hypothalamus, effect on, 105
insulin resistance, 105, 106
leptin, 105
lipoprotein lipase (LPL) activity, 105
metabolic rate, 105
pre-prescription, 106
prescription, 106–108
     see also individual considerations
thrombosis risk, 122
types, 107–108
weight management, 106
physiological effects, 101–103
     aerobic capacity/anaerobic threshold,
          101
     gallstones, 103
     heart/vasculature, 102
     insulin insensitivity, 102–103
     lipid metabolism, 101
     musculoskeletal problems, 103
     respiration, 103
     sex hormones, 102
     sodium-potassium pump, 102
     thermogenesis, 101–102
prevalence, 96
thrombosis risk, 118
treatment, 103–106
     diet control, 104
     pharmacological, 103
     physical activity/exercise, 104–106
          see also above
     surgical, 103–104
type 2 diabetes mellitus, 59
obesity-hypoventilation syndrome, 103
occupational asthma, 130
occupational dusts, COPD, 144
oedema, fluid, asthma, 128
oestradiol, physical activity/exercise, 183
oestrogen
     cancer and, 196
     osteoporosis, 179, 182
     thrombosis risk, 119
oestrogen therapy
     hyperlipidaemia aetiology, 44–45
     influence on functional ability, 231t
older adult, exercise and, 203–218
     aerobic exercise, 210–211
     balance/fall prevention training, 209–210
     barriers/facilitators, 212–213
     bone health exercise, 210
     cardiovascular health, 210–211
     endurance training, 210–211
     flexibility, 211–212
     functional capacity/quality of life,
          204–205
     interventions to promote, 213–214
     mental health/well being/quality of life,
          212
     muscle strength, 206–209
          changes in, 206
          functional/quality of life implications,
               206–207

muscle mass/quality, 206
power, 206
training for see strength training (below)
participation, 212
strength training, 207–208, 208–209
     exercise/sets required, 209
     how much is required?, 208–209
     interventions to promote, 213–214
see also age/ageing
one repetition maximum (1RM), older adult,
     207
     strength training in, 208
oral contraceptive, thrombosis risk,
     117–118
orlistat, influence on functional ability, 229
osteoarthritis, 161–163
     aetiology, 161–162
          non-inherited risk factors, 161t
     obesity, 103
     pathophysiology/symptoms, 161
     physical activity/exercise
          aetiology, 162
          considerations/contraindications, 169
          medication, 169
          pre-prescription, 167
          prescription, 167–169
          treatment, 162–163
          types, 168–169
     treatment, 162–163
osteoblasts, 175
     ageing, 179
osteoclasts, ageing, 179
osteocytes, 174
osteoporosis, 173–189
     aetiology, 178–181
          age, 178–179
          alcohol, 181
          body weight, 178
          calcium levels, 179–180
          gender, 178
          genetics, 179
          medications, 180
          physical activity levels, 180–181
          sex hormones, 179
          smoking, 181
          vitamin D levels, 180
     assessment, 177
     bone mineral density, 176–177
     bone structure, 174–175, 174f
     classification, 177
     pathology, 174
     physical activity/exercise, 182–183
          considerations, 185–186
          duration/frequency, 184
          intensity/impact, 184
          medications, 186
          pre-prescription, 183
          prescription, 183
          single vs. habitual, 183–184
          types, 184–185
     prevalence, 173–174
     prevention, 181–182
     treatment, 182–183
          influence on functional ability, 231
          non-pharmacological, 182–183
          pharmacological, 182

overweight adults *see* obesity
oxidative stress, COPD, 144
    physical activity/exercise, 154
oxygen (O$_2$)
    assessment/screening, 245
    saturation, COPD, 154
    supplementation, COPD, 153–154
oxygen free radicals, physical activity/
    exercise, 197

P

pacemakers, 17
palm oil, obesity aetiology, 99
pancreas, 59, 59f
    glucose regulation, 60
    hypertrophy, 102
pancreatic beta cells, hypertrophied, 102
pancreatic lipase, phospholipid, 37
paracetamol, glucose tests, 76–77
parathyroid hormone, 176
    influence on functional ability, 231t
    osteoporosis treatment, 182
peak expiratory flow rates (PEFR), asthma,
    128
percutaneous transluminal coronary
    angioplasty (PTCA), 17
peripheral adaptations, 3
    cardiovascular disease patients, 18
peripheral neuropathy, physical
    activity/exercise, 76
peripheral vascular disease (PVD), 17
    diabetes mellitus, 64, 76
peripheral vasculature, hypertension, 86
personal characteristics, older adults,
    212–213
pH (drugs), 222
phagocytes, 195
    rheumatoid arthritis, 164
pharmacodynamics, 220
    physical activity/exercise, 221–222
        external factors, 222
        internal factors, 221–222
pharmacokinetics, 220
    physical activity/exercise, 221–222
        external factors, 222
        internal factors, 221–222
pharmacological treatment *see* drug(s)
phospholipid, 37
    structure, 36f
physical activity/exercise, 1–7
    absolute contraindications, 26
    adaptations to, 3–4
    adverse cardiac events in response, 20–21
    age effects *see* age/ageing
    assessment/screening for prescription of
        see assessment/screening
    daily accumulation, 3
    dose-response in prescription, 23
    duration *see* duration of physical
        activity/exercise
    exercise stress test, 244
    frequency *see* frequency of physical
        activity/exercise
    guidelines, 2–3

hypoglycaemia, 67
intensity *see* intensity of physical
    activity/exercise
intermittent, 134–135
    osteoporosis aetiology and, 180–181
prescription *see* specific conditions
progression/progressive overload, 248
revascularized patients, 17
supervised, chronic heart failure, 18
T cells, 16
types *see* individual types
physical activity readiness questionnaire
    (PAR-Q), 237
physical fitness, 1–7
    aerobic, 2
        see also aerobic capacity (Vo$_2$max)
    obesity aetiology, 99
    thrombosis risk, 119, 121–122
physical inactivity, 2–3, 84
    cancer aetiology, 193
    obesity aetiology, 98–99
physical work, aerobic capacity, 4–5, 5f
pituitary, body weight influence, 97–98
plasma lipids, 35
platelet aggregation, physical
    activity/exercise
    physically unfit, 121–122
    single bout, 120
platelet plug formation, 114f, 115
platelets, 115
pneumonectomy, COPD, 149
power, age-related decline, 206
Prader–Willi syndrome, obesity
    aetiology, 100
pregnancy
    diabetes mellitus, 59
    thrombosis risk, 119
prekallikrein, 115
progesterone
    cancer, 196
    therapy, hyperlipidaemia aetiology,
        44–45
    thrombosis risk, 119
prostacyclin, 116
prostate tumours, 196
protein(s)
    dietary in hyperlipidaemia, 43
    insulin, 61
    see also specific types
protein albumin, drugs, 220
proteinases, COPD, 145
protein C, 116
proteolytic enzymes
    cancer, 193
    osteoarthritis, 161–162
prothrombin, 115
puberty, physical activity/exercise during
    and bone mineral density, 177
pulmonary embolism, 113
pulmonary endothelial cells, oxidative
    stress, 144
pulmonary function *see* lung function
pulmonary hypertension, COPD, 145–146
    cor pulmonale, 146
pulmonary rehabilitation, COPD, 149
pulmonary vascular changes, COPD, 145

pulse oximetry, assessment/screening, 245
pursed lip breathing, asthma attack, 134

Q

quadriceps, myopathy, 154
quality of life, older adults and exercise, 212
questionnaires, assessment/screening, 237,
    238–242t
quinapril, influence on functional ability,
    225

R

racial factors, hyperlipidaemia aetiology, 45
radiation, cancer aetiology, 192
radiation therapy, 194
    physical activity/exercise and, 199
rate pressure product (RPP)
    cardiovascular disease patients, 18
    hypertension, 88
ratings of perceived exertion (RPE)
    cardiovascular disease, 24
    hypertension, 90
    resistance/weight training, 24
    scales, exercise intensity, 247, 248t
renal excretion, blood pressure, 82–83
renal function, normal values, 63f
renin, 83
renin-angiotensin-aldosterone system
    blood pressure, 83
    diabetes mellitus, 68
    physical activity/exercise in hypertension,
        88
renin-angiotensin system, catecholamines, 20
resistance training
    arthritis, 168
    cancer patients, 198
    cardiac parameters, 19
    circuit training
        cardiovascular disease, 24–25
        COPD, 152
        hyperlipidaemia, 50
        hypertension, 90–91
        osteoporosis, 180, 183, 185
    hypertension, 89
    whole-body in older adult, 208
respiration
    obesity and, 103
    see also breathing
respiratory infections, COPD, 144
respiratory medications, influence on
    functional ability, 229–230
respiratory system, 140–141, 140f
    gas exchange, 141
    ventilation, 141
rest, rheumatoid arthritis, 166
retinopathy
    diabetes mellitus, 63
    hypertension, 86
    physical activity/exercise, 76
rheumatoid arthritis (RA), 163–167
    aetiology, 164–166
        autoimmunity, 164–166

endocrine system, 166
immune system, 164
complications, 160t
pathophysiology, 163–164
physical activity/exercise, 166–167
considerations/contraindications, 169
medication, 169
pre-prescription, 167
prescription, 167–169
types, 167, 168–169
treatment, 166–167
pharmacological, 166
physical activity/exercise, 166
rest, 166
rheumatoid factors (RFs), 163

S

schistosomiasis, cancer aetiology, 192
screening for prescription of physical
activity/exercise *see*
assessment/screening
scuba divers, osteoporosis aetiology, 180–181
seasonal variation, hyperlipidaemia aetiology,
45
sedentary lifestyle, 84
declines in physical capacity, 204
employment, 1
selective oestrogen-receptor modulators
influence on functional ability, 231t
osteoporosis, 182
self-confidence, strength training in older
adult, 208
sex hormones
hyperlipidaemia, 46
obesity, 102
osteoporosis aetiology, 179
sibutramine, influence on functional ability,
229
silent ischaemia, 17
'silent killer', 82
sit-ups, cardiovascular disease, 27
6-minute walk test, COPD, 151
skeletal adaptations, physical
activity/exercise, 3, 4
skeletal loading, osteoporosis aetiology,
178
skeletal muscle, insulin resistance, 69
smoke, COPD, 143–144
smoking cessation, COPD, 149
soccer players, osteoarthritis, 162
social factors, motivators to exercise, 213
socio-economic implications
ageing populations, 205–206
osteoporosis, 174
sodium intake, excess, hypertension, 84
sodium-potassium (Na⁺-K⁺), obesity, 102,
102f
spine, osteoporosis, 174, 174f
spirometry, COPD assessment, 148
spongy bone, 174–175
sputum production, COPD, 145
Starling mechanism
adaptation to physical activity/exercise, 4
in heart/vascular disease patients, 18–19

water-based activities, 25
Starling's law, physical activity/exercise in
hypertension, 88
steroids *see* corticosteroid(s)
strength training
assessment/screening, 245
cancer, 198
older adult *see* older adult, exercise and
rheumatoid arthritis, 167
Streptococcus, rheumatoid arthritis, 163
streptokinase, 117
influence on functional ability, 227, 229
stress fractures, physical activity/exercise in
osteoporosis, 185
stress hormones, thrombosis risk, 119
stretching, heart/vascular disease, 26
stroke
hypertension, 85–86
thrombosis, 114
stroke volume (SV), blood pressure, 82
submucous glands, 141
sudden cardiac death, exercise-induced, 20–21
in the physically unfit, 121–122
sulphonylureas
influence on functional ability, 227
type 2 diabetes mellitus, 68
supine exercise, heart/vascular disease, 27
surgical treatment
cancer, 194
physical activity/exercise, 199
COPD, 149
obesity, 103–104
sweating, hyperglycaemia in physical
activity/exercise, 74
sympathetic nervous system (SNS)
diabetes mellitus, 68
insulin, 64–65
physical activity/exercise in hypertension,
88
syndrome X, 10
synovial blood flow, joints, 166
synovial fluid, 160, 160t
rheumatoid arthritis, 164
synovial joints, 160
osteoarthritis, 161f
rheumatoid arthritis (RA), 163f
synovitis, 164
systolic blood pressure
catecholamines, 19–20
myocardial infarction, after, 16–17
systolic dysfunction, hypertension, 85

T

tai chi, older adults, 209
tar consumption, myocardial infarction risk,
10
T cells, 195
asthma, 131
COPD, 144
endothelium relationship, 16
exercise, 16
memory T cells, 195
physical activity/exercise, 195
rheumatoid arthritis, 164–165

10-metre shuttle walking test, 244, 244t
tenase complex, 116
testicular tumours, 196
testosterone
cancer, 196
osteoporosis aetiology, 179
Theraband (elasticated bands), older adults,
207
thermogenesis
body weight influence, 98
obesity, 101–102
thiazide diuretics, heart/vascular disease,
14
thiazolidinediones
influence on functional ability, 227
type 2 diabetes mellitus, 69
thrombin, 115
thrombosis, 113–114
classification, 113
high intensity, single bout, 120
lipoprotein A capacity for, 41
modified response-to-injury theory, 13
risk factors, 113–125, 114t, 117–119
ageing, 117–118
blood lipids, 118
cardiovascular disease, 118
diabetes mellitus, 118
hormones, 119
obesity, 118
physical activity/exercise, from,
121–122
physical fitness, 119
pregnancy, 119
smoking, 118
thromboxane A₂ (TXA₂), 115
thyroid disorders
hyperlipidaemia aetiology, 44, 46
thrombosis risk, 119
thyroid gland, body weight influence, 97–98
tidal breathing, COPD, 145, 146
time of day, in hypoglycaemia, 74
tissue damage, physical activity/exercise,
196–197
tissue plasminogen activator (tPA), 117
physical activity/exercise, regular, 121
total peripheral resistance (TPR), blood
pressure, 82
toxicity, drug interactions, 220
trabeculae, 175
trabecular bone, 175
training status, hyperlipidaemia, 48–49
treadmill walking
COPD assessment, 148
thrombosis risk, 122
triglyceride(s), 36
aerobic activity effects, 49–50
plasma concentration, thrombosis risk, 118
regular physical activity effects, 45
structure, 36f

U

ultrasound, osteoporosis assessment, 177
ultraviolet radiation, cancer aetiology, 192
upper body training, COPD, 151, 152

upright exercise, heart/vascular disease, 27
urine, glucose in, 68
USA, blood pressure classifications, 82

V

Valsalva manoeuvre, 24, 27
    hypertension, 90–91
vascular cell damage, hyperglycaemia, 67
vascular endothelium, function, 11
vasculature, obesity, 102
vasoconstriction, 11
    beta-blockers, 225
    coagulation systems, 114f
vasodilatation, 11
    exercise, 15
vasodilators, physical activity/exercise and, 91
vasopressin, thrombosis risk, 119
vasoregulation, 11
venous thrombosis, 113
    risk factors, 114t
ventilation, 141
ventilation/perfusion ratio (V_A/Q), mismatch, 146
ventilatory obstruction, adverse effects, 141
ventricular hypertrophy, adaptation to physical activity/exercise, 4
very low-density lipoproteins (VLDL), 39
    metabolism, 39
virus-associated cancer, 192
vitamin C, glucose tests, 77

vitamin D
    influence on functional ability, 231t
    metabolism, cigarette smoking, 181
    osteoporosis aetiology, 180
    osteoporosis treatment, 182
vitamin K, inhibition, 117
von Willebrand factor (vWF), 115

W

waist circumference, obesity diagnosis, 96
walking
    6-minute test, COPD, 151
    assessment, older adult, 211
    osteoarthritis, 162
warfarin, 117f
    influence on functional ability, 227, 228
warming up
    arthritis, 168–169
    asthma, 135
    cardiovascular disease, 25–26
    diabetes mellitus, 76
water-based activities
    arthritis, 168
    asthma, 134
    cardiovascular disease, 24, 25
    COPD, 152
    diabetes mellitus, 76
water immersion, cardiovascular changes, 25t
weight (body)
    hyperlipidaemia aetiology, 42
    influences on, 97–98
    osteoporosis aetiology, 178

reduction see weight loss
weight-bearing activities
    older adult, exercise and, 210
    osteoporosis, 183, 185
    rheumatoid arthritis, 167
weightlessness, osteoporosis aetiology, 180
weight lifters, osteoarthritis, 162
weight loss
    hypertension, 86
    lipid for changes due to PA/exercise, 48
    osteoarthritis, 163
    physical activity/exercise, 106
weights, ankle cuff, 209
weight training
    cardiovascular disease, 24–25
    COPD, 152
    hyperlipidaemia, 50
    hypertension, 90–91
Wellness Education group, older adults, 209–210
Western society, physical activity/exercise perception, 3
white coat syndrome, 82
women, hyperlipidaemia aetiology, 44–45
work time physical activity levels, 1
World Health Organization (WHO), osteoporosis, 177

X

X-ray absorptiometry, osteoporosis, 177